AF905727

Conventional Nuclear Medicine in Pediatrics

Maria Carmen Garganese
Giovanni Francesco Livio D'Errico
Editors

Conventional Nuclear Medicine in Pediatrics

A Clinical Case-Based Atlas

In collaboration with Milena Pizzoferro
and Maria Felicia Villani

Springer

Editors
Maria Carmen Garganese
Diagnostic Imaging Dept-Nuclear Med
IRCCS Bambino Gesù Paediatric Hospi
Rome
Italy

Giovanni Francesco Livio D'Errico
Diagnostic Imaging Dept-Nucl Med Un
Private Hospital "Pio XI"
Rome
Italy

ISBN 978-3-319-43179-6 ISBN 978-3-319-43181-9 (eBook)
DOI 10.1007/978-3-319-43181-9

Library of Congress Control Number: 2016959035

© Springer International Publishing Switzerland 2017
This work is subject to copyright. All rights are reserved by the Publisher, whether the whole or part of the material is concerned, specifically the rights of translation, reprinting, reuse of illustrations, recitation, broadcasting, reproduction on microfilms or in any other physical way, and transmission or information storage and retrieval, electronic adaptation, computer software, or by similar or dissimilar methodology now known or hereafter developed.
The use of general descriptive names, registered names, trademarks, service marks, etc. in this publication does not imply, even in the absence of a specific statement, that such names are exempt from the relevant protective laws and regulations and therefore free for general use.
The publisher, the authors and the editors are safe to assume that the advice and information in this book are believed to be true and accurate at the date of publication. Neither the publisher nor the authors or the editors give a warranty, express or implied, with respect to the material contained herein or for any errors or omissions that may have been made.

Printed on acid-free paper

This Springer imprint is published by Springer Nature
The registered company is Springer International Publishing AG Switzerland
The registered company address is Gewerbestrasse 11, 6330 Cham, Switzerland

To Professor Gianclaudio Ciofetta
who dedicated his life to pediatric nuclear medicine and has contributed
to our vocational education with humanity and scientific strength
Our work is a way to remember him and thank him for what he has given us
and all the young patients.

Preface

> That is a good book which is opened with expectation, and closed with delight and profit. (Amos Bronson Alcott)

When Professor D'Errico and I decided to write this book, myriad of thoughts and feelings went through my mind.

The first feeling was the delight of being able to share with him the writing of a work started when I was "young," and he was the first tutor when I was a resident in nuclear medicine: he asked me what I was able to do and I said "nothing at all"!

The second one was the sadness for the passing of Professor Gianclaudio Ciofetta, to whom this work is dedicated, who would have been proud to see his greatest wish realized.

The last one was the enthusiasm felt in translating in word a daily experience – made of kindness, of fears, of commitment, and of devotion to the children who pass every day through our unit – in order to create something that can help those who approach pediatric nuclear medicine and those who wish to find a hint or a method and an answer I hope, a tangle of possibilities that open up in front of a child and in front of a test to which a child is submitted.

Furthermore, the thoughts about the best and the most educational possible way to set up and to perform the various topics and the study of the various body districts, my wish is to provide to those who open the book, searching a help or an answer, more and more than they search, to find a case similar to his one and an adequate answer to his question.

The work was long and it would not have started without the help of my colleagues, Dr. Milena Pizzoferro and Dr. Maria Felicia Villani, who, with utmost care and great detail, have researched the clinical cases, have made the scintigraphic images for publication, and supplemented them with radiological images. They have left out no detail, no possible explanation, no images, and no texts. And all the iconographic documentation would not have been so complete and so made without the cooperation of the technical staff, Gaetano Masi, Stefano Chiapparelli, and Elisa Villanucci, and nurses – Consilia Lella and Filomena Petrucci –that, with professionalism and affection, have followed and cuddled the children and their parents during the execution of scintigraphic studies.

Performing quality studies on children without using anesthesia is a daily challenge; it is a goal that we try to achieve every day, keeping high our guard and also the commitment toward the standards that the "Bambino Gesù" Children Hospital child struggles to respect and to keep.

Dutiful thanks go to Professor Tomà and to all our fellow radiologists and clinicians in our hospital who actively participated in the drafting of the various chapters of the book but also to all those of which the name does not appear but who work and take part in our activities, collaborating in the good success, each one for his role.

Special thanks also go to the colleagues of the Medical Physics Unit – Dr. Vittorio Cannatà and Dr. Elisabetta Genovese – who are alongside us every day, helping us to respect the continued efficiency of our instruments and handling all aspects of dosimetry.

Affectionate thanks to Professor Paolo Caione with whom we have shared countless patients and numerous scientific discussions.

This book is the result of collaboration, and it is based on a daily teamwork. Each chapter is derived not only from our consolidated experience by now but also from the exchange of information and from the contact with the specialists who formulate the questions which we strive to answer in a complete, clear, and standardized way, making the interpretative doubts clear to them. It shows that we can and we must work well with humility. It strongly shows that conventional nuclear medicine can still give much if the studies are conducted properly and integrated with the supporting diagnostics.

We hope that the readers, who occasionally perform studies on children, find in the book what we have proposed they will find, and we hope that it is also useful to all the colleagues who deal with pediatric nuclear medicine as a part of their activities not dedicated to children.

Rome, Italy Maria Carmen Garganese

Preface

It was in the early 1980s that I get interested in pediatric nuclear medicine and, in particular, of pediatric nephro-urology. In the 1990s, the young doctor Garganese meets me and "pediatric nuclear medicine," and, since then, this field has represented her "great love."

Nuclear medicine, revealing the physiological processes in vivo, has had, in recent years, incredible progress, but, since the child is not a "young adult," it is not enough to adapt procedures performed in adults to the age and size of the child. Considerable progress has been made in the field of pediatric nuclear medicine due to the high capacity of earlier diagnosis, easier management of young patients, and treatment that have benefited children. Just to this reason, pediatric diagnostic paths have been developed internationally (e.g., health.wa.gov.au). The pediatric nuclear medicine has become an increasingly important tool both to follow the success of therapy and to assess the progression. In other words, the development of pediatric nuclear medicine is because it provides information about the condition of the child physiologically, fast, safe, sensitive, and minimally invasive.

The novelty of this work consists in providing a systematic approach, as a textbook, with the simplicity of consultation of an atlas, on a niche topic in nuclear medicine, so important and widespread as the pediatrics.

This book, entitled *Conventional Nuclear Medicine in Pediatrics: A Clinical Case-Based Atlas*, fills a gap in the literature of a reference tool "clinical case based" in pediatric nuclear medicine imaging, by a collection of richly illustrated teaching cases and problem-solving, dealing with clinical history, technical informations, workflows, image descriptions, and pitfalls.

Each chapter describes the diagnostic nuclear medicine molecular imaging based on the availability of sensitive and relatively specific radiopharmaceuticals tailored for different targets that can be expressed in this complex pediatric scenario.

Authors with different tasks (M. Pizzoferro, M.F. Villani, and M.C. Garganese as nuclear medicine physicians; G. Masi, S. Chiapparelli, and E. Villanucci as nuclear medicine technologists; and C. Lella and F. Petrucci as pediatric nurses) contributed by writing Chap. 1 about the need for a dedicated "teamwork" and several informations on the management of children such as reception, administration, and interaction with parents.

In Chap. 2 ("radiation exposure"), V. Cannatà, M. Longo, and E. Genovese provide information about the activities to be administered, according to dosimetric considerations.

The role of the nuclear medicine physician, in the usual pediatric clinical scenarios, is carefully covered, in Part 2, "Clinical Pediatric Practices," with the important contribution of many coauthors, skilled clinicians in each field.

N. Capozza, S. Nappo, G. Torino, E. Mele, G. Di Zazzo, G. Mosiello, M.L. Capitanucci, M. De Gennaro, and D. Barbuti, expert co-workers, treat, in Chaps. 3, 4, 5, 6, 7, 8, 9, and 10, the different aspects of nephro-urology.

Oncology was treated by F. Locatelli, L. Vinti, A. Mastronuzzi, A. Castellano, R. Lombardi, and D. Barbuti in Chaps. 11, 12, and 13, while gastroenterology was dealt by L. Dall'Oglio, T. Caldaro, P. De Angelis, R. Tambucci, F. Torroni, G. Angelino, L. Del Prete, F. Rea, V. Balassone, A.C.I. Contini, E.F. Romeo, F. De Peppo, G. Torre, M. Candusso, M.S. Basso, A. Pietrobattista, A. Infante, and L. Monti in Chaps. 14, 15, 16, 17, 18, and 19.

F. De Benedetti, A. Insalaco, and A. Krzysztofiak have contributed, in Chaps. 20 and 21, interesting clinical cases about inflammation–infection and rheumatology disease; L. Menchini, clinical cases about bronchopneumology (Chap. 27); and A. Grossi and G. Ubertini, clinical cases in endocrinology field (Chaps. 22, 23, 24, 25) and G. Natali and D. Barbuti, benign bone disease (Chap. 26).

We are very fortunate to have had the contributions of coauthors, also our colleagues, skilled clinicians in each field, whose experiences enrich this atlas, and therefore, we are deeply indebted to all of them.

Our close collaborators, Dr. M. Pizzoferro and Dr. M.F. Villani, deserve special acknowledgments for the care given to provide images and clinical cases.

Rome, Italy Giovanni Francesco Livio D'Errico

Contents

Contributors

Giulia Angelino Unit of Endoscopic Surgery, "Bambino Gesù" Children Hospital, Rome, Italy

Valerio Balassone Unit of Endoscopic Surgery, "Bambino Gesù" Children Hospital, Rome, Italy

Domenico Barbuti Imaging Department, "Bambino Gesù" Children Hospital, Rome, Italy

Maria Sole Basso Unit of Epathology, "Bambino Gesù" Children Hospital, Rome, Italy

Antonella Cacchione Oncoematology Department, "Bambino Gesù" Children Hospital, Rome, Italy

Tamara Caldaro Unit of Endoscopic Surgery, "Bambino Gesù" Children Hospital, Rome, Italy

Manila Candusso Unit of Epathology, "Bambino Gesù" Children Hospital, Rome, Italy

Vittorio Cannatà Unit of Medical Physics, "Bambino Gesù" Children Hospital, Rome, Italy

Maria Luisa Capitanucci Unit of Urology, Robotic Surgery and Urodynamic, "Bambino Gesù" Children Hospital, Rome, Italy

Nicola Capozza Unit of Urology, "Bambino Gesù" Children Hospital, Rome, Italy

Aurora Castellano Oncoematology Department, "Bambino Gesù" Children Hospital, Rome, Italy

Stefano Chiapparelli Nuclear Medicine Unit, Imaging Department, IRCCS "Bambino Gesù" Children Hospital, Rome, Italy

Anna Chiara Iolanda Contini Unit of Endoscopic Surgery, "Bambino Gesù" Children Hospital, Rome, Italy

Raffaele Cozza Oncoematology Department, "Bambino Gesù" Children Hospital, Rome, Italy

Luigi Dall'Oglio Unit of Endoscopic Surgery, "Bambino Gesù" Children Hospital, Rome, Italy

Paola De Angelis Unit of Endoscopic Surgery, "Bambino Gesù" Children Hospital, Rome, Italy

Fabrizio De Benedetti Unit of Rheumatology, "Bambino Gesù" Children Hospital, Rome, Italy

Mario De Gennaro Unit of Urology, Robotic Surgery and Urodynamic, "Bambino Gesù" Children Hospital, Rome, Italy

Debora De Pasquale Oncoematology Department, "Bambino Gesù" Children Hospital, Rome, Italy

Francesco De Peppo Unit of Pediatric Surgery, "Bambino Gesù" Children Hospital, Rome, Italy

Laura Del Prete Unit of Endoscopic Surgery, "Bambino Gesù" Children Hospital, Rome, Italy

Giacomo Di Zazzo Unit of Nephrology, "Bambino Gesù" Children Hospital, Rome, Italy

Simona Faraci Unit of Endoscopic Surgery, "Bambino Gesù" Children Hospital, Rome, Italy

Gaetano Masi Nuclear Medicine Unit, Imaging Department, IRCCS "Bambino Gesù" Children Hospital, Rome, Italy

Maria Carmen Garganese Nuclear Medicine Unit, Imaging Department, IRCCS "Bambino Gesù" Children Hospital, Rome, Italy

Elisabetta Genovese Unit of Medical Physics, "Bambino Gesù" Children Hospital, Rome, Italy

Armando Grossi Unit of Endocrinoly, "Bambino Gesù" Children Hospital, Rome, Italy

Amato Infante Imaging Department, "Bambino Gesù" Children Hospital, Rome, Italy

Antonella Insalaco Unit of Rheumatology, "Bambino Gesù" Children Hospital, Rome, Italy

Andrzej Krzysztofiak Unit of Infettivology, "Bambino Gesù" Children Hospital, Rome, Italy

Consilia Lella Nuclear Medicine Unit, Imaging Department, IRCCS "Bambino Gesù" Children Hospital, Rome, Italy

Franco Locatelli Oncoematology Department, "Bambino Gesù" Children Hospital, Rome, Italy

Roberta Lombardi Imaging Department, "Bambino Gesù" Children Hospital, Rome, Italy

Mariaconcetta Longo Unit of Medical Physics, "Bambino Gesù" Children Hospital, Rome, Italy

Angela Mastronuzzi Oncoematology Department, "Bambino Gesù" Children Hospital, Rome, Italy

Ermelinda Mele Unit of Urology, "Bambino Gesù" Children Hospital, Rome, Italy

Laura Menchini Imaging Department, "Bambino Gesù" Children Hospital, Rome, Italy

Evelina Miele Oncoematology Department, "Bambino Gesù" Children Hospital, Rome, Italy

Giuseppe Milano Oncoematology Department, "Bambino Gesù" Children Hospital, Rome, Italy

Lidia Monti Imaging Department, "Bambino Gesù" Children Hospital, Rome, Italy

Giovanni Mosiello Unit of Urology, "Bambino Gesù" Children Hospital, Rome, Italy

Simona Nappo Unit of Urology, "Bambino Gesù" Children Hospital, Rome, Italy

Gian Luigi Natali Imaging Department, "Bambino Gesù" Children Hospital, Rome, Italy

Filomena Petrucci Unit of Nuclear Medicine, "Bambino Gesù" Children Hospital, Rome, Italy

Andrea Pietrobattista Unit of Epathology, "Bambino Gesù" Children Hospital, Rome, Italy

Milena Pizzoferro Nuclear Medicine Unit, Imaging Department, IRCCS "Bambino Gesù" Children Hospital, Rome, Italy

Francesca Rea Unit of Endoscopic Surgery, "Bambino Gesù" Children Hospital, Rome, Italy

Erminia Francesca Romeo Unit of Endoscopic Surgery, "Bambino Gesù" Children Hospital, Rome, Italy

Annalisa Serra Oncoematology Department, "Bambino Gesù" Children Hospital, Rome, Italy

Renato Tambucci Unit of Endoscopic Surgery, "Bambino Gesù" Children Hospital, Rome, Italy

Paolo Tomà Imaging Department, "Bambino Gesù" Children Hospital, Rome, Italy

Giovanni Torino Unit of Urology, "Bambino Gesù" Children Hospital, Rome, Italy

Giuliano Torre Unit of Epathology, "Bambino Gesù" Children Hospital, Rome, Italy

Filippo Torroni Unit of Endoscopic Surgery, "Bambino Gesù" Children Hospital, Rome, Italy

Graziamaria Ubertini Unit of Endocrinoly, "Bambino Gesù" Children Hospital, Rome, Italy

Maria Felicia Villani Nuclear Medicine Unit, Imaging Department, IRCCS "Bambino Gesù" Children Hospital, Rome, Italy

Elisa Villanucci Nuclear Medicine Unit, Imaging Department, IRCCS "Bambino Gesù" Children Hospital, Rome, Italy

Luciana Vinti Oncoematology Department, "Bambino Gesù" Children Hospital, Rome, Italy

Part I

General Considerations

Paolo Tomà

1.1 Introduction to Pediatric Imaging in Multimodality Diagnostic Era

As a pediatric radiologist, I have seen the impact of SPECT and PET on the clinical care of children. Our imaging practice has had to change to accommodate the powerful nature of these new images.

Image fusion overlays two or more three-dimensional (3D) image sets of the same or different imaging modality that are in the same orientation in the same space. Anatomic and functional imaging is complementary; this is the metaphor of the relationships between radiologists and nuclear medicine physicians.

In my opinion, nuclear medicine is a crucial part of pediatric radiology.

Pediatric radiology has peculiar characteristics depending on anatomical development and specific clinical conditions related to the different stages of growth. Other peculiarities specifically related to pediatric radiology include radiation safety and the need of dedicated environments and approaches.

In both pediatric and adult patient care situations, there are family members with whom the imager must interact. However, in the pediatric setting, there are several unique features in the relationship among imager, patient, and family. Most of the complaints by parents and families are not related to technical errors; they are more commonly related to issues of professionalism and communication.

Providing child-friendly surroundings may help to ease a young child's anxiety and cause him or her to be more cooperative. Paintings on the walls and equipment and cartoonish figures in the examination rooms can be helpful. Eliminating or minimizing painful portions of the examination can also be very helpful in keeping a young child cooperative.

In general, the physicians who choose to go into pediatric subspecialties, as well as health care workers who choose to work at pediatric institutions in general, have to be nice, gentle people. Aggressive, power-hungry people cannot work with children.

This edition of the book comes at a very propitious time. Revolutions in medical imaging are modeling and quantification. Imaging of physiologic and cellular processes displays them in four dimensions (three-dimensional images over time).

The goal of the book is to provide a comprehensive text on the clinical applications of nuclear medicine in a pediatric population.

As some techniques have faded (e.g., scrotal scintigraphy), others have been added to the nuclear medicine arsenal. The most significant development has been the dissemination of positron emission tomography (PET) into pediatric practice.

Writing a book is a task that requires time and commitment from many people.

I express appreciation to MG, who has transformed their lives in a text. Her dedication is reflected in the high quality of the final product.

It is my sincere hope that readers will find this work to be a cornerstone of pediatric imaging and one that they will use frequently in their daily practices.

Management of the Pediatric Patient: A Teamwork

1

Milena Pizzoferro, Maria Felicia Villani, Maria Carmen Garganese, Gaetano Masi, Stefano Chiapparelli, Elisa Villanucci, Consilia Lella, and Filomena Petrucci

1.1 Introduction

Pediatric nuclear medicine refers to imaging examinations performed in babies, young children, and teenagers. Carrying out nuclear medicine procedure on children requires a completely different approach than on adults. The complexity of the examination varies depending on the age of the patient, the degree of cooperation, clinical conditions, and duration of scintigraphic acquisition. Depending on the increasing complexity of pediatric nuclear medicine studies, a higher level of department expertise is necessary for the delivery of good quality examination and safe patient care.

In a pediatric nuclear medicine department, all members must be proficient in performing their competencies according to their role, and a trained teamwork is the winning strategy to achieve the main goal, getting a diagnostic imaging that allows to accurately respond to specific clinical question.

Within a framework of a well-coordinated staff (including specialized training pediatric nurse, technician, and nuclear medicine physician), it is easier to create a positive atmosphere that serves to take the child cooperation, limiting the sedation in few selected children.

Pediatric patient management requires considering the special status of these patients in relation to age and medical condition depending on the underlying disease.

Working with pediatric population requires adequate awareness: in order to obtain appropriate acquisition standards, the team approach must be shaped to the child's mind-set, rather than fitting the child into the paradigm of adult examinations.

In fact, children are not miniature adults and, as well as the normal values of the vital parameters of infants and children are different than adults, even methods of communication should be adequate for their developmental age.

Besides, pediatric patients are children with special health care needs who could have any type of condition that may affect normal growth and development; this may include physical disability, acute or chronic illness, peculiar clinical condition (pain, technological dependency, etc.). During the diagnostic procedure, even when the staff use distraction techniques to hold child still and calm, health care professionals must be ready to manage a possible worsening of the patient's clinical status (Fig. 1.1).

Taking care of a pediatric patient includes parental management, and the attitude of all staff members must be positive toward the child and parent (or other family components). In "family-centered approach," the family's input is the major driving force to achieve a good cooperation of the child and a high degree of satisfaction of parents.

A department structured with colored paintings on the walls, playful environments (equipped with toys, books, video games, or DVDs) and child-friendly spaces could help foster a welcoming accommodation, but it does not replace the right atmosphere that the nuclear medicine staff must be able to create from the first patient approach.

M. Pizzoferro, MD, PhD (✉) • M.F. Villani, MD, PhD
M.C. Garganese, MD, PhD • G. Masi • S. Chiapparelli
E. Villanucci • C. Lella • F. Petrucci
Nuclear Medicine Unit, Imaging Department,
IRCCS "Bambino Gesù" Children Hospital,
Rome, Italy
e-mail: milena.pizzoferro@opbg.net

© Springer International Publishing Switzerland 2017
M.C. Garganese, G.F.L. D'Errico (eds.), *Conventional Nuclear Medicine in Pediatrics*, DOI 10.1007/978-3-319-43181-9_1

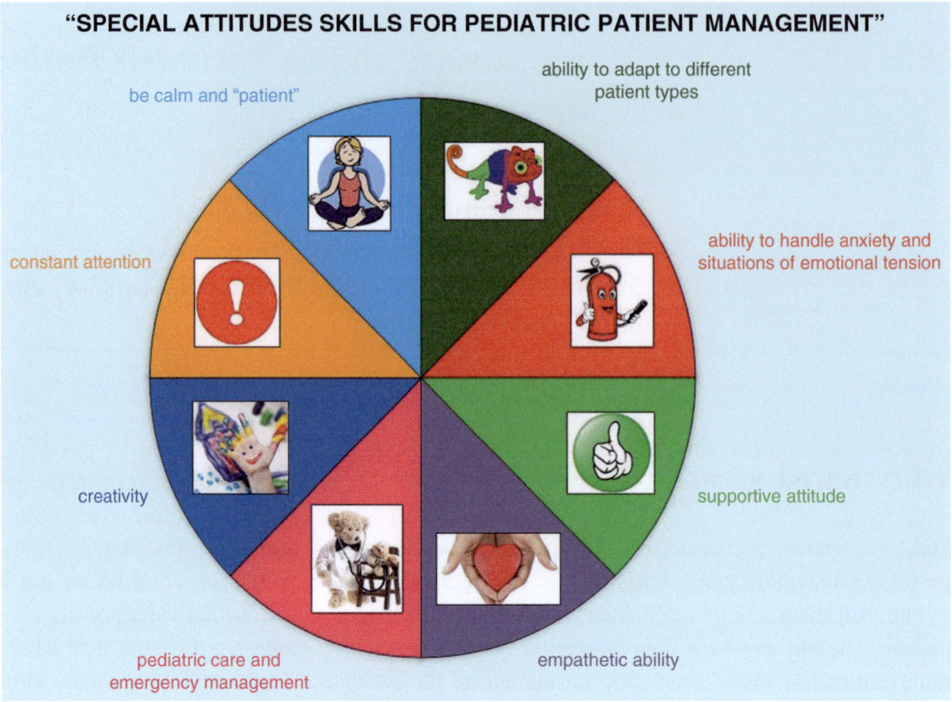

Fig. 1.1 Special attitudes and skills for pediatric patient management

1.2 Accommodate the Child and the Parents

Nurses usually handle the reception of the child and the parent. Based on a first quick observation, it is crucial to define an individual approach evaluating a child's personal features and familiar or sociocultural influences. In all cases, the first child approach must be slowly and calm in order to set the basis of a good relationship with all the nuclear medicine staff. The reception of pediatric patients must include an initial evaluation of clinical condition to set up an appropriate assistance and monitoring level in case of special health care needs.

From the first moment the child and parent enter the department, all members must be honest with both of them, in order to create a trusting relationship. In the case of both children and adolescents, the staff members must be able to adapt to different patient types, involving them in every moment and explaining the whole procedure in simple terms.

Starting from the first contacts, parents and children must be introduced into the department's environment by a specific education about correct paths within the department (with particular regard to the use of bathrooms and disposal of radioactive diapers) and explanation of the use of dedicated tools available in the waiting room (bottle warmer, electronic devices, etc.). To avoid the risk of accidental falls, it is necessary to enforce the standards of child safety, inviting the parents to buckle up the stroller and constantly monitoring the baby should not run or climb in the waiting room.

Parents are encouraged to stay with their children throughout every part of the examination (with the exception if the child's mother is pregnant), emphasizing the importance of their role in supporting the child for a good outcome of the examination. Generally, the idea to perform a scintigraphic examination generates fear in the child and the parent. Professionals in charge of the pediatric patient management have to be adequately trained handling anxiety and situations of emotional tension of child and the parents. This peculiar ability is closely related to a personal attitude (prone to a supportive and empathetic approach) as well as the capability to provide clear information.

To gain the trust of the child, put him at ease and reduce anxiety; one of the most used tricks in pediatrics is entertaining the patient speaking about his everyday life or family members before starting with the diagnostic procedure. Explaining same symptoms by metaphors could be useful to create a direct line of communication (i.e., we usually describe the puncture syringe similar to a mosquito bite or a little pinch).

Providing clear information is also the best form to reduce anxiety for parents. During the interview for the anamnesis and the acquisition of the written informed consent, nuclear medicine physician must explain the entire scintigraphic procedure, stressing the clinical utility within the global diagnostic–therapeutic iter. Providing instructions on how parents can collaborate together with staff is a helpful way to motivate them to be part of the team in order to improve the impact of diagnostic examination on their child.

One of the most difficult steps is minimizing and communicating radiation risk in pediatric nuclear medicine. Generally, parents can understand that their child will undergo an appropriate medical imaging test, but the explanation about radiation risk associated with nuclear medicine examination is always a critical point.

Nuclear medicine practitioners must be able to effectively communicate that the dose range associated with most nuclear medicine procedure results in a low radiation exposure and a very low risk of detrimental health effects. In case of scintigraphy, with a medium or high radiation exposure level, it is necessary to clarify that the potential risk associated to ionizing radiation remains still low compared with the benefits derived by the diagnostic information, unattainable using other imaging procedures.

Depending on the type of nuclear medicine exam, nuclear medicine physicians have to provide adequate radioprotection instructions to avoid undue radiation exposure of other children or pregnant women; in order to reduce global patient radiation exposure, proper indications should be suggested (good hydration with water or whatever is pleasing to the child and frequent urination).

1.3 Administration of Radiopharmaceutical

Depending on the type of nuclear medicine exam, the radiotracer is either injected into the body, swallowed, or inhaled as a gas in order to evaluate the functional information of the organ system being examined. Except for intravenous injections, most nuclear medicine procedures are painless and rarely associated with significant discomfort or side effects.

1.3.1 Endovenous Administration

If the tracer is given intravenously, a small needle is used to inject the radiotracer and removed immediately after. At times, an indwelling intravenous catheter may be used if it is already present, in case of multiple phases of administration or provocative examination (i.e., stress myocardial scintigraphy), when the patient is in poor clinical conditions. In oncological patients, the use of central venous catheter is limited only to certain types of scintigraphic examinations with proper antiseptic precautions.

For a successful intravenous injection, a team approach is necessary to distract the child, to properly immobilize the limb of the child, and to explain to the parent, as he may cooperate reassuring the child. During administration, a bed pad must be positioned under the injection site to limit potential contamination. Different immobilization techniques are used depending on the age of the child and administration site (Fig. 1.2).

1.3.2 Aerosol Administration

The radioaerosol can be inhaled through deep breaths, using a mask of appropriate size for age. In case of uncooperative patient, the radioaerosol can be adequately administered during the whole inspiration phase, even if the child cries. Immediately following the radioaerosol inhalation, the patients must rinse their mouth by gargling, when the child is able. Then, the patient is placed in the supine position, and a gamma camera detector is posteriorly positioned for acquiring lung radioactivity. After an initial qualitative evaluation, if a satisfactory distribution is not obtained, a number of extra inspirations must be performed. Measurement of the administered radioactivity dose can be performed calculating the ratio of first frame counts and a conversion ratio, specific for each gamma camera.

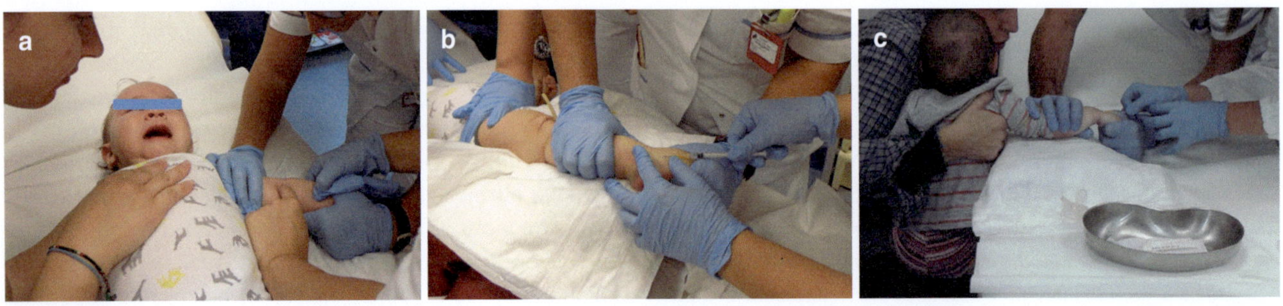

Fig. 1.2 The newborn is made to lie on the stretcher, the parent remains close to the head of the child, the nurse immobilizes the upper limb (arm or hand), while the doctor administers (**a**); in the case of administration to the foot, the use of sandbags is useful to facilitate the blocking of the contralateral leg (**b**). The child is seated on the parent's legs that blocks the baby's legs between his, the nurse immobilizes the child's arm or hand, while the doctor injects the radiopharmaceutical (**c**)

1.3.3 Meal Administration

1.3.3.1 Gastric Emptying Scintigraphy (GES) Protocol

For gastric emptying scintigraphy, radionuclide-labeled test meals are used. The test meal can be liquid, semiliquid, or semisolid, according to the normal meal that the patient under study would generally consume. When swallowed, the radiotracer has no taste. Labeled meals, milk scan as well as homogenized, yogurt or chocolate drinks, are used for gastric emptying studies in newborn, infants and children. The meal should have a pleasant taste to encourage a quick and complete recruitment of the meal, ensuring a good nutritional intake to obtain reliable functional information about gastric emptying parameters. A good amount of meal taken is also closely linked to the sensitivity of scintigraphy in detecting the presence of gastroesophageal reflux. Meals must be consumed within a 10-min period, after which the scintigraphy study must be started to avoid the beginning of intestinal progression of the meal from the stomach.

In case of oral feeding, one of the parents can administer the meal, so that the child does not notice the difference from the usual. The nurse provides instructions to parents to avoid contamination, supervises the administration, and supports the parent in case of difficulty. The necessary precautions to limit contamination in case of vomiting must be taken always.

In such a condition, the technique is completely noninvasive, whereas in evaluating children with feeding difficulties, the nurse can place a nasogastric tube which can be removed after meal administration. If a child is unable to feed orally, the nurse manages meal administration using nasogastric tube or percutaneous endoscopic gastrostomy when already positioned. Meal administration is with the patient lying on the bed of gamma camera and, by monitor persistence, nuclear medicine physician evaluates gastric filling according to the patient's capability. Habits of the patient and presence of indirect signs (as high grade of gastroesophageal reflux or the beginning of intestinal progression of the meal from the stomach) allow to determinate the right amount of meal (Fig. 1.3).

a b

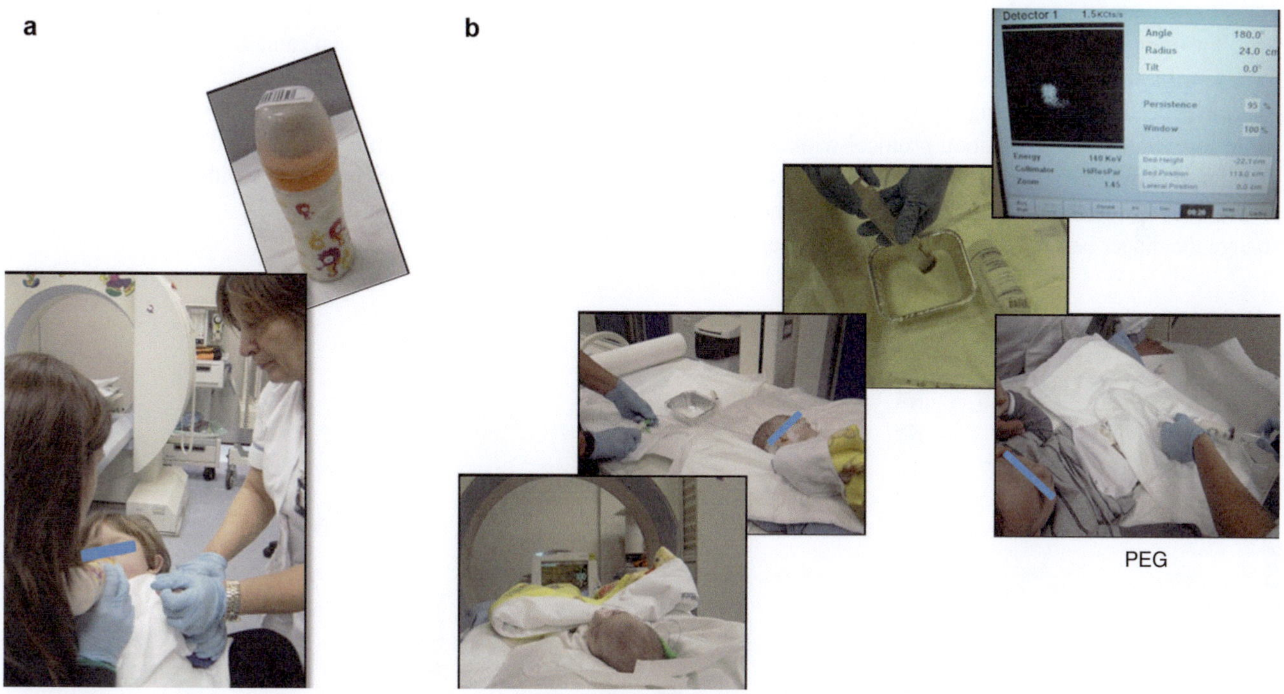

PEG

Oral Naso-gastric tube

Fig. 1.3 In case of oral feeding, one of the parents can administer the meal so that the child does not notice the difference from the usual. The nurse provides instructions to parents to avoid contamination, supervises the administration, and supports the parent in case of difficulty (**a**). If a child is unable to feed orally, the nurse manages meal administration using nasogastric tube or percutaneous endoscopic gastrostomy when already positioned (**b**). Meal administration is with the patient lying on the bed of gamma camera and, by monitor persistence, the nuclear medicine physician evaluates gastric filling according to the patient's capability. The right amount of meal is determined by the habits of the patient and by the presence of indirect signs as high grade of gastroesophageal reflux or the beginning of intestinal progression of the meal from the stomach

1.4 Acquisition of Images: Take the Child's Cooperation

Though nuclear imaging itself causes no pain, children may experience some discomfort from having to remain still during imaging, in particular for procedures of prolonged duration.

Approaching as much as possible the gamma camera to the patient is crucial to achieve good quality images using the recommended pediatric amounts of radioactivity, but it could be technically difficult when the child is frightened and does not cooperate. In a pediatric nuclear medicine department, drug sedation can be used only exceptionally using an alternative way, consisting in an adequate approach of the patient. Specific education of technologists is required, including proper handling of the child during the procedure and adequate psychological attitudes toward child and parents. Parents are encouraged to stay with their children to help them remain calm and still during imaging.

From a technical point of view, the way to get better results with less stress for the baby is to match the time of the acquisition with the natural sleep of the child. The importance of this simple method must be clearly explained to the parent who, knowing the habits of the child, is the major driving force to achieve this goal. In such a way, it can be possible to perform procedures of prolonged duration (as SPECT acquisition) or whole-body acquisition protocol without sedation. In order to avoid having scintigraphic images affected by the presence of radiourine, it is necessary to remind the parent to change the diaper before letting the child fall asleep.

Good image quality can be achieved even when the baby is awake with particular technical tricks. A whole-body acquisition can be divided in several static scans to give way to the child to relax between an image and the other, allowing staff to better block that part of the body. Sandbags are the most used means of restraint (Fig. 1.4).

Whenever possible, the camera should be rotated in the posterior view to ensure that the child does not feel "sandwiched" between the camera bed and the detector. With this arrangement of the gamma camera, the child can see and feel near to parents, and the team members can more easily block the patient, when necessary. In this position, the mother can actively collaborate for a good outcome of examination, also in newborns, breast-feeding the baby; this represents the best natural sedative. This setting with the gamma camera rotated in posterior view is also helpful for anterior acquisition, turning the child in prone position.

A practical tip to remember is that the most distressing acquisition view should be performed last on infants and younger children. Moreover, for particular scan views (like anterior skull acquisition), the parent can collaborate lying on the gamma camera bed next to the child, but turned on the contrary to bring his head to that of the child. In this way, even young children can remain calm and still during imaging (Fig. 1.5).

The use of books, toys, video games, or DVDs can be helpful to distract the child. A good staff is also able to take the patient's cooperation, interacting with him and capturing his interest by age (Fig. 1.6).

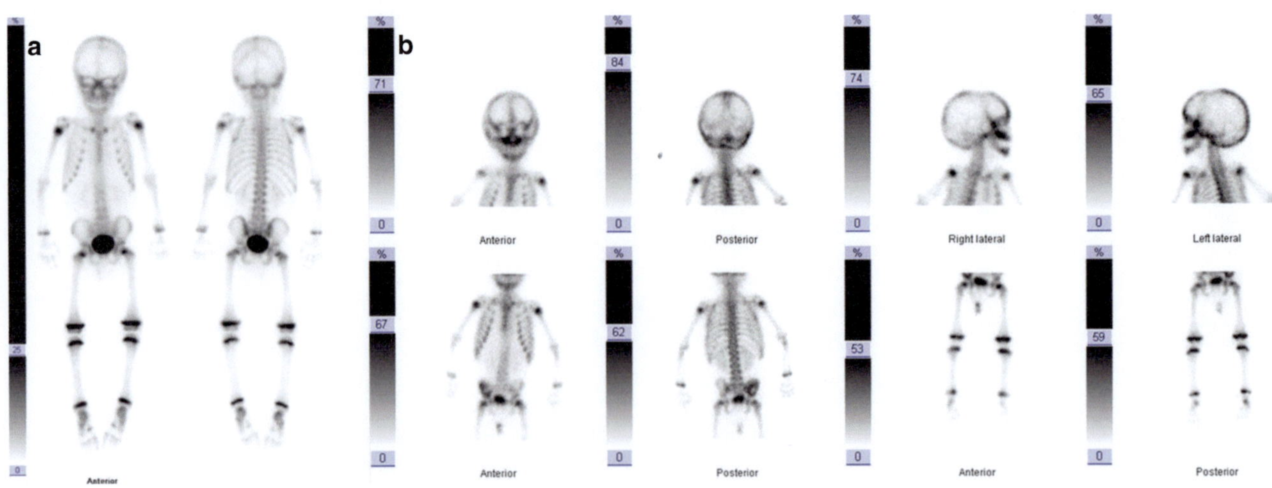

Fig. 1.4 If the child collaborates or sleeps, a whole-body acquisition protocol can be performed, using EANM procedural guidelines about speed scanning by age (**a**). In case of lack of cooperation of the child, the whole-body acquisition can be divided in several static scans to give way to the child to relax between an image and the other and allowing the staff to better block that part of the body (**b**)

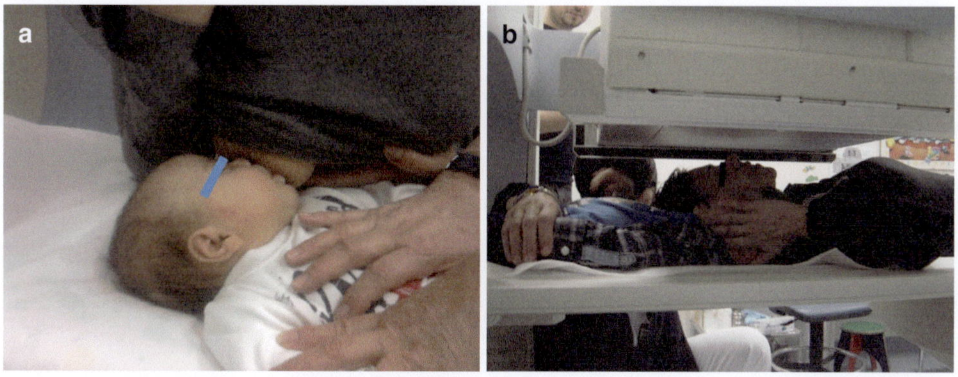

Fig. 1.5 In newborns, the mother can actively collaborate for a good outcome of examination, breast-feeding the baby; it is the best natural sedative for her child (**a**). The parent can also collaborate to perform distressing acquisition view, lying on the gamma camera bed next to the child but turned on the contrary to bring his head to that of the child (as represented in **b**)

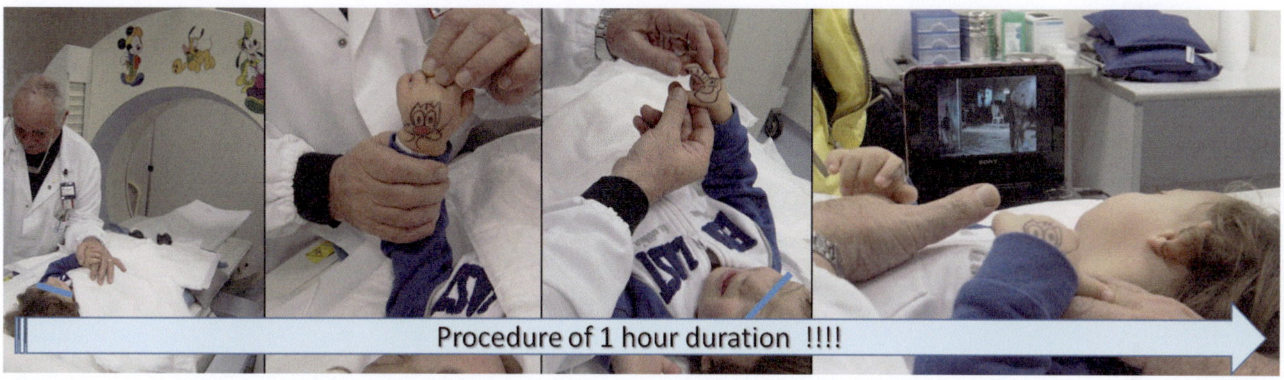

Fig. 1.6 For an adequate approach of the pediatric patient, it is necessary to create a positive atmosphere that serves to take the child's cooperation. Specific education of technologists is required, including proper handling of the child during the procedure and adequate psychological attitudes toward pediatric patient

Further Readings

1. Fahey FH, Treves ST, Adelstein SJ. Minimizing and communicating radiation risk in pediatric nuclear medicine. J Nucl Med Technol. 2012;40:13–24.
2. Gordon I. Issues surrounding preparation, information and handling the child and parent in nuclear medicine. J Nucl Med. 1998;39:490–4.
3. Pediatric nursing made incredibly easy!, Chap. 1–5. 1st ed. 2005. p. 1–50.

2 Radiation Risk

Vittorio Cannatà, Elisabetta Genovese, and Mariaconcetta Longo

2.1 Introduction

The practice of nuclear medicine leads to a potential risk of exposure for the patient. The activity of radiopharmaceutical should be administered in order to guarantee the correct balance between risks and benefits. In the last years, the introduction of technological advances, the increased availability of scanning equipment, and new radiopharmaceuticals lead to an intensified use of nuclear medicine examinations. On the one hand, these improvements involved in a remarkable progress in image quality; on the other hand, technological advances do not necessarily imply a decrease in patient exposure to ionizing radiation. The implementation of radiation protection practices aimed to limit radiation exposure in nuclear medicine exams is an utmost need. For pediatric patient, a more attention has to be paid as they have higher tissue radiosensitivity and longer life expectancy.

2.2 Effects of Ionizing Radiations

A type of radiation which has enough energy to eject electrons from atoms or molecules is defined as ionizing radiation. It is well known that the interaction between ionizing radiation and biological tissues or organs may cause changes in cells which may later cause them to become malignant or bring about other detrimental functional changes in irradiated tissues and organs. It is important to note that irrespective of the nature of the primary radiation (which may be composed of particles and/or electromagnetic waves), the energy transfer mechanism always occurs via the secondary electrons which are produced by interaction between the primary radiation beam and the biological targets. At the microscopic level, when incident rays or particles interact with orbital electrons within the atoms, two processes through which radiation interacts with matter can happen: one of these processes is the excitation, the other one is the ionization [14]. Excitation involves raising a bound electron to a higher energy state, leaving the atom in an excited state, while ionization happens when the electron receives sufficient energy to be ejected from its orbit and to leave the host atom. These physical interactions between radiation and specific structures within the cells can cause more or less serious biological damages. These latter are associated to the interaction of radiation with deoxyribonucleic acid (DNA) and can mainly occur through direct and indirect processes.

The direct interaction implies a direct damage of DNA structures after ionization of atoms or molecules, through a sequence of chemical events which can provoke the final biological damage. This is the dominant process for highly ionizing particles, i.e., heavy charged particles, proton and neutrons. On the contrary, the indirect interaction involves secondary electrons which are ejected during the ionization process. These secondary particles, energetic and unbound, are capable of migrating away from the site of their production giving up their energy to the surrounding medium, through a series of interactions with other atoms and molecules. This energy absorption process results in the formation of free radicals and other chemical species, i.e., more reactive molecules which are the true causatives of damages of critical targets in the cells [2].

For example, when the radiation interaction happens with water molecules, the created highly unstable free radicals, such as water ions (H_2O^+) and hydroxyl ($OH^{\cdot}$), can spread through the cell interacting even with distant cellular target. The indirect interaction and its consequently biological detriment are mainly caused by sparsely ionizing radiation, i.e., electrons or x-ray.

In the events timescale, the initial ionization event occurs instantaneously (~10^{-18} s) at the microscopic level, while the chemical changes may appear to operate over a timescale of about 10^{-5} s. Thus, the period during which the chemical damage is caused is relatively long on the microscopic scale.

V. Cannatà (✉) • E. Genovese • M. Longo
Unit of Medical Physics, Paediatric Bambino Gesù , Rome, Italy
e-mail: vittorio.cannata@opbg.net

© Springer International Publishing Switzerland 2017

M.C. Garganese, G.F.L. D'Errico (eds.), *Conventional Nuclear Medicine in Pediatrics*, DOI 10.1007/978-3-319-43181-9_2

These events are the precursors to a chain of subsequent events which may eventually lead to the clinical (macroscopic) manifestation of radiation damage. The clinically observable radiation effects, whose timescale may extend to years, are expressed as the results of the functional impairment after lethal damage inflicted to large numbers of cells or critical substructures [3].

Dealing with these macroscopic effects, an important distinction has to be made between low and high dose effects, whose consequences on biological tissues are really different. This concept is highlighted by the NCRP Report No. 136 [15] and by the BEIR VII Report [10] where a fundamental distinction is made: low to moderate doses encompass the values between 0 and 100 mSv, while high doses include values greater than 100 mSv.

Moreover, a distinction of the effects of ionizing radiation on biological tissues is often made according the required time for the effects to manifest. If an effect occurs within several hours or days after the exposure of the individual to extremely high doses, it is considered as an acute effect. Conversely, delayed or latent effects manifest several weeks or years after the exposure.

In some cases, the damaged component of the genetic material is essential for cell survival, and the cell may die or not be able to undergo proper mitosis. The removal of these cells will not contribute to late radiation effects such as carcinogenesis. Instead, late effects occur when the cell survives the initial genetic damage. The consequences of this damage manifest later, perhaps decades after the initial exposure; such late effects may result from genomic instability due to the initial radiation damage. In particular, cells that are growing rapidly and undergoing mitosis at a higher rate may be more susceptible to late radiation effects than those that are growing more slowly [9].

On the basis of these considerations, the radiation effects can also result in a radiation detriment, which is defined as the harm that would eventually be experienced by an exposed group and its descendants as a result of the group's exposure to a radiation source [11].

The radiation damage may be classified as being either deterministic or stochastic.

Deterministic effects are characterized by a threshold dose level. These effects manifest themselves in the form of harmful tissue reactions, i.e., cataract induction, general radiation syndromes, bone marrow ablation, which could manifest after an exposure to high radiation doses. Above the threshold dose level, the severity of the effect is linearly dependent with dose: if the amount of radiation dose is increased, the lesion severity also grows depending on the number of damaged cells [11].

Stochastic effects, which include both carcinogenic and hereditary effects, are those for which the likelihood of occurring is dose related, but the severity of the resultant condition is not related to the dose received. They may occur without a threshold dose, and for them, an increase on radiation dose will result in a growth of the probability of occurring [11].

In the field of Nuclear Medicine (NM) diagnostic uses, stochastic effects have to be predominantly considered as potential side effects while, for radionuclide therapy applications, the concerns relate to both stochastic and deterministic effects [12].

In addition, there are other parameters that influence the radiation effects and that need to be discussed. In fact, it is well established that the risk of ionizing radiation varies with both age and sex. In particular, for pediatric patients, the risk of radiation effect is higher than in adults. This behavior can be attributed to a twofold cause: on one hand, the tissues of younger subjects are more radiosensitive as they are actively growing and, on the other hand, life expectancy in young people is higher than in adults allowing a longer time for the risk to be realized. Moreover, girls demonstrated a higher risk for cancer induction than boys, which is, in large part, attributable to the excess risk of breast cancer in this population [9].

2.2.1 Evaluation of Radiation Exposure in Nuclear Medicine

Nuclear medicine procedures involve the use of radiopharmaceuticals that emit radiations such as γ-rays, α-particles, β-particles, and positron. These emissions expose the patient to ionizing radiation that might lead to detrimental health effects [11]. Nuclear Medicine offers the possibility to detect early stages diseases, and its noninvasive nature allows to use it as a powerful diagnostic tool in examinations involving children. The administered activities in nuclear medicine procedures are well established in many specialties including oncology, urology, cardiology, gastroenterology, and orthopedics. For pediatric patients, it is highly recommended that practitioners of pediatric nuclear medicine have to develop a knowledge in understanding radiation risk and dosimetry and how this risk may vary in children relative to adults. Using nuclear medicine procedures, expected clinical results can be guaranteed using the lowest possible administered activities and, thus, the minimum necessary risk for patients. To this purpose, as recommended by the Society of Nuclear Medicine and Molecular Imaging, the key to dose optimization is to perform the right test with the right dose on the right patient at the right time [8]. In order to estimate the dose received by organs and tissues during nuclear medicine procedures, the knowledge of bio-kinetic models about the incorporated radionuclides is needed.

The methodologies developed to assess dosimetric evaluations in nuclear medicine are mainly two: one of these models was developed by the International Commission on Radiological Protection (ICRP) [12], and the other one by the Medical Internal Radiation Dose (MIRD) Committee of the United States Society of Nuclear Medicine [16]. Based on the same theoretical considerations, MIRD model is focused on biological endpoints for which the knowledge of intake is necessary, while ICRP also gives an estimation of the radiation detriment.

The theoretical approach of both methods will be discussed in the following paying particular attention to how risk varies with age. Moreover, the radiation risk and dose calculation will be discussed later for pediatric nuclear medicine.

The calculation of the absorbed doses by the different organs or tissues is based on the definitions of sources and target organs. The target organs or tissues are those for whom the absorbed doses may arise as a result of radioactive decays occurring in other organs, the so-called source regions.

Thus, the absorbed dose in a particular organ or tissue is calculated as the sum of contributions from various sources, including the target organ or tissue itself.

In order to take into account the different radiosensitivity of organs or tissues, ICRP introduced a dosimetric quantity named effective dose. This definition allowed an overall cancer risk computation for a situation in which different organs receive different doses, with or without external irradiation of the whole body.

According to ICRP model, the mean absorbed dose $D(T \leftarrow S)$ to a target organ or tissue T is the sum of the contributions arising from nuclear transformations of the radionuclide in various source organs S and it is given by:

$$D(T \leftarrow S) = \tilde{A} \times \frac{1}{M_T} \sum_i E_i Y_i \varphi_i = \tilde{A} \times S(T \leftarrow S)$$

where $\tilde{A}$ is the time-integrated or cumulated activity, equal to the total number of nuclear transformations in S, and $S(T \leftarrow S)$ is the absorbed dose in T per unit of cumulated activity in S.

The other symbols have the following meaning: M_T is the mass of the target organ or tissue, E_i is the mean energy of radiation type i, Y_i is the yield of radiation type i per transformation, φ_i is the absorbed fraction of energy of radiation type i.

$\tilde{A}$ is the bio-kinetic component, $S(T \leftarrow S)$ represents the physical-geometrical component, as it depends on the radiation type, on the energy emitted per transformation, on the mass of the target organ, and on the geometry of the mathematical phantoms representing the adult and children of various ages.

This model is essential to estimate the dose absorbed by the different target organs or tissues. However, if we wish to compare different procedures and the resulting patient doses for assessment of risk versus benefit, the more appropriate parameter to be consider is the effective dose, as it takes into account the different organs sensitivities. ICRP 106 also reports, for each radionuclide, the bio-kinetic model, the bio-kinetic data, the absorbed dose, and the correspondent effective dose per unit of activity administered for different ages (Adult and 15, 10, 5, 1 years old) [12].

The MIRD Committee follows the same theoretical dosimetric approach described above for ICRP. For each source organ, the radiation dose is calculated and summed to determine the total dose to the target organ.

For pediatric patients, the radiopharmaceutical dose varies from that to an adult as organ masses of children differ from those of adults because they are smaller and closer together. S values for patients of different ages can be used to estimate the radiation dose to children. However, both ICRP and MIRD methods do not take into account individual differences in anatomy and physiology from the standard models. The patient's body may vary from the standard with respect to size, weight, shape, organ orientation, and distances from other organs. These models also make assumptions with respect to the amount of source organ radioactivity, including rates for uptake and clearance of the radiopharmaceutical from that organ. These methods were developed for estimating the average dose to a population and should not be used to estimate the dose to a specific patient [11].

Even though models have traditionally used simple shapes representing the organs, more realistic voxel-based models have been developed with the aim to provide more accurate dose estimations [4]. Using these methods, the radiation dose to organs of patients of different sizes and ages can be estimated.

The software code Organ Level INternal Dose Assessment/EXponential Model (OLINDA/EXM) [17] has been developed to facilitate automated and standardized internal dose calculations for nuclear medicine applications. The OLINDA/EXM code uses the same technical basis (phantoms, organ masses, equations, relationships assumed, and other details) reported by MIRD [16].

2.2.2 Radiation Protection Principles and Considerations on Diagnostic Reference Levels

The ionizing properties of radiation and the correspondent biological effects have to be taken into account in order to implement some radiation protection measures. The ICRP on its 2007 Publication [11] states that practices involving the use of ionizing radiation are regulated by three fundamental principles of radiological protection: justification, optimization, and limitation of doses.

According to the first principle, any medical practice involving patient exposures must be justified: any decision that alters the radiation exposure situation should do more good than harm [11]. It should be in the right balance between risk and benefit, taking into account social, economic, and technical factors involving the realization of the procedure itself.

The second principle states that once the exposure to ionizing radiation is justified, each examination must be performed so that individual doses should all be kept as low as reasonably achievable (ALARA), taking into account economic and societal factors [11].

Dose limits are established to ensure that no individual is exposed to radiation risk level exceeding the appropriate limits recommended by the ICRP. Medical exposure is not subjected to the third principle but to the first two only [5].

In 1997, the European Council of Ministers, following the recommendation of the ICRP in its Publication 73 [13], issued the Medical Exposure Directive (MED) [5] which introduced the Diagnostic Reference Levels (DRLs) for diagnostic exams.

DRLs are part of the quality assurance program and are defined as the dose levels in medical diagnostic practices or, in case of radiopharmaceuticals, levels of activity, for typical examinations for groups of standard-sized patients or standard phantoms for broadly defined types of equipment [5]. DRLs are primarily intended to offer benchmark values as a rough guideline for appropriate practice and can be considered as a useful tool to help physicians in realizing best practices [1]. These levels are expected not to be exceed for standard procedures when good and normal practice regarding diagnostic and technical performance is applied.

In diagnostic nuclear medicine, DRLs are expressed in terms of administered activity. This latter is based on the administered activity necessary for a good image during a standard procedure. DRLs can be used for diagnostic examinations in clinical practice to different aims: set standards to identify average doses, compare local practice with peer institutions and national levels, provide required protocol settings for local practices, and provide legal justification in event of malpractice law suit. However, as administered activity is not expected to be exceeded in standard procedures, it should be approached as closely as possible to produce optimized images [6]. This is the reason because in nuclear medicine an "optimum" value for DRL is used. On the basis of the experience of the professional groups, it is recommended to nationally set reference levels for administered activities of radionuclides with the aim to obtain information for standard groups of patients (adults and children).

In therapeutic nuclear medicine, where all exposure of target tissues should be specially planned for each patient, so that the doses are as low as possible in nontarget tissues, a system of reference levels is not applicable.

The administered activities are highly dependent on the procedures used. Poorly functioning gamma camera or other chain imaging equipment, the calibration of the activity-meter, the nuclear medicine staff expertise can influence DRL values. Therefore, not only it is highly difficult to compare administered activities without knowing precisely the protocol used, but also there is a large variation between DRLs given by different countries. Not all European Member States have still recommended DRLs for nuclear medicine [7].

Only the 64 % of the European countries set DRLs for NM exams, while the 33 % have no DRLs and the data of the remaining 3 % are unknown (Fig. 2.1).

Most European countries provided optimal values for almost all types of examinations produced by the professional groups and approved by the competent authorities, giving national DRLs for NM procedures [7]. The existence of specific guidance showed that some countries had included references for the DRLs such as published guidance, reports or results of national surveys.

It should be noted that DRLs are based on administered activities used for normal size patients (70 kg). If the adult patients are of a nonstandard size, the injected activities need to be correspondently adjusted. A pro-rata adjustment by patient weight is the simplest method to allow for patient size variation [6].

Regarding pediatric patients, it is highly important to give guidance for a dosage and the following effective dose.

For children the administered activity has to be a fraction of that for adults: this can be assessed on the basis of child weight or by age. Basing the evaluation simply on weight, the resulted activity uptake is comparable to that for adults of less weight, but for children aged under 10, it could not be the right strategy due to children smaller organ masses or to a shorter retention times. The European Association of Nuclear Medicine's Task Group on Pediatrics has produced a list of fractions of adult activity (Table 2.1) which gives an acceptable image quality using nomograms for surface area [6].

These fractions are suitable for most nuclear medicine examinations. Both methods require a minimum activity of 1/10th of the adult value and should be used to ensure that imaging times are acceptable in young children (see Table 2.2) [6].

The employment of DRLs in nuclear medicine clinical practice can ensure the right balance between image quality for a specific diagnostic task and the administered activity, especially for pediatric patients.

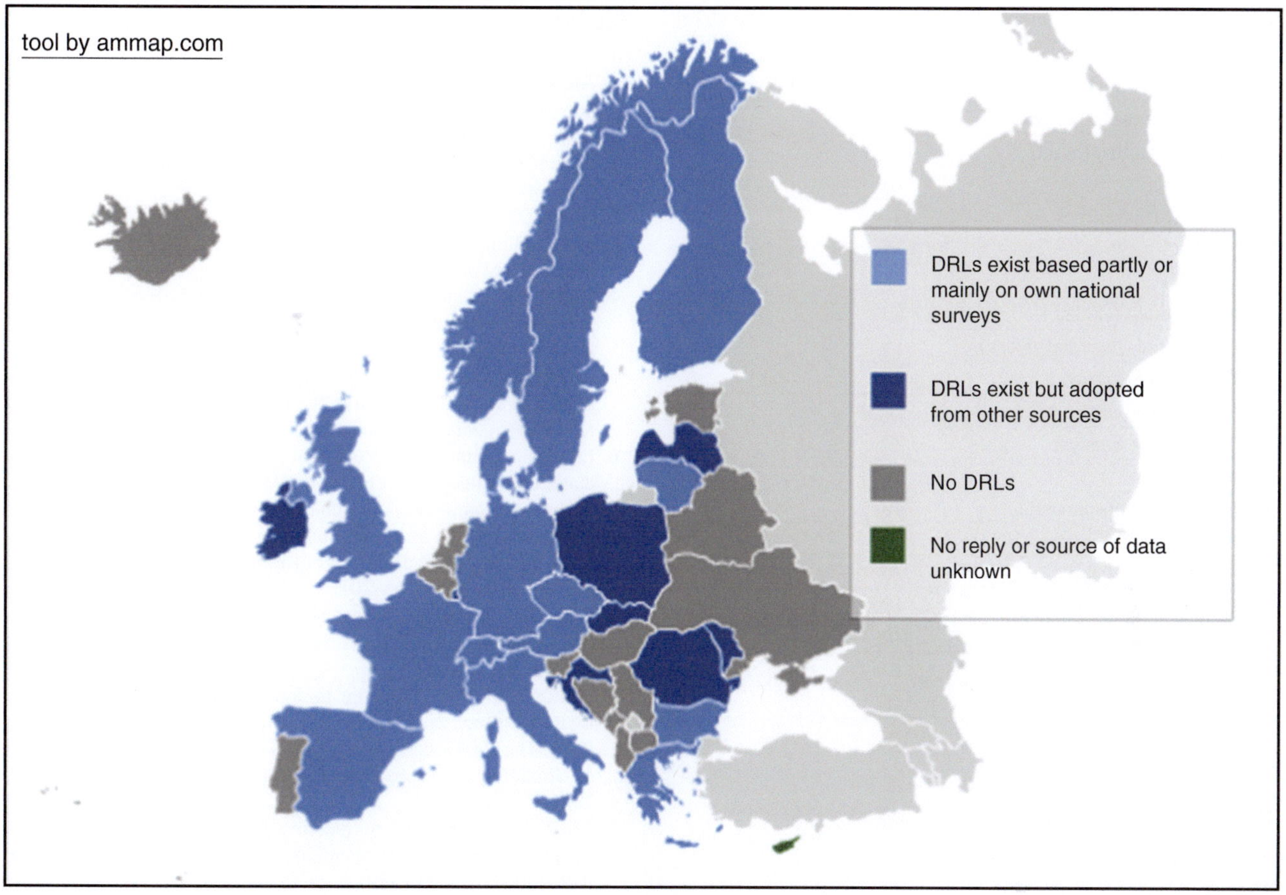

Fig. 2.1 Adoption of national Diagnostic Reference Levels for NM examinations in European countries [7]

Table 2.1 Fraction of adult administered activity for different age groups of children recommended by the Pediatric Task Group of the European Association of Nuclear Medicine [6]

kg	Fraction of adult administered activity	kg	Fraction of adult administered activity	kg	Fraction of adult administered activity
3	0.1	22	0.50	42	0.78
4	0.14	24	0.53	44	0.80
6	0.19	26	0.56	46	0.82
8	0.23	28	0.58	48	0.85
10	0.27	30	0.62	50	0.88
12	0.32	32	0.65	52–54	0.90
14	0.36	34	0.68	56–58	0.95
16	0.40	36	0.71	60–62	1.00
18	0.44	38	0.73	64–66	
20	0.46	40	0.76		

Table 2.2 Minimum amounts of administered activities for children [6]

Radiopharmaceutical	Minimum administered activity for children (MBq)
Gallium-67-citrate	10
I-123-Amphetamine (brain)	18
I-123-Hippuran	10
I-123-Iodide (thyroid)	3
I-123-MIBG	35
I-131-MIBG	35
Tc-99m-albumin (cardiac)	80
Tc-99m-colloid (liver and spleen)	15
Tc-99m-colloid (marrow)	20
Tc-99m-colloid (gastric reflux)	10
Tc-99m-DTPA (kidneys)	20
Tc-99m-DMSA	15
Tc-99m-MDP (phosphonate)	40
Tc-99m-spleen (denatured RBC)	20
Tc-99m-HIDA (biliary)	20
Tc-99m-HMPAO (brain)	100
Tc-99m-HMPAO (WBC)	40
Tc-99m-MAA or microspheres	10
Tc-99m-MAG3	15
Tc-99m-pertechnetate (micturating-cystography)	20
Tc-99m-pertechnetate (first pass)	80
Tc-99m-pertechnetate (Meckel's diverticulum/ectopic gastric mucosa)	20
Tc-99m-pertechnetate (thyroid)	10
Tc-99m-RBC (blood pool)	80

Bibliography

1. Alessio AM, Farrell MB, Fahey FH. Role of reference levels in nuclear medicine: a report of the SNMMI dose optimization task force. J Nucl Med. 2015;56(12):1960–4.
2. Attix FH. Introduction to radiological physics and radiation dosimetry. New York: Wiley; 1986.
3. Bailey DL, Humm JL, Todd-Pokropek A, Van Aswegen A. Nuclear medicine physics: a handbook for teachers and students. Vienna: International Atomic Energy Agency; 2014.
4. Bolch WE, et al. MIRD pamphlet no. 17: the dosimetry of non-uniform activity distributions: radionuclide S values at the voxel level. J Nucl Med. 1999;40(Suppl):11S–36.
5. Council directive 97/43/EURATOM of 30 June 1997 on health protection of individuals against the dangers of ionising radiation in relation to medical exposure. Off J Eur Comm, No L 180.
6. European Commission. Radiation protection n. 109. Guidance on diagnostic reference levels (DRLs) for medical exposures. 1999.
7. European Commission. Radiation protection n. 180. Diagnostic reference levels in thirty-six European countries. 2014.
8. Fahey FH, Stabin M. Dose optimization in nuclear medicine. Semin Nucl Med. 2014;44:193–201.
9. Fahey FH, Treves ST, Adelstein SJ. Minimizing and communicating radiation risk in pediatric nuclear medicine. J Nucl Med. 2011;52(8):1240–51.
10. Health risks from exposure to low levels of ionizing radiation: BEIR VII Phase 2. 2006.
11. ICRP. The 2007 recommendations of the International Commission on Radiological Protection. ICRP publication 103. Ann ICRP. 2007;37(2–4):1–332.
12. ICRP. Radiation dose to patients from radiopharmaceuticals – addendum 3 to ICRP publication 53. ICRP publication 106. Ann ICRP. 2008;38(1–2):1–197.
13. ICRP. Radiological protection and safety in medicine. ICRP publication 73. Ann ICRP. 1996;26(2).
14. Johns HE, Cunningham JR. The physics of radiology. 4th ed. Springfield: Charles C. Thomas; 1983.
15. National Council on Radiation Protection and Measurements, Report No. 136. Evaluation of the linear-nonthreshold dose-response model for ionizing radiation. 2001.
16. Siegel JA, et al. MIRD pamphlet no. 16: techniques for quantitative radiopharmaceutical biodistribution data acquisition and analysis for use in human radiation dose estimates. J Nucl Med. 1999;40:37S–61.
17. Stabin MG, Sparks RB, Crowe E. OLINDA/EXM: the second-generation personal computer software for internal dose assessment in nuclear medicine. J Nucl Med. 2005;46:1023–7.

Part II

Clinical Pediatric Practice

3 Focus on Children with Nephrological and Urological Problems

Nicola Capozza and Giacomo Di Zazzo

3.1 Introduction

Pediatric urology in recent decades has made fundamental progress in the field of minimally invasive. The development of laparoscopic and endoscopic surgical techniques went hand in hand with the adoption of minimally invasive diagnostic methods.

Especially nuclear medicine and ultrasound have become the methods of choice for the diagnosis and management of urological problems of childhood, completely replacing the urography and limiting the use of other more invasive imaging studies.

The main advantage of nuclear medicine is the possibility of obtaining functional data, which are of fundamental importance in pediatric urology.

The studies of nuclear medicine do not require sedation, fasting, or bowel preparation. Rarely, urinary catheterization is necessary. These characteristics, in addition to the low dose of radiation, have contributed to the spread of these methods, generally performed on an outpatient basis.

3.1.1 Main Nuclear Medicine Procedures in Pediatric Urology

3.1.1.1 DMSA Scan

The DMSA renal scintigraphy is the preferred radiotracer for imaging of the renal cortex and has its main indication in the search of renal scarring. The radiopharmaceutical is closely linked to the renal tubules, providing the best visualization of the renal cortex without any interference due to dilatation of the renal pelvis. It also provides functional data correlated with GFR separately for each kidney. At some centers, DMSA scan is also used for the diagnosis of acute pyelonephritis [6]. Other indications are made by the confirmation of multicystic kidney, dysplasia, agenesis, or ectopia. Especially in the neonatal period, ultrasound may sometimes be insufficient to differentiate multicystic kidney from hydronephrosis; in these cases, renal scintigraphy can give a definitive answer. In case of ectopic kidneys, renal scintigraphy is also able to identify minimally functional parenchyma residues.

3.1.1.2 MAG3 Scan

MAG3 is the radiotracer of first choice currently utilized for dynamic renal scintigraphy in pediatric population. The sequential renal scintigraphy is the gold standard in the study of congenital abnormalities of the urinary tract.

The study, carried out according to clearly defined guidelines, provides useful information on separate renal functions (angiographic phase), the excretion and urinary drainage. In case of suspected urinary obstruction, the examination is supplemented by orthostatic and diuretic tests [5].

3.1.1.3 Radionuclide Cystography

Radionuclide cystography is an alternative to voiding cystourethrography (VCUG) for detection of vesicoureteral reflux (VUR). There are two distinct methods of radionuclide cystography: direct and indirect.

The direct radionuclide cystography, initially proposed by Winter in 1959 and modified by Conway in 1972, is performed instilling the radiopharmaceutical directly into the bladder [4, 14]. Reflux is identified when there is the appearance of radioactivity in the kidney and ureter. The indirect cystography is obtained at the end of the sequential renal scintigraphy. When the patient is asked to empty the bladder, reflux causes the reappearance of the radioactivity in the kidney and ureter.

N. Capozza (✉)
Unit of Urology, "Bambino Gesù" Children Hospital, Rome, Italy
e-mail: nicola.capozza@opbg.net

G. Di Zazzo
Unit of Nephrolgy, "Bambino Gesù" Children Hospital, Rome, Italy

© Springer International Publishing Switzerland 2017

M.C. Garganese, G.F.L. D'Errico (eds.), *Conventional Nuclear Medicine in Pediatrics*, DOI 10.1007/978-3-319-43181-9_3

3.1.2 Main Pediatric Nephrological and Urological Problems

3.1.2.1 Congenital Anomalies of the Kidney and Urinary Tract (CAKUTs) and Inherited Kidney Disease

CAKUTs occur in 3–6 per 1000 live births and are responsible for 34–59 % of chronic kidney disease (CKD) and for 31 % of all cases of end-stage kidney disease (ESKD) in children in the United States. All children with ESKD require renal replacement therapy, and up to 70 % of them develop hypertension. CAKUTs comprise a wide range of structural and functional malformations of renal system that occur at the level of the kidney (e.g., hypoplasia and dysplasia, horseshoe kidney, and renal agenesia), collecting system (e.g., hydronephrosis and megaureter), bladder (e.g., ureterocele and vesicoureteral reflux), or urethra (e.g., posterior urethral valves). With improved prenatal screening, many cases of CAKUT are diagnosed by antenatal ultrasonography performed on the fetus of 18–20 weeks of gestation. Most common antenatal manifestations of CAKUT include oligohydramnios or variations in gross morphology of the kidney, ureter, or bladder. Postnatal manifestations of CAKUT may include presence of palpable abdominal mass or single umbilical artery, feeding difficulties, decreased urine output, deficient abdominal wall musculature, and undescended testes in a male infant or multiorgan birth defects. Renal scintigraphy using DMSA is accepted for evaluating renal cortical damage associated with vesicoureteral reflux. Diuretic renography using MAG3 is widely accepted for evaluating differential renal function and/or the shape of the diuretic curve associated with obstructive uropathy. Renal scintigraphy is also a complementary imaging modality in the workup of patients with inherited kidney disease as polycystic kidney disease, tuberous sclerosis complex, medullary cystic kidney disease (MCKD), and nephronophthisis. DMSA is a highly sensitive tracer for detecting functioning renal cortical tissue, and there have been several reports about its utility in different forms of parenchymal and tubulointerstitial diseases.

3.1.2.2 Hydronephrosis

Generally, the ultrasound diagnosis of hydronephrosis has been known since prenatal age and, if it is confirmed in the first weeks of life, the question arises of whether this is due to a real stenosis of ureteropelvic junction. At our center, we perform the renal scintigraphy in cases of hydronephrosis with anteroposterior diameter greater than 15 mm, usually after 2 months of age. The renal scintigraphy provides useful information on whether the obstruction is significant (positive diuretic test) and if there is a decrease in kidney function. This information, supplemented by clinical and ultrasound (worsening of dilation?), let ultimately assess which patients need surgery or just conservative follow-up [11].

Primary hydronephrosis has an incidence of approximately 1:1250 newborns, with a male/female ratio of 3–2/1, mainly interesting the left side. In the newborn and in the infant, there are no symptoms; only sometimes there is a palpable abdominal mass. As mentioned above, the diagnosis is frequently made prenatally. Ultrasound and renal scintigraphy have a key role in the follow-up, to select the correct surgical indications, whereas prenatal hydronephrosis resolves spontaneously in the postnatal period, as long as 80 %. In cases operated with pyeloplasty, renal scintigraphy allows to verify the success of the surgical procedure in most cases. However, in some patients, postoperative renal scintigraphy shows a persistent obstruction, even when a real stenosis can be excluded with endourological procedure. The scintigraphic and ultrasound monitoring of these cases will prevent unnecessary repetition of surgery, showing a gradual resolution of hydronephrosis and stable renal function.

3.1.2.3 Megaureter

The primary megaureter, in order of frequency, is the second cause of obstruction in pediatric urology.

Some authors have proposed as definition of megaureter a dilation larger than 5 or 7 mm. In our experience, we take care of megaureter only when the dilation exceeds 10 mm [8, 9]. The voiding cystourethrography (VCUG) is necessary to differentiate between refluxing and nonrefluxing megaureter. In this second case, the next step is the distinction between obstructive and nonobstructive megaureter. For these assessments, as for hydronephrosis, ultrasound and renal scintigraphy are the methods of choice.

The initial management of obstructive megaureter is usually conservative, but surgical or endourological treatment is indicated in case of symptoms, increase of dilation, or progressive kidney damage [7]. This last point is still debated, but it must be noted and communicated to parents of children that a possible kidney damage is still unpredictable and irreversible. In our center, the selection of patients for surgery/endourology is based on the complex of clinical, scintigraphic, and ultrasound data. Patients with a ureteral dilation >15 mm are investigated with MAG3 renal scintigraphy. The regions of interest are kidney and ureter, getting a renogram and a ureterogram. The examination is almost always completed by the diuretic test. An obstructive pattern, with no decrease in kidney function, is not an absolute indication for treatment. If ureteral dilatation persists or tends to increase at follow-up ultrasound, the renal scintigraphy is repeated and compared with the previous study, allowing to assess the evolution of megaureter and to decide for a treatment [13].

3.1.2.4 Vesicoureteral Reflux

Vesicoureteral reflux is the most frequent problem in pediatric urology (1–2 % of the pediatric population).

Nuclear medicine has a key role in the diagnosis of the so-called reflux nephropathy. Actually, as recently well-known, in most cases, the nephropathy is simply associated to the reflux (CAKUT). According to the known theory of Mackie and Stephens, the ectopic ureteral bud is at the basis of both vesicoureteral reflux (intramural ureteral tract shorter than normal) and anomalous induction of renal blastema, with the result of different grades of renal dysplasia [10]. However, the real acquired reflux nephropathy can intervene subsequently as a result of episodes of pyelonephritis that determine renal scarring [1]. From the clinical point of view, the distinction between congenital dysplasia and acquired nephropathy is very important. The first, if unilateral, is usually compensated by hyperplasia (improperly defined hypertrophy by some authors) of the contralateral kidney, without affecting the total renal function. On the contrary, acquired nephropathy can reduce the function of the affected kidney, but especially the presence of scars may be associated with hypertension and proteinuria in the following years [12].

DMSA scan defines very well the presence of renal scarring, providing essential information for the clinical management of vesicoureteral reflux [15].

Nuclear medicine also has a role in the diagnosis of vesicoureteral reflux, traditionally entrusted to voiding cystourethrography.

Both methods of radionuclide cystography, direct and indirect, can be used.

The advantage of radionuclide cystography is the lower radiation dose compared to VCUG. The indirect cystography also has the advantage of not requiring catheterization of the bladder, although it requires the active cooperation of the patient, who has to be toilet-trained; this technique is therefore reserved for children over the age of 2–3 years. Another advantage of indirect radionuclide cystography is to allow a simultaneous evaluation of renal function and reflux. The main disadvantage of this kind of cystography (direct and indirect) is the less morphological definition, with the ability to classify reflux in three grades, instead of five of that of VCUG.

In our center, we use the indirect radionuclide cystography in the follow-up of vesicoureteral reflux according to our minimally invasive commitment to our young patients [2, 3].

In the follow-up of vesicoureteral reflux treated endoscopically, we consider three groups of patients: (A) children of any age with mild-to-moderate reflux, (B) children with severe reflux under the age of 3 years, and (C) children with severe reflux over the age of 3.

In group A, we do not perform any routine control cystography, because success rate of endoscopic treatment in mild and moderate reflux approaches 100%. In group B, we still perform VCUG, 6 months after treatment. In group C, we have completely replaced VCUG with indirect radionuclide cystography.

3.1.2.5 Renovascular Disorders

Renovascular hypertension refers to hypertension caused by renal hypoperfusion, which is usually the result of renal artery stenosis. The stenosis may be unilateral or bilateral and may involve one or more branches of the renal artery. Therefore, the angiographic demonstration of stenosis in a hypertensive patient does not prove that the stenosis caused the hypertension. The prevalence of renovascular hypertension varies with the nature of the hypertensive population that has also been recognized in neonates and children.

Renal infarction is a rare disease and results from interruption of the normal blood supply to part of or to the whole kidney. Most often, it is secondary to a known underlying disease or appears as idiopathic. The causes of renal infarction include thromboembolism, trauma, polycythemia vera, dissection of artery, aneurysm, connective tissue disease, and primary antiphospholipid syndrome. This condition should be suspected in cases of sudden flank or upper abdominal pain. DMSA is useful to detect cortical defects in the kidney.

3.1.2.6 Renal Transplant

Ultrasound (US) and Doppler US are the primary imaging modalities for evaluation of the renal transplant. US can identify post-transplant complications, obstruction, and mass lesions. Doppler US can detect vascular disease after kidney transplant. Radionuclide imaging is useful when US does not provide an explanation for graft dysfunction. Absence of flow to the kidney occurs with arterial or venous obstruction or with hyperacute rejection. In contrast, a graft with acute tubular necrosis (ATN) has normal renal perfusion, but delayed or no excretion. Radionuclide imaging is useful for demonstrating urinary obstruction or that a perinephric fluid collection is due to a urine leak.

Bibliography

1. Arant Jr BS. Medical management of mild and moderate vesicoureterl reflux: followup studies of infants and young children. A preliminary report of the Southwest Pediatric Nephrology Study Group. J Urol. 1992;148:1683–7.
2. Capozza N, Caione P. Dextranomer/hyaluronic acid copolymer implantation for vesico-ureteral reflux: a randomized comparison with antibiotic prophylaxis. J Pediatr. 2002;140(2):230–4.
3. Capozza N, Lais A, Matarazzo E. Treatment of vesicoureteral reflux: a new algorithm based on parental preference. BJU Int. 2003;92(3):285–8.
4. Conway JJ, King LR, Belman AB, et al. Detection of vesicoureteral reflux with radionuclide cystography. Am J Roentgenol Radium Ther Nucl Med. 1972;115:720–7.
5. Conway JJ, Maizels M. The "well tempered" diuretic renogram: a standard method to examine the asymptomatic neonate with hydronephrosis or hydroureteronephrosis. A report from combined meetings of The Society for Fetal Urology and members of The Pediatric Nuclear Medicine Council – The Society of Nuclear Medicine. J Nucl Med. 1992;33:2047–51.

6. Elison BS, Taylor D, Van der Wall H, et al. Comparison of DMSA scintigraphy with intravenous urography for the detection of renal scarring and its correlation with vesicoureteric reflux. Br J Urol. 1992;69:294–302.
7. Farrugia MK, Steinbrecher HA, Malone PS. The utilization of stents in the management of primary obstructive megaureters requiring intervention before 1 year of age. J Pediatr Urol. 2011;7:198–202.
8. King LR. Megaloureter: definition, diagnosis and management. J Urol. 1980;123:222–3.
9. Liu HY, Dhillon HK, Yeung CK, et al. Clinical outcome and management of prenatally diagnosed primary megaureters. J Urol. 1994;152:614–7.
10. Mackie GG, Awang H, Stephens FD. The ureteric orifice: the embryologic key to radiologic status of duplex kidneys. J Pediatr Surg. 1975;10:473–81.
11. Mandell GA, Cooper JA, Leonard JC, et al. Procedure guideline for diuretic renography in children. J Nucl Med. 1997;38:1647–50.
12. Smellie J, Edwards D, Hunter N. Vesico-ureteric reflux and renal scarring. Kidney Int. 1975;8(4):565–72.
13. Torino G, Collura G, Mele E, Garganese MC, Capozza N. Severe primary obstructive megaureter in the first year of life: preliminary experience with endoscopic balloon dilation. J Endourol. 2012;26(4):325–9.
14. Winter CC. A new test for vesicoureteral reflux: an external technique using radiosotopes. J Urol. 1959;81:105–11.
15. Yen TC, Chen WP, Chang SL, et al. Technetium-99m-DMSA renal SPECT in diagnosing and monitoring pediatric acute pyelonephritis. J Nucl Med. 1996;37:1349–53.

Hydronephrosis

4

Maria Felicia Villani, Milena Pizzoferro, Simona Nappo, and Maria Carmen Garganese

4.1 Introduction

Hydronephrosis, which is the dilatation of the renal pelvis, is the most common urological anomaly. In the vast majority of cases, hydronephrosis is nowadays detected prenatally and is therefore asymptomatic. A limited number of cases are still diagnosed during childhood or adolescence after symptoms (urinary tract infection, hematuria, and pain), and their management is straightforward surgical in order to relieve symptoms and obstruction.

Congenital hydronephrosis is detected from 1 to 5 % of all pregnancies. These patients offer a unique dilemma, since over 50–75 % of them will undergo resolution either prenatally or postnatally. The goals of treatment are therefore the early identification of patients at risk of significant uropathy and prevention of renal damage, avoiding at the same time overmedicalization of children not at risk.

How should patients with hydronephrosis be evaluated prenatally and postnatally and who should be candidate to surgery have been the objects of intense debate over the past 20 years.

4.1.1 Prenatal Diagnosis

Prenatal hydronephrosis is one of the most common findings on prenatal ultrasound, with an incidence of 1–5 % of pregnancies. The most common clinically significant etiology of hydronephrosis is ureteropelvic junction obstruction (UPJO), which has an incidence of 1/1000–1/1250.

There is no clear consensus defining the entity of prenatal dilatation and which should be considered clinically significant, and therefore requires postnatal investigation.

The first and most common system of classification of hydronephrosis is by measuring the anteroposterior diameter (APD) of the renal pelvis. In the original work by Corteville, an APD >4 mm at 33 weeks and >7 mm at 40 weeks of gestational age were considered threshold for postnatal evaluation. Other studies have proposed clinically significant hydronephrosis as being >10 mm in the second trimester and >15 mm in the third trimester: such cutoff values are associated with a >50 % likelihood of UPJO in the postnatal age. However, one should keep in mind that dilatation also depends on gestational age, bladder fullness, and maternal hydration status.

A second classification system of hydronephrosis was proposed by the Society of Fetal Urology (SFU) in 1993, based not only on the pyelic diameter but also on the global appearance of the renal collecting system. The SFU system goes from grade 1, with normal parenchymal thickness and/or renal pelvis splitting, to grade 4 hydronephrosis, in which distension of pelvis and calyces goes together with parenchymal thinning. The SFU grading correlates with the potential for postnatal resolution of the hydronephrosis, with >50 % grade 1 and only 3 % grade 4 hydronephrosis resolving spontaneously. However, similarly, hydronephrosis with APD <15 mm seldom requires surgery, while almost 100 % of those with APD >40 mm will definitely need surgery.

When facing a hydronephrosis, in addition to defining the grade of pyelocalyceal dilatation, the ultrasonography must also assess other issues: presence and morphology of contralateral kidney, visualization of dilated ureter, visualization of the distended bladder and bladder cycling, and in the fetus, amount of amniotic fluid, fetal growth, and other organ system abnormalities. These additional findings will guide prenatal counseling and postnatal differential diagnosis (Table 4.1).

M.F. Villani • M. Pizzoferro
Nuclear Medicine Unit, Imaging Department, "Bambino Gesù" Children Hospital, Rome, Italy

S. Nappo (✉)
Unit of Urology, "Bambino Gesù" Children Hospital, Rome, Italy
e-mail: simona.gerocarni@opbg.net

M.C. Garganese
Department of Diagnostic Imaging-Nuclear Medicine, IRCCS Bambino Gesù Paediatric Hospital, Rome, Italy

© Springer International Publishing Switzerland 2017
M.C. Garganese, G.F.L. D'Errico (eds.), *Conventional Nuclear Medicine in Pediatrics*, DOI 10.1007/978-3-319-43181-9_4

Other postnatal obstructive uropathies than PUJO can be associated with prenatal or neonatal hydronephrosis, such as posterior urethral valves (PUV) or ureterovescical junction obstruction (UVJO), and are more often associated with higher grades of hydronephrosis. Vesicoureteric reflux (VUR) is present in 5–15 % of prenatal hydronephrosis and, differently from the aforementioned obstructive uropathies, does not appear to be related to the severity of the dilatation, which is obvious if one thinks to the intermittent nature of VUR. As a consequence, postnatal imaging could be warranted even in the setting of mild prenatal hydronephrosis.

Table 4.1 Differential diagnosis of antenatal/postnatal hydronephrosis

Etiology	Incidence (%)	US findings	Diagnostic exams
Transient hydronephrosis	50–70	Isolated hydronephrosis (mild)	US
UPJO	10–30	Isolated hydronephrosis (DAP >15 mm)	MAG3
VUR	10–40	Intermittent hydronephrosis, ureteric dilatation, small kidney	VCUG/DMSA
UVJU	5–10	Ureteric dilatation	VCUG/MAG3
MCDK	1–5	Random renal cyst, little or no hyperechoic parenchima	DMSA
PUV	2–5	Thickened bladder wall, hydronephrosis, hyperechoic kidney, ureteric dilatation, oligoidramnios (fetal), key-hole sign (fetal)	VCUG/MAG3

4.1.2 Postnatal Management

There is general consensus that moderate to severe prenatal hydronephrosis should undergo routine postnatal imaging: in such cases, the risk of postnatal pathological finding ranges from 45 to 80 % of cases (the more severe hydronephrosis is, the higher is the risk). In infants with mild hydronephrosis, the role of postnatal imaging is less clear; however, up to 10 % of these cases may have significant uropathies. Therefore, even in infants with mild or disappeared hydronephrosis, at least a single postnatal imaging seems of benefit.

Renal ultrasonography (US) is the principal imaging technique used in both postnatal and in prenatal life, due to the easy availability, low cost, and absence of radiation exposure; however, it is operator-dependent.

Postnatal ultrasonography should be performed at 3–7 days of life, in order to avoid underestimation or incorrect assessment due to physiological disidratation occurring in the very first days of life.

Differential diagnosis of postnatal hydronephrosis based on US findings is shown in Table 4.1.

When dilatation of calyces and pelvis is isolated and not associated with any other abnormal finding, up to 50–70 % of these cases will be transient, and will gradually disappear spontaneously without any clinical sequelae or renal impairment. The remaining 30 % of prenatal hydronephrosis will require further postnatal investigation other than ultrasonography.

4.1.3 Diagnostic Investigations

Since the vast majority of hydronephrosis will gradually disappear, periodic urinary tract ultrasonography (every 2–3 months in the first year of life) is mandatory in order to assess the evolution of the urinary dilatation.

In cases of hydronephrosis associated with ureteric dilatation, and in patients presenting with symptomatic UTI, international guidelines recommend the execution of VCUG in order to rule out the presence of VUR, as in the chapter on VUR. Otherwise, in asymptomatic isolated hydronephrosis, routine VCUG may not be needed: in this instance, infact VUR prevalence is low (15 %), with VUR being of low grade in most cases and clinically not significant.

In the absence of VUR, and when periodic ultrasonography shows persistence or worsening of hydronephrosis, the presence of UPJO has to be suspected. Dynamic renal scan is the imaging investigation of choice.

The most popular dynamic scan in cases of suspected obstruction uses Tc-mercaptoacetyltriglycine (MAG3) as radiotracer. Briefly, MAG3 is primarily excreted by secretion from the proximal tubule. As a result, it can allow evaluation of both split renal function and urine progression to the bladder.

Renal immaturity prompts us to perform nuclear medicine exams before the infant is 1 month old, for the risk otherwise to underestimate split renal function. For the same reason, the child must be adequately fed and well hydrated. IV fluids are however considered unnecessary to the vast majority of cases. Sedation is not required, and the placement of a bladder catheter should be reserved to much selected cases.

4.1.4 Particular Cases

4.1.4.1 Symptomatic Hydronephrosis

Symptomatic hydronephrosis is a totally different entity from congenital asymptomatic hydronephrosis. It generally occurs in a school-age child or adolescent, which presents with intermittent abdominal pain, sometimes together with vomiting. Urinary tract infection may or may not be present. Perinatal US may be negative, or a previous hydronephrosis may have solved spontaneously. Children as young as 3 years may present with colicky pain due to hydronephrosis. In the vast majority of symptomatic cases, aberrant vessels may be found going to the lower pole of the kidney and causing intermittent compression of the UPJ. In situation of hyperdiuresis, the UPJ is compressed and the pelvis gets distended; this in turn determines reduction of diuresis and reduction of the hydronephrosis. The pain is therefore intermittent, as is the US finding of hydronephrosis, Nonetheless, this mechanism can lead to significant loss of kidney function. Grade of hydronephrosis can be extremely variable at US. MAG3 scan can be nonobstructive. The treatment is straightforward surgical.

4.1.4.2 Hydronephrosis in Renal Anomalies

Three peculiar cases are possible: hydronephrosis in duplex system, hydronephrosis in ectopic kidney, and in horseshoe kidney. In most cases of renal anomalies, an anatomical defect of UPJ is present and spontaneous resolution of obstruction is less plausible.

Hydronephrosis in horseshoe kidney occurs more commonly than in normal kidneys. Vascular anomalies with aberrant vessels may be present as well as the anomalies of the UPJ with very high insertion of the ureter on the pelvis. The surgical approach must be decided, keeping in mind the abnormal position of the renal pelvis (anterior and medial to the kidney), and a laparoscopic transperitoneal approach should be considered nowadays the surgical approach of choice. Section of the hystums is no longer an option.

Hydronephrosis in the ectopic kidney can be associated with reduced function due to renal hypoplasia. At US, the pelvis is generally malrotated. Evaluation of UPJO and indication to surgery may not be so evident.

Hydronephrosis in the duplex kidney is the less common. It generally occurs in the lower pole. Compression by aberrant vessels to the lower pole can be a possible cause. Hypoplasia of UPJ in case of incomplete duplex system (two pelvis draining in a single ureter) is also a possible occurrence.

4.2 The Surgical Treatment

Surgical correction of UPJO consists of excision of the obstructed tract at the UPJ and a pyeloureteral anastomosis, as described by Anderson–Hynes technique. Surgery can be performed in an open fashion, through a lumbar lateral, anterior or posterior incision. In the last decade, minimally invasive approaches have become popular, which means by small open-fashioned incisions in infants and young children, laparoscopy-assisted procedures in infants and young children, laparoscopic trans-or retroperitoneal in grown-up children, or robotics-assisted procedures. These procedures have gained wide acceptance due to the reduced pain, quicker recovery, and similar results as in traditional open surgery.

In children and adolescents with aberrant vessels, cephalad mobilization of the vessel (so-called "vascular hitch"), according to Hellstrom technique, can be as effective as the dismembered Anderson–Hynes pyeloplasty in selected patients.

4.3 The Follow-Up

Periodical US is recommended after surgery. Significant reduction of the hydronephrosis is expected, but it may take months or years to take place. Persistent dilatation of the renal pelvis is a possible occurrence even in the absence of obstruction, especially when very large hypotonic pelvis and calyces were observed before surgery. MAG3 scan should be repeated at 6–12 months follow-up, or earlier if dilatation persists. In this latter case, definition of persistent obstruction from large hypotonic pelvis with dilated calyces can be particularly challenging for the nuclear medicine specialist.

4.4 Dynamic Renal Scintigraphy

Dynamic renal scintigraphy allows to assessing renal function and drainage, evaluating both renal excretion and differential renal function (DRF).

Most common indications in pediatric population include determination of DRF and drainage in hydronephrosis and megaureter, in diagnostic phase, after surgical repair (when performed), and during follow-up.

4.4.1 Study Technique and Interpretation

The patient, adequately hydrated, receives ^{99m}Tc-MAG3 (mercaptoacetyltriglycine) as a bolus injection contextually with the starting of 30-min dynamic acquisition The administered activity of radiotracer is adjusted to the patient's weight, according to EANM dosage card and to the national regulations.

Region-of-interest (ROI) around the heart, the kidneys, and the area around the kidneys ("background") are drawn on a summed image of dynamic frames using a dedicated software; thus, time/activity curves are obtained, of expression of perfusion (flow T/A) and of renal function and drainage (renograms), respectively. In renograms, the ascending part represents the parenchymal phase (single kidney function) and the descending part reflects renal transit and emptying; with the same method, differential renal function (DRF or split function) is also determined.

If renal drainage is impaired at the end of the dynamic study, an additional image after 5 min standing upright is acquired ("gravity-assisted drainage," GAD1). In case of still poor drainage (cutoff = 30 %), a 1 mg/kg dose of furosemide is given intravenously and an additional 20-min dynamic acquisition follows. If pyelic drainage is still incomplete (half-time >20 min, drainage <30 %), a second "gravity-assisted drainage" test (GAD-2) is also performed. The drainage is classified as impaired on the basis of all the previous mentioned three tests.

4.4.2 Teaching Cases

4.4.2.1 Case 4.1 Normal Ultrasonographic and Scintigraphic Pattern After Left Pyeloplasty

A 5-year-old boy came to Emergency for recurrent left lumbar pain. On ultrasonography, grade 3 left hydronephrosis was detected. No urinary tract dilatation was referred at prenatal ultrasound. Dynamic renal scintigraphy showed symmetrical split function with obstructive urinary drainage at diuretic test. Pyeloplasty for correction of UPJO was performed with complete ultrasonographic resolution of the left hydronephrosis. MAG3 scan was repeated at 1-year follow-up after pyeloplasty (Fig. 4.1).

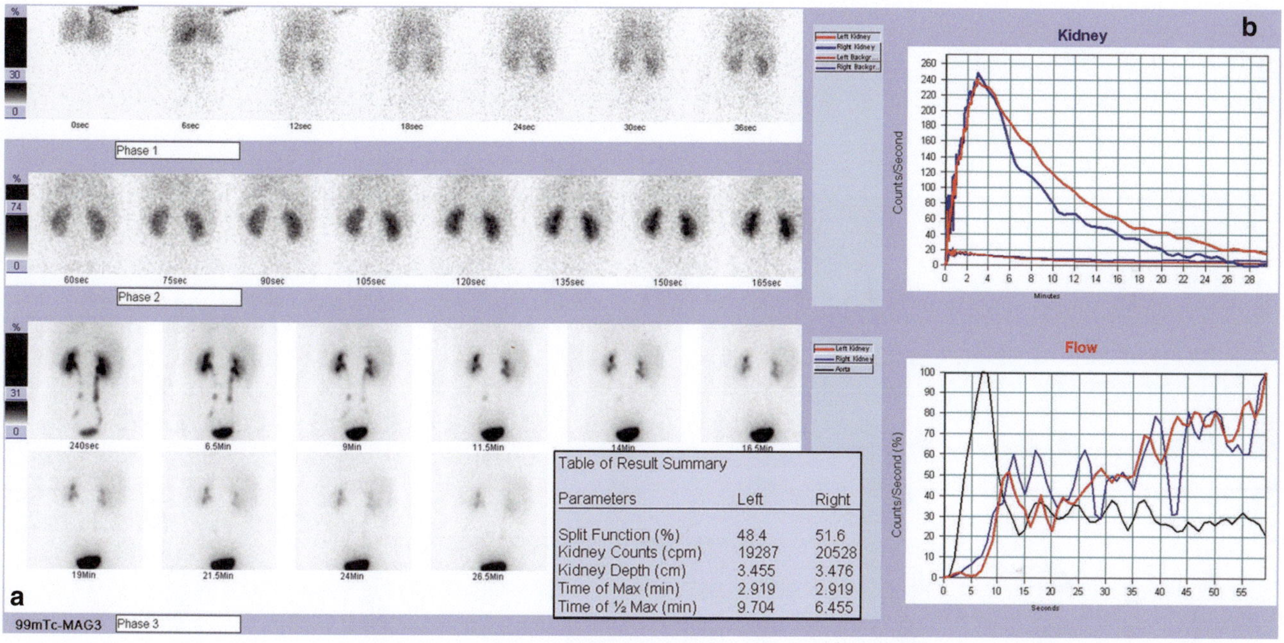

Fig. 4.1 MAG3 dynamic renal scan (after pyeloplasty): dynamic images (**a**) show good and homogeneous radiotracer uptake and normal drainage in both kidneys; renograms (**b**) confirm normal function and drainage of both kidneys (left DRF: 48 %; right DRF: 52 %); flow T/A curves (**b**) show synchronous and symmetrical perfusion

4.4.2.2 Case 4.2 Persistent nonobstructive Left Hydronephrosis with Normal Split Function

A boy of 3 years was followed for prenatal diagnosis of bilateral hydronephrosis, stable during pregnancy and confirmed at birth with an anteroposterior diameter (APD) of 15 mm. After birth, progressive decrease of right pyelic dilatation and persistent left hydronephrosis was found. One episode of acute pyelonephritis occurred at 3 months with subsequent cystography (VCUG) negative for vesicoureteric reflux. No further episodes of urinary tract infections (UTI). At the age of 3 years, he presented persistent left hydronephrosis with anteroposterior (AP) pyelic diameter of 24 mm and good parenchymal thickness, asymptomatic. MAG3 scan showed normal left split renal function and adequate urinary drainage after GAD-1 test. No surgical indication. Ultrasonographic follow-up was recommended (Fig. 4.2).

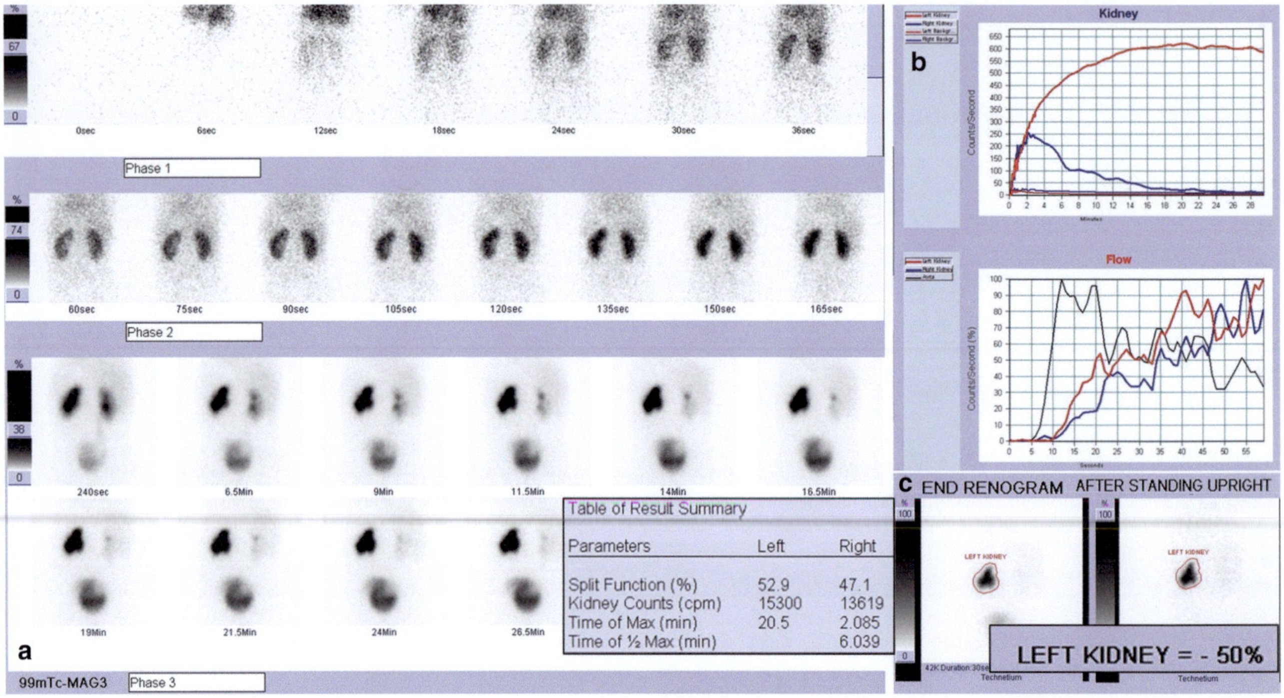

Fig. 4.2 MAG3 dynamic renal scan: dynamic images (**a**) show good radiotracer uptake and nonhomogeneous intraparenchymal distribution in left kidney; an area devoid of tracer corresponding to dilated renal pelvis is evident and drainage is poor; right kidney presents good and homogeneous radiotracer uptake and normal drainage; renograms (**b**) confirm normal function but poor drainage of left kidney ("plateau pattern") and normal function and drainage of right kidney (left DRF: 53 %; right DRF: 47 %); flow T/A curves show synchronous and symmetrical perfusion. Gravity-assisted drainage-1 test shows significant emptying of left kidney, excluding a significant obstacle in the upper pyelic junction (**c**)

4.4.2.3 Case 4.3 Prenatal Diagnosis of Right Hydronephrosis with Worsening of Dilatation at Follow-Up

A girl of 4 years was seen for prenatal diagnosis of right hydronephrosis, confirmed at birth and stable at follow-up. No UTI were referred. Toilet training was attained at the age of 2, with no lower urinary tract symptoms. At 4 years, ultrasonography showed increase of right hydronephrosis with AP diameter of 28 mm and calyceal dilatation. The girl was asymptomatic. Dynamic renal scintigraphy showed normal right split function and adequate urinary drainage after diuretic test. No surgical indication. Ultrasonographic follow-up was recommended (Fig. 4.3).

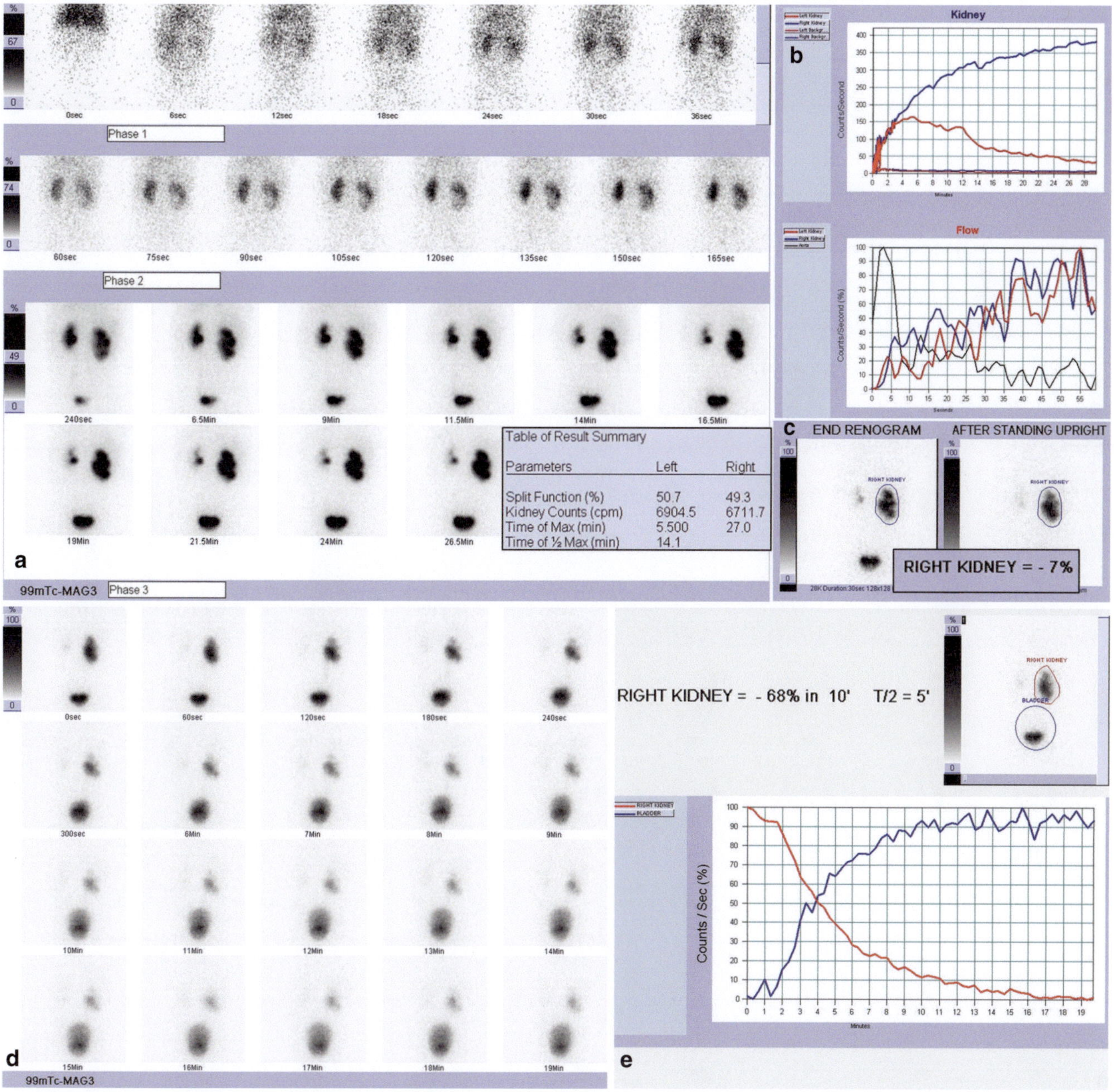

Fig. 4.3 MAG3 dynamic renal scan: dynamic images (**a**) show good and homogeneous radiotracer uptake and normal drainage in left kidney; right kidney shows good radiotracer uptake and nonhomogeneous intraparenchymal distribution. A large area devoid of tracer corresponding to right dilated renal pelvis and collecting system is evident, and urinary drainage is poor. Renograms (**b**) confirm normal function and drainage of left kidney and normal function but poor drainage of right kidney ("rising curve") (left DRF: 51 %; right DRF: 49 %); flow T/A curves (**b**) show synchronous and symmetrical perfusion. Gravity-assisted drainage-1 test shows no significant improvement in right kidney drainage (**c**). Diuretic dynamic images (**d**) and diuretic renogram (**e**) show prompt and significant renal washout after administration of furosemide, ruling out a significative obstructive pattern

4.4.2.4 Case 4.4 Persistent Left Calyceal Dilatation at 10 Years Follow-Up After Pyeloplasty with Preserved Split Renal Function

A case of a boy with Noonan syndrome is presented. Left pyeloplasty was performed at 1 year of age for UPJO. During follow-up, at 13 years of age, the boy was asymptomatic, and ultrasonography and MAG3 renal scan were performed; ultrasonography showed persistent calyceal dilatation, stable over time, without significant pyelic dilatation (AP diameter 9 mm). Dynamic renal scintigraphy showed normal split renal function and slow but significant urinary drainage after diuretic test. Delayed transit time at diuretic test may be found in calyceal dilatation, but significant washout at diuretic test and preserved split renal function support the thesis of absence of significant obstruction. Since left kidney split function was preserved at 12 years follow-up, ultrasonographic surveillance every 3–5 years is suggested (Fig. 4.4).

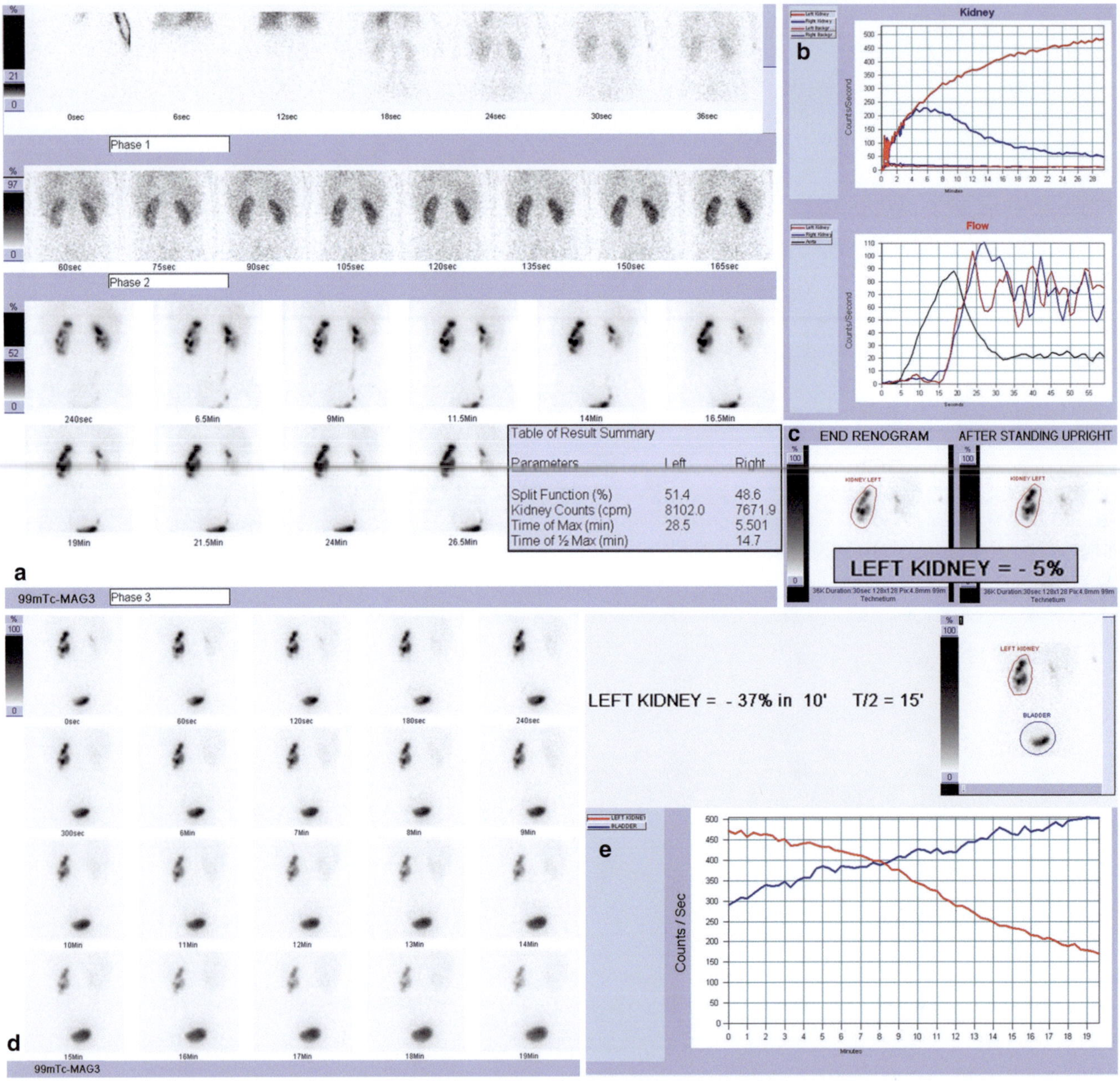

Fig. 4.4 MAG3 dynamic renal scan: dynamic images (**a**) show good radiotracer uptake and nonhomogeneous intraparenchymal distribution in left kidney; an area devoid of tracer corresponding to dilated renal pelvis and collecting system is evident, and drainage is poor; right kidney presents good and homogeneous radiotracer uptake and normal drainage. Renograms (**b**) confirm normal function but poor drainage of left kidney ("rising curve") and normal function and drainage of right kidney (left DRF: 51 %; right DRF: 49 %); flow T/A curves (**b**) show synchronous and symmetrical perfusion. Gravity-assisted drainage-1 test shows no significant improvement in left kidney drainage (**c**). Diuretic dynamic images (**d**) and diuretic renogram (**e**) show slow response to furosemide in left kidney, but significant washout

4.4.2.5 Case 4.5 Persistent Left Hydronephrosis with Delayed Urinary Drainage After Pyeloplasty

After prenatal finding of bilateral grade 3 hydronephrosis, with postnatal progressive worsening of dilatation on the left side, a girl of 3 years of age underwent left pyeloplasty for UPJO. At follow-up, persistent grade 3–4 hydronephrosis was found. MAG3 scan was performed 6 months after pyeloplasty and showed preserved split function and urinary drainage after GAD-2 test; based on the scintigraphic scan, the ultrasonographic finding of persistent high-grade hydronephrosis was interpreted as hypotonic dilated pelvis in the absence of significant obstruction. Repeated surgery was not indicated. Strict ultrasonographic surveillance was scheduled (Fig. 4.5).

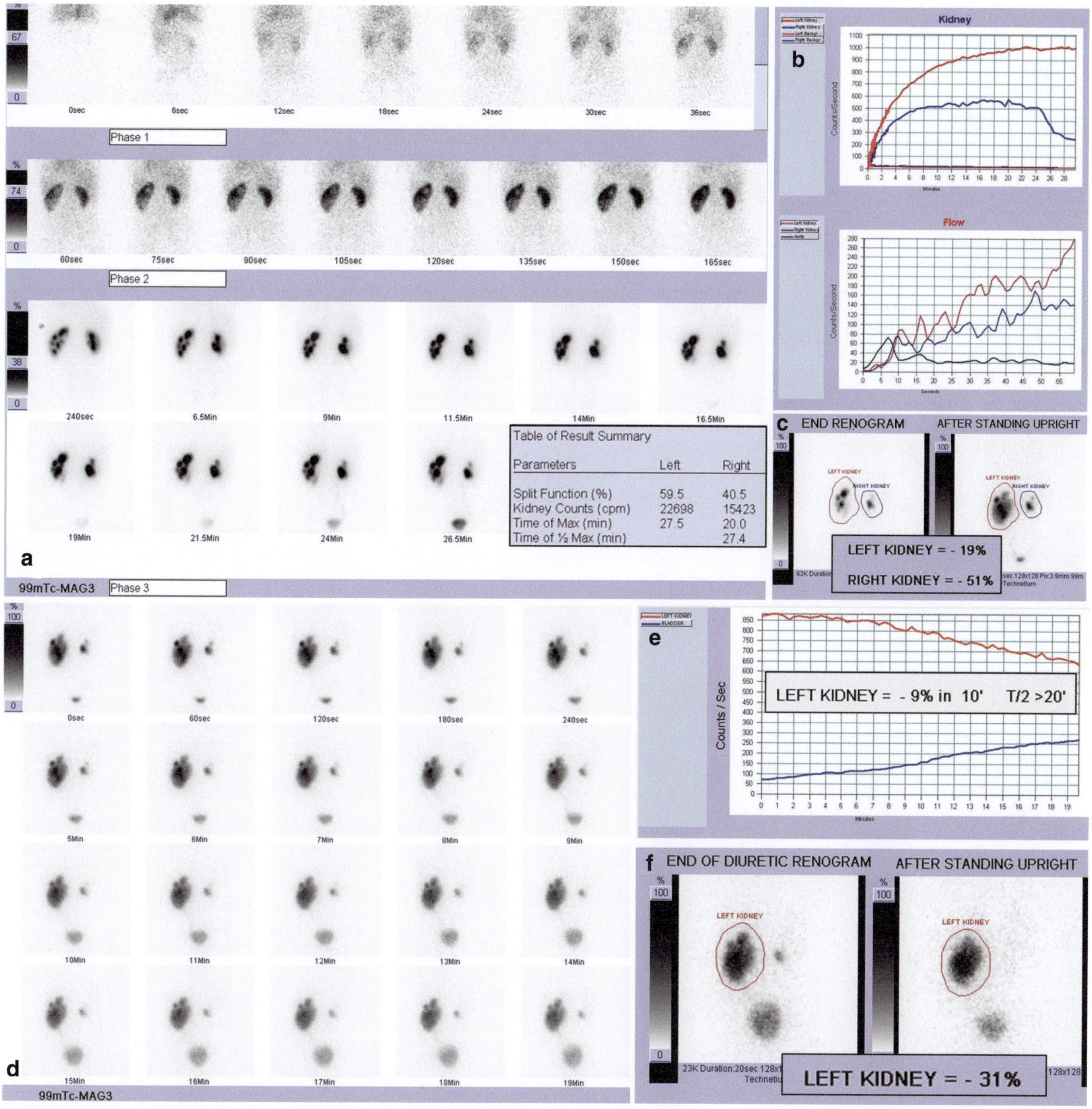

Fig. 4.5 MAG3 dynamic renal scan: dynamic images (**a**) show good radiotracer uptake and nonhomogeneous intraparenchymal distribution in left kidney; an area devoid of tracer corresponding to dilated renal pelvis and collecting system is evident, and drainage is poor; right kidney presents good and homogeneous radiotracer uptake and mildly poor drainage; renograms (**b**) show normal function and impaired drainage of left kidney ("rising curve") and normal function of right kidney with partial radiotracer washout during the last minutes of the study (left DRF: 59.5 %; right DRF: 40.5 %); flow T/A curves (**b**) show synchronous but mildly asymmetrical perfusion (reduced in right kidney, due to reduced size of the kidney). Gravity-assisted drainage-1 test shows further improvement in right kidney drainage, but no significant improvement in left kidney drainage (**c**). Diuretic dynamic images (**d**) and diuretic renogram (**e**) show slow response to furosemide and no significant improvement in drainage in left kidney. Gravity-assisted drainage-2 test (**f**) shows significant washout in left kidney

4.4.2.6 Case 4.6 Prenatal Hydronephrosis: Normal Split Function

A boy of 7 months of age was seen after prenatal diagnosis of left hydronephrosis. Postnatally, progressive increase of left hydronephrosis was found, with most recent ultrasonography showing grade 4 hydronephrosis and AP diameter of 32 mm with calyceal dilatation. No UTI occurred. MAG3 scan showed symmetrical split function with insufficient urinary drainage after all scintigraphic tests. Pyeloplasty was scheduled. At surgery confirmation of intrinsic UPJO was found. Postoperative follow-up was uneventful with minimal residual dilatation at ultrasonography at 6 months follow-up (Fig. 4.6).

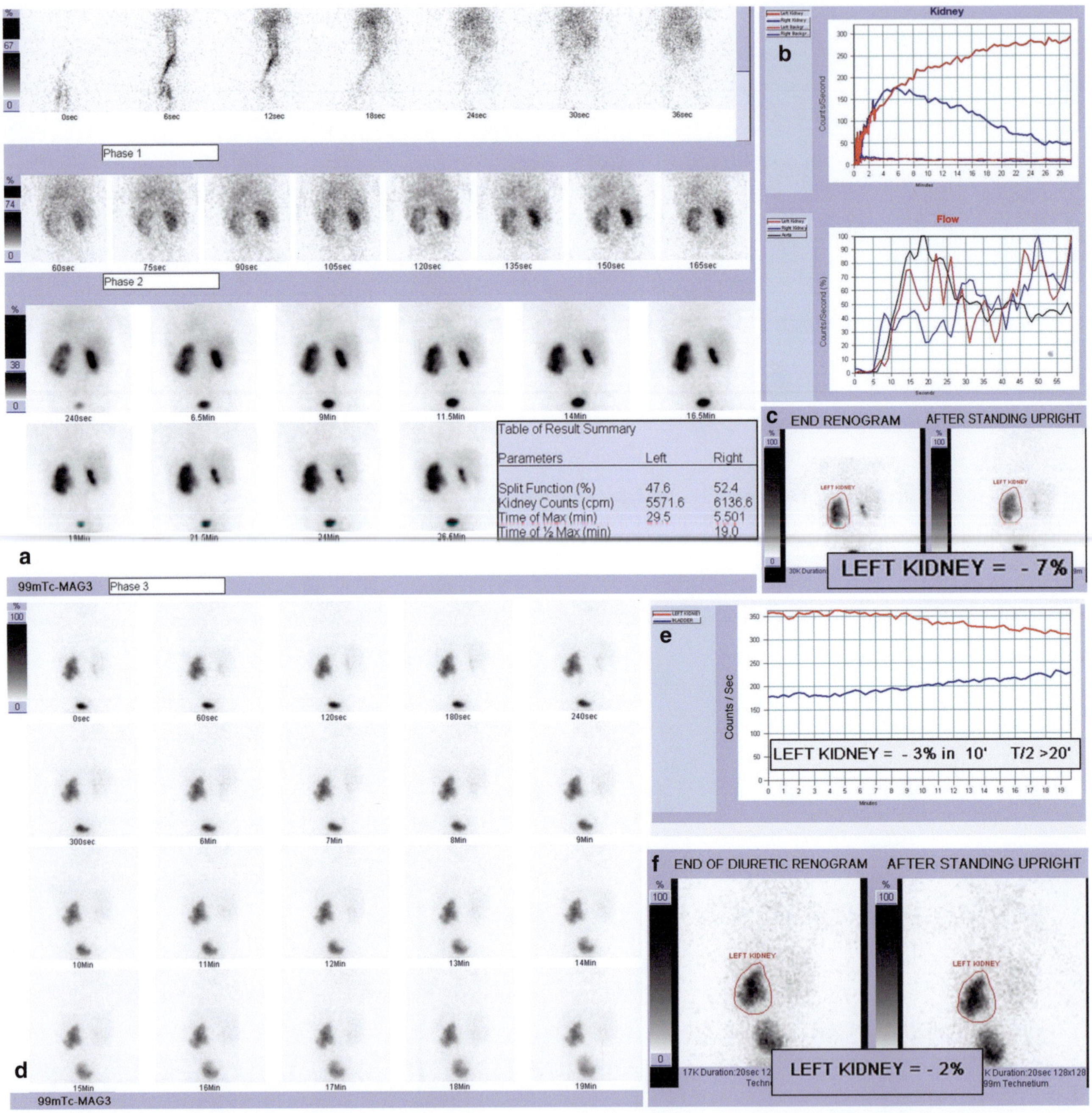

Fig. 4.6 MAG3 dynamic renal scan: left kidney is larger than the other one, with good radiotracer uptake and nonhomogeneous intraparenchymal distribution; a large area devoid of tracer corresponding to dilated renal pelvis and collecting system is evident, and drainage is poor; right kidney presents good and homogeneous radiotracer uptake and normal drainage (dynamic images, **a**); renograms (**b**) confirm normal function but poor drainage of left kidney ("rising curve") and normal function and drainage of right kidney (left DRF: 48 %; right DRF: 52 %); flow T/A curves (**b**) show synchronous and symmetrical perfusion. Gravity-assisted drainage-1 test shows no significant improvement in left kidney drainage (**c**). Diuretic dynamic images (**d**) and diuretic renogram (**e**) show very slow response to furosemide and no significant improvement in drainage in left kidney. Finally, left kidney drainage remains still poor even after gravity-assisted drainage-2 test (**f**)

4.4.2.7 Case 4.7 Late Diagnosis of Right Hydronephrosis: Reduced Split Function

An 8-year-old girl came to Emergency for acute lumbar pain and vomiting. Ultrasonography showed right grade 4 hydronephrosis. In the history, prenatal detection of bilateral hydronephrosis was reported, which was improved at 1 year of age. The patient was then lost at follow-up. Considering the diagnosis of hydronephrosis, a MAG3 scan was performed in order to assess split function and urinary drainage, and showed severe hypofunction and poor drainage of right kidney. Based on the results of MAG3 scan, laparoscopic pyeloplasty was performed confirming UPJ obstruction without aberrant vessels. At 1 year follow-up, ultrasonographic reduction of dilatation was found, together with mild increase of split function at MAG3 scan (left split function 27 %) and improvement of urinary drainage (Fig. 4.7).

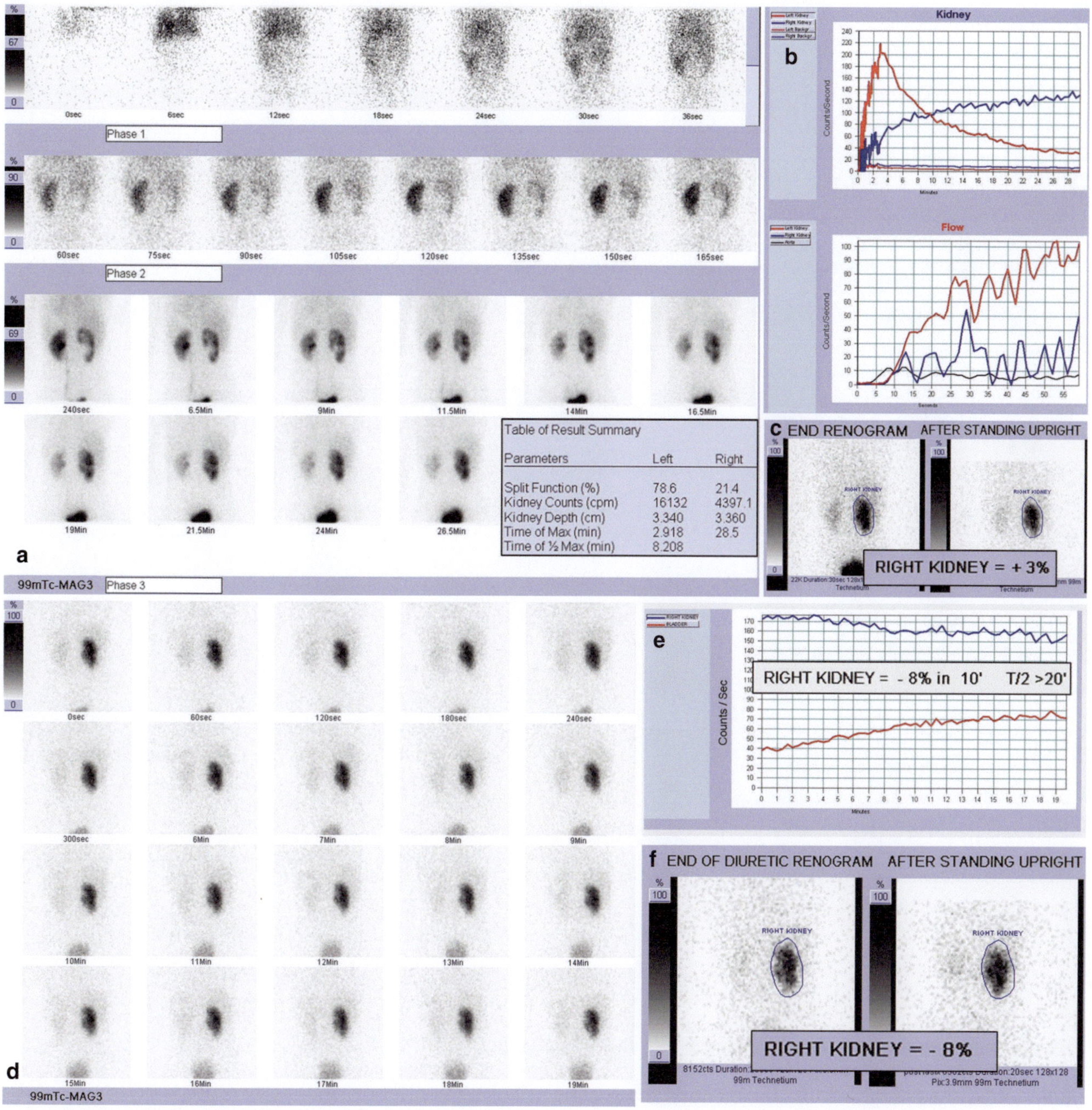

Fig. 4.7 MAG3 dynamic renal scan: dynamic images (**a**) show good and homogeneous radiotracer uptake and normal drainage in left kidney; right kidney shows globally reduced radiotracer uptake and nonhomogeneous intraparenchymal distribution with a large area devoid of tracer corresponding to dilated renal pelvis and collecting system, and drainage is poor; renograms confirm normal function and drainage of left kidney and severe hypofunction and poor drainage of right kidney ("rising curve") (left DRF: 79 %; right DRF: 20 %); flow T/A curves (**b**) show synchronous but asymmetrical perfusion (reduced in right kidney). Gravity-assisted drainage-1 test shows no significant improvement in right kidney drainage (**c**). Diuretic dynamic images (**d**) and diuretic renogram (**e**) show very slow response to furosemide and no significant improvement in drainage in right kidney. Right kidney drainage remains still poor even after gravity-assisted drainage-2 test (**f**)

4.4.2.8 Case 4.8 Bilateral Prenatal Hydronephrosis with Nonobstructive Pattern

A male newborn was seen with prenatal diagnosis of bilateral grade 4 hydronephrosis, normal amniotic fluid, and normal intrauterine growth. Postnatal ultrasonography showed grade 2 right hydronephrosis with APD 9 mm and grade 4 left with APD 28 mm. Based on MAG3 scan showing mildly reduced left function with an adequate urinary drainage after diuretic test, a strict ultrasonographic follow-up was scheduled. At 6 months follow-up, right hydronephrosis (APD 5 mm) appeared significantly improved while left hydronephrosis was severely worsened with APD of 38 mm. Left pyeloplasty was scheduled (Fig. 4.8).

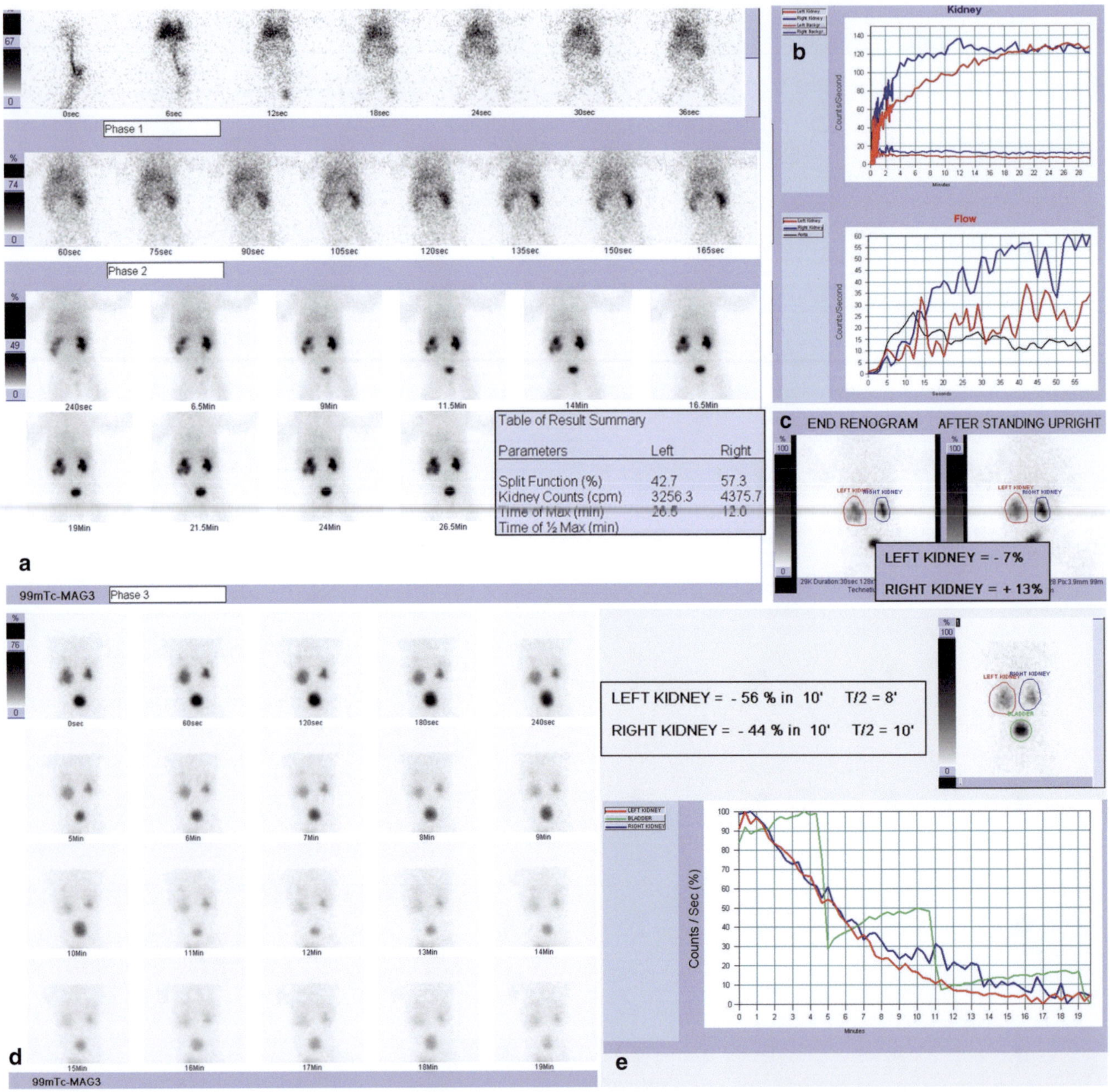

Fig. 4.8 MAG3 dynamic renal scan: left kidney is larger than the other one, with irregular shape; radiotracer uptake is globally reduced, and intraparenchymal distribution is nonhomogeneous, with a large area devoid of tracer corresponding to dilated renal pelvis and collecting system; drainage is poor; right kidney shows good and homogeneous radiotracer uptake and normal drainage (dynamic images, **a**); renograms confirm mild hypofunction and impaired drainage of left kidney ("plateau pattern") and normal function of right kidney with poor drainage ("rising curve") (left DRF: 43 %; right DRF: 57 %); flow T/A curves (**b**) show synchronous but asymmetrical perfusion (reduced in left kidney). Gravity-assisted drainage-1 test (**c**) shows no significant improvement in drainage in both kidneys, but diuretic dynamic images (**d**) and diuretic renogram (**e**) show prompt and significant renal washout after administration of furosemide in both kidneys

4.4.2.9 Case 4.9 Hydronephrosis in Lower Pole of Complete Duplex System

A 10-year-old boy was seen at Emergency for acute abdominal pain in the left upper quadrant. Previous history was uneventful, in particular prenatal ultrasonography was referred as normal and no UTI were reported. Ultrasonography showed bilateral duplex system with grade 2 hydronephrosis of the left lower system. MAG3 scan was asked in order to enquire split function of the lower and upper poles, together with the evaluation of urinary drainage (Fig. 4.9).

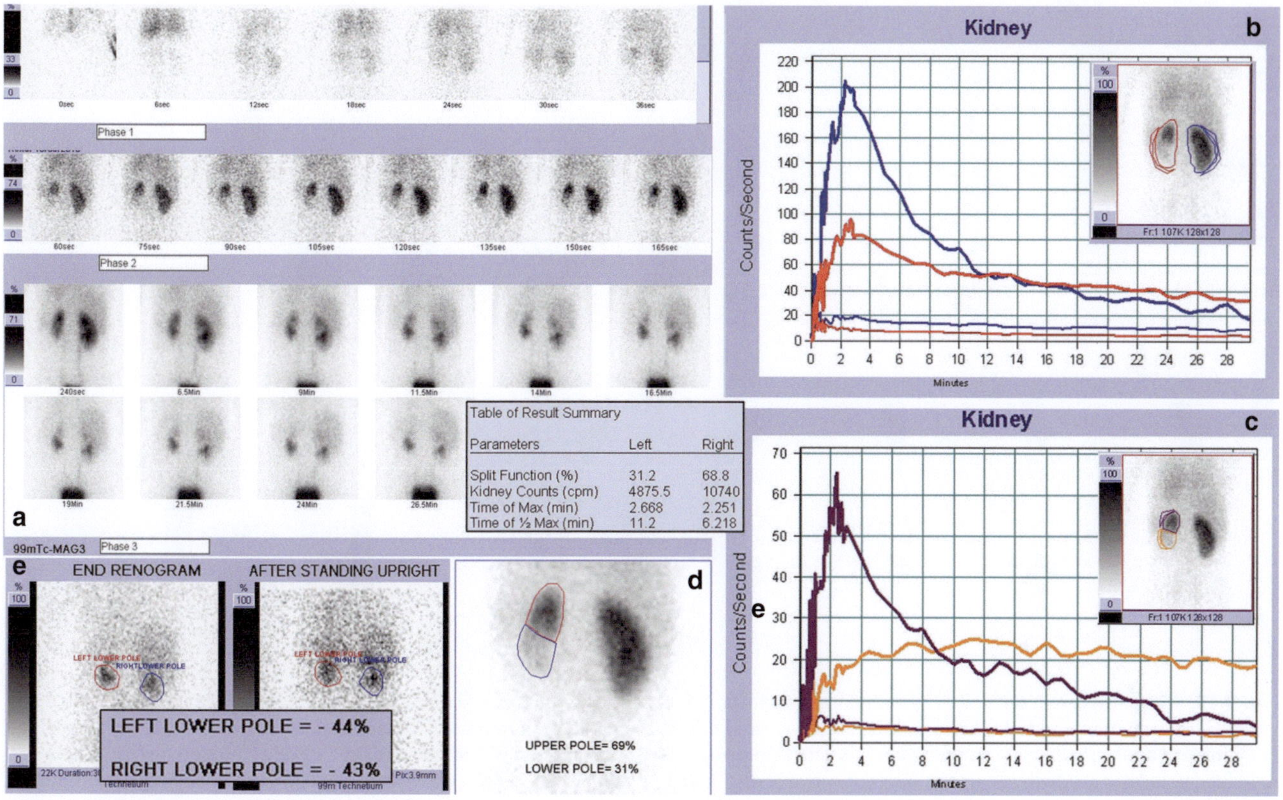

Fig. 4.9 MAG3 dynamic renal scan: dynamic images (**a**) show duplex system in left kidney, which is smaller than the other one, with irregular shape; radiotracer uptake is good and homogeneous, and drainage is normal in upper pole; lower pole shows reduced uptake and nonhomogeneous intraparenchymal distribution, with an area devoid of tracer corresponding to dilated system and poor drainage; right kidney also shows a duplex system, with good and homogeneous radiotracer uptake in both systems; drainage is normal in upper system and mildly poor in lower one; renograms (**b**) confirm mild hypofunction and preserved drainage of left kidney and normal function and drainage of right kidney (left DRF: 31 %; right DRF: 69 %). T/A curves of duplex systems of left kidney (**c**) show normal function and drainage of upper system and moderate hypofunction and poor drainage of lower system. DRF of duplex systems calculated on a composite image extracted from parenchymal phase (**d**) shows: upper system DRF: 69 %; lower system DRF: 31 %. Gravity-assisted drainage-1 test (**e**) shows significant improvement in drainage in lower systems of both kidneys

4.4.2.10 Case 4.10 Hydronephrosis in Ectopic Kidney

A boy was followed after prenatal diagnosis of right pelvic kidney. At birth, ultrasonography confirmed the renal ectopia, showing grade 2 hydronephrosis. VCUG did not show any VUR. At the age of 10 years, worsening of the right hydronephrosis was detected with grade 3 hydronephrosis and APD of 22 mm. MAG3 scan was asked in order to assess renal split function and urinary drainage (Fig. 4.10).

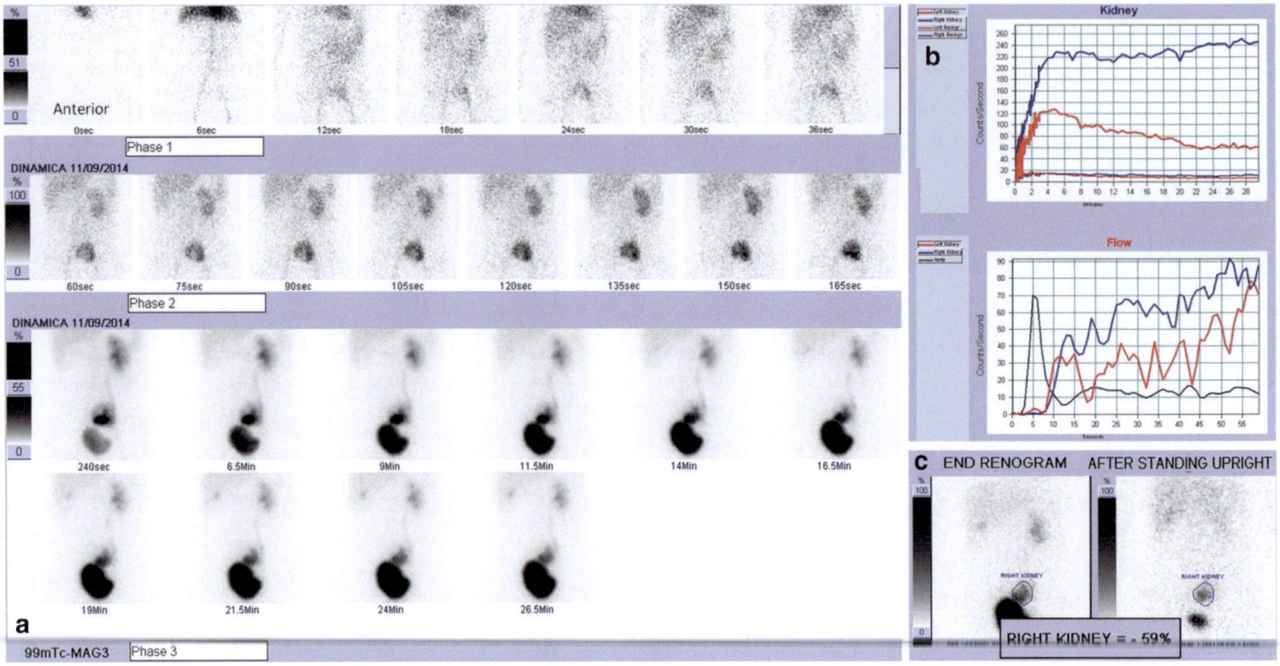

Fig. 4.10 MAG3 dynamic renal scan (anterior view): left kidney is located in its own proper site and shows good and homogeneous uptake of radiotracer and normal drainage; right kidney is ectopic pelvic, with round shape and good radiotracer uptake; intraparenchymal distribution is nonhomogeneous, with an area devoid of tracer corresponding to dilated renal pelvis, and drainage is poor (dynamic images, **a**); renograms (**b**) show normal function and drainage of left kidney and normal function but poor drainage of right kidney ("plateau pattern"); flow T/A curves (**b**) show synchronous and symmetrical perfusion. Gravity-assisted drainage-1 test shows significant emptying of right kidney (**c**)

4.4.2.11 Case 4.11 Hydronephrosis in Horseshoe Kidney: Nonobstructive Pattern with Preserved Renal Function

A 7-year-old boy was seen after recurrent abdominal pain. Ultrasonography was suspicious for horseshoe kidney with bilateral grade 2 hydronephrosis. MAG3 scan was asked in order to confirm renal fusion and assess urinary drainage (Fig. 4.11).

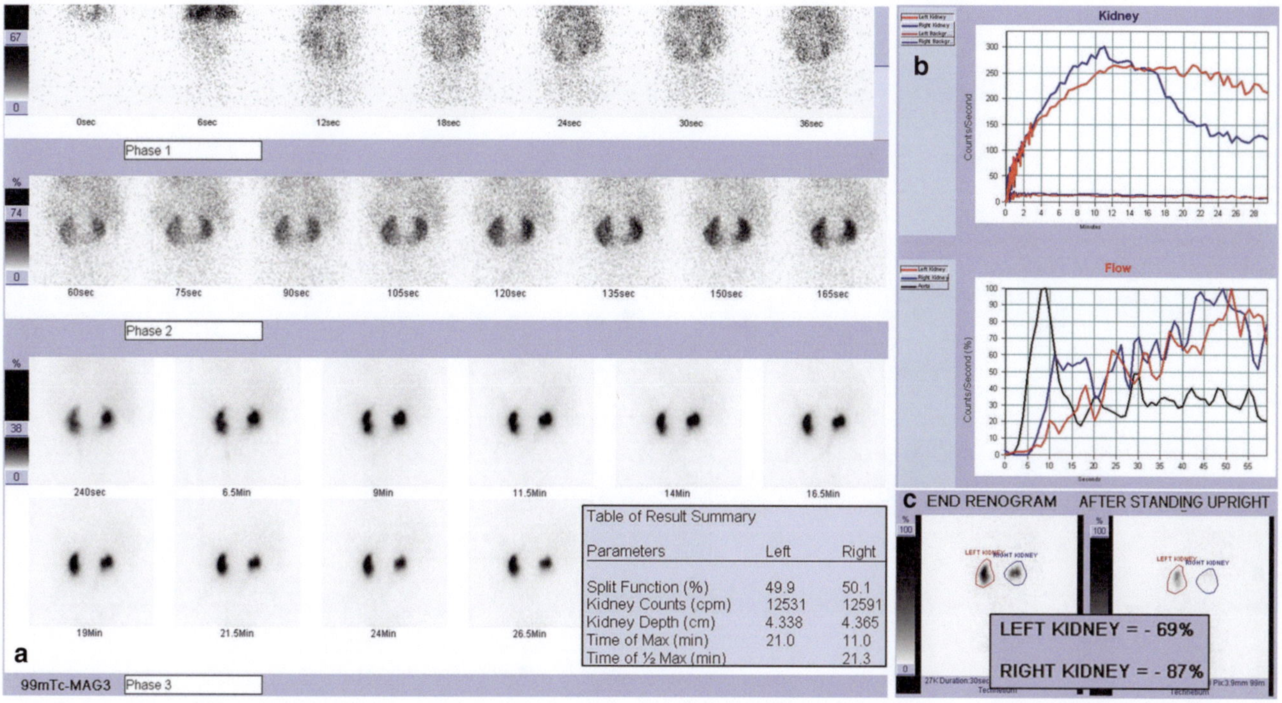

Fig. 4.11 MAG3 dynamic renal scan: dynamic images (**a**) show horseshoe kidney, with good radiotracer uptake and poor drainage in both kidneys; renograms (**b**) show normal function (left DRF: 50 %; right DRF: 50 %) and impaired drainage with delayed excretion phase in both kidneys, in particular, in the left one; flow T/A curves (**b**) show synchronous and symmetrical perfusion. Gravity-assisted drainage-1 test (**c**) shows significant improvement in drainage in both kidneys

4.4.2.12 Case 4.12 Hydronephrosis in Horseshoe Kidney: Obstructive Pattern with Renal Function Impairment

A 14-month-old girl was seen for prenatal diagnosis of left hydronephrosis. At postnatal follow-up, progressive worsening of the left hydronephrosis was observed (grade 4 hydronephrosis with pyelic APD of 33 mm). No UTI occurred. MAG3 scan was asked in order to confirm surgical indication (Fig. 4.12).

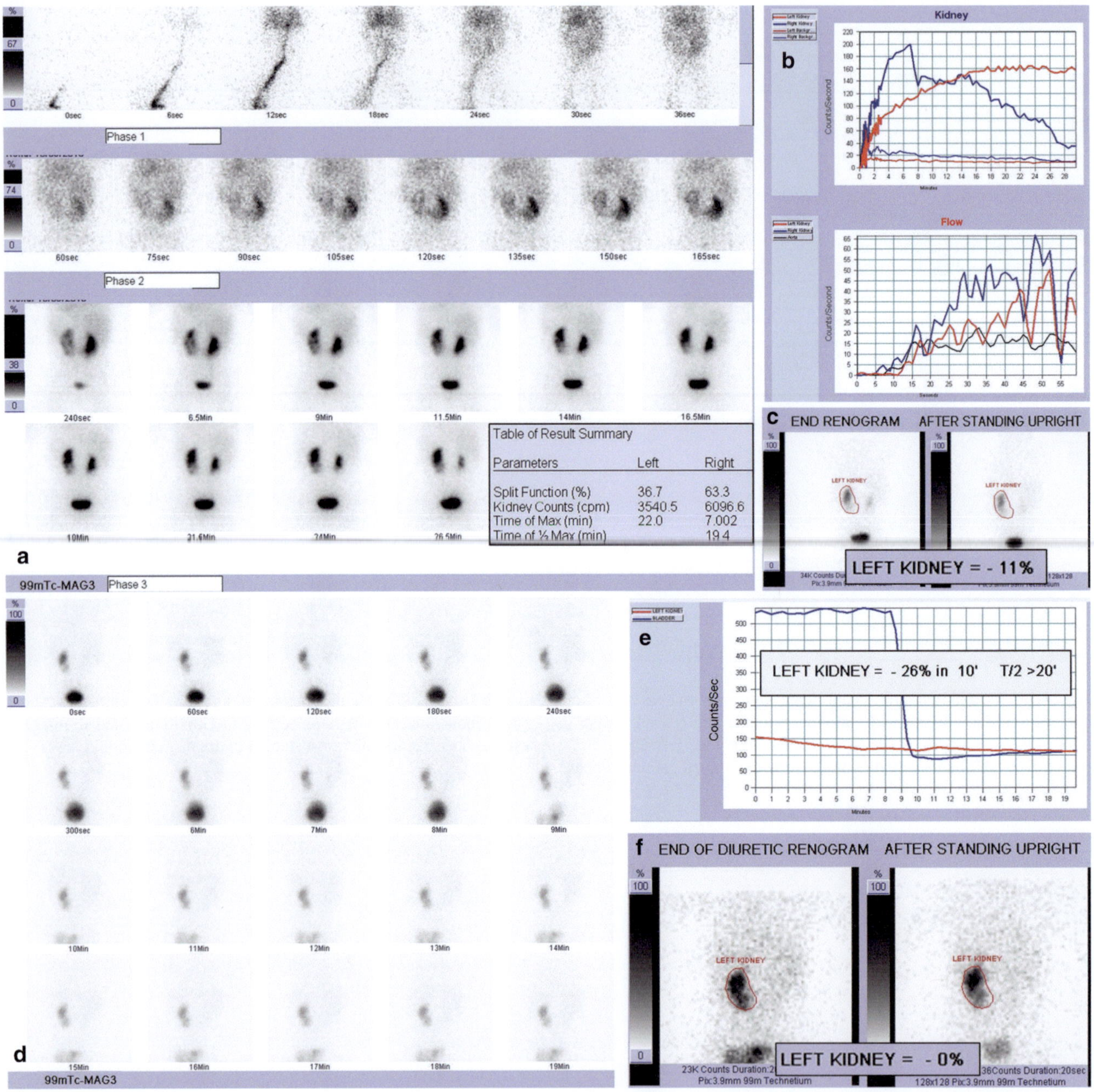

Fig. 4.12 MAG3 dynamic renal scan: dynamic images (**a**) show a horseshoe kidney; in left kidney, radiotracer uptake is reduced and intraparenchymal distribution is nonhomogeneous, with an area devoid of tracer corresponding to dilated renal pelvis and collecting system; drainage is poor; right kidney shows good and homogeneous radiotracer uptake and normal drainage; renograms (**b**) show moderate hypofunction and impaired drainage of left kidney ("plateau pattern") and normal function and drainage of right kidney (left DRF: 37 %; right DRF: 63 %); flow T/A curves (**b**) show synchronous but asymmetrical perfusion (mildly reduced in left kidney). Gravity-assisted drainage-1 test (**c**) shows no significant improvement in drainage in left kidney. Diuretic dynamic images (**d**) and diuretic renogram (**e**) show very slow response to furosemide and no significant improvement in drainage in left kidney. Drainage remains still poor even after gravity-assisted drainage-2 test (**f**)

4.4.2.13 Case 4.13 Poor Drainage in Very Dilated Renal Pelvis: A Potential Scintigraphic Pitfall

A girl was first seen at the age of 6 years for recurrent abdominal pain since 3 years of age. Ultrasonography showed grade 4 right hydronephrosis with pyelic APD of 60 mm. Pyeloplasty was performed. At follow-up, gradual decrease of ADP was first seen, with a minimum APD of 20 mm. Then progressive increase of right hydronephrosis occurred. MAG3 scan was asked in order to assess renal split function and urinary drainage and showed normal function of right kidney and poor drainage. Ascending pyelogram did not show any kinking or recurrent obstruction at the pyeloureteric junction. The girl remained asymptomatic. Split renal function was stable (Fig. 4.13).

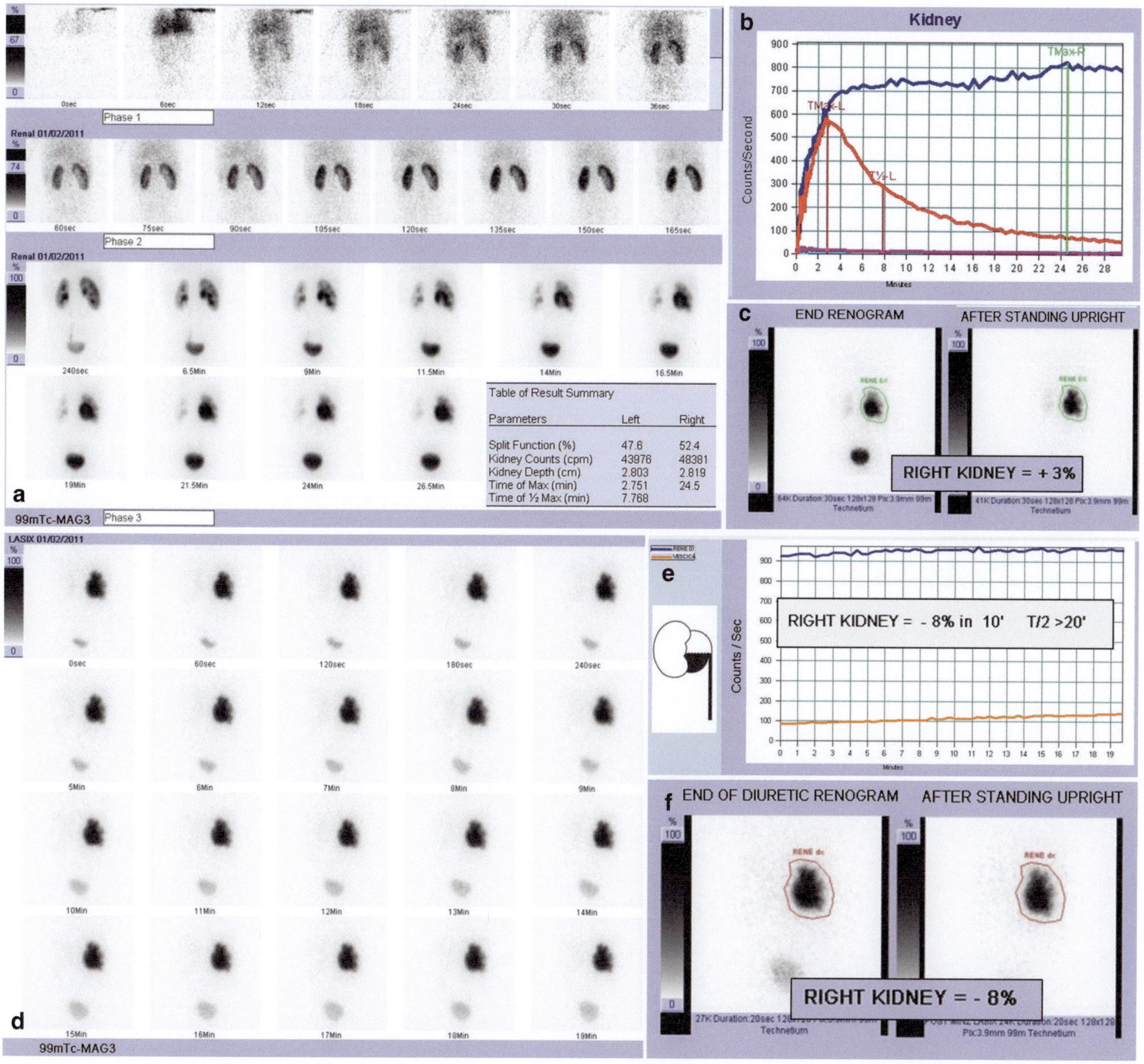

Table of Result Summary

Parameters	Left	Right
Split Function (%)	47.6	52.4
Kidney Counts (cpm)	43976	48381
Kidney Depth (cm)	2.803	2.819
Time of Max (min)	2.751	24.5
Time of ½ Max (min)	7.768	

Fig. 4.13 MAG3 dynamic renal scan: dynamic images (**a**) show good and homogeneous radiotracer uptake and normal drainage in left kidney; right kidney is larger than the other one, with good radiotracer uptake and nonhomogeneous intraparenchymal distribution; a large area devoid of tracer corresponding to very dilated renal pelvis and collecting system is evident, and drainage is poor; renograms (**b**) confirm normal function and drainage of left kidney and normal function but poor drainage ("plateau pattern") of right kidney (left DRF: 48 %; right DRF: 52 %). Gravity-assisted drainage-1 test shows no improvement in right kidney drainage (**c**). Diuretic dynamic images (**d**) and diuretic renogram (**e**) show very slow response to furosemide and no significant improvement in drainage in right kidney. Right kidney drainage remains still poor even after gravity-assisted drainage-2 test (**f**). Persistence of a very dilated pelvis after pyeloplasty may represent a potential pitfall in interpretation of scintigraphic findings, because some renal scintigraphies could show a persistent poor drainage even in the absence of anatomical pyeloureteric junction obstruction. In our experience, this could be probably explained with the analogy of the "bathtub": it takes long time to empty a bathtub when the plug has been removed, because of the dimension of the bathtub related to the small drainage hole. In the same way, emptying of very dilated pelvis can be very slow, even in the absence of an anatomical obstacle. In this group of patients, when renal function remains stable over the time, periodical clinical evaluation and ultrasonographic monitoring are recommended

Bibliography

1. Castagnetti M, Novara G, Beniamin F, et al. Scintigraphic renal function after unilateral pyeloplasty in children: a systematic review. BJU Int. 2008;102:862–8.
2. Corteville JE, Gray DL, Crane JP. Congenital hydronephrosis: correlation of fetal ultrasonographic findings with infant outcome. Am J Obstet Gynecol. 1991;165:384–8.
3. Eskild-Jesen A, Gordon I, Piepsz A, Froakier J. Interpretation of the renogram: problems and pitfalls in hydronephrosis in children. BJU Int. 2004;94:887–92.
4. Gordon I, Piepsz A, Sixt R. Guidelines for standard and diuretic renogram in children. Eur J Nucl Med Mol Imaging. 2011;38:1175.
5. Ismaili K, Hall M, Donner C, et al. Results of systematic screening for minor degrees of fetal renal pelvis dilatation in an unselected population. Am J Obstet Gynecol. 2003;188:242–6.
6. Lee R, Cendron M, Kinnamon D, Nguyen H. Antenatal hydronephrosis as a predictor of postnatal outcome: a meta-analysis. Pediatrics. 2006;118:586–93.
7. Matsui F, Shimada K, Matsumoto F, Takano S. Late recurrence of symptomatic hydronephrosis in patients with prenatally detected hydronephrosis and spontaneous improvement. J Urol. 2008;180:322.
8. Nguyen HY, Herndon CDA, Cooper C, et al. The Society for Fetal Urology consensus statement on the evaluation and management of antenatal hydronephrosis. J Pediatr Urol. 2010;6:212–31.
9. Piepsz A. The predictive value of the renogram. Eur J Nucl Med Mol Imaging. 2009;36:1661.
10. Piepsz A. Antenatal detection of pelviureteric junction stenosis: main controversies. Semin Nucl Med. 2011;41:11–9.
11. Piepsz A, Gordon I, Brook J, Koff S. Round table on the management of renal pelvic dilatation in children. J Pediatr Urol. 2009;5:437–44.
12. Piepsz A, Sixt R, Gordon I. Performing renography in children with antenatally detected pelvi-ureteric junction stenosis: errors, pitfalls, controversies. Q J Nucl Med Mol Imaging. 2010;54:350–62.
13. Ulman I, Jayanthi V, Koff S. The long term followup of newborns with severe unilateral hydronephrosis initially treated nonoperatively. J Urol. 2000;164:1101.
14. Vemulakonda V, Wilcox DT. Prenatal hydronephrosis: postnatal evaluation and management. Curr Urol Rep. 2014;15:430–7.
15. Yamacake KGR, Nguyen HT. Current management of antenatal hydronephrosis. Pediatr Nephrol. 2013;28:237–43.

5 Megaureter

Maria Felicia Villani, Milena Pizzoferro, Giovanni Torino, and Maria Carmen Garganese

5.1 Dynamic Renal Scintigraphy

Study technique has been reported in Chapter 4.

5.1.1 Interpretation of Ureteral Time/Activity Curves

Ureteral time/activity (T/A) curves are obtained from ROI drawn on both ureters on dynamic renal study and diuretic sequence (when performed). T/A curves may present three different patterns:

- A normal pattern, with horizontal trend;
- A dilated nonobstructive pattern, with an initial ascending tract and a following horizontal tract;
- An obstructive pattern, with rising trend.

5.1.2 Teaching Cases

5.1.2.1 Case 5.1: Transient Secondary Left Megaureter by Bladder Diverticulum

A 6-year-old boy was referred to our outpatient clinic due to nonfebrile urinary tract infections and one hematuria episode.

No urological abnormality was detected during the pregnancy and the first 6 years of age of the child.

The urinary tract ultrasonography, at 6 years of age, revealed a left hydroureteronephrosis (pelvic anteroposterior diameter of 11 mm; distal ureteral dilation of 12 mm); for this reason, the voiding cystourethrography was performed, and it showed the absence of vesicoureteral reflux and the presence of left paraureteral bladder diverticulum (maximum diameter of 60 mm during the voiding phase).

M.F. Villani • M. Pizzoferro • M.C. Garganese
Nuclear Medicine Unit, Imaging Department, "Bambino Gesù" Children's Hospital and Research Institute, Rome, Italy

G. Torino (✉)
Paediatric Urology Unit, "Bambino Gesù" Children's Hospital and Research Institute, Rome, Italy
e-mail: giovanni.torino@opbg.net

© Springer International Publishing Switzerland 2017
M.C. Garganese, G.F.L. D'Errico (eds.), *Conventional Nuclear Medicine in Pediatrics*, DOI 10.1007/978-3-319-43181-9_5

The following technetium-99m-labeled mercaptoacetyltriglycine (MAG-3) renography detected a normal split renal function with no evidence of urinary tract dilation and normal urinary drainage without diuretic injection.

At the last day hospital follow-up, the patient remained asymptomatic, and the ultrasound scan confirmed the presence of left paraureteral bladder diverticulum but it described the absence of left hydroureteronephrosis.

The patient is actually awaiting to remove with the surgery the bladder diverticulum (Fig. 5.1).

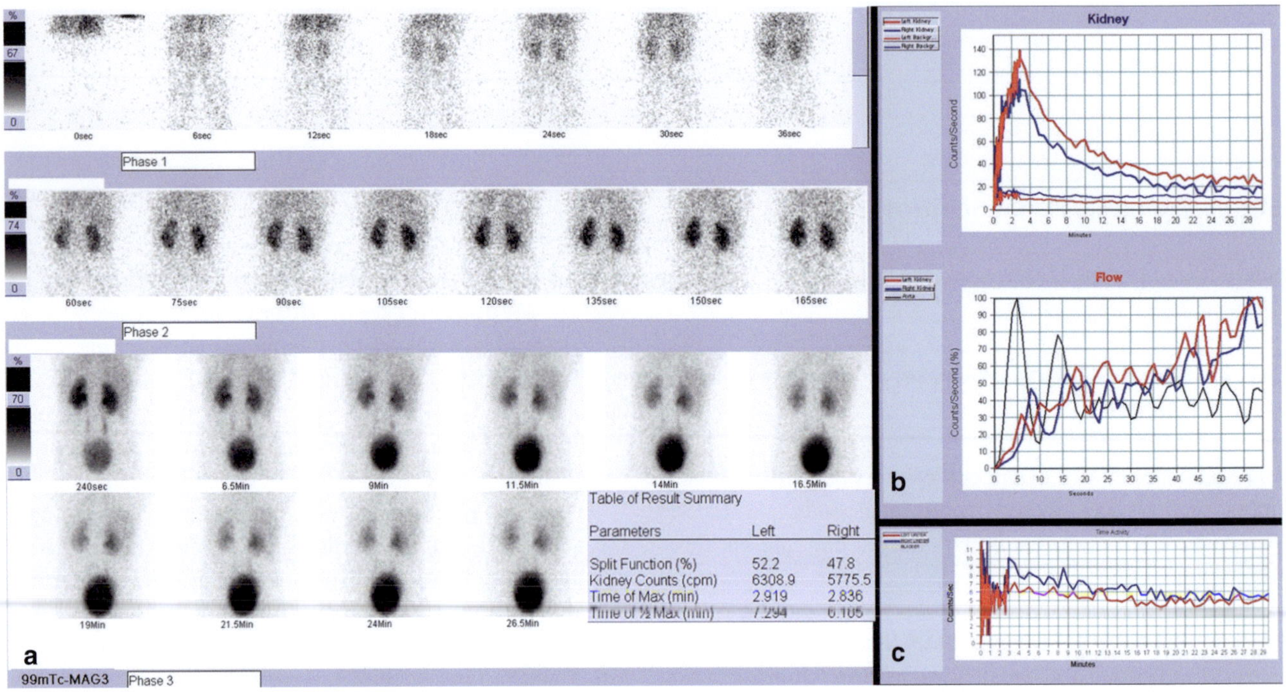

Fig. 5.1 MAG3 dynamic renal scan: dynamic images (**a**) show good and homogeneous radiotracer uptake and normal drainage in both kidneys, with mild and transient radioactivity in both ureters; renograms (**b**) confirm normal function and drainage of both kidneys; flow T/A curves (**b**) show synchronous and symmetrical perfusion. Ureter T/A curves (**c**) show normal pattern

5.1.2.2 Case 5.2: Nonrefluxing and Nonobstructive Primary Right Megaureter with Normal Split Renal Function

Female patient affected by prenatally detected right uropathy.

At 1 month of life, the ultrasonographic scan showed a right urinary tract dilation (pelvic anteroposterior diameter of 6 mm; distal ureteral dilation of 5 mm).

At the follow-up, the patient had a febrile urinary infection and a worsening of the right ureteral dilation (up to 10 mm); for this reason, the voiding cystourethrography was performed, but it revealed the absence of urinary pathologies.

The following technetium-99m-labeled mercaptoacetyltriglycine (MAG-3) renography detected a normal split renal function with evidence, at the right side, of the megaureter and slow urinary drainage but absence of obstructive urinary pattern (no diuretic injection was necessary).

At the last clinical checkup, the patient remained asymptomatic and the ultrasonographic scan showed the stability of the right megaureter (diameter of 10 mm).

The management of the patient is actually based on wait-and-see strategy associated to serial ultrasonographic evaluations (Fig. 5.2).

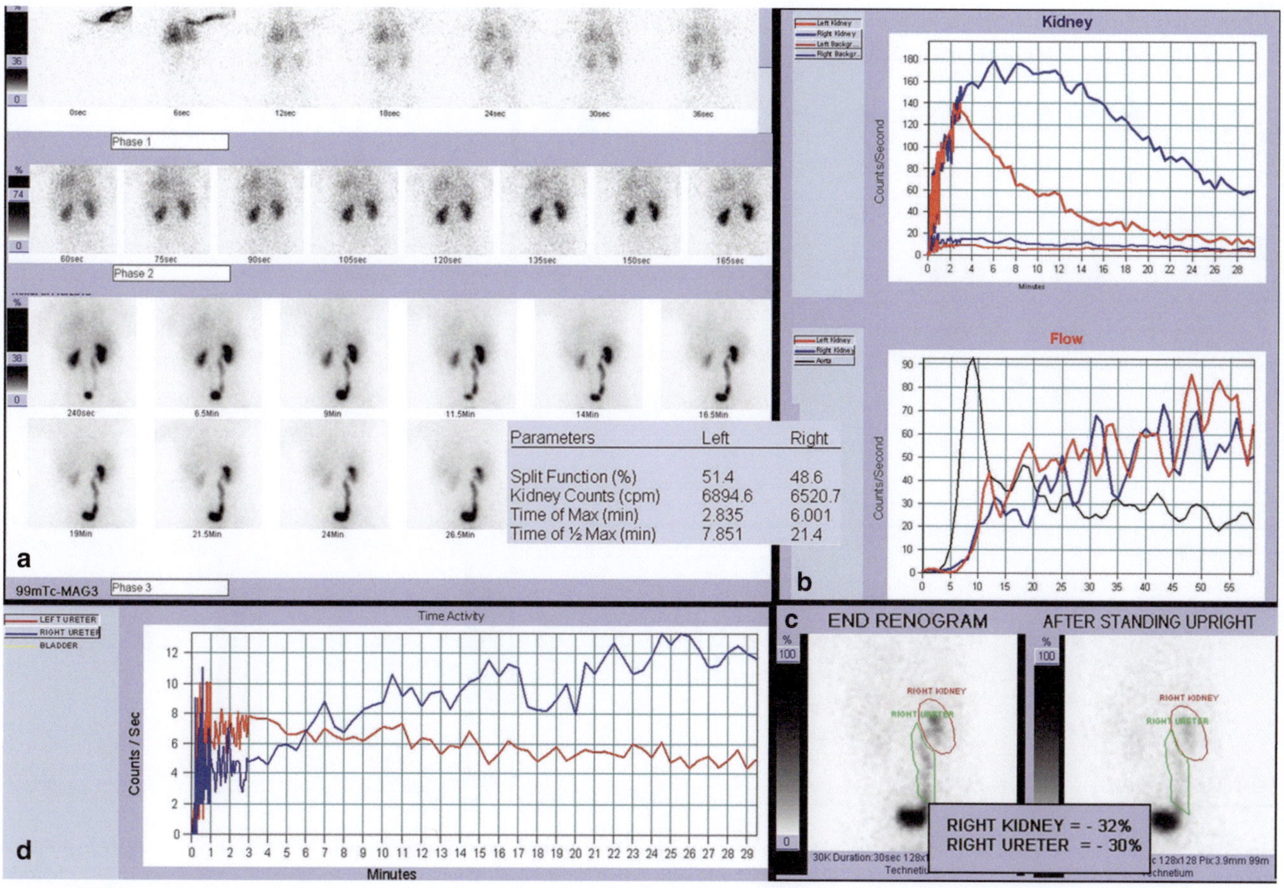

Fig. 5.2 MAG3 dynamic renal scan: dynamic images (**a**) show good and homogeneous radiotracer uptake and normal drainage of left kidney; right kidney presents good and homogeneous radiotracer uptake; pyelic drainage is poor, and persistent radioactivity stasis is evident also in ipsilateral dilated ureter; renograms confirm normal function and drainage of left kidney, and normal function, prolonged transit time, and delayed excretion of right kidney; flow T/A curves (**b**) show synchronous and symmetrical perfusion. Gravity-assisted drainage-1 test shows significant emptying of right kidney and right ureter (**c**). This finding is confirmed by ureter T/A curves (**d**): normal pattern of left ureter and dilated nonobstructive pattern of right ureter

5.1.2.3 Case 5.3: Nonobstructive Right Megaureter with Low Right Split Renal Function, Autosomal Dominant Bilateral Polycystic Kidney Disease, and Bilateral Urinary Microlithiasis

A 15-year-old girl with history of acute renal pain episodes, bilateral urinary microlithiasis, and poor right renal function was admitted to our hospital.

The initial ultrasonographic scan showed right kidney hypoplasia, bilateral urinary microlithiasis, bilateral polycystic kidney disease, and right urinary tract dilation.

The following technetium-99m-labeled mercaptoacetyltriglycine (MAG-3) renography revealed a poor right split renal function and right kidney hypoplasia with evidence at the right side of megaureter and slow urinary drainage but absence of obstructive urinary pattern (no diuretic injection was necessary).

At the last clinical follow-up, the patient remained asymptomatic.

The management of the patient is actually based on clinical and ultrasonographic evaluations (Fig. 5.3).

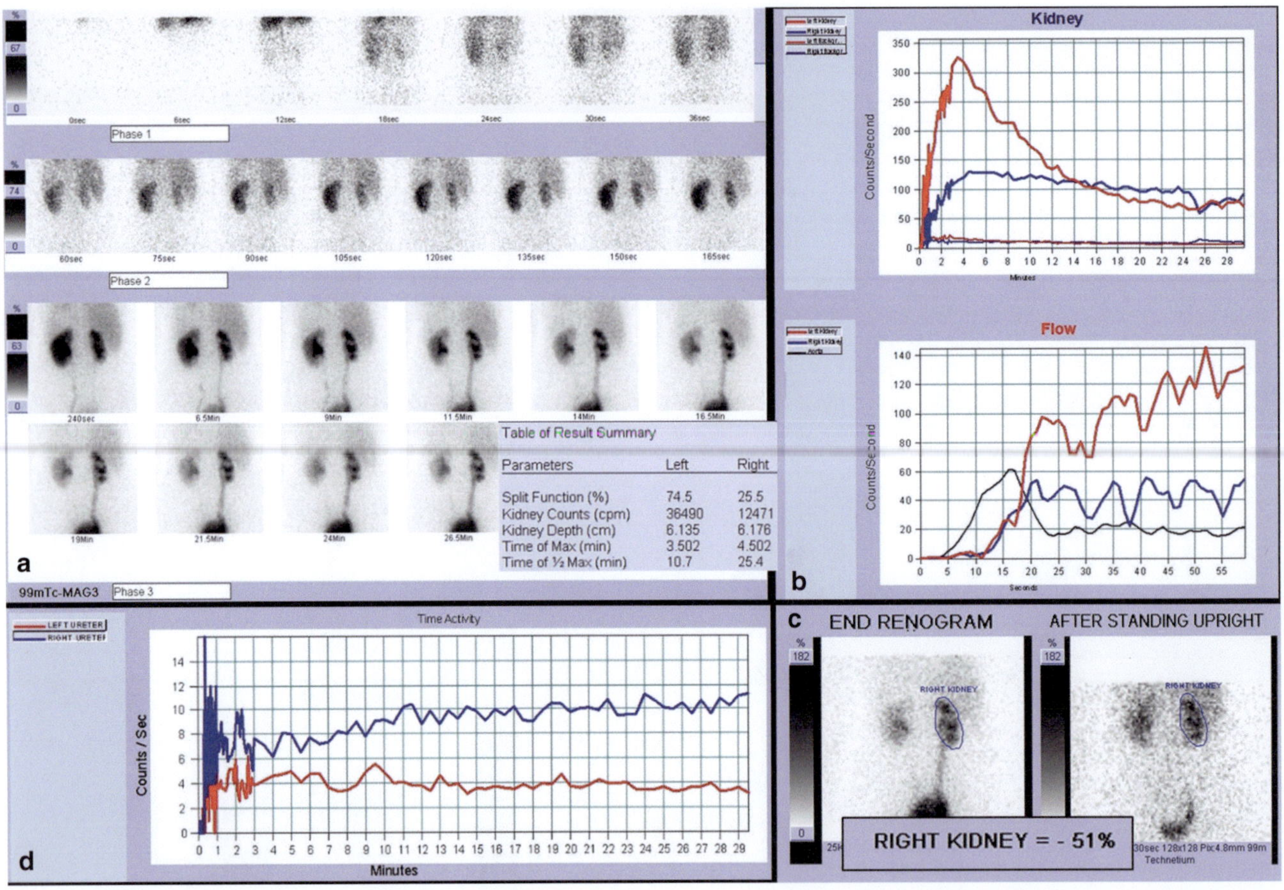

Fig. 5.3 MAG3 dynamic renal scan: dynamic images (**a**) show good and homogeneous radiotracer uptake and normal drainage of left kidney; right kidney is smaller than the other one, with irregular shape; right kidney presents reduced radiotracer uptake with nonhomogeneous intraparenchymal distribution due to an area devoid of tracer corresponding to dilated collecting system, and the drainage is poor; persistent radioactivity is also evident in ipsilateral ureter. Renograms (**b**) show normal function and drainage of left kidney and severe hypofunction, prolonged transit time, and delayed excretion phase of right kidney; flow T/A curves (**b**) show synchronous but asymmetrical perfusion (reduced in right kidney). Gravity-assisted drainage-1 test shows significant emptying of right kidney and right ureter (**c**). This finding is confirmed by ureter T/A curves (**d**): normal pattern of left ureter and dilated nonobstructive pattern of right ureter

5.1.2.4 Case 5.4: Secondary Left Megaureter by Posterior Urethral Valves

Male infant affected by prenatally detected left uropathy.

During the first month of life, the initial ultrasonographic scan showed a left urinary tract dilation (pelvic anteroposterior diameter of 7.5 mm; distal ureteral dilation of 16 mm) and a bladder wall hypertrophy.

The voiding cystourethrography was performed, and it revealed the absence of vesicoureteral reflux but the presence of posterior urethral valves; for this reason, at 6 months of life, the patient was submitted to endoscopic ablation of posterior urethral valves.

The ultrasonographic scan at 2 months postoperative follow-up confirmed the stability of the preoperative left megaureter.

The following technetium-99m-labeled mercaptoacetyltriglycine (MAG-3) renography showed a normal split renal function with left ureteral dilation and poor urinary drainage that required the diuretic injection; no obstructive urinary pattern was detected after the diuretic injection.

At the last day hospital follow-up, the patient remained asymptomatic, and the ultrasonographic scan revealed the reduction of the left megaureter (diameter of 8 mm).

Conservative management is actually the utilized strategy for the patient (Fig. 5.4).

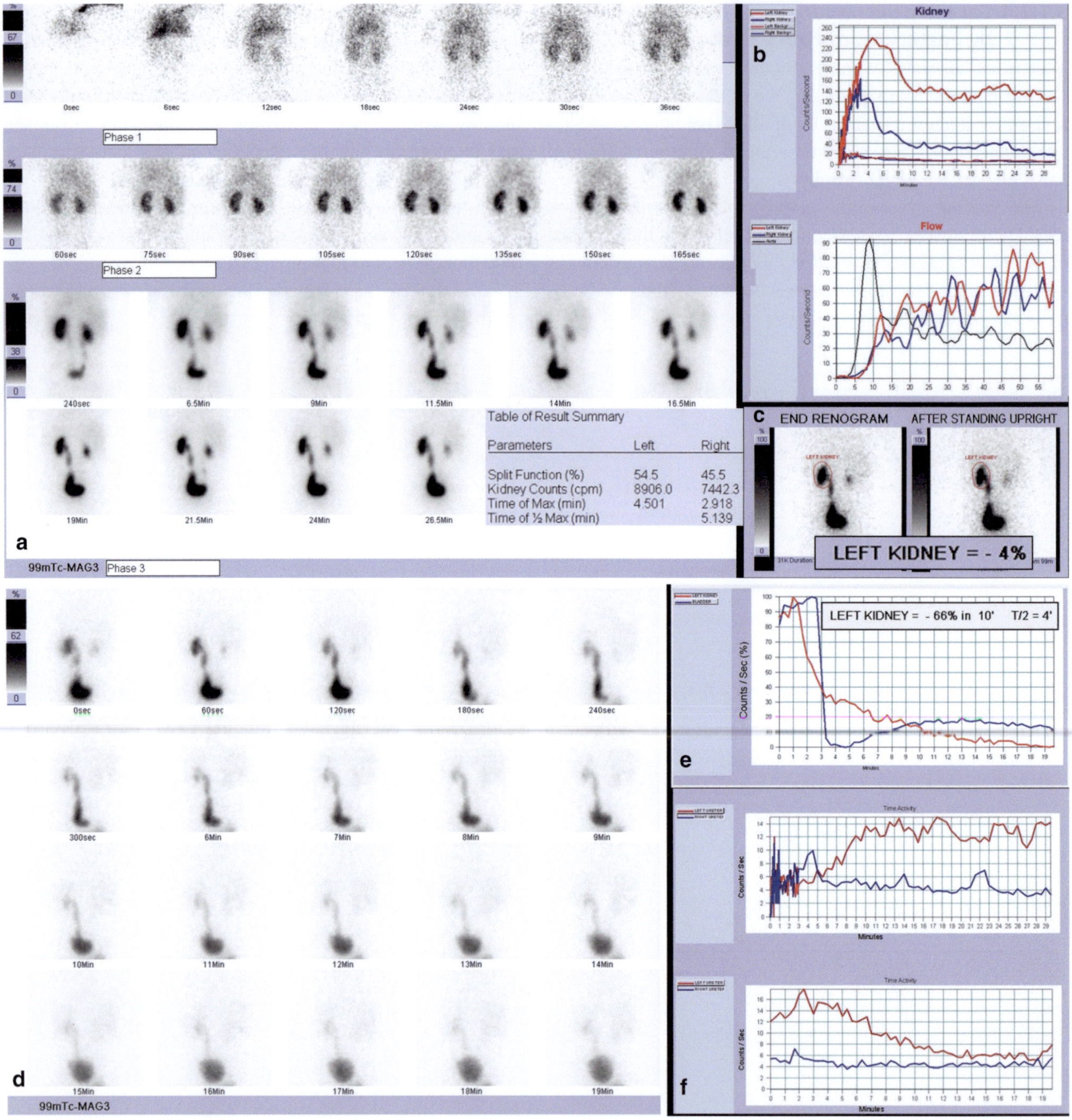

Fig. 5.4 MAG3 dynamic renal scan: dynamic images (**a**) show good radiotracer uptake in left kidney with nonhomogeneous intraparenchymal distribution due to an area devoid of tracer corresponding to dilated renal pelvis and collecting system; drainage is poor, with persistent radioactivity also in left ureter, in particular in its distal tract; right kidney presents good and homogeneous radiotracer uptake and normal drainage; renograms (**b**) confirm normal function but mildly delayed excretion phase of left kidney, and normal function and drainage of right kidney; flow T/A curves (**b**) show synchronous and symmetrical perfusion. Gravity-assisted drainage-1 test shows no significant washout of left kidney and left ureter (**c**). Diuretic dynamic images (**d**) and diuretic renogram (**e**) show prompt and significant washout in both left kidney and left ureter after administration of furosemide. Ureter T/A curves (**f**) show: normal pattern of right ureter and dilated nonobstructive pattern of left ureter during dynamic renal scan (*upper graph*); normal pattern of right ureter and prompt washout of left ureter during diuretic scintigraphy (*lower graph*)

5.1.2.5 Case 5.5: Nonobstructive Right Megaureter and Left Renal Agenesis

A male newborn affected by right urinary tract dilation (pelvic anteroposterior diameter of 10 mm; distal ureteral dilation of 9 mm) and left renal agenesis as showed by the ultrasonographic scan at 6 days of life.

At 4 months of life, the technetium-99m-labeled mercaptoacetyltriglycine (MAG-3) renography confirmed the absence of the left kidney and the right megaureter, but it showed a poor urinary drainage that required the diuretic injection; no obstructive urinary pattern was detected after the diuretic injection.

At the last follow-up (at 16 months of life), the patient remained asymptomatic, and the ultrasonographic scan revealed a stability of the right megaureter.

The management of the patient is actually based on wait-and-see strategy associated to serial ultrasonographic evaluations (Fig. 5.5).

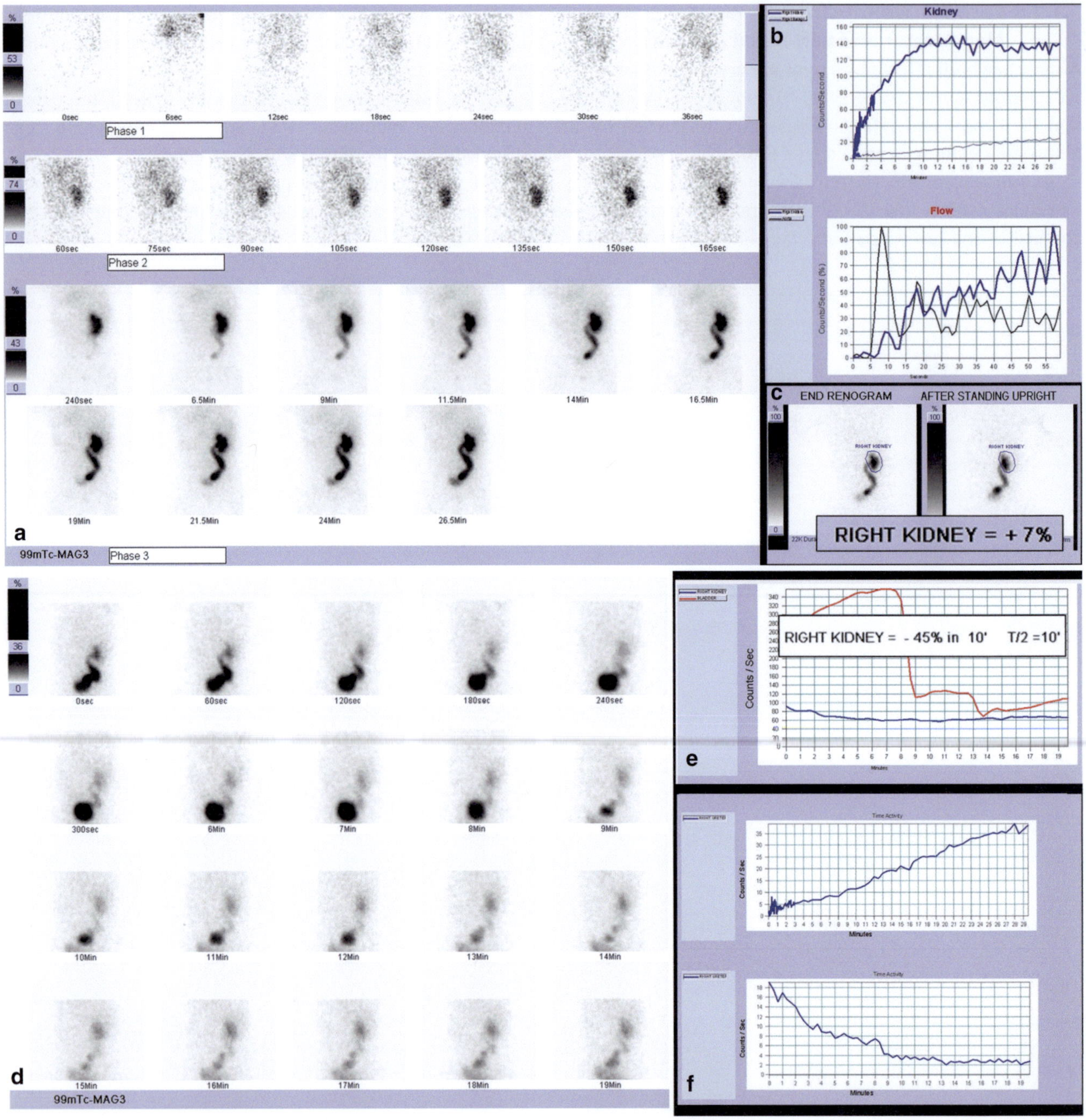

Fig. 5.5 MAG3 dynamic renal scan: dynamic images (**a**) show good and homogeneous radiotracer uptake in right kidney; drainage is poor and stasis of radiourine is evident in dilated pelvis; persistent radioactivity is also present in dilated and tortuous right ureter; there is no visualization of left kidney. Renogram (**b**) shows good slope of parenchymal phase and poor drainage of right kidney ("plateau pattern"); flow T/A curves (**b**) show regular perfusion of right kidney. Gravity-assisted drainage-1 test shows no significant washout of right kidney and ureter (**c**). Diuretic dynamic images (**d**) and diuretic renogram (**e**) show slow but significant renal washout after administration of furosemide. Ureter T/A curves (**f**) show: "rising curve" during dynamic renal scan (*upper graph*); prompt washout during diuretic scintigraphy (*lower graph*)

5.1.2.6 Case 5.6: Secondary Obstructive Left Megaureter by Surgical Treatment of Anorectal Malformation in Child with Valve Bladder

Male patient affected by valve bladder (endoscopically treated posterior urethral valves) and surgically treated anorectal malformation.

During the follow-up, the patient developed an intermittent left megaureter as shown by serial ultrasonographic scans associated with urinary incontinence and incomplete bladder emptying.

The first technetium-99m-labeled mercaptoacetyltriglycine (MAG-3) renography detected a poor left split renal function with evidence at the left side of megaureter and slow urinary drainage, but absence of obstructive urinary pattern (no diuretic injection was necessary); during the same examination, the indirect MAG-3 cystography revealed the absence of vesicoureteral reflux.

During the following period was observed an increase of left megaureter up to 25 mm diameter; for this reason, the patient underwent magnetic resonance urography (MRU) that showed a distal ureteral stricture at the left side.

The patient was submitted to surgical operation with extravesical approach: removal of left distal ureter, left ureteral tapering, and its reimplantation for distal ureteral stenosis caused by the previous surgical treatment of the anorectal malformation.

During the postoperative period was highlighted an initial improvement of the left megaureter, but after 2 years follow-up, a worsening of the left ureteral dilation (up to 27 mm diameter) associated with urinary incontinence and incomplete bladder emptying was detected.

The following MAG-3 renography showed a poor left split renal function with left megaureter and poor urinary drainage that required the diuretic injection; no obstructive urinary pattern was detected at upright position with emptied bladder at the end of diuretic test.

The additional MRU observed a left megaureter with absence of strictures and normal urinary drainage.

Based on the results of the last MAG-3 renography and MRU, the patient has been until now treated with toilet training and alpha-blocking agent, and he has up to now remained asymptomatic with stable left megaureter (Fig. 5.6).

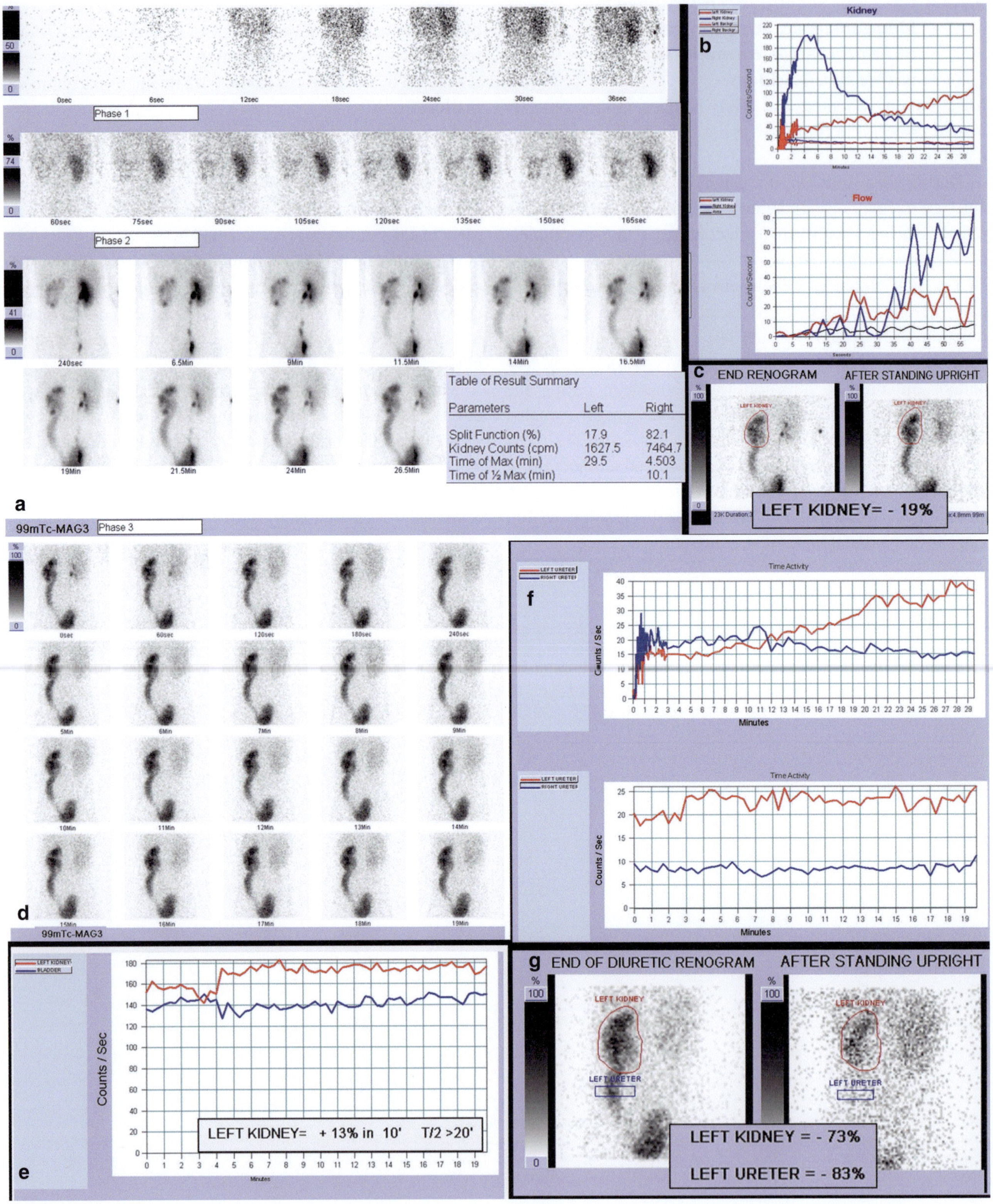

Fig. 5.6 MAG3 dynamic renal scan, after surgery: dynamic images (**a**) show severe reduction of uptake in left kidney, with nonhomogeneous intraparenchymal distribution due to an area devoid of tracer corresponding to dilated renal pelvis and collecting system; shape is irregular and drainage is poor; persistent radioactivity is evident also in dilated left ureter; right kidney presents good and homogeneous radiotracer uptake and normal drainage; renograms (**b**) confirm severe hypofunction and poor drainage of left kidney ("rising curve"), and normal function and drainage of right kidney; flow T/A curves (**b**) show synchronous but asymmetrical perfusion (severely reduced in left kidney). Gravity-assisted drainage-1 test shows no significant washout of left kidney and ureter (**c**). Diuretic dynamic images (**d**) and diuretic renogram (**e**) show very slow response to furosemide and no significant improvement in drainage in left kidney. Ureter T/A curves (**f**) show: "rising curve" of left ureter and normal pattern of right ureter during dynamic renal scan (*upper graph*); no significant washout during diuretic scintigraphy in left ureter (*lower graph*). Only after micturition and further gravity-assisted drainage-2 test (**g**), significant washout in both left kidney and ureter is evident

5.1.2.7 Case 5.7: Partial Obstructive Primary Left Megaureter

Male infant affected by prenatally detected left uropathy.

At 7 days of life, the ultrasonographic scan revealed a left urinary tract dilation (pelvic anteroposterior diameter of 18 mm; distal ureteral dilation of 14 mm).

At 9 days of life, the patient was admitted to the hospital for febrile urinary tract infection; for this reason, the voiding cystourethrography was performed, and it showed the absence of vesicoureteral reflux with normal urethra and bladder.

The following technetium-99m-labeled mercaptoacetyl-triglycine (MAG-3) renography detected a normal split renal function with evidence at the left side of hydronephrosis without ureteral dilation and poor urinary drainage out of the left pelvis that normalized itself during the diuretic phase (demonstrating no obstructive renal pattern); on the contrary, during the diuretic phase, a left megaureter was observed with poor urinary drainage out of the left ureter until the end of the diuretic scintigraphy (demonstrating a partial obstructive ureteral pattern).

At the last day hospital follow-up (at 7 months of life), the patient remained asymptomatic, and the ultrasonographic scan revealed a stability of the left megaureter.

The management of the 7-month-old patient is actually based on clinical and ultrasonographic serial evaluations (Fig. 5.7).

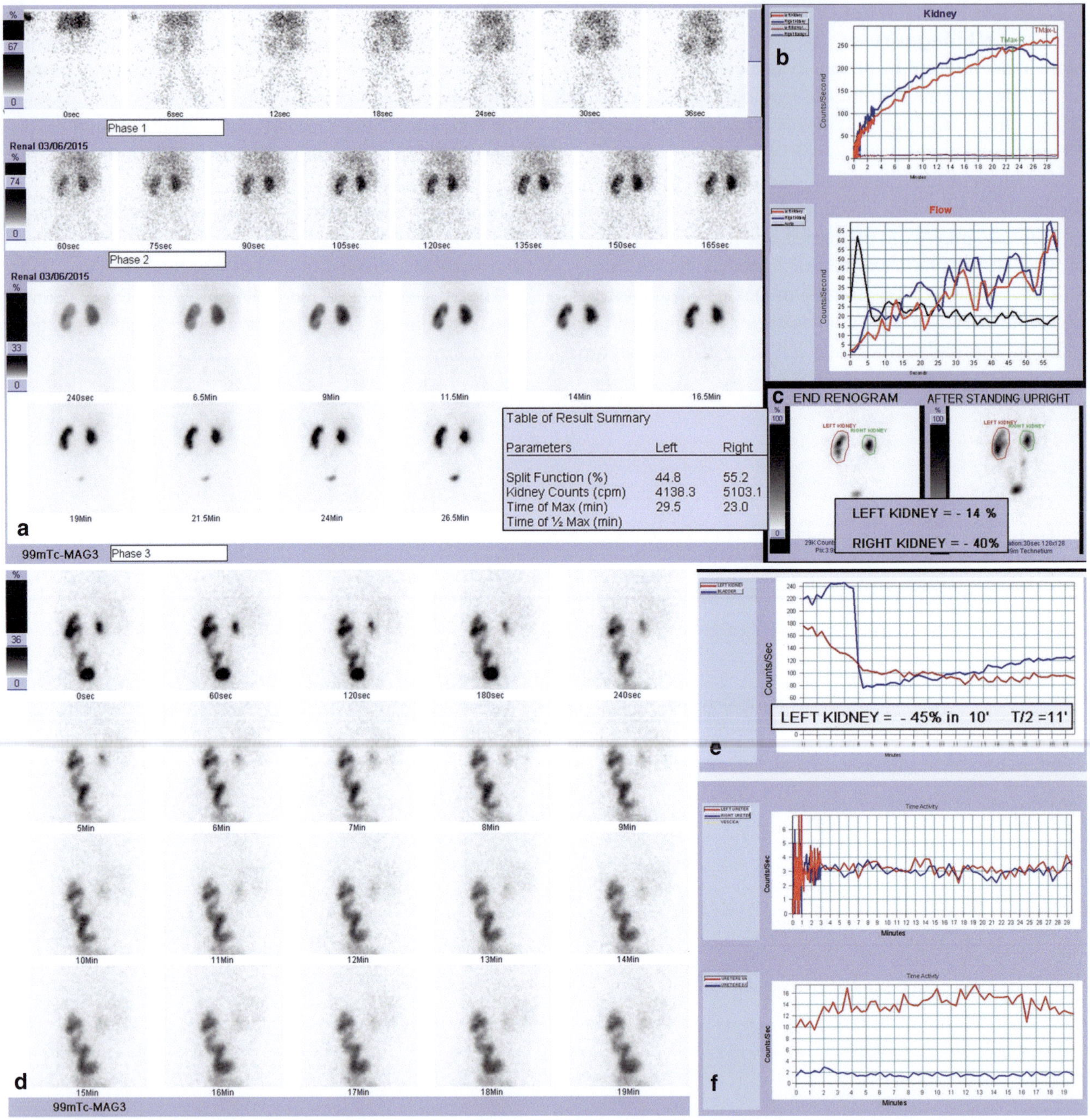

Fig. 5.7 MAG3 dynamic renal scan: dynamic images (**a**) show good and nonhomogeneous radiotracer uptake in left kidney with an area devoid of tracer corresponding to dilated renal pelvis and collecting system, and drainage is poor; right kidney presents good and homogeneous radiotracer uptake and poor drainage; renograms (**b**) confirm normal function and impaired drainage of left kidney ("rising curve"), and normal function and impaired drainage of right kidney; flow T/A curves (**b**) show synchronous and symmetrical perfusion. Gravity-assisted drainage-1 test shows no significant washout of left kidney, but improved drainage of right kidney (**c**). Diuretic dynamic images (**d**) and diuretic renogram (**e**) show prompt response to furosemide and significant improvement in drainage in left kidney, but also show dilated and tortuous left ureter, not evident at basal renal scan. Ureter T/A curves (**f**) show: normal pattern of both ureters during dynamic renal scan (*upper graph*); during diuretic scintigraphy, left ureterogram shows a rising phase until 13th minute of the study, followed by a mild decrement of activity in the last minutes (*lower graph*); pattern of right ureter is normal

5.1.2.8 Case 5.8: Primary Obstructive Right Megaureter: Treatment with Endoscopic High-Pressure Balloon Dilation

A right urinary tract dilation (pelvic anteroposterior diameter of 26 mm; distal ureteral dilation of 17 mm) was accidentally detected by the ultrasonographic scan in a male infant after a febrile urinary tract infection that required admission to hospital.

The voiding cystourethrography was performed, and it showed the absence of vesicoureteral reflux with normal urethra and bladder.

The following technetium-99m-labeled mercaptoacetyl-triglycine (MAG-3) renography revealed a normal split renal function with, at the right side, megaureter and poor urinary drainage that required the diuretic injection; an obstructive urinary pattern was observed during the diuretic phase, and it was confirmed at upright position at the end of the diuretic scintigraphy.

Because of the age (<12 months of life), the patient was submitted to mini-invasive treatment of the primary obstructive right megaureter: endoscopic high-pressure balloon dilation of the vesicoureteral junction was performed.

At 6 postoperative months, the MAG-3 renography confirmed a normal split renal function with right megaureter, but it showed an improvement of the urinary drainage with nonobstructive urinary pattern (no diuretic injection was necessary).

During the postoperative follow-up, the patient has remained asymptomatic, and the serial ultrasonographic scans have revealed an improvement of the right megaureter up to 8 mm diameter.

The management of the patient is actually based on the conservative treatment (Fig. 5.8).

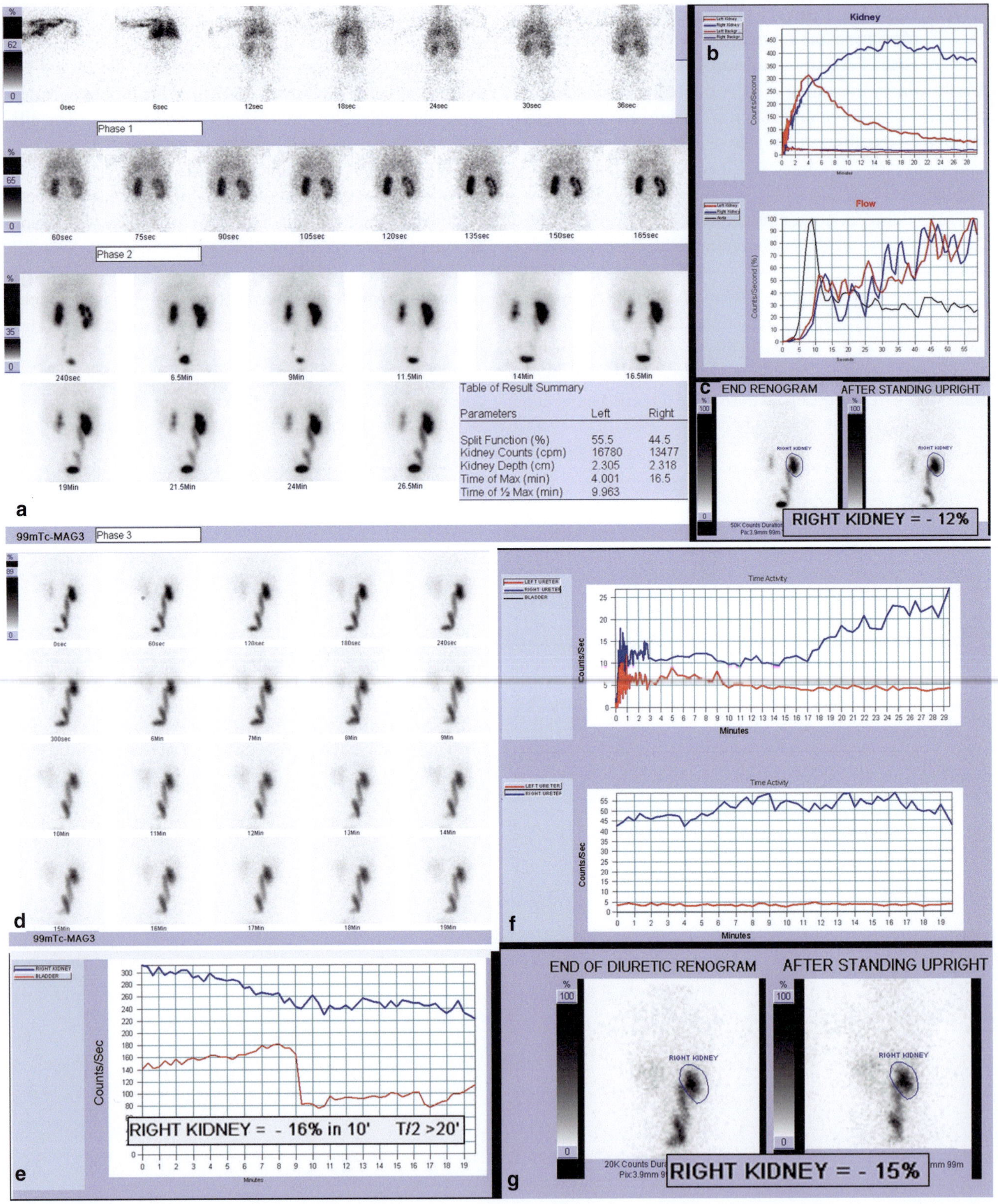

Fig. 5.8 MAG3 dynamic renal scan: dynamic images (**a**) show good and homogeneous radiotracer uptake and normal drainage in left kidney; right kidney presents good radiotracer uptake with nonhomogeneous intraparenchymal distribution due to an area devoid of tracer corresponding to dilated renal pelvis and collecting system; drainage is poor, with persistent radioactivity also in tortuous and dilated right ureter; renograms (**b**) confirm normal function and drainage of left kidney, and normal function and poor drainage of right kidney ("plateau" pattern); flow T/A curves (**b**) show synchronous and symmetrical perfusion. Gravity-assisted drainage-1 test shows no significant washout of right kidney and ureter (**c**). Diuretic dynamic images (**d**) and diuretic renogram (**e**) show very slow response to furosemide and no significant improvement in drainage in right kidney. Gravity-assisted drainage-2 test confirms poor drainage of right kidney and ureter (**g**). Ureter T/A curves (**f**) show: normal pattern of left ureter and "rising curve" of right ureter during dynamic renal scan (*upper graph*); no significant washout during diuretic scintigraphy in right ureter (*lower graph*)

5.1.2.9 Case 5.9: Transplanted Kidney Affected by Nonrefluxing and Nonobstructive Megaureter

A 16-year-old boy was submitted to kidney transplant, because he was affected by nephropathy associated to vesicoureteral reflux.

A urinary increasing dilation (pelvic anteroposterior diameter up to 19 mm; distal ureteral dilation up to 16 mm) of the renal graft associated with a progressive increase of the creatinine was observed during the post-transplant follow-up.

For this reason, the technetium-99m-labeled mercaptoacetyltriglycine (MAG-3) renography was performed, and it showed a small reduction of the renal graft function (at the upper pole) with evidence, at the renal graft, of megaureter associated with slow urinary drainage but absence of obstructive urinary pattern (no diuretic injection was necessary); during the same examination, the indirect MAG-3 cystography revealed the absence of vesicoureteral reflux.

During the postrenography follow-up, the patient has remained asymptomatic with normalization of the creatinine, and the serial ultrasonographic scans have revealed a spontaneous decrease of the megaureter up to 8 mm diameter.

For this reason, the management of the patient is actually based on wait-and-see strategy associated to clinical and ultrasonographic serial evaluations, in addition to repeated blood tests (Fig. 5.9).

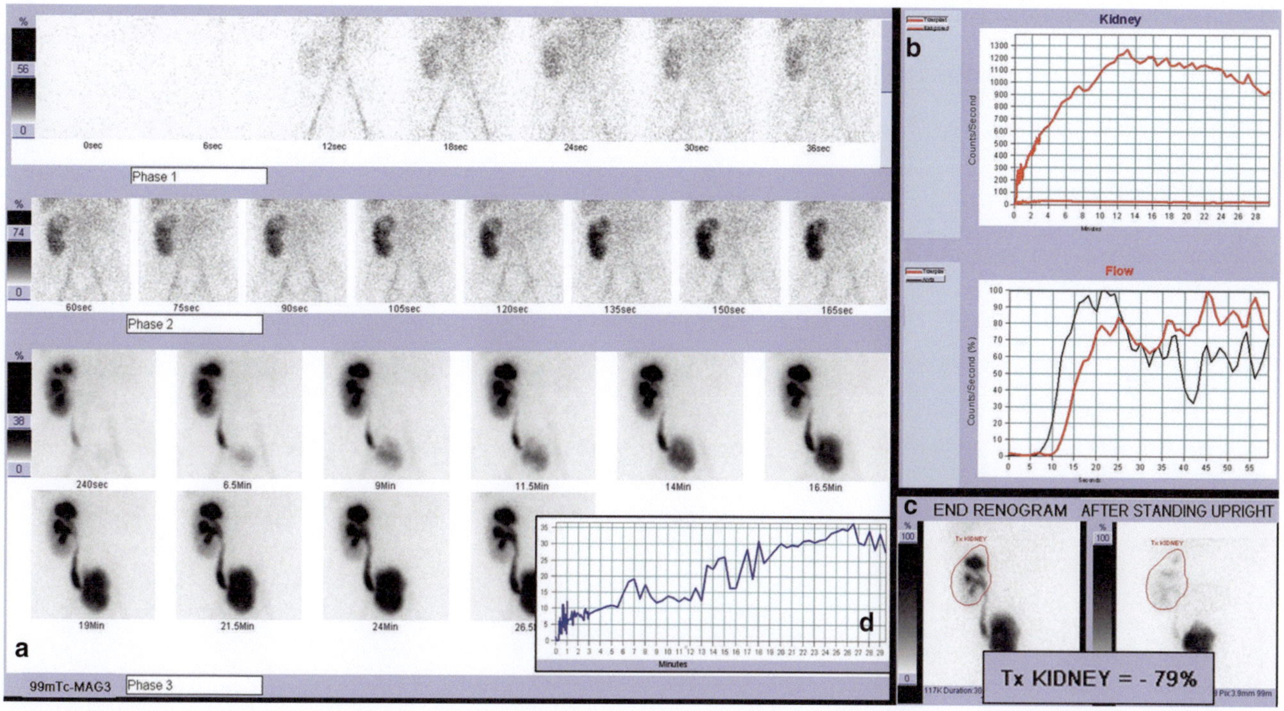

Fig. 5.9 MAG3 dynamic renal scan: dynamic images (**a**) show transplanted kidney in right iliac fossa; the kidney presents mildly reduced radiotracer uptake, in particular in the upper pole; intraparenchymal distribution is not homogeneous due to an area devoid of tracer corresponding to dilated collecting system; drainage is poor, and persistent radioactivity is present in the ureter too; a moderately low target/background ratio is also evident. Renogram (**b**) shows mildly reduced slope of parenchymal phase and poor drainage of transplanted kidney. Gravity-assisted drainage-1 test shows significant emptying of transplanted kidney and ureter (**c**). Ureter T/A curves (**d**) confirm a dilated nonobstructive pattern. In the presence of a dilated ureter, when the obstructive pattern has been ruled out, it could be useful (in toilet-trained patients) to perform an indirect cystoscintigraphy, in order to verify the possible presence of vesicoureteral reflux responsible for dilatation

Bibliography

1. Jamar F, Piret L, et al. Influence of ureteral status on kidney washout during technetium-99m-DTPA diuresis renography in children. J Nucl Med. 1992;33:73–8.

Nephrourology: Vesicoureteral Reflux

6

Milena Pizzoferro, Maria Felicia Villani, Ermelinda Mele, and Maria Carmen Garganese

6.1 Indirect Radionuclide Cystogram

6.1.1 Study Technique and Interpretation

Indirect radionuclide cystogram (IRC) is a radionuclide technique that gives the possibility of detecting vesicoureteral reflux (VUR) without a bladder catheter (micturition is studied under physiological conditions) with a low effective radiation dose. Furthermore, the IRC is done following a dynamic renogram (early, after, or whenever the child wishes to void). In such a way, a unique tracer administration allows to achieve the overall function of the kidneys, drainage data from the upper tracts (by dynamic renogram) followed by VUR, and micturition evaluation under normal physiological conditions (by IRC). If necessary, IRC can be performed also after diuretic test, achieving better technical conditions: improving urinary drainage and bladder filling (i.e., helpful in case of megaureter).

The unique preparations required for this test are good hydration, and children must be toilet-trained.

IRC is recorded by fast dynamic scintigraphy (0.5 s/frame) by posterior view registration (with gamma camera centered on pelvic and abdominal region). Well-trained staff (nurse and technician) must be extremely careful to start registration before bladder voiding (avoiding to fail micturition phase), limiting patient's movement (critical for mild VUR assessment).

Dedicated software for movement correction could be useful, but sometimes can introduce possible artifacts in relation to low activity dose and fast dynamic acquisition. Nuclear medicine staff have to be kind with the child and must be also able to perform several micturition attempts in case of uncooperative child or particular clinical conditions.

Results can be described as reframed dynamic series or by means of activity/time curves obtained in multiple regions (kidneys, ureters, and bladder).

6.1.2 Teaching Cases

6.1.2.1 Indirect Radionuclide Cystogram in Vesicoureteral Reflux Detection

Case 6.1 Urinary Tract Infections not Associated with Vesicoureteral Reflux in a Child with Normal Renal Function and Bilateral Renal Microlithiasis

Child followed for previous acute pyelonephritis, bilateral renal microlithiasis (composed by 70 % ammonium phosphate and 30 % calcium), and mild hydronephrosis. At 8 months of life, a cystography performed after the first acute event showed neither pathological finding nor vesicoureteral reflux (VUR). The child was followed up with periodic urinalysis and ultrasonography scans until the age of 10 years old when the baby had an acute pyelonephritis. During hospitalization, he underwent a MAG3 dynamic study that showed a normal renal function, and an indirect radioisotope cystography (IRC) confirmed the absence of voiding reflux. After excluding suspicion of VUR predisposing to urinary infections, clinical condition improved by a better hydration and more correct voiding habits.

M. Pizzoferro • M.F. Villani
Nuclear Medicine Unit, Imaging Departement – "Bambino Gesù" Children Hospital, Rome, Italy

E. Mele (✉)
Unit of Urology, "Bambino Gesù" Children Hospital, Rome, Italy
e-mail: ermelinda.mele@opbg.net

M.C. Garganese
Diagnostic Imaging Department of Nuclear Medicine, IRCCS Bambino Gesù Paediatric Hospital, Rome, Italy

© Springer International Publishing Switzerland 2017

M.C. Garganese, G.F.L. D'Errico (eds.), *Conventional Nuclear Medicine in Pediatrics*, DOI 10.1007/978-3-319-43181-9_6

Case 6.2 Urinary Tract Infections Associated with Low-Grade Vesicoureteral Reflux (Grade I) Without Nephropathy

A 3-year-old child with a urinary tract infection episode. Having acquired the control of urination, a renal scintigraphy with IRC was performed. The scintigraphic study showed a left kidney slightly smallest compared with the contralateral one with a normal renal function and a low-grade reflux on the left side. As the child had a unilateral low-grade VUR without nephropathy, he was followed on surveillance by periodic urinalysis and ultrasonography scans, and he is currently asymptomatic. In general, in fact, low-grade refluxes (Grades I–II) have high rates of spontaneous resolution (usually more than 80 %) in young children (Fig. 6.1).

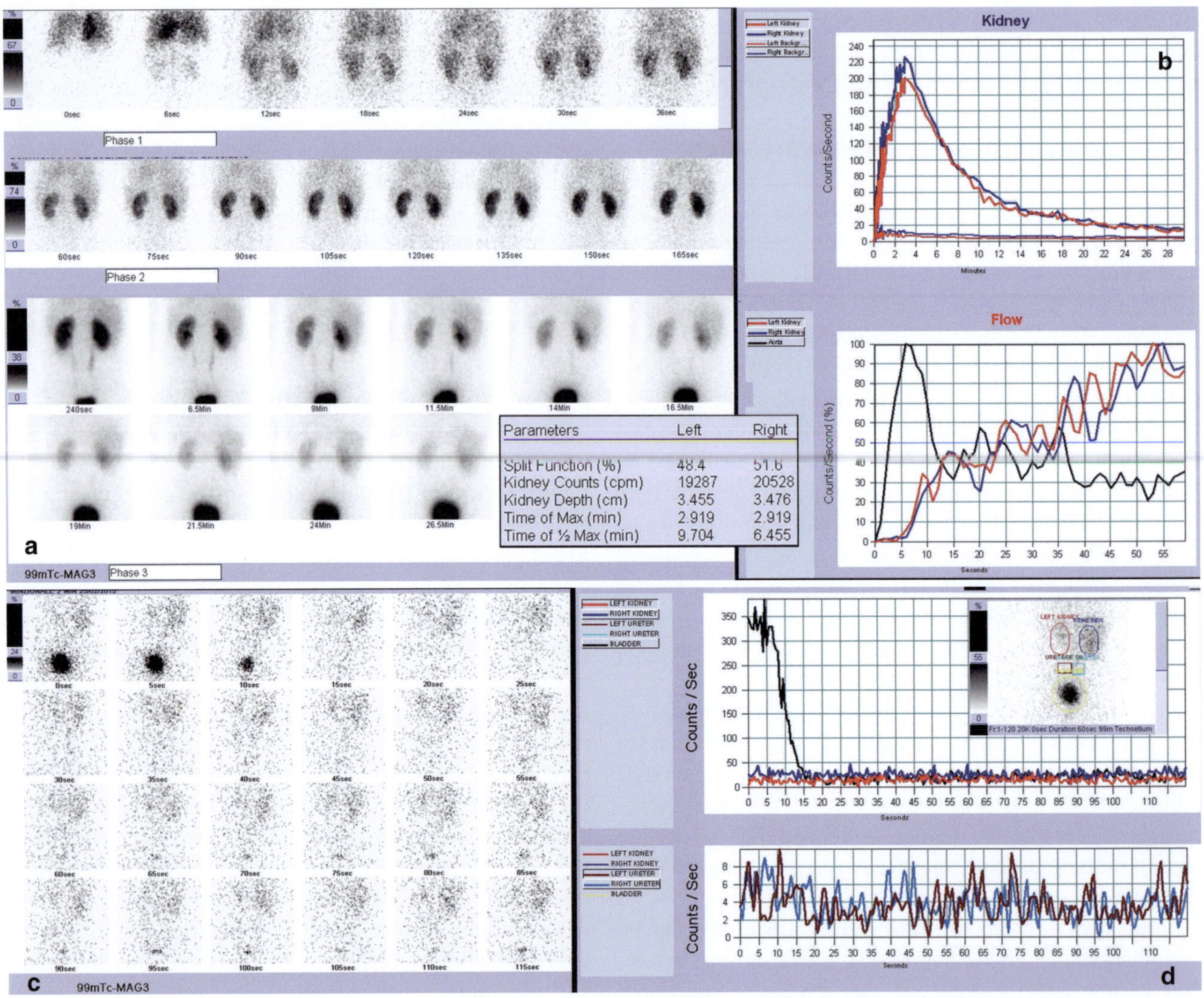

Fig. 6.1 (**a**, **b**) The qualitative analysis of basic dynamic study reveals an intense concentration of tracer in the renal parenchyma and rapid washout of both kidneys (**a**). Renogram curves confirm qualitative interpretation of the study, showing normal tracer uptake in both kidneys, bilateral regular transit with rapid urinary excretion; the basic renogram also provides a symmetrical measurement of relative renal function (**b**). IRC images show a complete bladder voiding in the absence of VUR (**c**). Time-activity curves of bladder and kidneys confirm a regular and complete bladder voiding without radioactivity increment corresponding to kidneys and ureters (**d**)

Case 6.3 Asymptomatic Residual Monolateral Reflux (Grade II) After Endoscopic Correction of Bilateral Vesicoureteral Reflux

A 2-year-old girl referred to our center for recurrent pyelonephritis. An IRC showed a bilateral vesicoureteral reflux (Grade II); thus, we performed an endoscopic treatment of VUR, followed by antibiotic prophylaxis for 1 month. During follow-up, the child has presented urinary tract infection no longer, but an IRC performed after about 1 year of treatment, as control treatment effectiveness, documented persistence of left-sided vesicoureteral reflux (Fig. 6.2c, d). Therefore, the child underwent ureteral reimplantation, and currently she is asymptomatic.

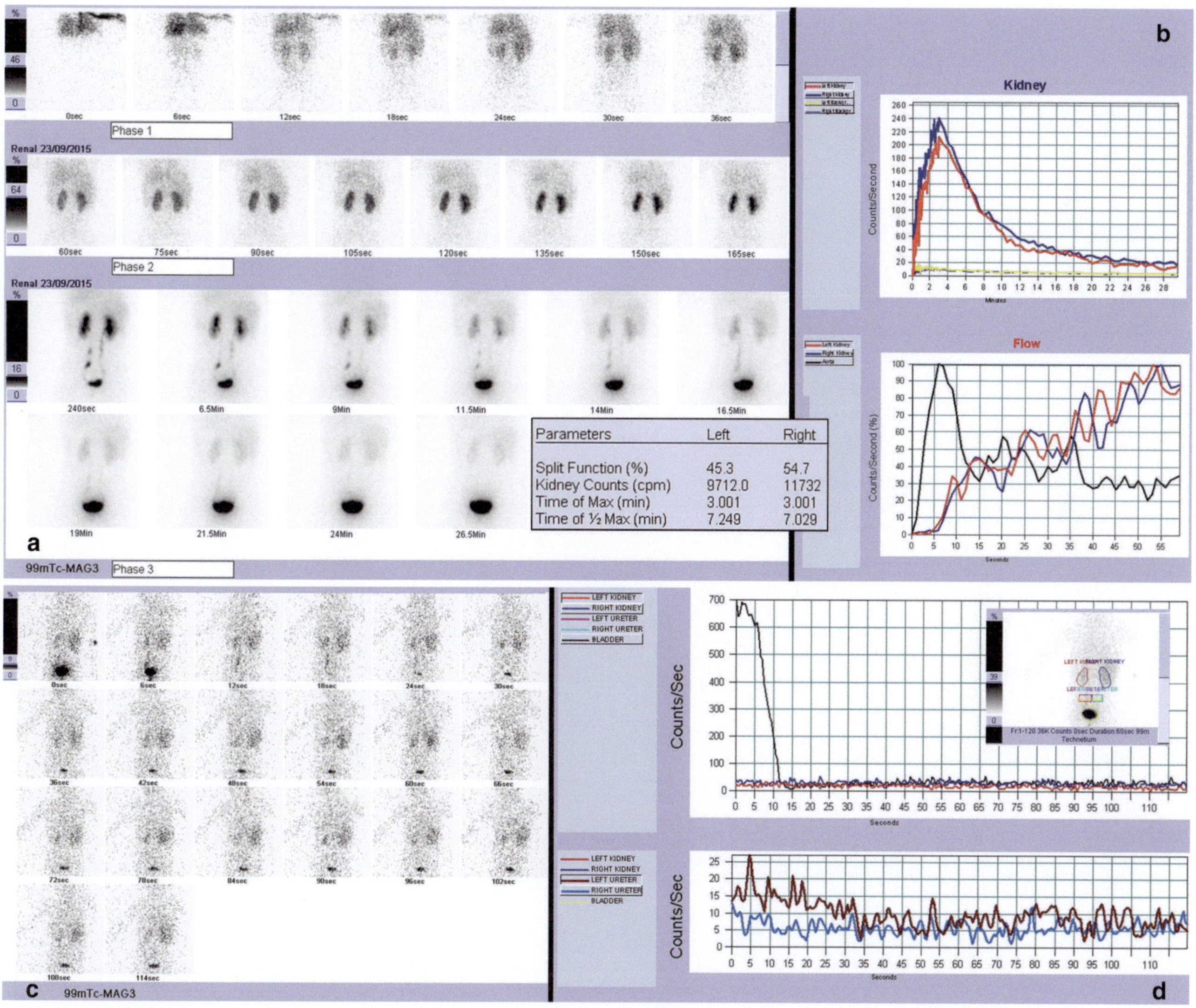

Fig. 6.2 (**a**, **b**) A 3-year-old child with a urinary tract infection episode. Having acquired the control of urination, a renal scintigraphy with IRC was performed. The scintigraphic study showed a left kidney slightly smaller than the contralateral one with a normal renal function and a low-grade reflux on the *left side*. As the child had a unilateral low-grade VUR without nephropathy, he was followed on surveillance by periodic urinalysis and ultrasonography scans, and he is currently asymptomatic. In general, in fact, low-grade refluxes (Grades I–II) have high rates of spontaneous resolution (usually more than 80 %) in young children. By the qualitative assessment of scintigraphic images, both kidneys are located in their own proper sides with regular perfusion. Left kidney is slightly smaller than the contralateral one, even if both kidneys show normal morphology, renal uptake, and urinary excretion. (**a**) Both renogram curves show normal slope of parenchymal phase and regular elimination of tracer from the kidneys (left curve is slightly less wide in relation to the size of the kidney). The split renal function is sufficiently symmetric (**b**). (**c**, **d**) During bladder voiding (regular and complete), a synchronous radiourine reflux limited to left ureter is observed (Grade I) (**c**). This scintigraphic finding is confirmed by time-activity curve of the left ureter without radioactivity increment corresponding to homolateral kidney (**d**)

Case 6.4 Persistent Urinary Tract Infections Secondary to Residual Bilateral Reflux (Grade II–III) After Endoscopic Correction in Bilateral Duplex Collecting System

A 1-year-old baby with right high-grade vesicoureteral reflux in double system. She was treated with antibiotics for several episodes of pyelonephritis in the first months of life. During follow-up, a DMSA scan showed double bilateral system with good function of both kidneys, even if renal scars were bilaterally present in lower systems. The child continued to present febrile urinary infection after endoscopic treatment of vesicoureteral reflux, and a cystography showed persistence of VUR (in both systems of left kidney and in the upper right system). Therefore, a new endoscopic treatment of reflux was performed at 18 months of life, but next IRC showed persistence of bilateral vesicoureteral reflux. Due to the close proximity of the ureteral orifices, endoscopic correction of vesicoureteral reflux in duplicated collecting systems is challenging to be effective, avoiding secondary obstructive megaureter.

Case 6.5 Relapse of High-Grade Vesicoureteral Reflux (Grade II–III) After Acquisition of Bladder-Voiding Control in Child with Reflux Nephropathy and Retensionist Habit

A 3-year-old child with previous recurrent pyelonephritis, followed for bilateral high-grade VUR (treated endoscopically at 18 months) and bilateral nephropathy (at 2 months of life, a DMSA scan showed bilateral renal scarring with greater impairment of the right kidney).

After acquisition of bladder-voiding control, the child had a retentionist attitude, and he had an acute pyelonephritis, despite a time-urination management. An IRC was performed revealing a bilateral vesicoureteral reflux (obtained with high bladder filling), with a severe reflux nephropathy at the right side. VUR highlighted by the scintigraphic study was confirmed by a subsequent cystography, and patient underwent ureter reimplantation (Figs. 6.3, 6.4, and 6.5).

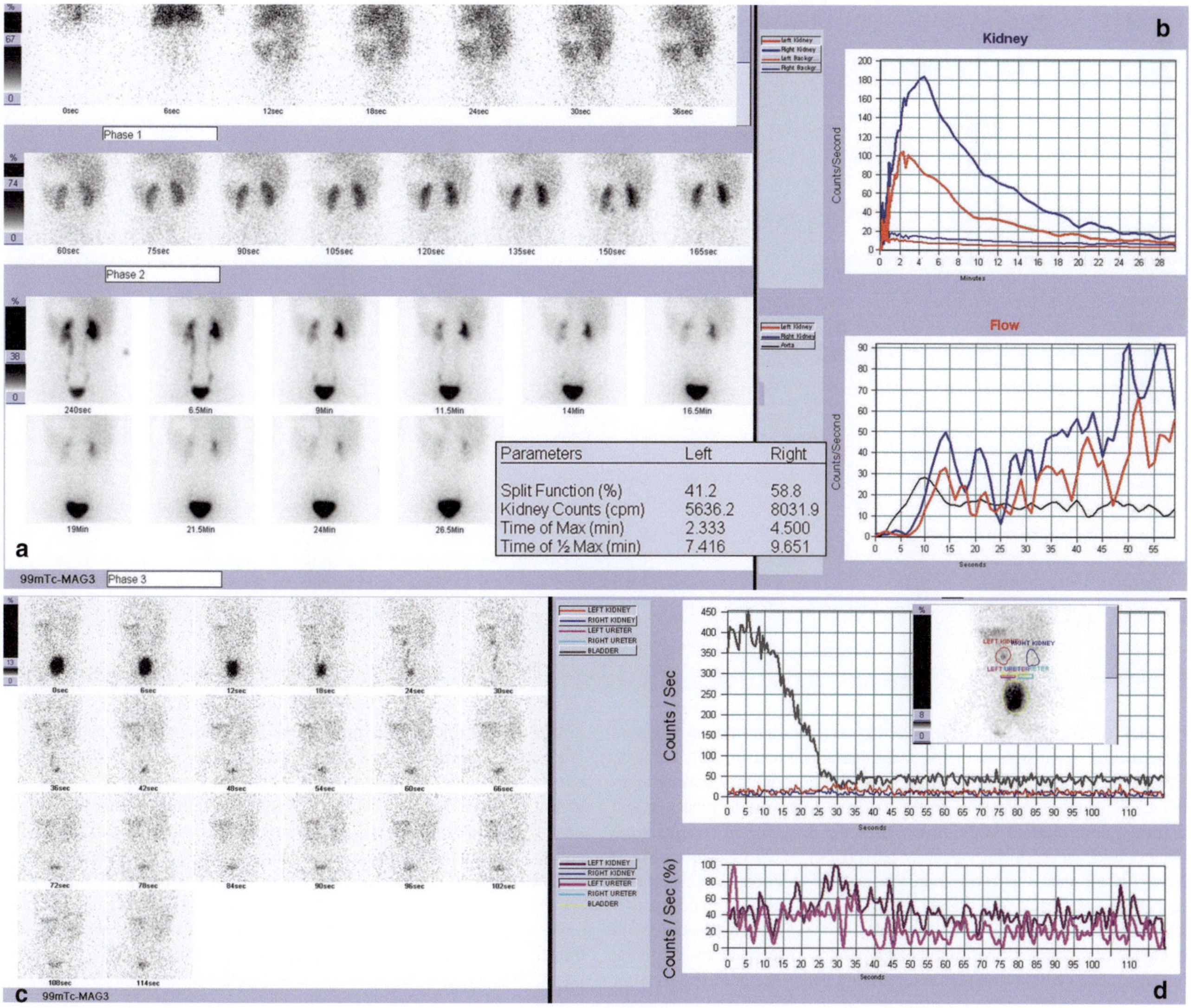

Fig. 6.3 By qualitative assessment of scintigraphic images, both kidneys are located in their own proper sides with synchronous but asymmetrical perfusion (reduced on the *left side*). Left kidney is small with a slightly irregular morphology; left renal uptake is preserved, and urinary excretion is normal. Right kidney shows an intense concentration of tracer in the renal parenchyma and a rapid washout (**a**). Left renogram curve (less wide than the contralateral one) shows preserved slope of parenchymal phase and regular elimination of tracer. The shape of the right renogram curve is normal in all phases. The split renal function is slightly asymmetric (relatively reduced on the left) (**b**). (**c, d**) IRC images show a complete and regular bladder voiding. During bladder voiding, a synchronous radiourine reflux is present on the *left side* that reaches the renal pelvis without dilatation (Grade II) (**c**). Time-activity curves of bladder and kidneys reveal a regular and complete bladder voiding, with a radioactivity increment corresponding to left ureter and kidney (**d**)

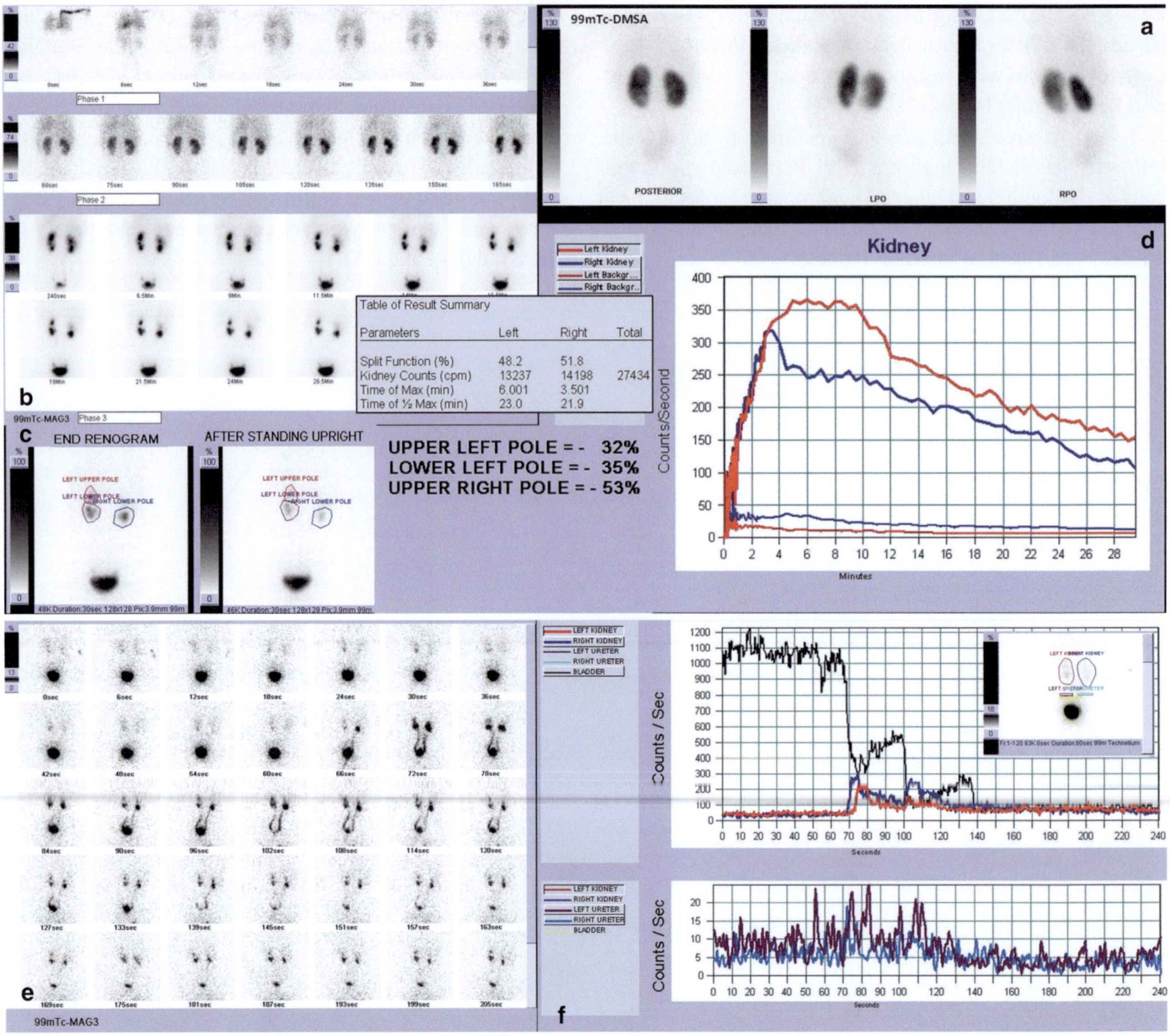

Fig. 6.4 (**a**) At 8 months of life, a DMSA scan shows a double bilateral system with good uptake of the radiopharmaceutical in both kidneys; tracer concentration is regular in the upper systems, while a nonhomogeneous distribution is detected in the lower systems due to focal cortical defects (more marked scars on the left). No evidence of parenchymal defects is observed in the upper systems.(**b**, **c**) At 26 months of life, a MAG3 renal scan is performed showing a good function of the right kidney (both systems) and a double left kidney district with hypofunction and scars of the lower system. Bilaterally, urinary excretion is slow with evidence of moderate stasis of radiourine (in the lower systems and in the left upper one) which tended to resolve itself and to further improve after orthostatism, excluding the presence of lower or upper pole pelviureteric junction obstruction in duplicated collecting systems (**b**). Both renogram curves show normal slope of parenchymal phase and mildly slow elimination of tracer from the kidneys. Overall, the split renal function is sufficiently symmetric. (**d**, **e**) IRC study (qualitative images and time-activity curves) shows irregular but complete bladder emptying: for three times, a sudden interruption of urination is observed with bilateral VUR and subsequent refilling of the bladder. Time-activity curves of ureters and kidneys reveal a bilateral radioactivity increment corresponding to the bilateral ureter and kidney (reaching up the renal pelvis with a mild dilatation, these kinds of VUR are classified as II–III scintigraphic grade)

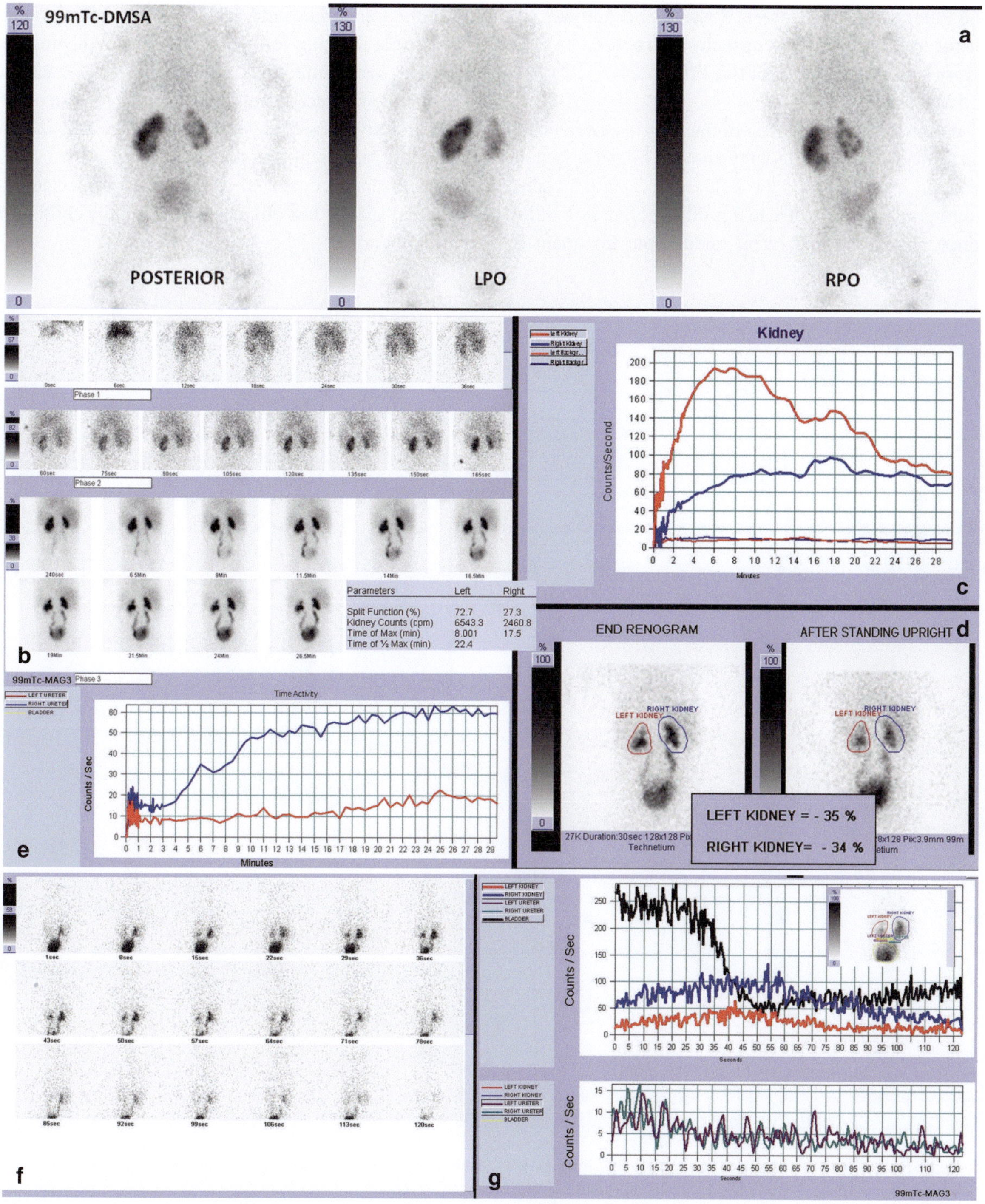

Fig. 6.5 (**a**) At 2 months of life, a DMSA scan is performed after recurrent pyelonephritis. Scintigraphic imaging shows radiopharmaceutical uptake preserved in the left kidney and markedly reduced in the right one. Bilaterally, tracer distribution is not homogeneous due to multiple focal cortical defects with greater impairment of the right kidney (split renal function of right kidney was 29 %). Background signal is increased as for global insufficient renal function. At 18 months of life, a MAG3 renal scan confirms bilateral renal scars with preserved parenchymal function in the left kidney and severe hypofunction in the right one. Urinary excretion is mildly delayed in the left kidney, delayed and slow on the right, with evidence of radiotracer stasis which tended to resolve itself (**b**) and to further improve after orthostatism (gravity-assisted drainage test-1, **d**). Bilateral tracer accumulation is observed in the ureters, but both ureterograms show nonobstructive pattern. (**e**). Left renogram curve shows preserved slope of parenchymal phase and mildly slow elimination of tracer. Right renogram curve has a low width, showing reduced slope of parenchymal phase, delayed transit, and slow urinary excretion (**c**). The basic renogram shows a poor right split renal function, steady if compared to the previous DMSA scan. (**f–g**) IRC study is obtained only after several attempts, with a high filling bladder: performing an IRC study can sometimes be difficult due to poor child cooperation, but it is of crucial importance. In the IRC images, in fact, we can observe a regular and complete bladder emptying with bilateral VUR, more severe on the *right side* (**f**). Time-activity curves of kidneys reveal a bilateral radioactivity increment, synchronous with the bladder emptying, especially on the right (II–III scintigraphic grades on the left and III scintigraphic grade on the *right*) (**g**)

Case 6.6 Relapse of Monolateral Passive and Active Vesicoureteral Reflux Endoscopically Corrected, Secondary by Displacement of the Previously Injected Material

Female infant followed by pediatricians for suspected urinary tract infection. A cystography showed bilateral vesicoureteral reflux (Grade IV on the left, Grade I on the right), and a scintigraphic scan revealed a mild hypofunction of the left kidney. Thus, she underwent endoscopic treatment of vesicoureteral reflux, and baby was always asymptomatic with normal imaging follow-up. At 3 years of life, the child presented new infections of the urinary tract, and a radionuclide indirect cystography showed relapse of left passive and active vesicoureteral reflux (Fig. 6.6c, d). A new endoscopic treatment was performed, and at the cystoscopy, an evident displacement of the previously injected material was found. At the last clinical follow-up, the child remained asymptomatic.

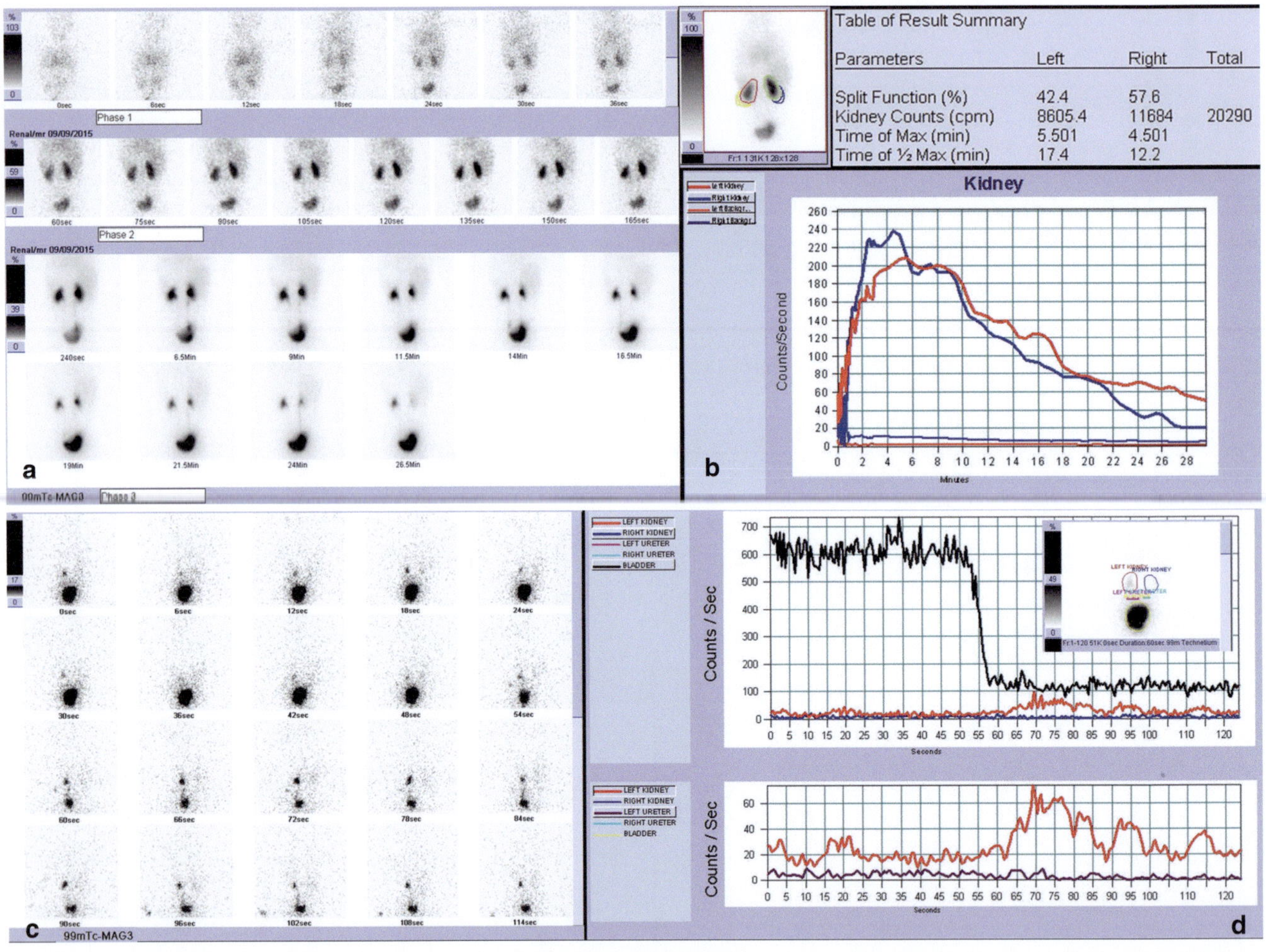

Fig. 6.6 (**a**, **b**) By qualitative assessment of scintigraphic images, left kidney is smaller than normal with a slightly reduced renal uptake. Transit and urinary excretion of radiotracer from the kidney are slightly delayed and slow with evidence of mild pelvic stasis which tends to resolve itself during basal study. Right kidney shows an intense concentration of tracer in the renal parenchyma and a rapid washout (**a**). Left renogram curve (less wide than the contralateral one) shows preserved slope of parenchymal phase, transit slightly prolonged, and elimination of tracer from the kidney mildly slow. The shape of the right renogram curve is normal in all phases. The split renal function is slightly asymmetric (mildly reduced on the left) (**b**). (**c**, **d**) In order to obtain a diagnostic examination with improving sensitivity, IRC study was performed after oral hydration awaiting a better filling bladder and a further left pelvic stasis resolution. In the IRC images, we can observe persistence of left pelvic stasis, which slightly decreases and increases before bladder emptying. After a regular but incomplete bladder emptying (about 15% of residual postvoiding activity), a high-grade VUR was detected on the *left side* (**c**). Time-activity curves of kidneys confirm a left radioactivity increment previously and synchronous with bladder emptying (passive and active VUR, II and III scintigraphic grades, respectively) (**d**). A good technical IRC performing is crucial to avoid false-negative findings or movement artifacts (especially when residual urine stasis is present)

Case 6.7 Indirect Radionuclide Cystography Evaluation After Endoscopic Vesicoureteral Reflux Treatment: Absence of Residual Reflux in Asymptomatic Child with Nephropathy

Female infant with febrile urinary tract infections. Renal ultrasonography previously performed showed no abnormalities while a cystography revealed bilateral vesicoureteral reflux (Grade III). A renal DMSA scintigraphy was performed showing multiple scarring in both kidneys, with greater impairment of the right one (split renal function of right kidney was mildly reduced). At 3 years of life, the child underwent endoscopic treatment of reflux. A control IRC was performed 1 year later, showing a steady hypofunction of right kidney and absence of residual reflux. Currently, she is asymptomatic.

Case 6.8 Indirect Radionuclide Cystography Evaluation After Endoscopic Vesicoureteral Reflux Treatment: Persistent Low-Grade Monolateral Reflux in Asymptomatic Child with Nephropathy

Female infant with febrile urinary tract infections. Renal ultrasound was normal. Given the presence of periodic urinary tract infections, a cystography was performed showing bilateral vesicoureteral reflux (Grade III).

At 6 months of age, the child underwent endoscopic treatment for vesicoureteral reflux. About a year later, the child underwent a new endoscopic treatment for persistence of reflux detected by cystography. An ultrasound also showed left kidney mildly small (57 mm) with cortical thinning. At 4 years of life, a MAG3 renal scan was performed, showing a severe impairment of left kidney function, and an IRC revealed persistence of left vesicoureteral reflux (Grade II). The child remained asymptomatic since the last endoscopic reflux correction, and conservative management is actually the utilized strategy for the patient (followed on surveillance by periodic urinalysis, blood pressure measurements, and ultrasonography scans).

Case 6.9 Bilateral High-Grade Vesicoureteral Reflux Detected by Indirect Radionuclide Cystography in Severe Left Kidney Hypodisplasia (Secondary to Monolateral Reflux Endoscopically Treated)

A 9-year-old boy, followed for severe left kidney hypodysplasia and monolateral VUR (Scintigraphic Grade II), endoscopically treated at 7 years of age. He had no infections with mild hypertension.

Case 6.10 Renal Ectopia with Abdominal Pain and Kidney Lithiasis

A 3-year-old girl with family history of kidney stones and renal ectopia. During an episode of abdominal pain, an ultrasound scan was performed revealing right kidney in lumbar ectopia without ureteral dilatation but with the presence of small lithiasic formations (diameter of about 2 mm); right kidney size was smaller than contralateral ones with reduced parenchymal thickness and five renal cysts in the lower pole (5–7 mm). To obtain a functional renal evaluation, a MAG3 scan was performed showing a mild-moderate hypofunction of right kidney, and an IRC excluded the presence of vesicoureteral reflux associated with renal ectopia.

Case 6.11 Single Kidney in Ectopic Region with Vesicoureteral Reflux Endoscopically Corrected

Male patient followed since birth for single kidney ectopic in pelvic region and vesicoureteral reflux endoscopically corrected at 6 months of life. The child no longer has presented urinary tract infection, and renal function remained normal. At 7 years of life, an ultrasonographic scan showed mild pelvis dilatation without ureter dilatation. A MAG3 scan was performed to evaluate renal function end urinary drainage; an IRC control was also achieved showing no vesicoureteral reflux.

Case 6.12 Vesicoureteral Reflux Detection in Transplanted Kidney

An 8-year-old boy followed for kidney transplantation secondary to chronic renal insufficiency for posterior urethral valves. Numerous infections of urinary tract occurred despite endoscopic correction of vesicoureteral reflux, and an IRC control was performed showing persistent VUR. For this reason, a surgical VUR correction was performed with subsequent clinical resolution of urinary tract infections.

6.1.2.2 Complication of Endoscopical Reflux Correction

Case 6.13 Infection of Injected Material in Vesicoureteral Reflux, Endoscopic Treatment

A 6-year-old girl with left vesicoureteral reflux associated to reflux nephropathy underwent endoscopic treatment in two different occasions. After 2 years from the last reflux correction, the child developed bladder voiding disorders (urinary retention), and an ultrasonographic scan showed a significant dilation of left pelvis and ureter. A new renal scintigraphy was performed confirming poor left split renal function and showing a significant obstruction of the ureterovesical junction. Radionuclide cystography was not achieved because the child could not empty the bladder despite the urge to urinate and numerous voiding attempts.

For this reason, the child underwent ureteral left reimplantation, and an infection of previous injected material for reflux correction was histologically detected. The child is actually asymptomatic, and the last functional imaging follow-up showed renal function stability and left residual nonrefluxing and nonobstructive hydroureteronephrosis.

Case 6.14 Right Obstructive Megaureter Secondary to Endoscopic Reflux Correction

A male patient affected by posterior urethral valves endoscopically treated with bilateral vesicoureteral reflux underwent endoscopic treatment in two different occasions. During postoperative follow-up, ultrasonographic scan revealed a significant dilation of bilateral ureters.

A MAG3 scan showed normal function of both kidneys with nonobstructive left megaureter and obstructive pattern on the right. For this reason, the child underwent meatoplasty on the left and ureteral right reimplantation.

6.1.2.3 Technical Teaching Cases

Case 6.15 Beware of Indirect Radionuclide Cystography Evaluation in Case of Residual Renal Stasis

A 12-year-old boy, followed since birth by nephrologists for moderate chronic renal failure secondary to bilateral renal hypoplasia and vesicoureteral reflux endoscopically corrected at the age of 1 year. At radionuclide cystography control, no more vesicoureteral reflux was detected.

The last ultrasonographic follow-up showed right hypodysplastic kidney (a small echogenic mass with some simple peripheral cysts) and left kidney with irregular thinning of cortical parenchyma (characterized by hyperechoic structure with almost absent corticomedullary differentiation) and dilatation of calyces and pelvis in the middle and inferior renal third (pelvic anteroposterior diameter of 22 mm). At the last clinical surveillance, creatinine level remained steady, but an acute febrile urinary tract infection occurred, and a MAG3 scan with IRC study was performed to evaluate renal function and to detect possible VUR relapse.

Case 6.16 Compare Indirect Radionuclide Cystography Imaging to Basal Renal Study

A 5-year-old girl with prenatal diagnosis of bilateral renal double system. A postnatal ultrasound revealed dilated lower systems, and several acute pyelonephritis episodes occurred. The cystography showed a bilateral high-grade vesicoureteral reflux. No evidence of scars was detected by DMSA renal scan. Two endoscopic reflux treatments were performed, and an IRC control (after 8 months from the last treatment) showed persistent bilateral reflux. Therefore, the child was proposed for surgical correction of vesicoureteral reflux.

Case 6.17 Perform Several Attempts to Achieve a Complete Bladder Voiding

An 11-year-old boy followed for left renal dysplasia (markedly poor left renal function, equal to 2 %) secondary to vesicoureteral reflux, and the child underwent endoscopic correction at 10 years of life. Last renal ultrasound showed right kidney in compensatory hypertrophy and did not display left kidney. A subsequent episode of cystitis occurred, and a radionuclide cystography showed a mild residual left vesicoureteral reflux. Until now, the management is based on conservative treatment (Figs. 6.7, 6.8, 6.9, 6.10, 6.11, 6.12, 6.13, 6.14, 6.15, 6.16, and 6.17).

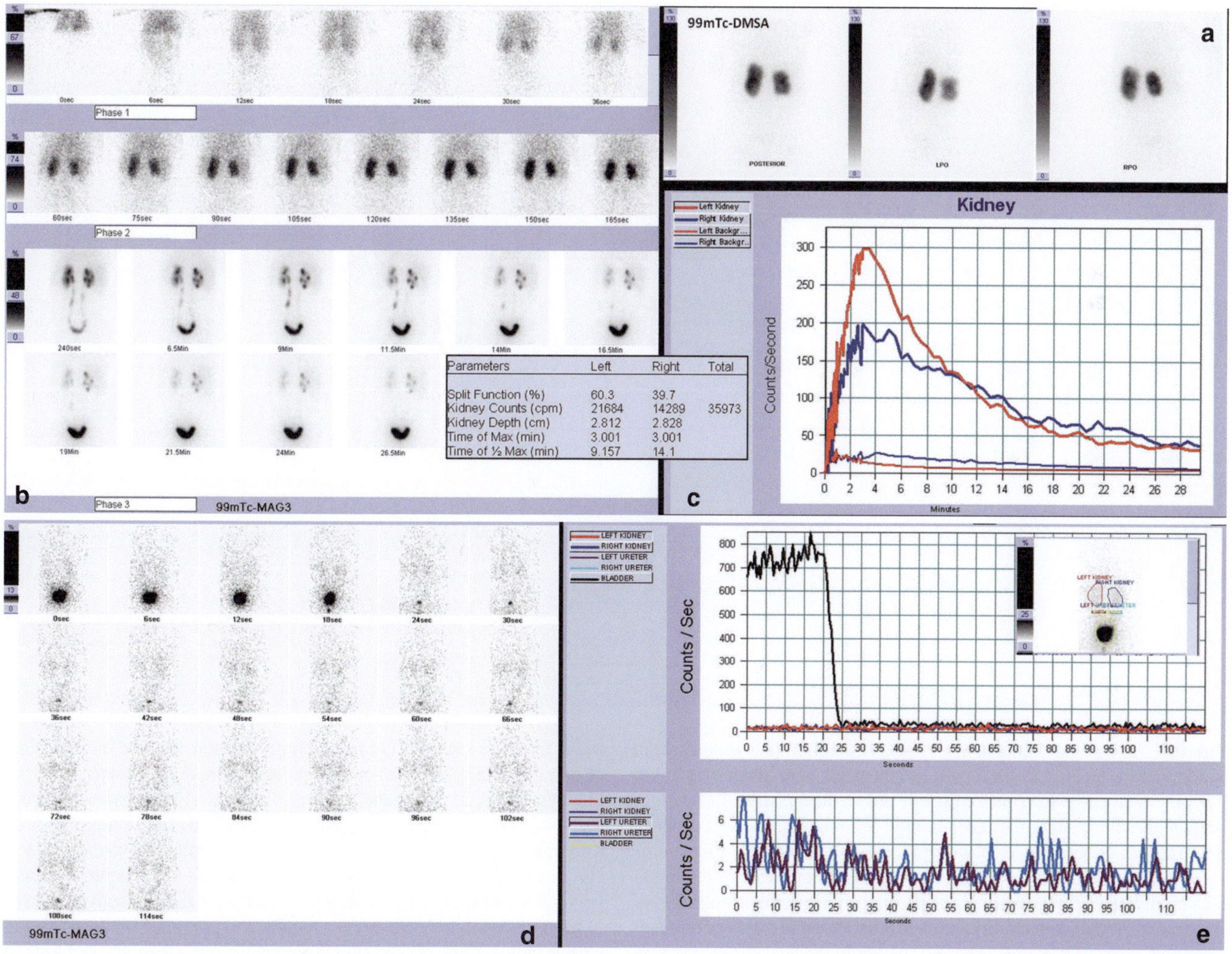

Fig. 6.7 (**a**) At 2 years of life, a DMSA scan is performed. Scintigraphic imaging shows radiopharmaceutical uptake preserved in both kidneys; bilaterally, tracer distribution is not homogeneous due to multiple focal cortical defects with more serious impairment of the right kidney. As we can observe in posterior and left posterior oblique views, parenchymal defects are evident in the left kidney in correspondence of *upper pole*, medial *lower pole* and the *middle* third (anterior face). Right kidney is smaller than normal with multiple scars and split renal functions mildly reduced is detected (Right Differential Renal Function: 41 %). (**b**, **c**) At 3 years of life, a MAG3 renal scan confirms bilateral renal scars with preserved parenchymal function in left kidney and mild hypofunction in the right one. Urinary excretion is normal in the left while the right kidney tracer transit is slightly extended without evidence of significant residual stasis at the end of basal registration. (**c**). Left renogram curve shows normal slope of parenchymal phase and regular elimination of tracer. Right renogram curve is less wide than the contralateral kidney showing mildly reduced slope of parenchymal phase, slightly prolonged transits and quite normal urinary excretion. The basic renogram confirms a mildly reduced split renal function of right kidney, quite steady if compared to the previous scintigraphic DMSA study (**d**). (**d**, **e**) IRC images shows a complete bladder voiding in absence of VUR (**d**). Time-activity curves of bladder and kidneys confirm a regular and complete bladder voiding without radioactivity increment corresponding to kidneys and ureters (**e**)

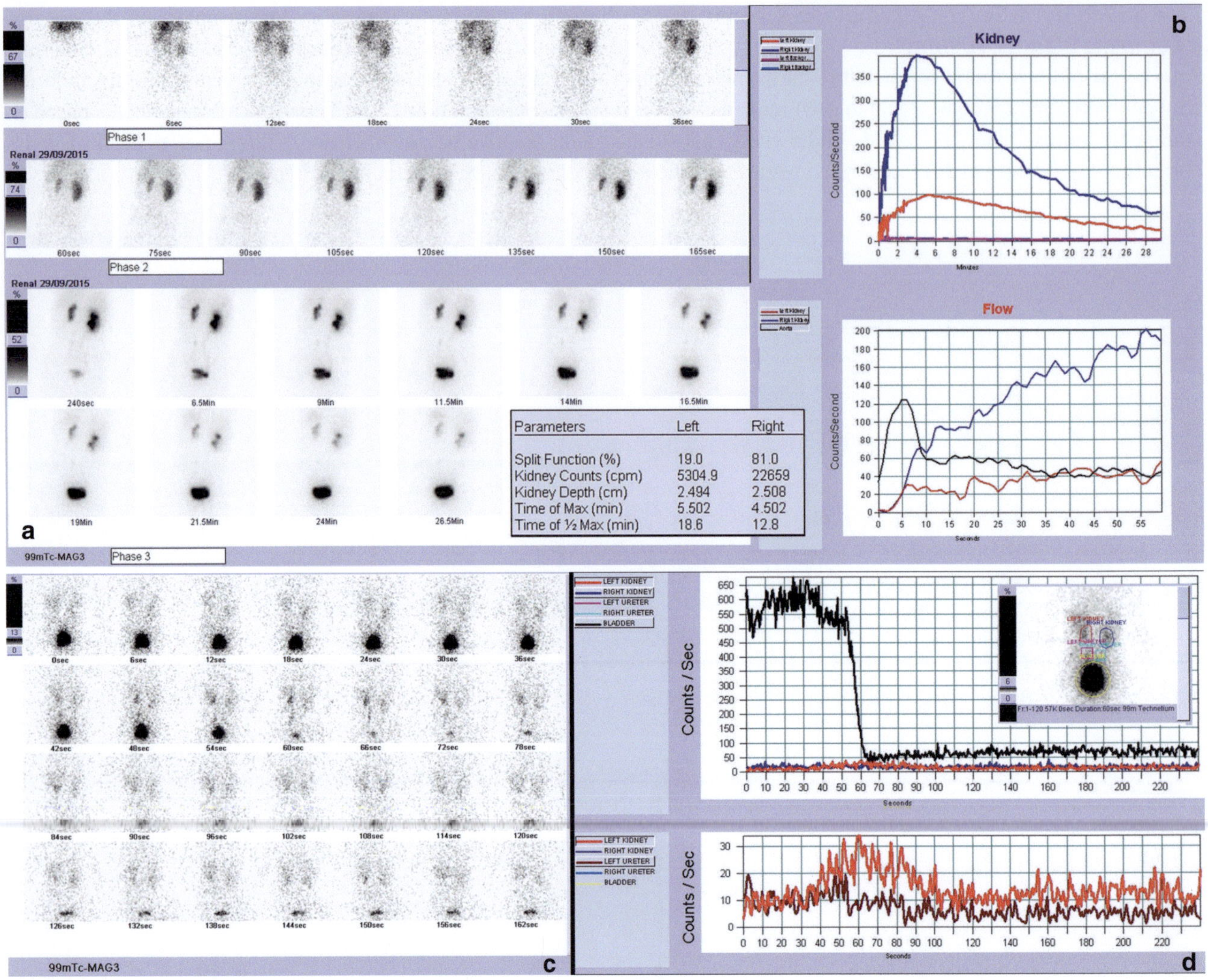

Fig. 6.8 (**a**, **b**) By qualitative assessment of scintigraphic images, both kidneys were located in their own proper sides with synchronous but asymmetrical perfusion (markedly reduced on the *left side*). Left *kidney* was small with an irregular morphology; left renal uptake was reduced and tracer distribution was inhomogeneous due to multiple focal cortical defects. Radiotracer transit was prolonged, and urinary excretion was moderately slow. Right kidney showed an intense concentration of tracer in the renal parenchyma and a sufficiently rapid washout (**a**). Left renogram curve (little wide) showed markedly reduced slope of parenchymal phase, prolonged transit, and moderately slow elimination of tracer from the kidneys. The right renogram curve showed normal slope of parenchymal phase and quite regular elimination of tracer from the kidneys. The split renal function was markedly asymmetric with a very low left renal split function (equal to 19 %). (**b–d**) IRC images showed a complete and regular bladder voiding. During bladder voiding, a synchronous radiourine reflux was present on the left that reaches the renal pelvis without significant dilatation (Grade II) (**c**). Time-activity curves of bladder and kidneys revealed a regular and complete bladder voiding with a radioactivity increment corresponding to left ureter and kidney (**d**)

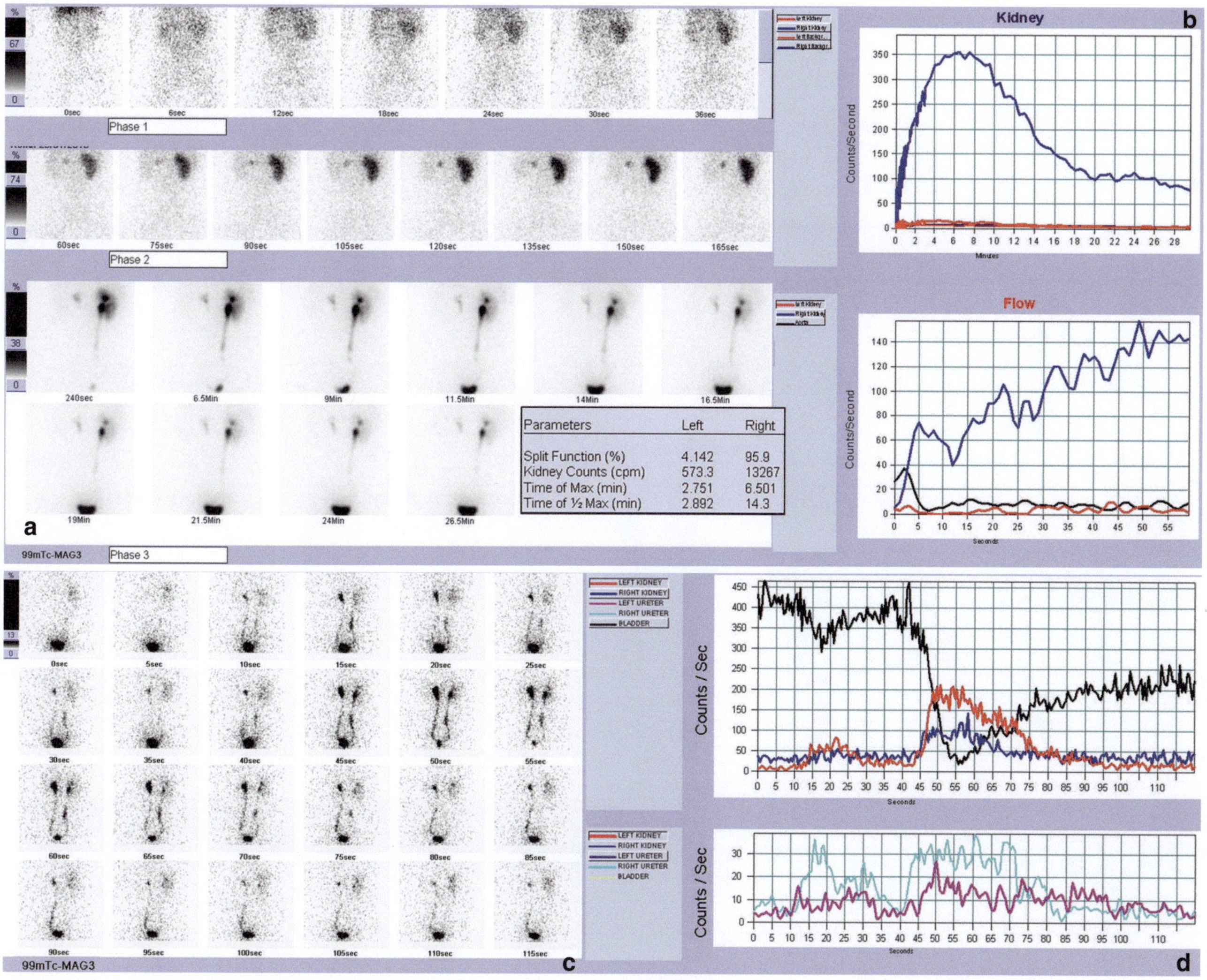

Fig. 6.9 (**a**, **b**) By the qualitative assessment of scintigraphic images, left kidney is late displayed and hypoperfused with small size and irregular shape. The parenchymal uptake was poor, and urinary excretion was slow. Right kidney showed an intense concentration of tracer in the renal parenchyma, and urinary excretion was mildly delayed with slight and transient stasis (**a**). Left renogram curve (very little wide) appeared flattened. The right renogram curve showed normal slope of parenchymal phase, and elimination of tracer from the kidneys mildly delayed. The split renal function was markedly asymmetric (left renal split function was severely reduced, equal to 4 %). (**b**). IRC study (qualitative images and time-activity curves) showed irregular but complete bladder emptying: for two times, a sudden interruption of urination was observed with bilateral VUR and subsequent refilling of the bladder. (**c**). Time-activity curves of ureters and kidneys reveal a bilateral radioactivity increment corresponding to ureters and kidneys (reaching up the renal pelvis more markedly on the left, III scintigraphic degree on the *left* and II scintigraphic degree on the *right*) (**d**)

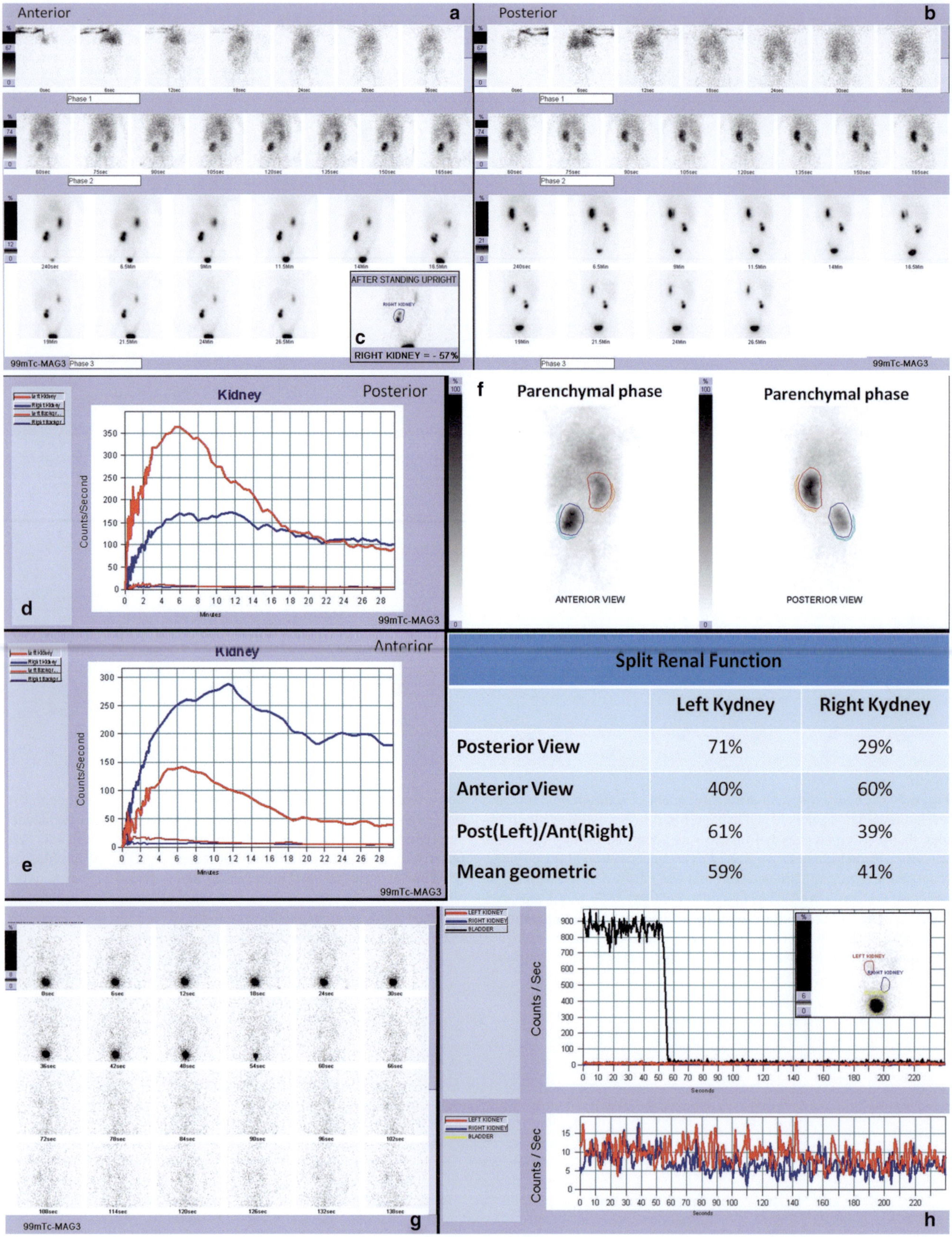
Anterior
a
Posterior
b
Phase 1
Phase 2
Phase 3
AFTER STANDING UPRIGHT
RIGHT KIDNEY
c
RIGHT KIDNEY = - 57%
99mTc-MAG3
Kidney
Posterior
Counts/Second
Minutes
d
f
Parenchymal phase
ANTERIOR VIEW
POSTERIOR VIEW
Kidney
Anterior
e
Split Renal Function
Left Kydney
Right Kydney
Posterior View 71% 29%
Anterior View 40% 60%
Post(Left)/Ant(Right) 61% 39%
Mean geometric 59% 41%
LEFT KIDNEY
RIGHT KIDNEY
BLADDER
Counts / Sec
Seconds
g
h

Fig. 6.10 (**a**–**c**) The imaging was performed posteriorly and anteriorly, in the supine position, by a double-head gamma camera. Left kidney was located in its own side and therefore was analyzed in posterior projection. By visually evaluating, dynamic images showed an intense concentration of tracer in the renal parenchyma and a rapid washout from the kidney. Right kidney was confirmed in lumbar ectopia with smaller size and slightly irregular morphology. By qualitative evaluation of images in anterior view, tracer uptake was slightly reduced, and transit was mildly prolonged with a moderately slow elimination of tracer from the kidneys (**a**). Left renogram curve in the posterior view showed normal slope of parenchymal phase and regular elimination of tracer from the kidneys. Right renogram curve in the anterior projection showed mildly reduced slope of parenchymal phase, slightly prolonged transits, and slow urinary excretion (**d**). The split renal function should be calculated, considering the different distance of each kidney from the detectors to avoid errors that may lead to inadequate assessment of renal function. As we reported in (**f**), measurement of split renal function can be extremely variable according to the considered projection. Measurement of relative renal function exclusively performed in the posterior view leads to a significant underestimation of ectopic split renal function. Measurement of relative renal function is accurate if performed in posterior view for the normal positioned kidney and in anterior projection for the ectopic kidney. Split renal function calculated by geometric mean is a precise method too. (**g**, **h**) After a full resolution of residual urine stasis, IRC was performed showing a complete bladder voiding in the absence of VUR (**g**). Time-activity curves of bladder and kidneys confirmed a regular and complete bladder voiding without radioactivity increment corresponding to the kidneys and ureters (**h**)

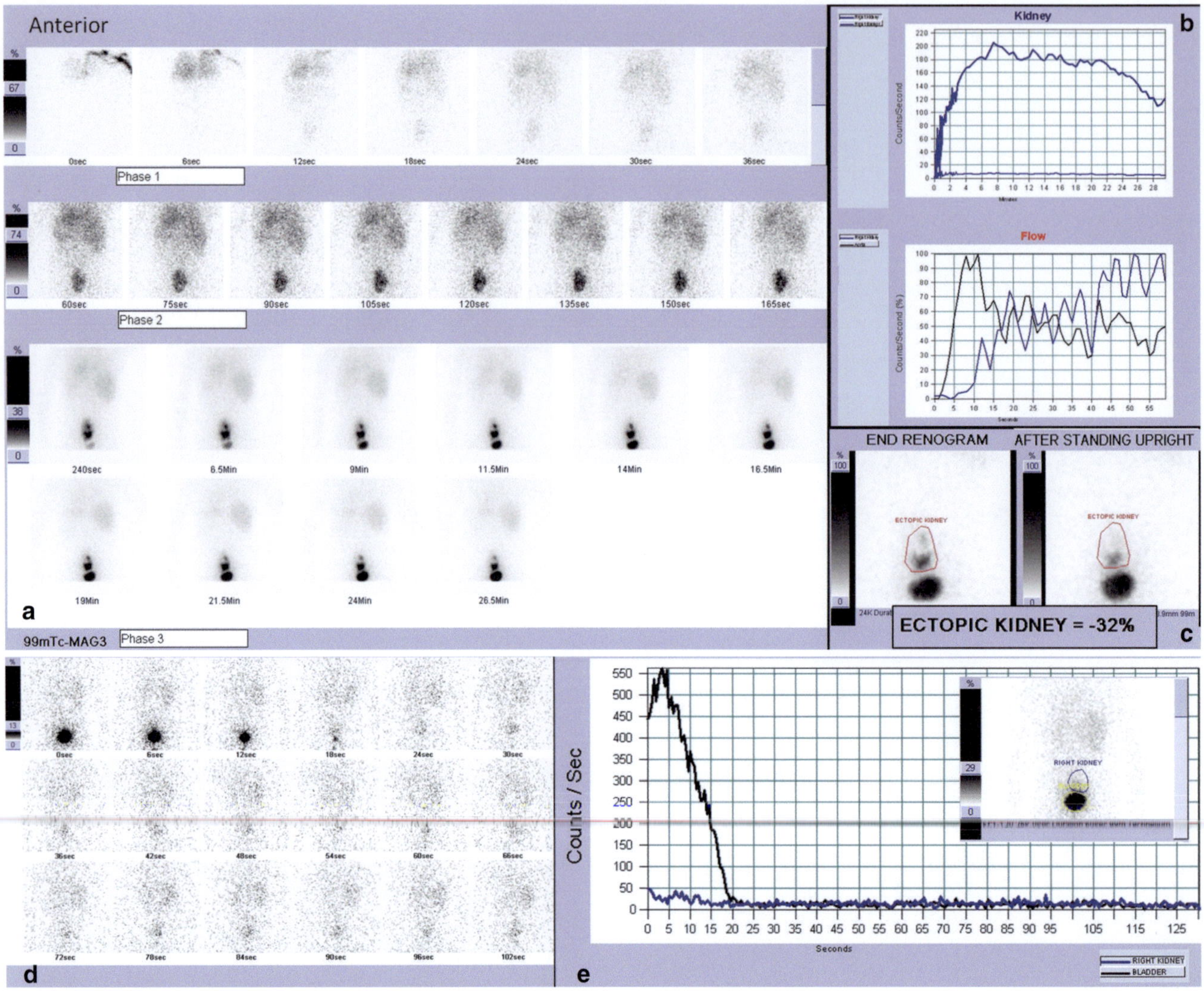

Fig. 6.11 (**a–c**) The imaging was performed anteriorly including the pelvic area within the field of view of the camera (extremely important in case of pelvic kidney). By simple visual observation of the parenchymal phase, a single kidney in the pelvic region was observed. Renal uptake of the tracer was preserved, and intraparenchymal distribution was inhomogeneous due to an area devoid of tracer corresponding to the medial renal side (as for calyces and pelvis dilatation). Urinary excretion was delayed and was slow, with the evidence of radiotracer stasis, which tended to resolve itself during basal study (**a**) and to further improve after orthostatism. (**c**). Renogram curve showed preserved slope of parenchymal phase and slow elimination of tracer from the kidney. Renogram curve showed preserved slope of parenchymal phase, prolonged transit, and slow urinary excretion. (**b**). IRC imaging showed a complete bladder voiding without any radioactivity increment in supravesical region, corresponding to the kidney side (**d**). Time-activity curves of the bladder and kidney confirmed qualitative IRC evaluation (**e**)

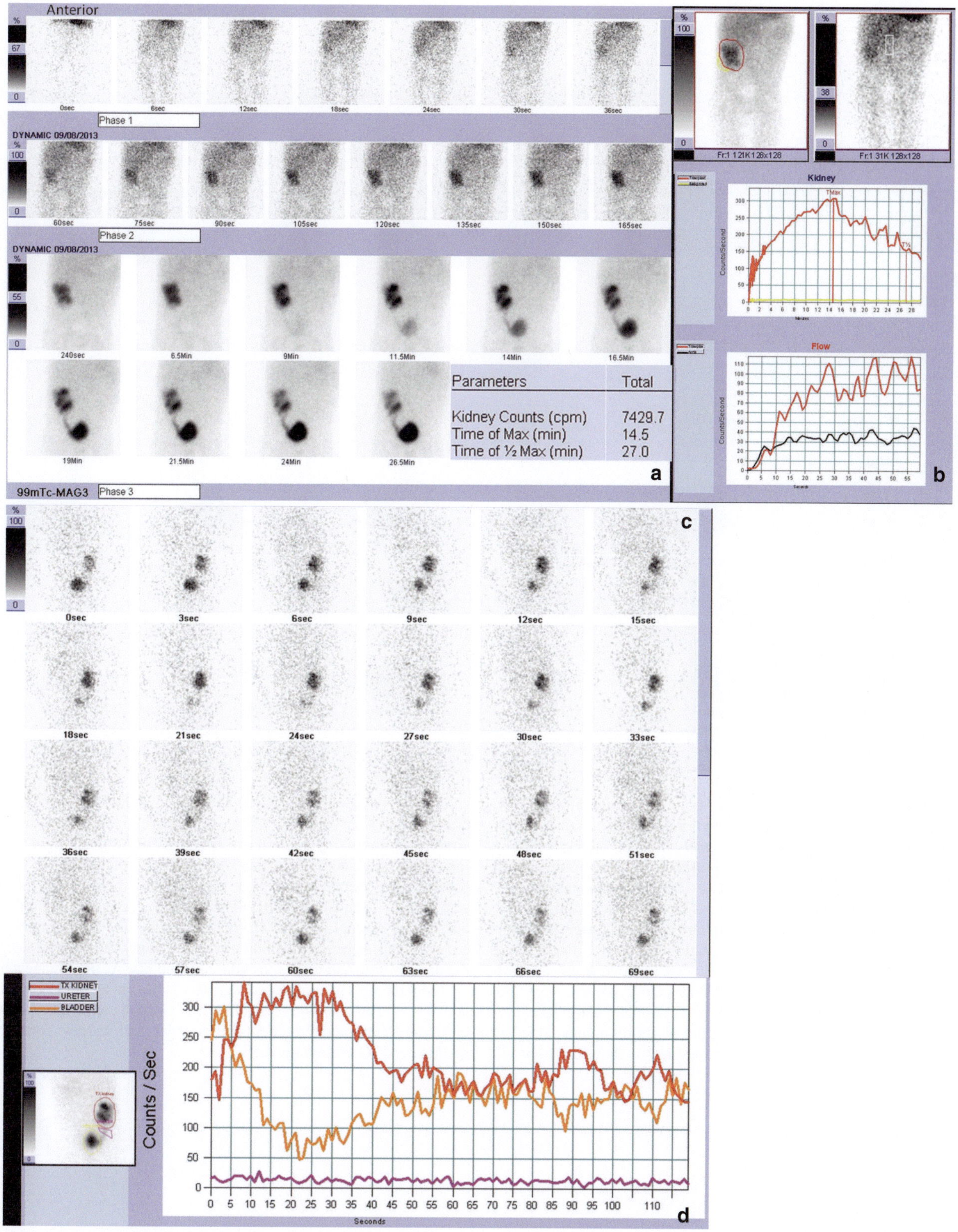

Fig. 6.12 The imaging was performed anteriorly including the pelvic area within the field of view of the camera. By simple visual observation of the parenchymal phase, a single kidney in the pelvic region was observed. Transplanted kidney showed moderately reduced uptake of the tracer (with slight increased background activity) and inhomogeneous intraparenchymal distribution due to cortical focal defects. Urinary excretion was delayed and was slow, with evidence of radiotracer stasis corresponding to pelvis and ureter, which tended to resolve itself during basal study (**a**). Renogram curve showed moderately reduced slope of parenchymal phase, prolonged transit, and slow urinary excretion. (**b**). IRC imaging showed a quite complete bladder voiding with high radioactivity increment corresponding to the transplanted kidney (**c**). Time-activity curves of bladder and kidney confirmed qualitative IRC evaluation (**d**)

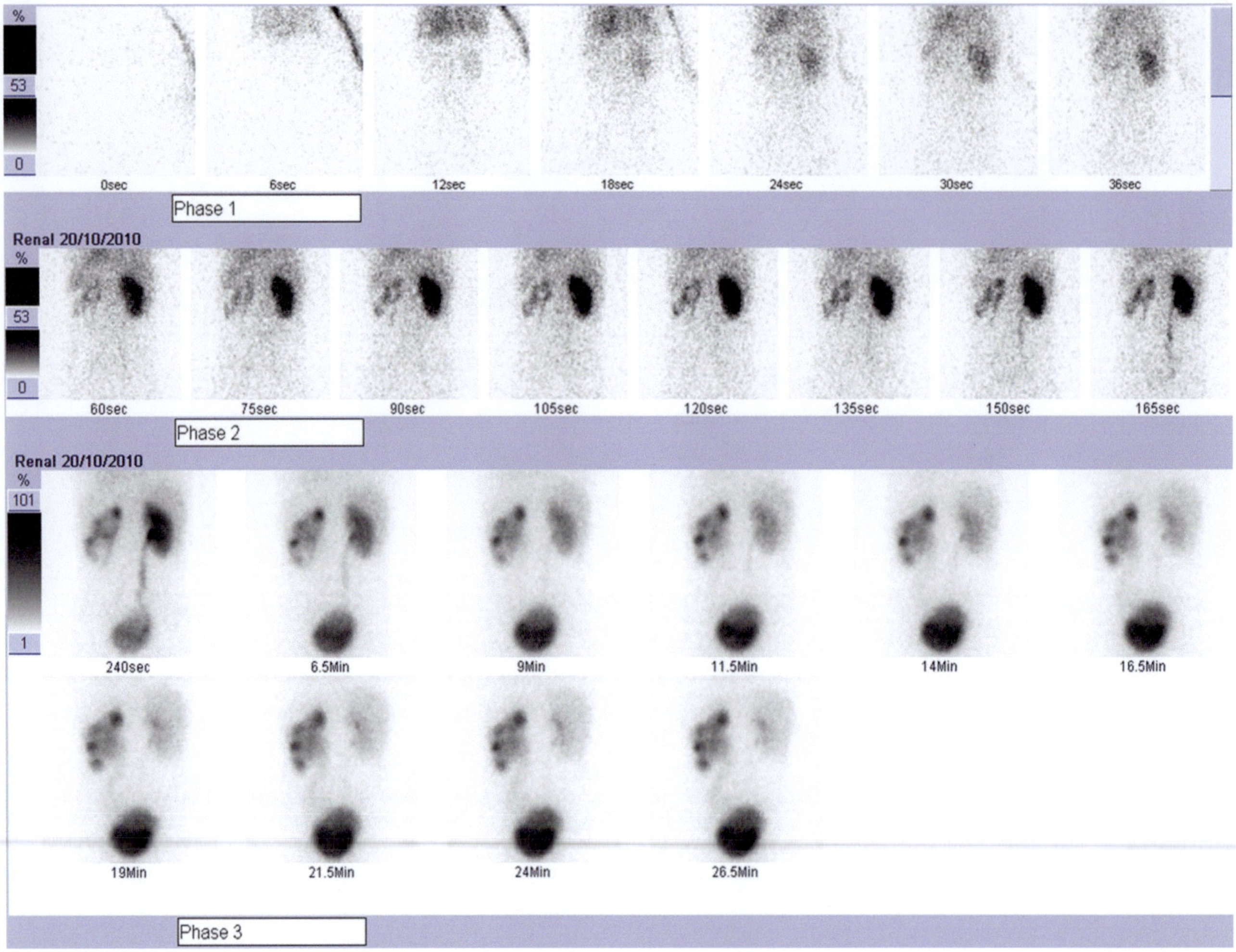

Fig. 6.13 (**a**–**c**) By qualitative assessment of scintigraphic images, both kidneys were located in their own proper sides with synchronous but asymmetrical perfusion (severely reduced on the *left side*). Left kidney was small with irregular morphology. Radiotracer uptake was poor, and tracer distribution was markedly inhomogeneous due to photodeficient area (depending on calyces dilatation) and multiple focal cortical defects. Urinary pelvis and ureter drainage was slow with persistent radioactivity after standing upright. Right renal uptake was intense, tracer distribution was homogeneous, and urinary drainage was normal (**a-c**). Left renogram curve had very little width, showing markedly reduced slope of parenchymal phase, prolonged transits, and low urinary excretion. Right renogram curve had normal shape of all phases. The basic renogram showed a poor left split renal functions (**b**). (**d**–**g**) Diuretic dynamic images (**d**) and diuretic renogram (**e**) show very slow response to furosemide without significant improving in drainage in left kidney after upright standing. Ureter T/A curves showed "rising curve" of left ureter during basal dynamic renal scan without significant washout during diuretic scintigraphy (persisting a slight radioactivity increment). Right ureter showed normal pattern (**f**). (**h**, **i**) Radionuclide cystography was not achieved, because the child could not empty the bladder despite the urinary urge and numerous voiding attempts. At IRC images, hindered by the presence of residual urinary stasis, no evidence of radioactivity increment corresponding to kidneys and ureters was observed. Time-activity curves of bladder and kidney confirmed qualitative IRC evaluation (**h**)

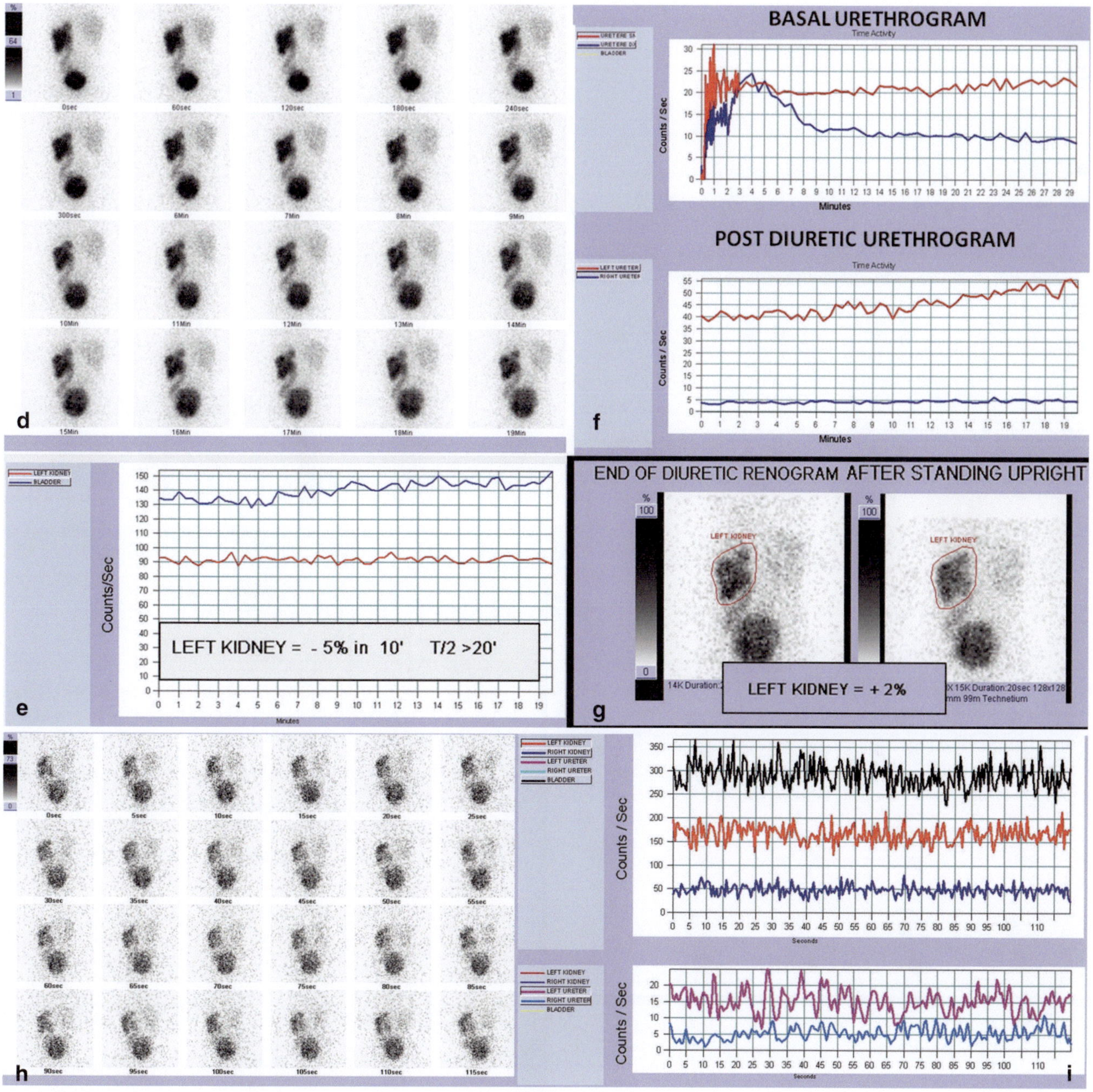

Fig. 6.13 (continued)

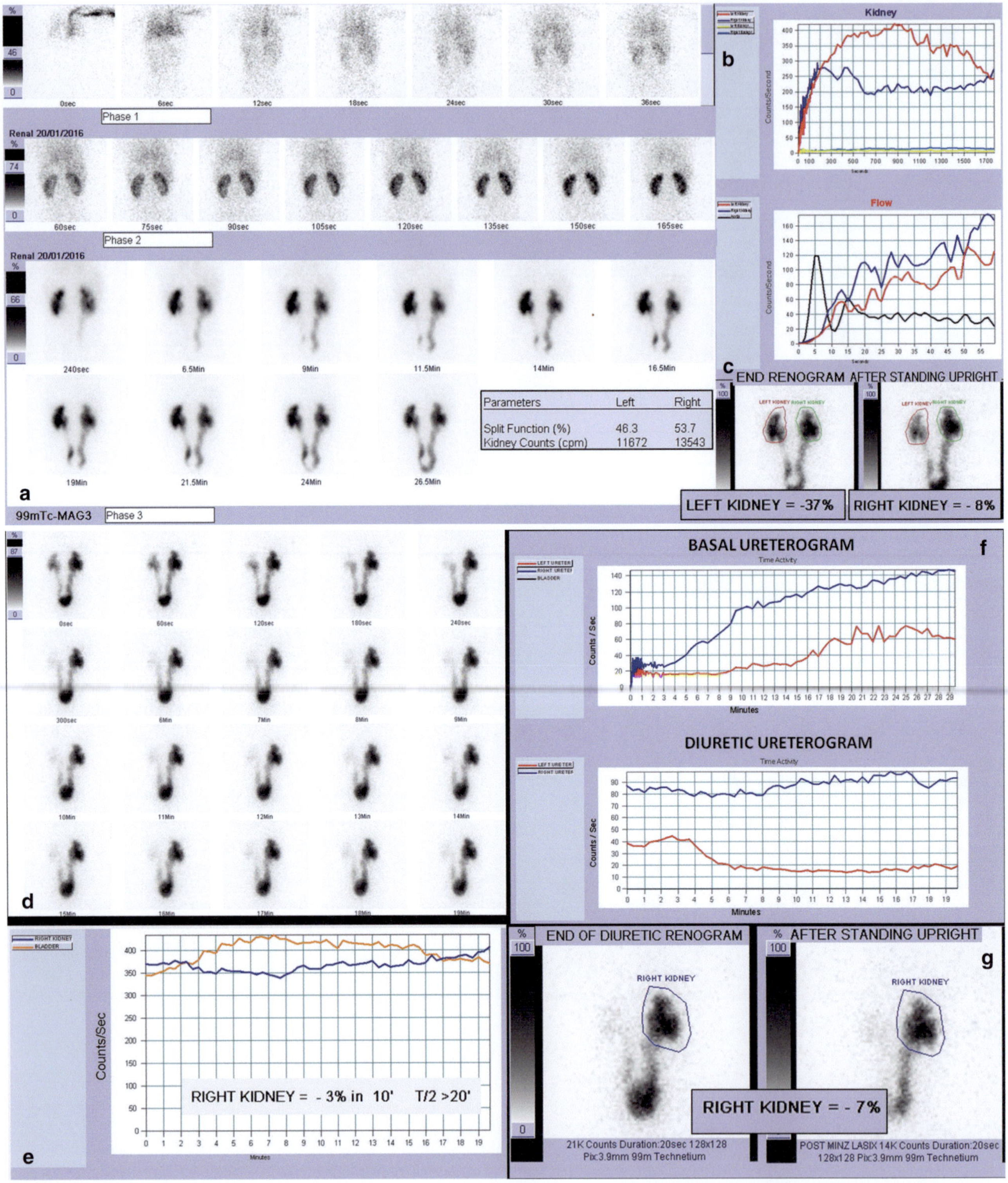

Fig. 6.14 (**a–c**) MAG3 dynamic renal scan showed normal function of both kidneys and bilateral impaired urinary drainage (worst on the *right side*); persistent radioactivity stasis was also detected in both dilated ureters (**a**). After gravity-assisted drainage-1 test, there was improved drainage in left kidney but no significant improvement in the right one (**c**). Both renogram curves showed normal slope of parenchymal phase, prolonged transit, and low urinary excretion. The basic renogram showed symmetric split renal functions (**d**). Diuretic dynamic study (images and time/activity curves) showed complete resolution of left ureter stasis and very slow response to furosemide of right kidney without significant improvement in ureter drainage too (**d, e**). Ureter T/A curves (**f**) showed: normal pattern of left ureter and "rising curve" of right ureter during dynamic renal scan; no significant washout was detected during diuretic scintigraphy in the right ureter

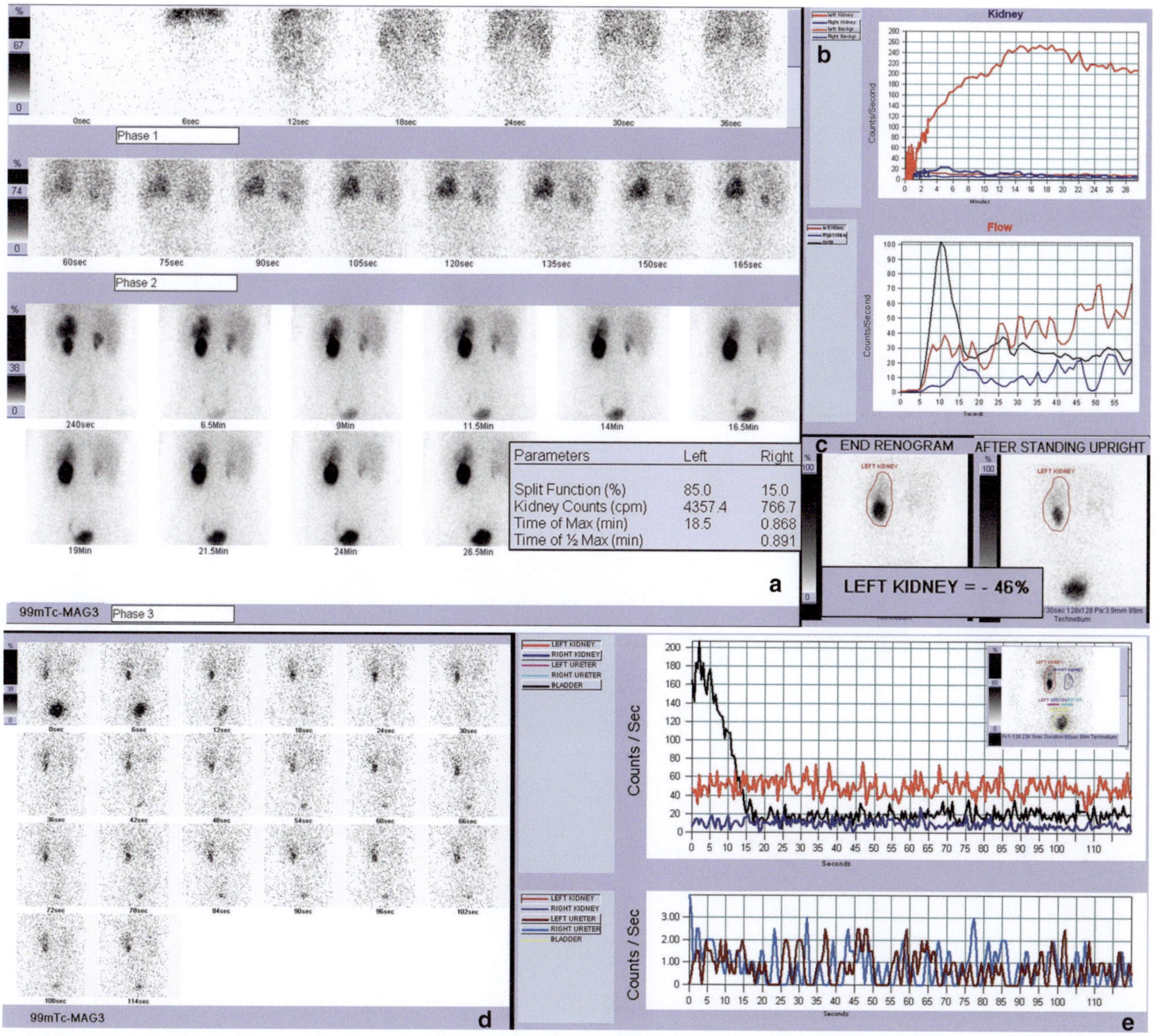

Fig. 6.15 (**a–c**) MAG3 renal scan showed left kidney with increased size and irregular morphology. Tracer distribution was markedly inhomogeneous with limited uptake in the upper renal third and a wide area devoid of tracer in the middle and inferior renal third (corresponding to ultrasonography-detected dilatation). On the left, urinary excretion was delayed and was slow, with the evidence of an intense radiotracer stasis in the middle-inferior renal third, which tends to resolve itself and to further improve after upright standing. Right kidney was small with an irregular morphology; right renal uptake was reduced, and tracer distribution was inhomogeneous due to multiple focal cortical defects. Radiotracer transit was prolonged, and urinary excretion was sufficiently rapid (**a**). Left renogram curve showed mildly reduced slope of parenchymal phase, and elimination of tracer from the kidney was delayed and slow. Right renogram curve had very little width showing markedly reduced slope of parenchymal phase, prolonged transits, and quite rapid urinary excretion. The basic renogram showed a poor right split renal function (**b**). (**d, e**) When the child has voiding stimulus, it is not possible waiting for a complete urine stasis resolution. In this technical condition, avoiding patient movement is crucial to not have artifactual increment and decrement of renal activity. IRC images showed a complete bladder voiding in the absence of VUR. In fact, considering the first IRC frame, a mild residual stasis was observed in the left pelvis without increment during bladder emptying (**d**). Time-activity curves of bladder and kidneys confirmed a regular and complete bladder voiding without radioactivity increment corresponding to the kidneys and ureters (**e**)

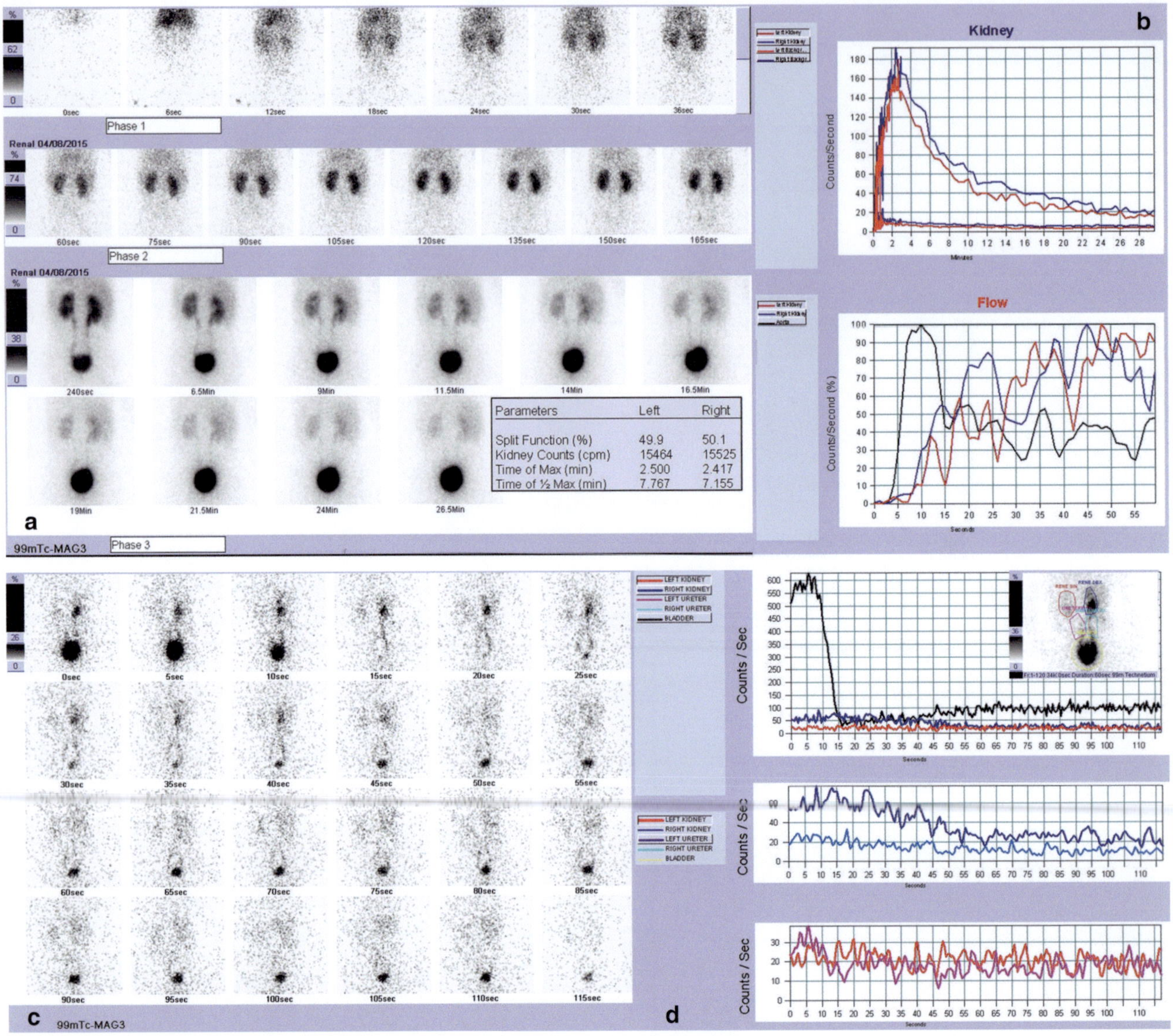

Fig. 6.16 (**a**, **b**) The qualitative analysis of basic dynamic study revealed a bilateral intense concentration of tracer in the renal parenchyma (in upper and lower systems) and a rapid washout from both the kidneys (**a**). Renogram curves confirmed the qualitative interpretation of the study, showing a normal tracer uptake in both kidneys, a bilateral regular transit with a rapid urinary excretion; the basic renogram also provides a symmetrical measurement of relative renal function (**b**). (**c**, **d**) In these clinical cases, IRC images showed a complete bladder voiding with a slight radioactivity increment corresponding to the left ureter. In the first IRC frame, a urinary stasis was observed on the *right side* with just a mild radioactivity increment in the upper part during bladder voiding; afterward, a progressive decrement was detected after bladder emptying. The first IRC image, however, must be compared to the last frame of basal dynamic study, revealing a high-grade passive reflux in the lower right system (**c**). By time-activity curves (of bladder and kidneys) evaluation, a regular and complete bladder voiding was confirmed with evidence of low-grade radioactivity increment corresponding to the left ureter and right kidney (**d**). Interpretation of IRC images must include a careful comparative evaluation of basal dynamic study, especially when residual tracer stasis in the renal collecting system was present.

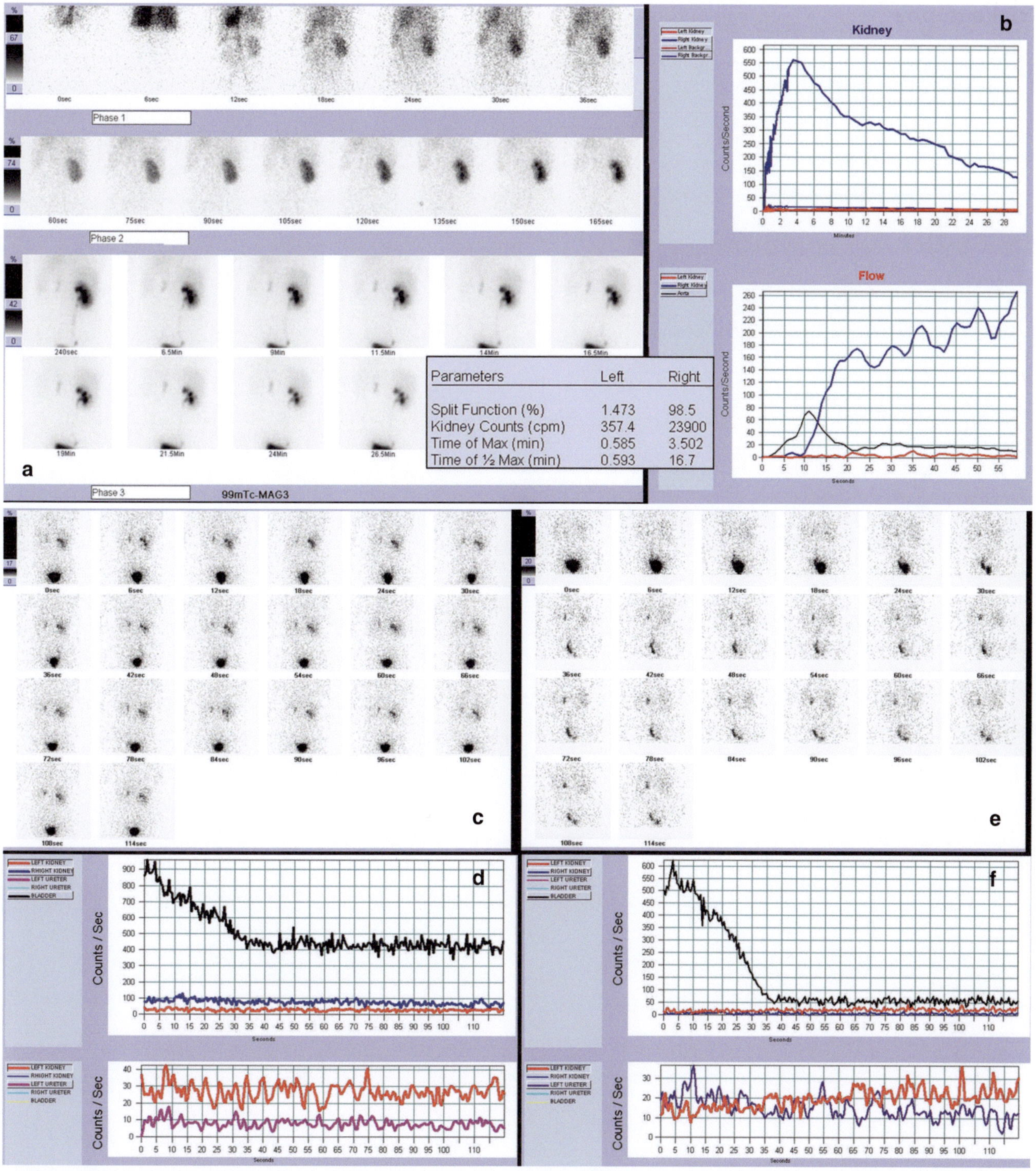

Fig. 6.17 (**a**, **b**) The qualitative analysis of basic dynamic study revealed a small left kidney with severely impaired blood flow, poor tracer uptake, and delayed intrarenal transit. Right kidney showed normal morphology, an intense concentration of tracer in the renal parenchyma, and a mildly slow urinary excretion (**a**). The pattern of the left renogram curve was flat. Right renogram curve showed normal slope of parenchymal phase, and elimination of tracer from the kidney was mildly slow. The basic renogram showed an extremely poor left split renal function (**b**). (**c**, **d**) IRC images showed an incomplete bladder voiding (about 50 % of postvoiding residual radioactivity in bladder) without significant activity in increment corresponding to the kidneys and ureters. In these technical conditions, IRC study has a low sensibility of VUR detection, and other bladder-emptying attempts are mandatory. (**e**, **f**) A second bladder-emptying attempt was performed after oral hydration to obtain a good bladder refill. The first IRC frame showed a bilateral complete resolution of tracer stasis in the renal collecting system, and a complete bladder voiding was achieved. In these proper technical conditions, an exiguous VUR was detected on the *left side* (**e**) and confirmed by time-activity curves (**f**)

Bibliography

1. Gordon I, Colarinha P, et al. Guidelines for indirect radionuclide cystography. Eur J Nucl Med. 2001;28(3):BP16–20.

Nephrourology: Nephrological Problems

7

Maria Felicia Villani, Milena Pizzoferro, Giacomo Di Zazzo, Domenico Barbuti, and Maria Carmen Garganese

7.1 Teaching Cases

In this chapter are reported several teaching cases in which scintigraphic evaluation was helpful in clinical assessment of nephrological disease and its complications.

7.1.1 Case 7.1 DMSA Scan in Differential Diagnosis Between Renal Hypoplasia and Renal Hypodysplasia

In patients with ultrasonographic finding of "small" kidney, DMSA scan allows to differentiate renal hypoplasia from renal hypodysplasia. In the presence of renal functional impairment, renal scan assesses the severity of impairment, selecting patients eligible for nephrectomy.

7.1.2 Case 7.2 DMSA Scan in Case of Ultrasonographic Finding of Multiple Hypoechoic Round Areas

In patients with ultrasonographic finding of multiple hypoechoic round areas, DMSA scan allows to confirm diagnosis of multicystic kidney, to differentiate multicystic from polycystic kidney, and to assess renal function in severe hydronephrosis eligible for surgery.

7.1.3 Case 7.3 Functional and Drainage Assessment in Tuberous Sclerosis Syndrome with Hydronephrosis

A 3-year-old girl with tuberous sclerosis (TSC2/PKD1 contiguous gene syndrome). She has hamartomatous lesions in various organs (including brain, skin, heart, eyes, and kidney) with a typical phenotype of TSC and early-onset renal polycystic disease. She also had a prenatal diagnosis of right hydronephrosis with progressive increase of pyelic dilatation (last US showed right renal pelvis diameter of 23.1 mm and left pelvis of 7.5 mm, respectively). Therefore, she underwent a dynamic renal scan, which showed severe hypofunction and poor drainage of right kidney. The girl then underwent right pyeloplasty and is actually on clinical ultrasonographic follow-up.

7.1.4 Case 7.4 Functional Assessment in Tuberous Sclerosis Syndrome with Pyelonephritis

A 14-year-old boy with tuberous sclerosis. He presented large angiomyolipomas, benign tumors consisting of fatty tissue associated with an elevated risk of bleeding when the diameter is over 4 cm. Therefore, several transcatheter-selective arterial embolizations were carried out electively since he was 11 years old. He presented a renal abscess, treated with antibiotic therapy, and 6 months later a DMSA renal scan was performed in order to assess renal function and to evaluate kidney damage.

M.F. Villani • M. Pizzoferro
Nuclear Medicine Unit, Imaging Departement – "Bambino Gesù" Children Hospital, Rome, Italy

G. Di Zazzo (✉)
Unit of Nephrolgy, "Bambino Gesù" Children Hospital, Rome, Italy
e-mail: giacomo.dizazzo@opbg.net

D. Barbuti
Imaging Department, "Bambino Gesù" Children Hospital, Rome, Italy

M.C. Garganese (✉)
Diagnostic Imaging Department of Nuclear Medicine, IRCCS Bambino Gesù Paediatric Hospital, Rome, Italy
e-mail: mcarmen.garganese@opbg.net

© Springer International Publishing Switzerland 2017

M.C. Garganese, G.F.L. D'Errico (eds.), *Conventional Nuclear Medicine in Pediatrics*, DOI 10.1007/978-3-319-43181-9_7

7.1.5 Case 7.5 Chronic Renal Failure in a Child with Surgically Treated Neuroblastoma and Contralateral Duplex System

A 3-month-old baby with chronic renal failure, right duplex system, and previous left nephrectomy-adrenalectomy for neuroblastoma. A DMSA renal scan was performed in order to assess renal function, in a child with complicate clinical and therapeutic management.

7.1.6 Case 7.6 DMSA Scan in the Assessment of Kidney Damage Secondary to Ischemia

DMSA renal scan is helpful in the assessment of renal function and in the evaluation of kidney damage, secondary to renal ischemia; comparative evaluation of radiological and scintigraphic imaging is necessary to add functional data to anatomical imaging and to read scintigraphic imaging by anatomical backup.

7.1.7 Case 7.7 Metabolic Assessment of Skeletal Involvement in Primary Hyperoxaluria: Bone Scintigraphy Pattern

Type 1 primary hyperoxaluria is an autosomal recessive disorder due to the deficiency of glyoxylate aminotransferase; it is characterized by hyperoxaluria, calcium oxalate urinary lithiasis, nephrocalcinosis, and renal failure; oxalate precipitates in the skin, blood vessels, and bone.

The case of a 3-year-old baby, with type 1 primary hyperoxaluria, chronic renal failure in dialytic therapy, and liver transplantation, is reported.

7.1.8 Case 7.8 Functional Assessment in Newborn with Drug-Resistant Hypertension and Thrombosis of Multiple Arteries: Additional Value of SPECT-CT Fused Images

A 5-month-old baby refers to our Emergency for severe drug-resistant hypertension. She had multiple hospitalizations since her birth, and her medical history included thrombosis of multiple arteries (abdominal aorta, renal arteries, and celiac tripod), thrombophilia, left ventricular hypertrophy, left cerebral hemisphere ischemia, respiratory distress, and klebsiella infection.

Because of the presence of thrombosis of renal arteries, a renal hypertension is hypothesized and a therapeutic nephrectomy is considered. Therefore, a renal scintigraphy with ^{99m}Tc-DMSA is performed in order to evaluate functional assessment.

Static images of abdomen are acquired 3 h after radiotracer injection. Single photon emission computed tomography (SPECT) images are also obtained and manually fused with computed tomography (CT) (Fig. 7.1, 7.2, 7.3, 7.4, 7.5, 7.6, 7.7, and 7.8).

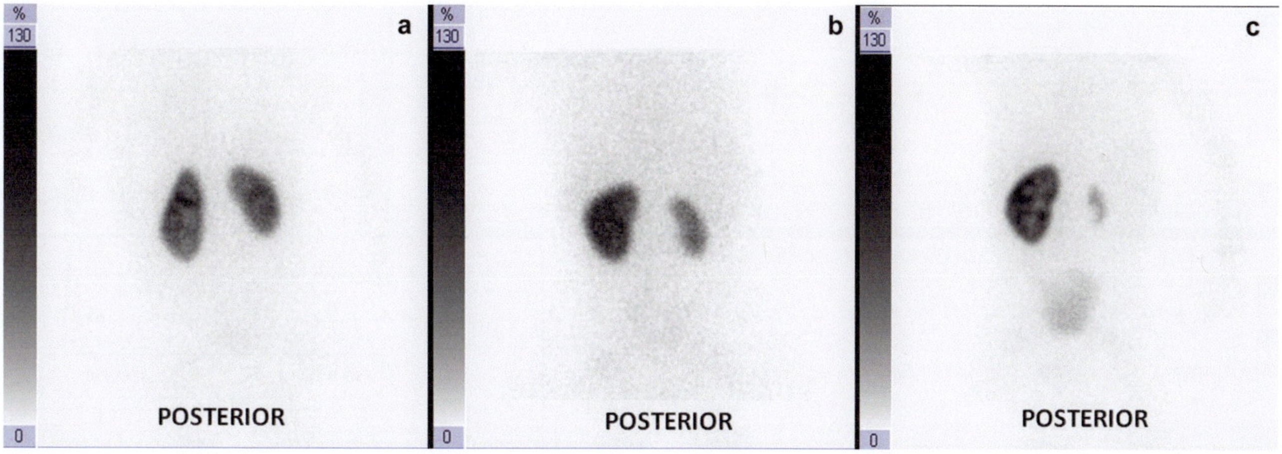

Fig. 7.1 In the DMSA renal scan, posterior view, are displayed three patients with normal *left kidney* and ultrasonographic finding of small *right kidney*: (**a**) *right kidney* is smaller than the other one, but shows good and homogeneous uptake of radiotracer without evidence of cortical defect; *right kidney* DRF is 39 %, as seen in hypoplastic kidneys; (**b**) *right kidney* is smaller than the other one, with moderate-severe reduction of radiotracer uptake (*right kidney* DRF: 21 %, "moderate-severe hypodysplasia"); (**c**) *right kidney* is markedly smaller than the other one, with severe reduction of the radiotracer uptake (*right kidney* DRF: 5 %, "severe hypodysplasia")

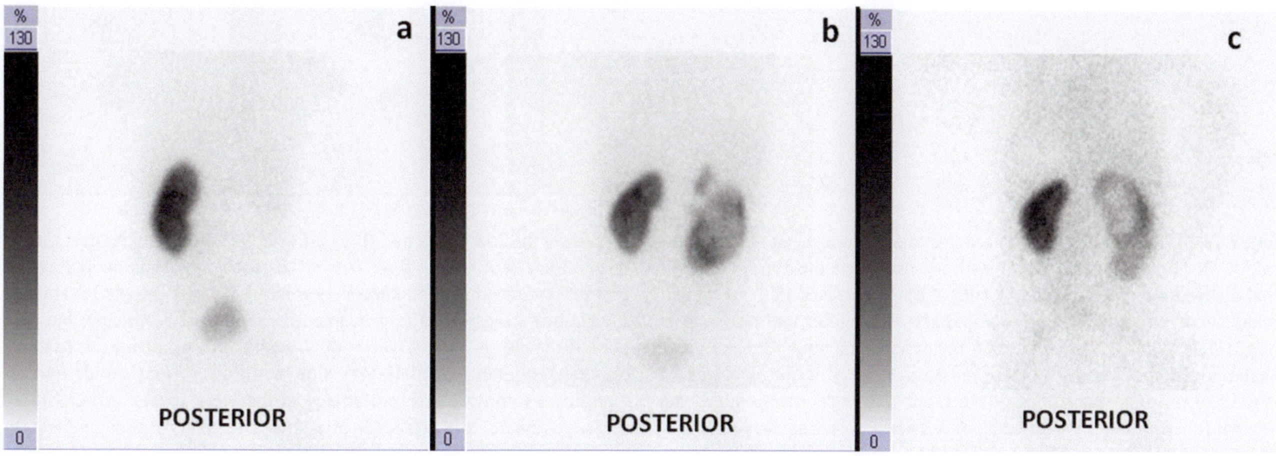

Fig. 7.2 In the DMSA renal scan, posterior view, are displayed three patients with normal *left kidney* and ultrasonographic finding of multiple hypoechoic round areas in right kidney: (**a**) DMSA renal scan in a 8-month-old boy with prenatal diagnosis of multicystic kidney: there is no visualization of *right kidney* (multicystic dysplastic kidney is not able to uptake radiotracer, because there is no functioning parenchyma); (**b**) DMSA renal scan in a 3-year-old boy with prenatal diagnosis of renal cystic dysplasia: *right kidney* is larger than the other one and shows irregular shape, with nonhomogenous intraparenchymal radiotracer distribution and multiple focal areas of reduced uptake, especially in the upper pole, associated with cortical defects, related to the presence of cystic lesions (polycystic dysplasia); (**c**) DMSA renal scan, in a 5-year-old boy with severe hydronephrosis: *right kidney* is larger than the other one, with irregular shape; moderate reduction of radiotracer uptake is evident associated with multiple areas devoid of tracer corresponding to dilated collecting system, surrounded by thin parenchyma without cortical defects (right DRF: 35 %). DMSA renal scan is considered the gold standard for split renal function assessment, even if MAG3 renal scan allows an analog split function evaluation and adds definition of urinary drainage, useful in follow-up after surgery

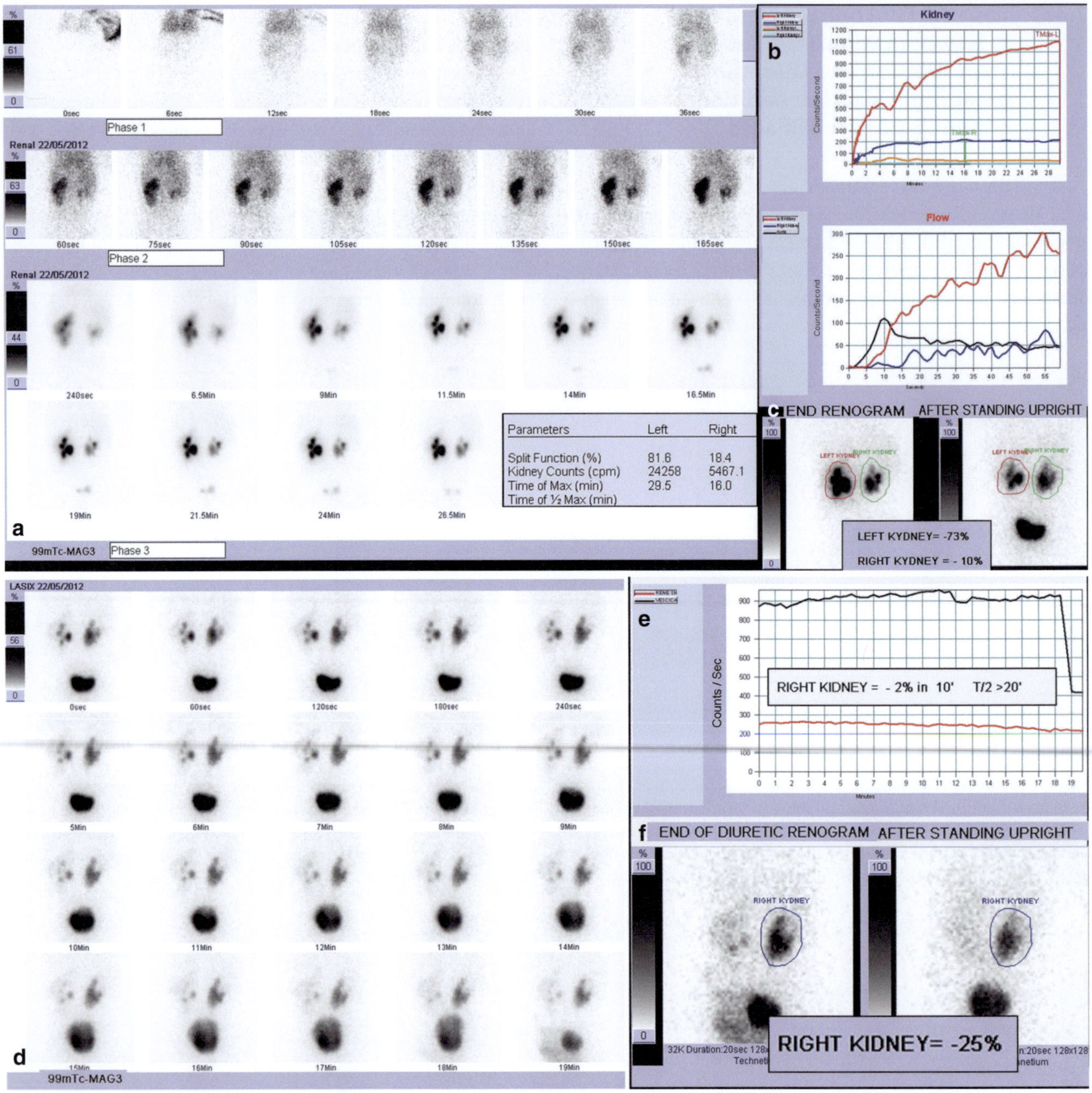

Fig. 7.3 MAG3 dynamic renal scan: dynamic images (**a**) show good radiotracer uptake in *left kidney* with nonhomogeneous intraparenchymal distribution due to an area devoid of tracer corresponding to dilated renal pelvis and collecting system; shape is irregular and drainage is poor; *right kidney* is smaller than the other one, with very irregular shape, severe reduction of uptake, and poor drainage; radiotracer uptake is evident only in lower third of the kidney. (**b**) *Left renogram* shows normal function but poor drainage of *left kidney* ("rising curve"); *right renogram* has low width and shows severe hypofunction of *right kidney* with impaired drainage; flow T/A curves show synchronous but asymmetrical (reduced in *right kidney*) perfusion. Gravity-assisted drainage-1 test shows significant improvement in *left kidney* drainage, but still poor drainage of *right kidney* (**c**). Diuretic dynamic images (**d**) and diuretic renogram (**e**) show very slow response to furosemide and no significant improvement in drainage in the *right kidney. Right kidney* drainage remains still poor even after gravity-assisted drainage-2 test (**f**)

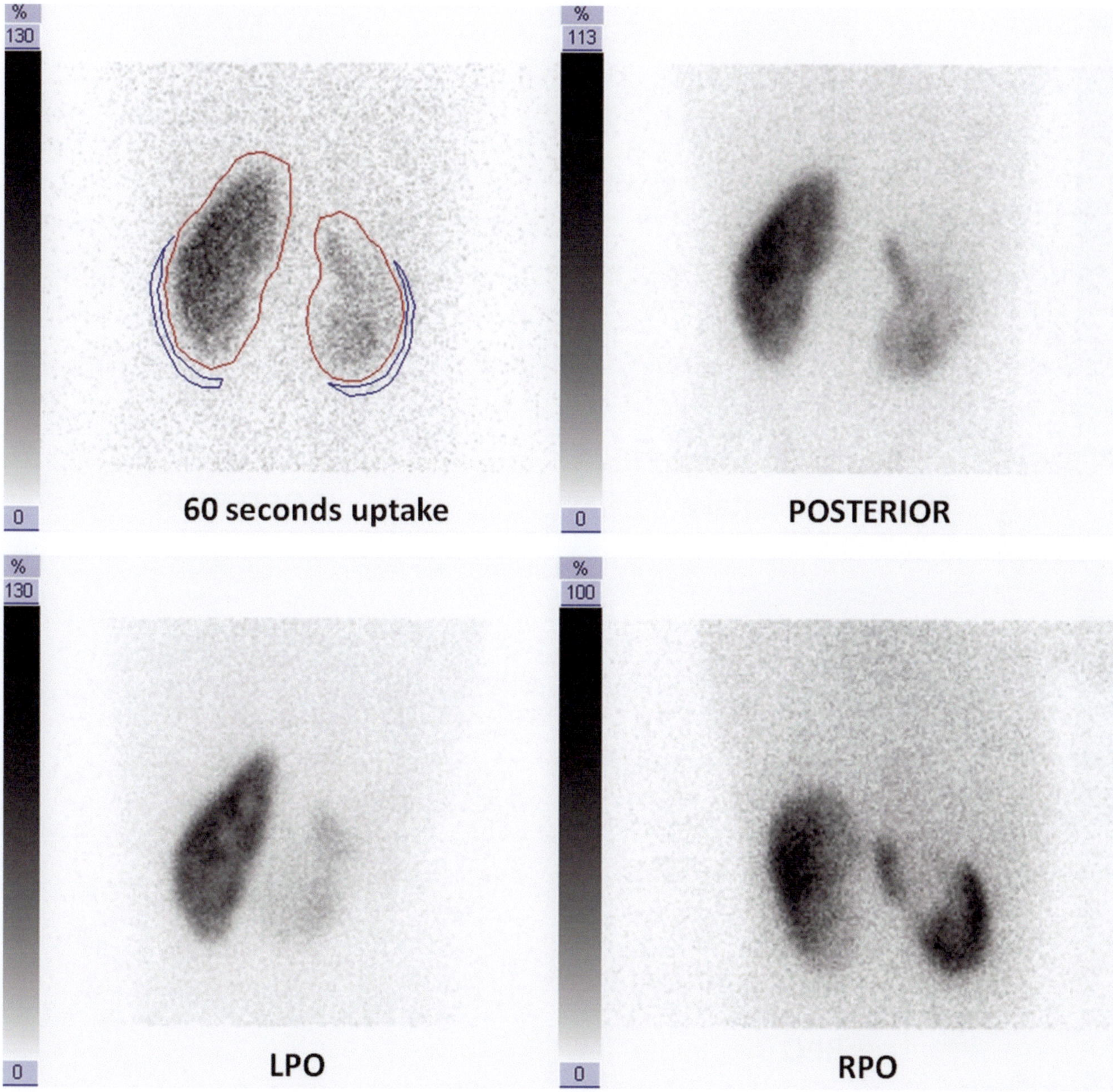

Fig. 7.4 DMSA renal scan (60 s uptake image, posterior view, LPO view, and RPO view): *left kidney* shows good uptake of radiotracer, with homogeneous intraparenchymal distribution; *right kidney* is smaller than *left* one, with irregular shape; radiotracer uptake is good in *lower third* of the kidney, but very much reduced in the *upper and middle two-thirds*, with cortical defects

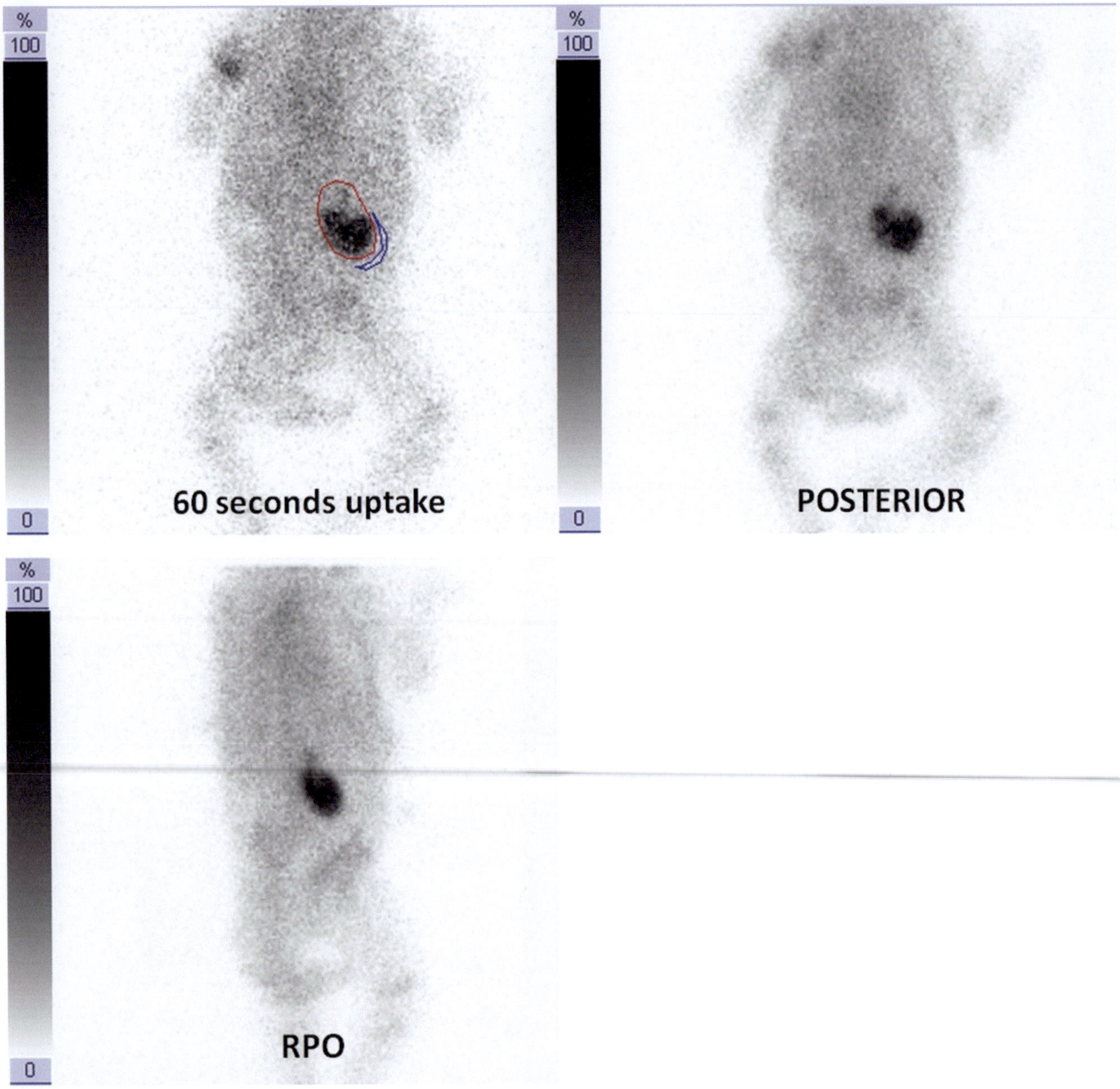

Fig. 7.5 DMSA renal scan (60 s uptake image, posterior view and RPO view): there is no visualization of *left kidney* (previous nephrectomy); *right kidney* shows global reduction of radiotracer uptake and evidence of a large hypoactive area with cortical defect in the upper system. A very low target/background ratio is also evident

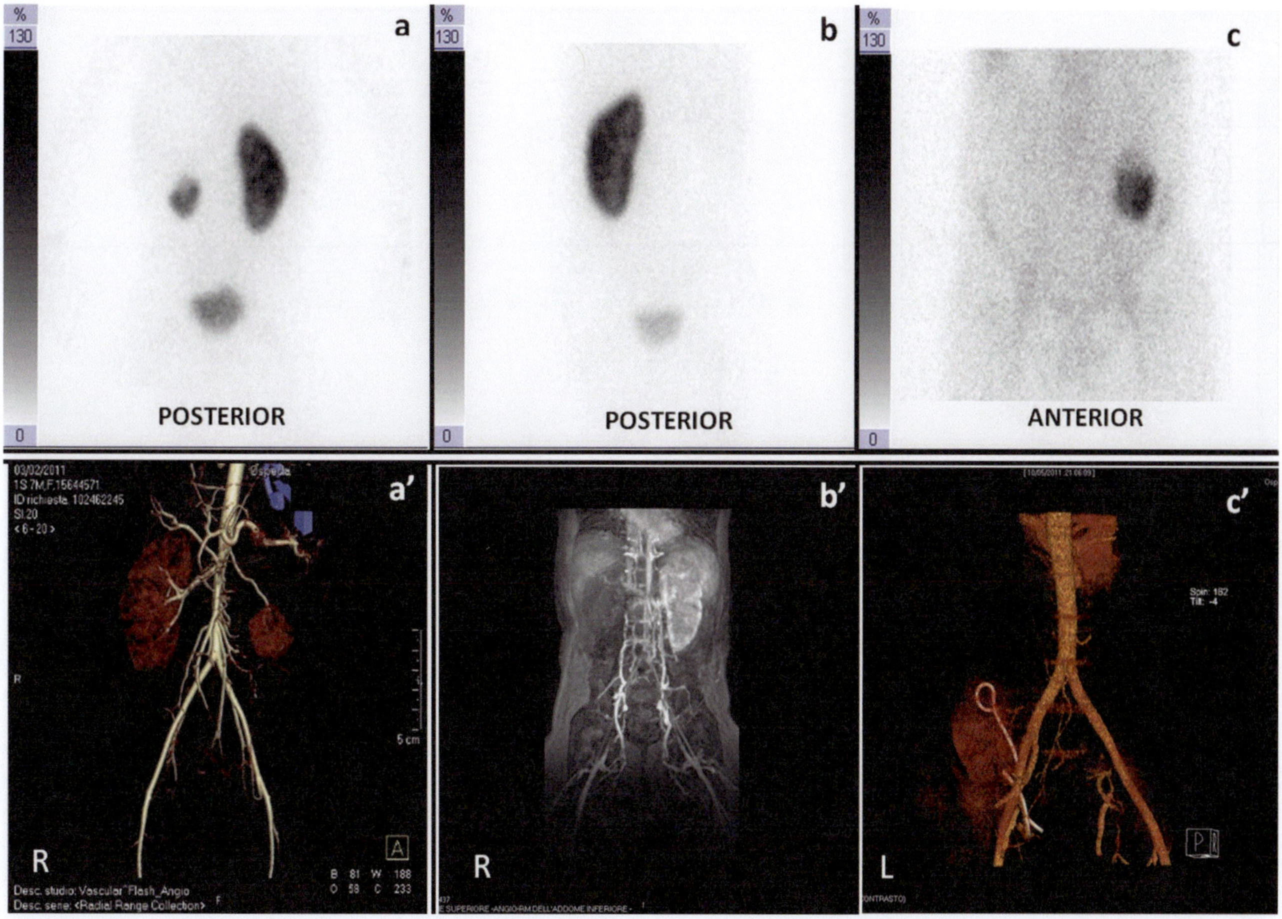

Fig. 7.6 *Thrombosed aneurysm of upper pole left renal artery, surgically treated,* in an 18 month-old infant with hypertension DMSA renal scan, posterior view. (**a**) *Left kidney* is very small, with evidence of radiotracer uptake only in *lower third*, but not in *upper and middle two-thirds* (previous infarction); *right kidney* shows good uptake of radiotracer with homogeneous intraparenchymal distribution and no evidence of scars. Computed tomography angiography. (**a'**) *Left kidney* presents reduced volume, showing parenchymal hypoperfusion in upper and middle portions. *Perinatal right renal artery thrombosis* in a 9-year-old girl with congenital thrombophilia (antithrombin III deficit) and right renal artery thrombosis: DMSA renal scan, posterior view. (**b**) *Left kidney* shows good uptake of radiotracer, with homogeneous intraparenchymal distribution; no visualization of *right kidney*. Magnetic resonance angiography. (**b'**) No evidence of gadolinium enhancement in *right kidney*, due to known right renal artery thrombosis. *Renal infarction* in a 14-year-old boy who underwent *renal transplantation*, complicated by renal arterial stenosis. DMSA renal scan, anterior view. (**c**) Transplanted kidney is located in the *left* iliac fossa; it is small and shows global reduction of radiotracer uptake; intraparenchymal distribution is not homogeneous, and two hypoactive areas with cortical defects are evident: the larger one in the *upper pole* and a small focal one in the *lower pole*, respectively (renal infarction). A very low target/background ratio is also evident. Computed tomography angiography (**c'**) shows reduced renal parenchymography with nonhomogeneous enhancement in the *upper* and *lower poles*.

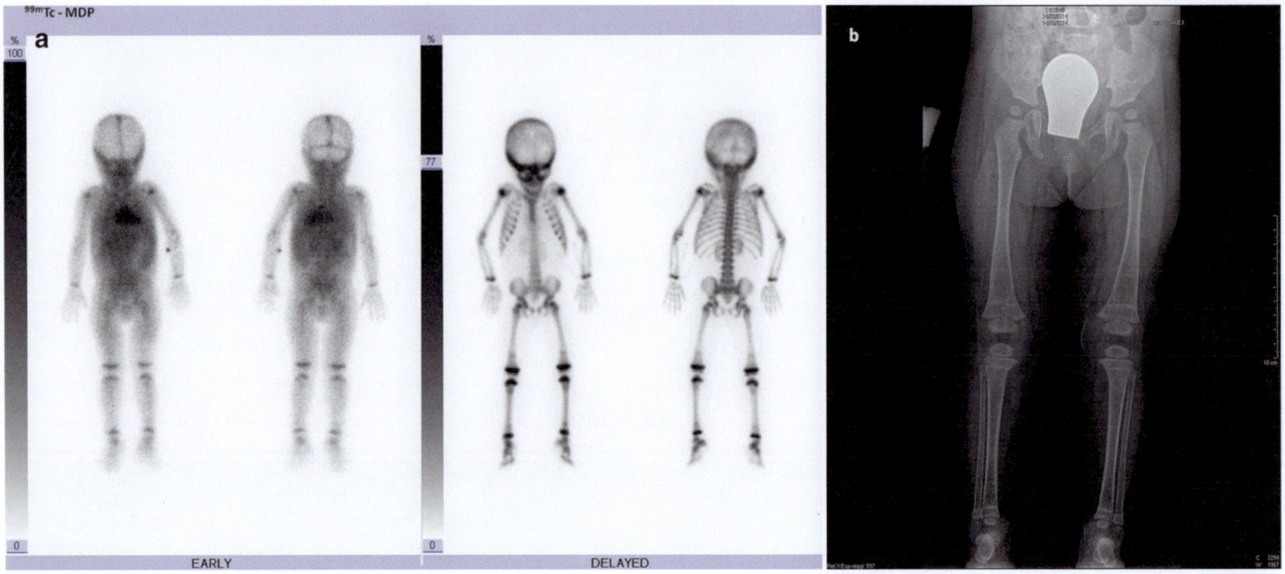

Fig. 7.7 (**a**) Bone scan, early phase (*left image*): no pathological radiotracer uptake in soft tissue in whole body blood pool image. Bone scan, delayed phase (*right image*): delimited and linear radiotracer uptake, symmetrically located in distal metadiaphyses of both femurs and in proximal and distal metadiaphyses of both tibiae. These characteristic findings are typical features of scintigraphic pattern of skeletal involvement in primary hyperoxaluria; corresponding radiological images are reported in (**b**) showing typical skeletal changes of oxalosis characterized by marked translucent metaphyseal bands with sclerotic margins in lower limbs

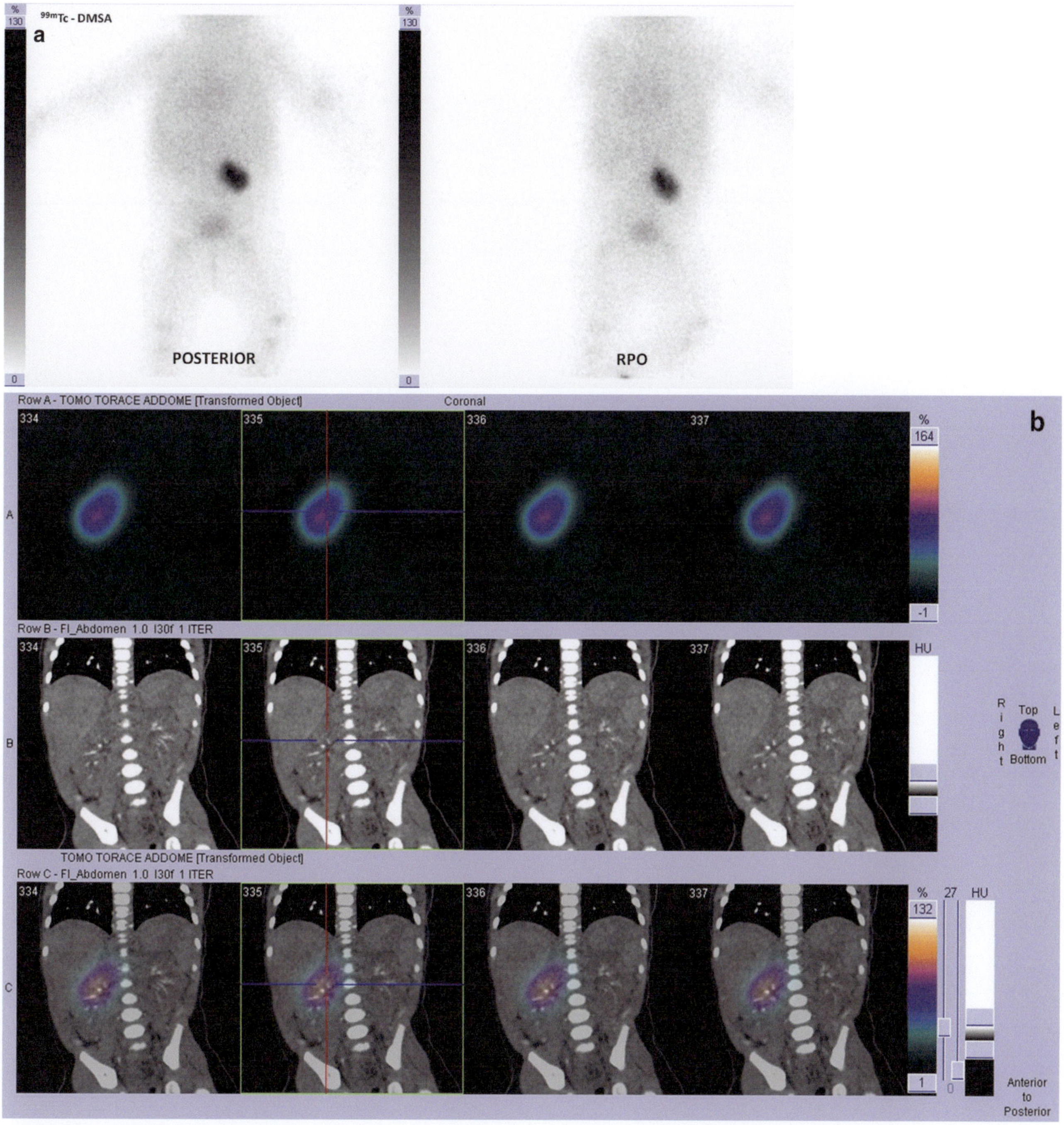

Fig. 7.8 (**a**) Static images show absence of radiotracer uptake in *left* renal lodge and uptake in *right* kidney. Only SPECT-CT images (**b**) allow to better define which portion of *right* kidney is actually functioning, that is, the upper half of the kidney. In this case, SPECT images and in particular SPECT-CT fused images are essential to detect renal functioning parenchyma. Planar images alone, in fact, did not allow a correct identification of kidneys for the lack of morphological definition of scintigraphic images, especially in abdomen of small size

8 Nephrourology: Urinary Tract Infections

Maria Felicia Villani, Milena Pizzoferro, Giacomo Di Zazzo, and Maria Carmen Garganese

8.1 Static Renal Scintigraphy

8.1.1 Study Technique and Interpretation

Static images in posterior, left posterior oblique (LPO), and right posterior oblique (RPO) views are acquired at least 4 h after ^{99m}Tc-DMSA (dimercaptosuccinic acid) injection; administered activity of radiotracer is adjusted to the patient's weight, according to EANM dosage card and to the national regulations.

When kidneys are ectopic or when a congenital kidney abnormality is suspected, additional and adequate static views are required (i.e., anterior view, left anterior oblique view).

A 60 s image, reflecting kidney uptake, is also registered in all patients. Using ROI technique method, with a dedicated software, global uptake and differential renal function are calculated.

M.F. Villani • M. Pizzoferro
Nuclear Medicine Unit, Imaging Departement – "Bambino Gesù" Children Hospital, Rome, Italy

G. Di Zazzo (✉)
Unit of Nephrology, "Bambino Gesù" Children Hospital, Rome, Italy
e-mail: giacomo.dizazzo@opbg.net

M.C. Garganese
Diagnostic Imaging Department of Nuclear Medicine, IRCCS Bambino Gesù Paediatric Hospital, Rome, Italy

© Springer International Publishing Switzerland 2017
M.C. Garganese, G.F.L. D'Errico (eds.), *Conventional Nuclear Medicine in Pediatrics*, DOI 10.1007/978-3-319-43181-9_8

8.1.2 Teaching Cases

8.1.2.1 DMSA Renal Scan: Normal Pattern (Fig. 8.1)

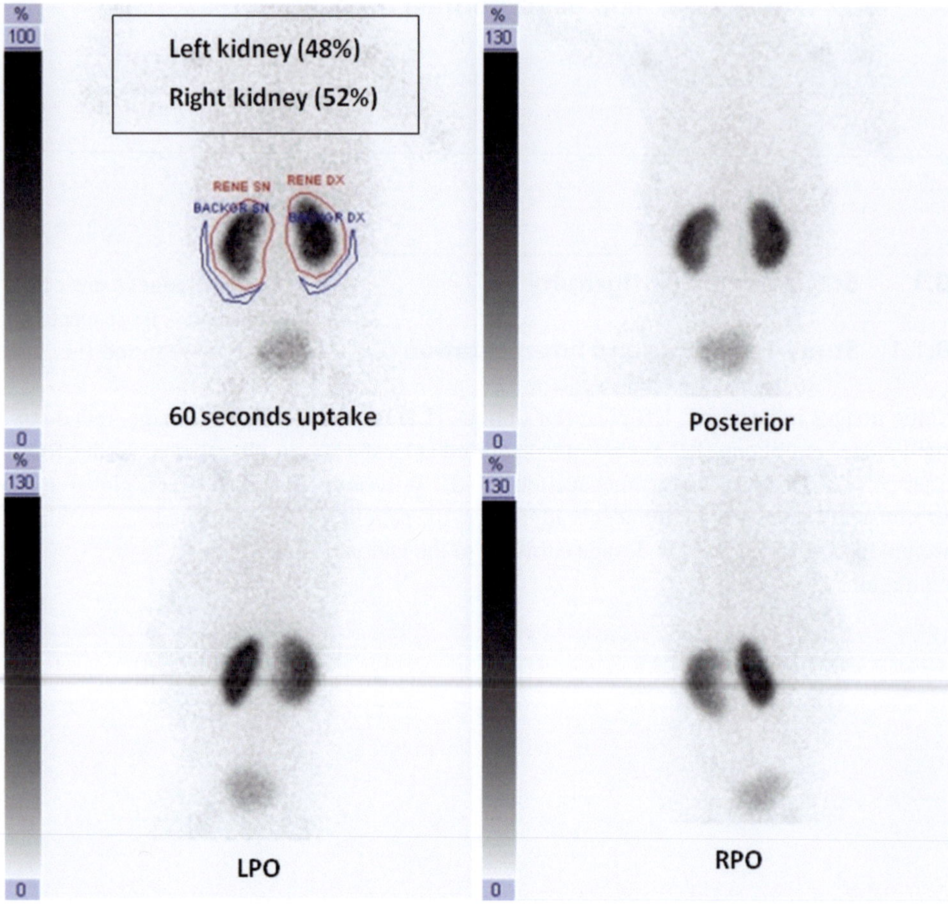

Fig. 8.1 (60 s uptake image, posterior view, *LPO* view, and *RPO* view): both kidneys show good uptake of radiotracer, with homogeneous intraparenchymal distribution; no cortical defects are evident in both kidneys

8.1.2.2 DMSA Renal Scan in Acute Pyelonephritis

DMSA renal scan in a 4-month-old baby, with diagnosis of acute pyelonephritis. No evidence of pathological findings was detected by ultrasonography, while DMSA scan showed a characteristic acute pyelonephritis pattern. Cystography performed after 1 month revealed bilateral high-grade vesicoureteral reflux (VUR). DMSA renal scan in acute pyelonephritis allows an early detection of kidney damage and is characterized by a high prognostic value in identifying children with higher risk of renal impairment (Fig. 8.2a, b).

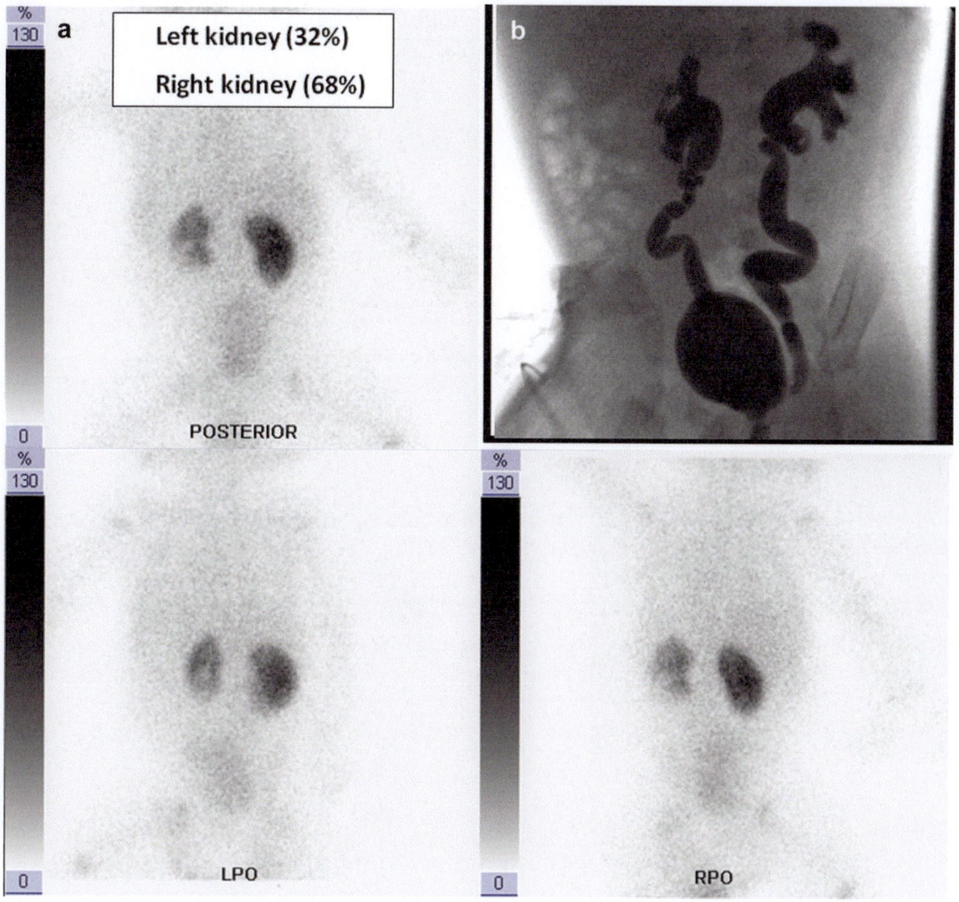

Fig. 8.2 (**a**) DMSA renal scan (posterior view, *LPO* view, and *RPO* view): *left kidney* is smaller than the other one, with global reduction of radiotracer uptake (acute flogosis); two cortical defects are evident, one in the *upper pole* and the larger one in the *lower pole*, respectively; *right kidney* shows good uptake of radiotracer with decreased uptake in *upper* and *lower poles*, without cortical defects. A very low target/background ratio is also evident. (**b**) Cystography: bilateral high-grade vesicoureteral reflux (Grade IV)

8.1.2.3 DMSA Renal Scan in Follow-up ofVUR: Evaluation of Stable Scars

DMSA renal scan in an 8-year-old child with renovascular hypertension and treated bilateral VUR (Fig. 8.3).

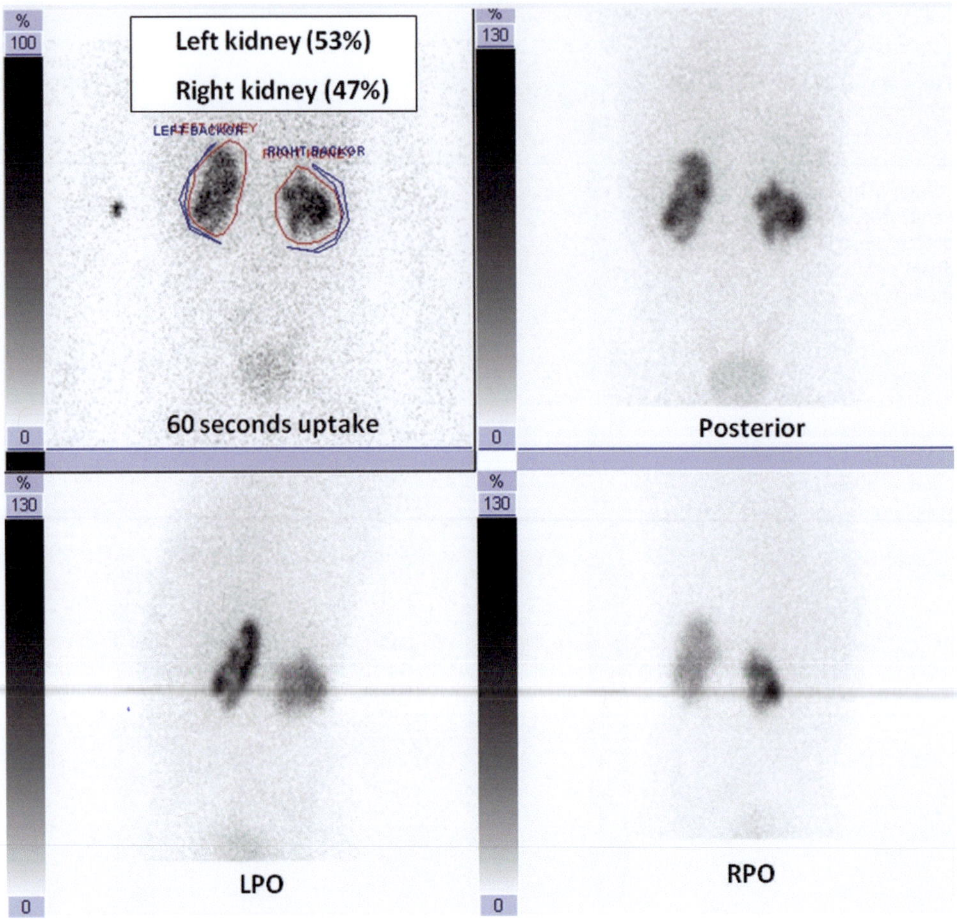

Fig. 8.3 (60 s uptake image, posterior view, *LPO* view, and *RPO* view): radiotracer uptake is reduced in both kidneys with bilateral multiple cortical defects, in particular, in the right one. A low target/background ratio is also evident

8.1.2.4 DMSA Renal Scan in Diagnosis of Renal Scars in High-Grade VUR

Severity of VUR is not always proportional to kidney damage, as it is showed in the following cases (Fig. 8.4).

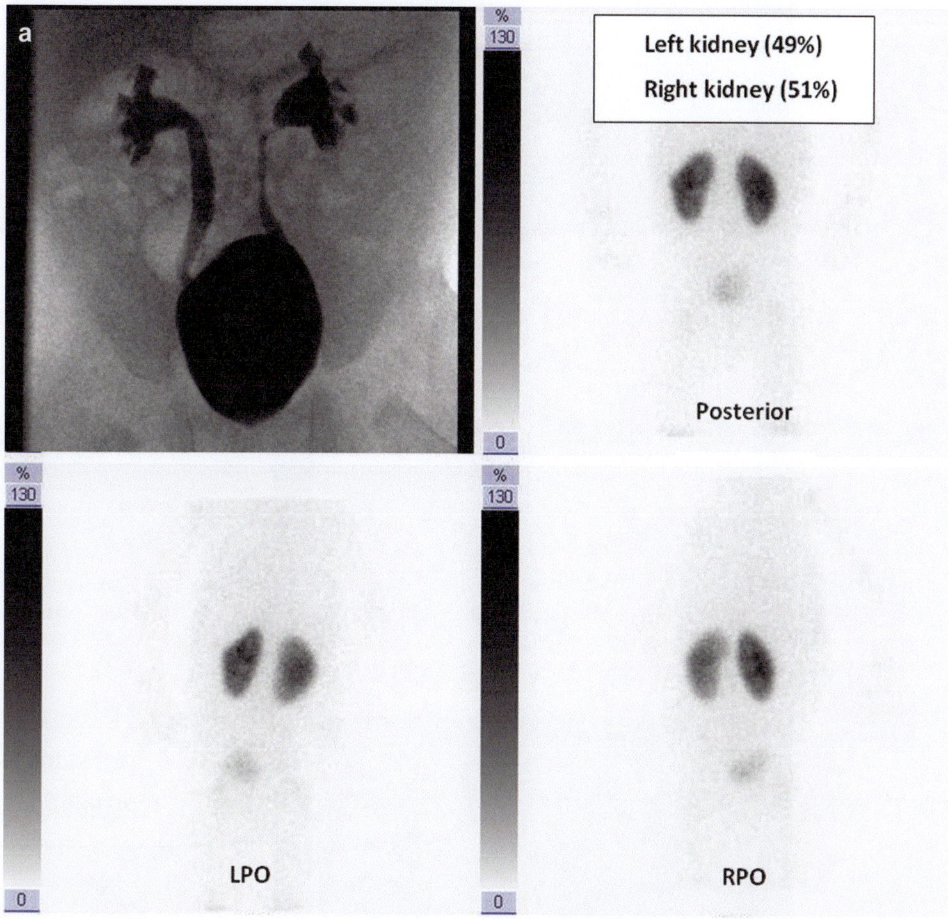

Fig. 8.4 (**a**) No evidence of scars in relation to high-grade VUR. DMSA renal scan (posterior view, *LPO* view, and *RPO* view): both kidneys show good uptake of radiotracer, with homogeneous intraparenchymal distribution; no cortical defects are evident in both kidneys. (**b**) Evidence of a small scar in relation to high-grade VUR. DMSA renal scan (posterior view, *LPO* view, and *RPO* view): *left kidney* is smaller than the other one, with globally reduced radiotracer uptake and a central area devoid of tracer corresponding to dilated renal pelvis; a small focal cortical defect is evident in the upper pole. *Right kidney* shows good uptake of radiotracer with homogeneous intraparenchymal distribution and no evidence of cortical defects. (**c**) Evidence of multiple bilateral scars. DMSA renal scan (posterior view, *LPO* view, and *RPO* view): both kidneys are small with irregular shape; radiotracer intraparenchymal distribution is nonhomogeneous, and multiple cortical defects are evident in both kidneys, in particular, in the left one. A very low target/background ratio is also evident.

Fig. 8.4 (continued)

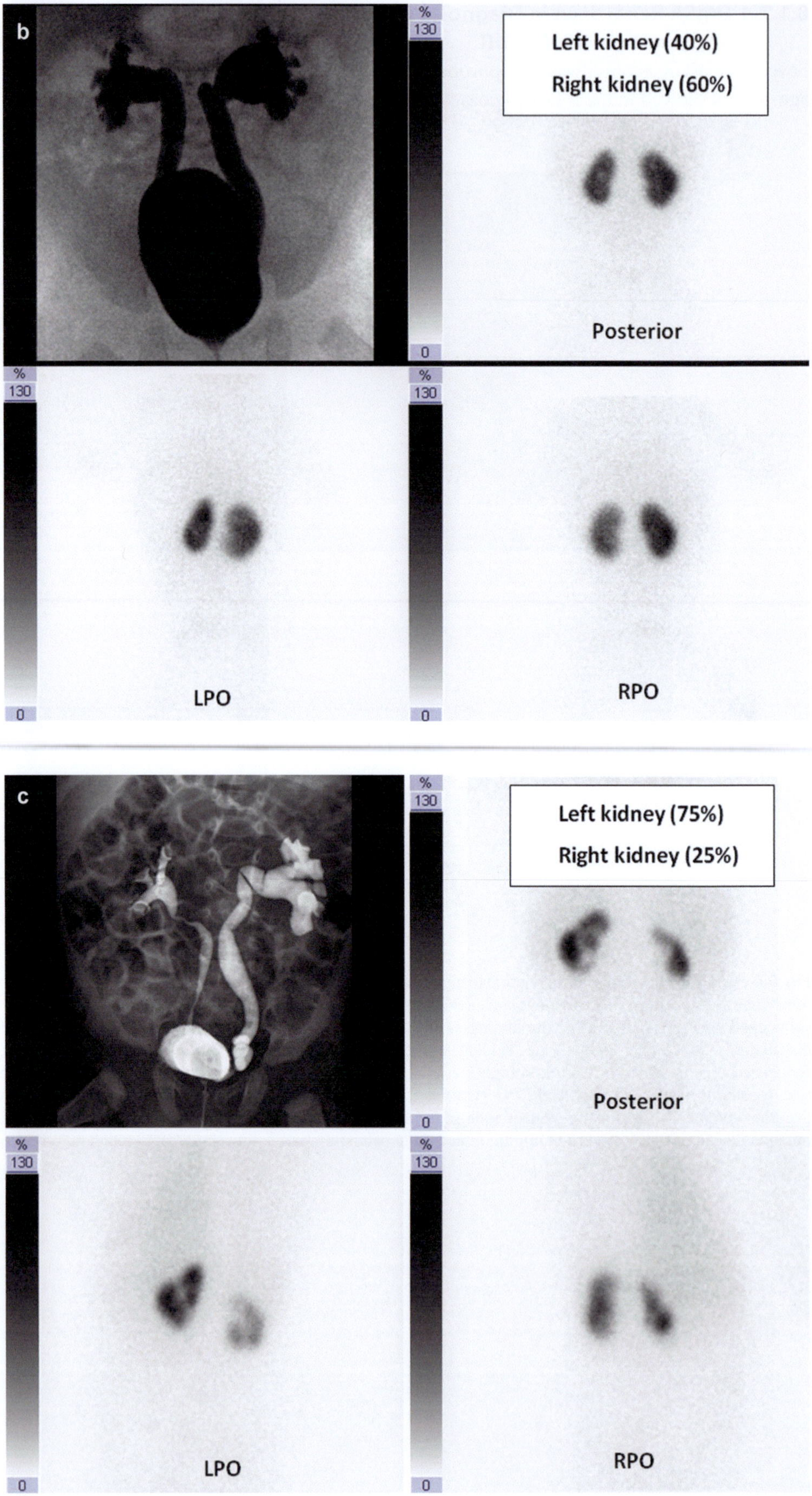

8.1.2.5 DMSA Renal Scan in Assessment of Renal Function and in Diagnosis of Cortical Defects in Posterior Urethral Valves

A 6–month-old baby, with chronic renal failure secondary to posterior urethral valves.

(a) Cystography: bilateral high-grade vesicoureteral reflux (V grade on the left, IV grade on the right) with dilated proximal urethra and radiological signs of posterior urethral valves.
(b) DMSA renal scan (posterior view, LPO view): no visualization of right kidney; left kidney has got an irregular shape and shows globally reduced uptake of radiotracer with nonhomogeneous intraparenchymal distribution. A very low target/background ratio is also evident.

8.1.2.6 DMSA Renal Scan in Obstructive Uropathy (With or Without Scars)

(a) DMSA renal scan (posterior view) in left hydronephrosis with no evidence of cortical defects. Left kidney is very much enlarged, with mildly irregular shape; it shows nonhomogeneous intraparenchymal distribution of radiotracer, with the evidence of a large area dilated renal pelvis; renal parenchyma is thin, with no cortical defects. Radiourine is evident in dilated pelvis. Right kidney shows good uptake of radiotracer, with homogeneous intraparenchymal distribution and no evidence of cortical defects (left DRF: 55 %; right DRF: 45 %).
(b) DMSA renal scan (posterior view) in right hydroureteronephrosis with no evidence of cortical defects. Left kidney shows good uptake of radiotracer, with homogeneous intraparenchymal distribution. Right kidney shows good uptake of radiotracer with nonhomogeneous intraparenchymal distribution for the presence of an area devoid of tracer corresponding to dilated renal pelvis; no cortical defects are evident in both kidneys (left DRF: 48 %; right DRF: 52 %).
(c) DMSA renal scan (posterior view) in right kidney hydronephrosis with renal impairment and multiple cortical defects. Left kidney shows good uptake of radiotracer, with homogeneous intraparenchymal distribution and no evidence of cortical defects. Right kidney shows reduced uptake of radiotracer, with the evidence of a large area devoid of tracer corresponding to dilated renal pelvis and collecting system; renal parenchyma is thin, and multiple cortical defects are evident (left DRF: 71 %; right DRF: 29 %).
(d) DMSA renal scan (posterior view) in staghorn calculi of left kidney with low renal function. Left kidney is smaller than the other one, with irregular shape, and shows severe reduction of radiotracer uptake. Intraparenchymal distribution is not homogeneous, and many areas devoid of tracer (corresponding to renal litiasis) are evident with multiple focal cortical defects. Right kidney shows good uptake of radiotracer, with homogeneous intraparenchymal distribution and no evidence of cortical defects (left DRF: 28 %; right DRF: 72 %).

8.1.2.7 Urinary Tract Malformations: Duplex Kidney

(a) DMSA renal scan (posterior view): both kidneys show good uptake of radiotracer, with homogeneous intraparenchymal distribution; no cortical defects are evident in both kidneys. There is evidence of duplex system in the left kidney, with regular uptake of radiotracer in both systems.
(b) DMSA renal scan (posterior view): left kidney shows good uptake of radiotracer, with homogeneous intraparenchymal distribution. There is evidence of duplex system in right kidney, with reduction of radiotracer uptake in upper system and evidence of dilated renal pelvis; good uptake in lower system is evident. No cortical defects are evident in both kidneys. Using ROI technique method, it is possible to calculate DRF and function of each system too.
(c) DMSA renal scan (posterior view): evidence of duplex system in left kidney, with good radiotracer uptake in upper system and severe reduction of uptake in lower system. Right kidney shows good uptake of radiotracer with homogeneous intraparenchymal distribution without cortical defects.

8.1.2.8 Renal Congenital Abnormalities with No Evidence of Cortical Defects

(a) DMSA renal scan (posterior view): horseshoe kidney, with bilateral good uptake of radiotracer and homogeneous intraparenchymal distribution. No cortical defects are evident in both kidneys.
(b) DMSA renal scan (anterior view): visualization of a single kidney, round-shaped (as seen in "pancake kidney"), with good uptake of radiotracer and mildly nonhomogeneous intraparenchymal distribution. No cortical defects are evident.
(c) DMSA renal scan (posterior view): right kidney is in its own proper site and shows good uptake of radiotracer, homogeneous intraparenchymal distribution, and no evidence of cortical defects. Left kidney is located in the abdomen, is malrotated, and its upper pole is fused with the medial border of the lower pole of the right one (as seen in cross-fused ectopic kidneys or sigmoid kidney). Intraparenchymal tracer distribution of left ectopic kidney is mildly nonhomogeneous (decreased uptake in both poles), with no evidence of significant cortical defects.

8.1.2.9 Renal Congenital Abnormalities: Horseshoe Kidney

(a) DMSA renal scan (posterior view, anterior view, LPO view, and RPO view): horseshoe kidney, with good uptake of radiotracer and homogeneous intraparenchymal distribution in both kidneys without cortical defects.
(b) DMSA renal scan (posterior view, anterior view, LPO view, and RPO view) in horseshoe kidney. Left kidney shows reduction of radiotracer uptake and nonhomogeneous intraparenchymal distribution (due to an area devoid of tracer corresponding to dilated renal pelvis and collecting system) and multiple cortical defects. Right kidney shows good uptake of radiotracer, homogeneous intraparenchymal distribution, and no evidence of cortical defects.

8.1.2.10 Renal Congenital Abnormalities: Fused Ectopic Kidneys

(a) DMSA renal scan (anterior view) in ectopic pelvic kidneys fused on their medial border. Left kidney shows good and homogeneous uptake of radiotracer, with no evidence of cortical defects. Right kidney shows irregular shape, with nonhomogeneous radiotracer uptake; two small cortical defects are evident in the upper and middle two-thirds of the kidney, on the medial and lateral border.
(b) DMSA renal scan (anterior view): as displayed by drawing, a single ectopic kidney is located in the abdomen on the left paramedian line, showing good and homogeneous uptake of radiotracer without evidence of cortical defects.
(c) DMSA renal scan (anterior view): as displayed by drawing, a single ectopic pelvic kidney is evident, showing good uptake of radiotracer with two cortical defects in the upper and lower poles, respectively.

8.1.2.11 Renal Congenital Abnormalities: Nonfused Ectopic Kidneys (Cortical Defects and Renal Pelvis Dilatation)

(a) DMSA renal scan (posterior view, anterior view, LAO view, and RPO view) shows left ectopic kidney located in the pelvis, with irregular shape and mild reduction of radiotracer uptake; a cortical defect is evident in the upper pole. Right kidney is located in its own proper site and shows good uptake of radiotracer, homogeneous intraparenchymal distribution, and no evidence of cortical defects.
(b) DMSA renal scan (posterior view, anterior view, LAO view, and RPO view) shows left kidney located in its own proper site with good uptake of radiotracer, homogeneous intraparenchymal distribution, and no evidence of cortical defects. Right ectopic kidney is located in the pelvis with irregular shape and mild reduction of radiotracer uptake. Intraparenchymal distribution is nonhomogeneous, with an area devoid of tracer corresponding to dilated renal pelvis and no cortical defects (Figs. 8.5, 8.6, 8.7, 8.8, 8.9, 8.10, and 8.11).

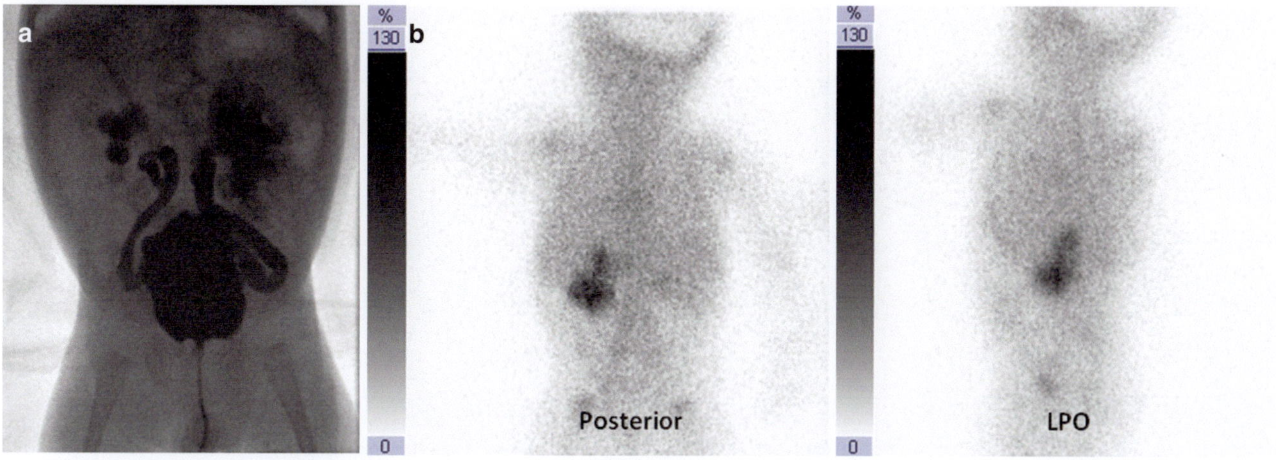

Fig. 8.5 A 6–month-old baby, with chronic renal failure secondary to posterior urethral valves. (**a**) Cystography: bilateral high-grade vesicoureteral reflux (V grade on the left, IV grade on the *right*) with dilated proximal urethra and radiological signs of posterior urethral valves. (**b**) DMSA renal scan (posterior view, *LPO* view): no visualization of *right kidney*; *left kidney* has got an irregular shape and shows globally reduced uptake of radiotracer with nonhomogeneous intraparenchymal distribution. A very low target/background ratio is also evident

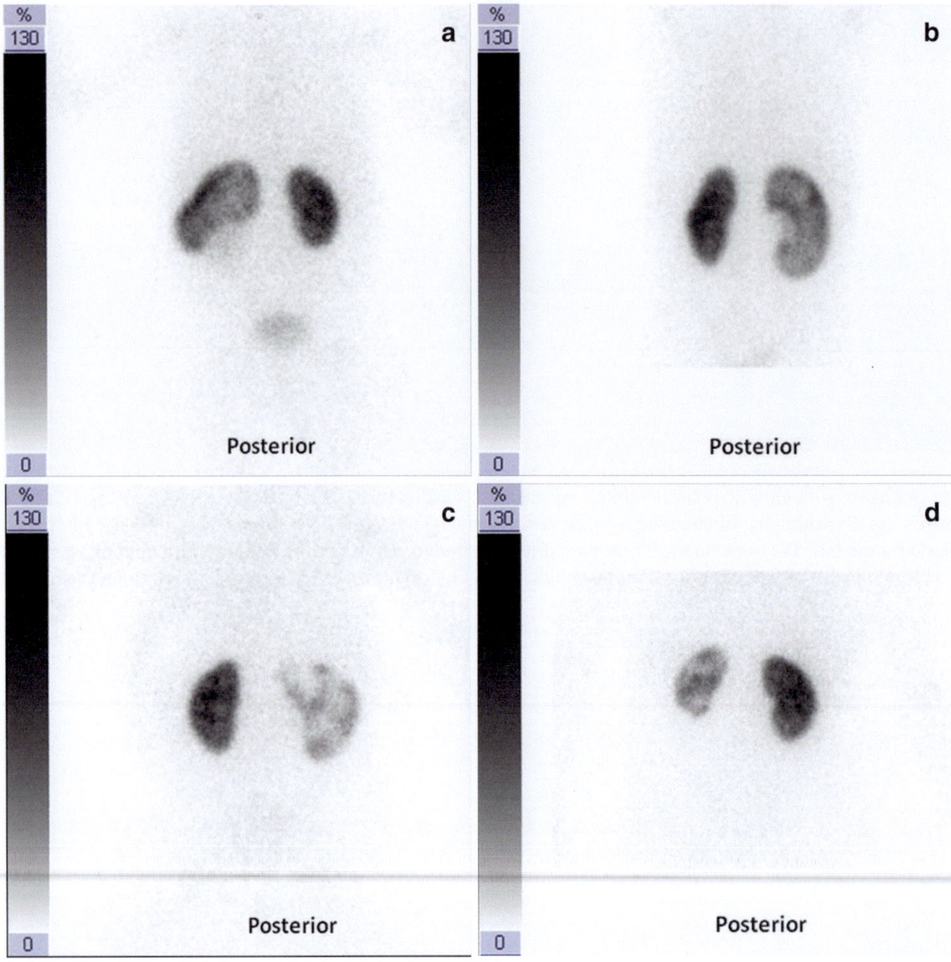

Fig. 8.6 (**a**) DMSA renal scan (posterior view) in *left* hydronephrosis with no evidence of cortical defects. *Left kidney* is very much enlarged, with mildly irregular shape; it shows nonhomogeneous intraparenchymal distribution of radiotracer, with the evidence of a large area dilated renal pelvis; renal parenchyma is thin, with no cortical defects. Radiourine is evident in dilated pelvis. *Right kidney* shows good uptake of radiotracer, with homogeneous intraparenchymal distribution and no evidence of cortical defects (left DRF: 55 %; right DRF: 45 %). (**b**) DMSA renal scan (posterior view) in right hydroureteronephrosis with no evidence of cortical defects. *Left kidney* shows good uptake of radiotracer, with homogeneous intraparenchymal distribution. *Right kidney* shows good uptake of radiotracer with nonhomogeneous intraparenchymal distribution for the presence of an area devoid of tracer corresponding to dilated renal pelvis; no cortical defects are evident in both kidneys (left DRF: 48 %; right DRF: 52 %). (**c**) DMSA renal scan (posterior view) in *right kidney* hydronephrosis with renal impairment and multiple cortical defects. *Left kidney* shows good uptake of radiotracer, with homogeneous intraparenchymal distribution and no evidence of cortical defects. *Right kidney* shows reduced uptake of radiotracer, with the evidence of a large area devoid of tracer corresponding to dilated renal pelvis and collecting system; renal parenchyma is thin, and multiple cortical defects are evident (left DRF: 71 %; right DRF: 29 %). (**d**) DMSA renal scan (posterior view) in staghorn calculi of *left kidney* with low renal function. *Left kidney* is smaller than the other one, with irregular shape, and shows severe reduction of radiotracer uptake. Intraparenchymal distribution is not homogeneous, and many areas devoid of tracer (corresponding to renal litiasis) are evident with multiple focal cortical defects. *Right kidney* shows good uptake of radiotracer, with homogeneous intraparenchymal distribution and no evidence of cortical defects (left DRF: 28 %; right DRF:72 %)

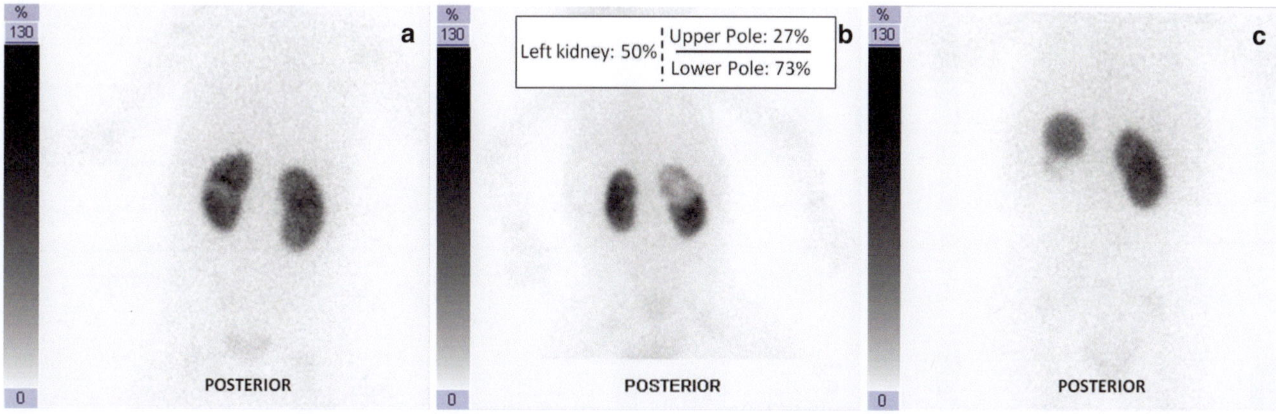

Fig. 8.7 (**a**) DMSA renal scan (posterior view): both kidneys show good uptake of radiotracer, with homogeneous intraparenchymal distribution; no cortical defects are evident in both kidneys. There is evidence of duplex system in the *left kidney*, with regular uptake of radiotracer in both systems. (**b**) DMSA renal scan (posterior view): *left kidney* shows good uptake of radiotracer, with homogeneous intraparenchymal distribution. There is evidence of duplex system in *right kidney*, with reduction of radiotracer uptake in upper system and evidence of dilated renal pelvis; good uptake in lower system is evident. No cortical defects are evident in both kidneys. Using ROI technique method, it is possible to calculate DRF and function of each system too. (**c**) DMSA renal scan (posterior view): evidence of duplex system in *left kidney*, with good radiotracer uptake in upper system and severe reduction of uptake in lower system. *Right kidney* shows good uptake of radiotracer with homogeneous intraparenchymal distribution without cortical defects

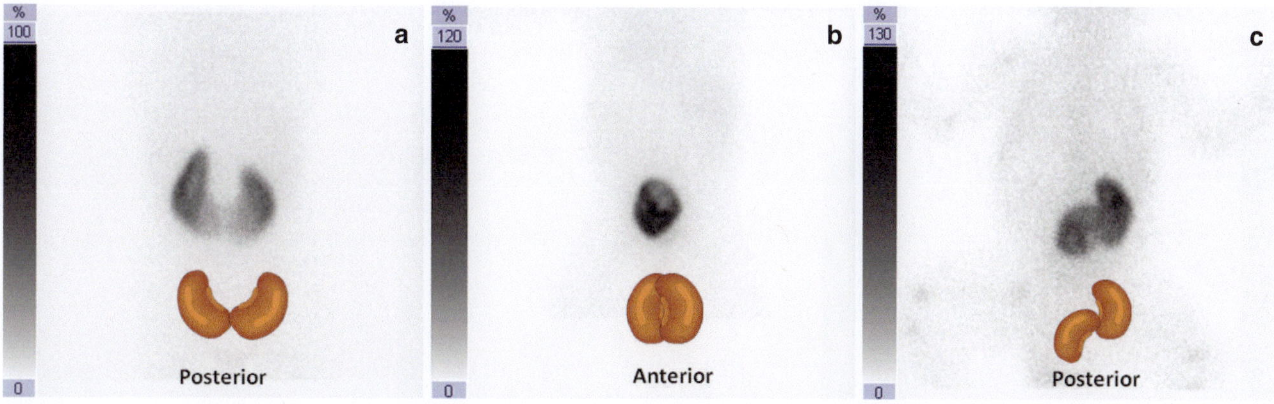

Fig. 8.8 (**a**) DMSA renal scan (posterior view): horseshoe kidney, with bilateral good uptake of radiotracer and homogeneous intraparenchymal distribution. No cortical defects are evident in both kidneys. (**b**) DMSA renal scan (anterior view): visualization of a single kidney, round-shaped (as seen in "pancake kidney"), with good uptake of radiotracer and mildly nonhomogeneous intraparenchymal distribution. No cortical defects are evident. (**c**) DMSA renal scan (posterior view): *right kidney* is in its own proper site and shows good uptake of radiotracer, homogeneous intraparenchymal distribution, and no evidence of cortical defects. *Left kidney* is located in the abdomen, is malrotated, and its upper pole is fused with the medial border of the lower pole of the right one (as seen in cross-fused ectopic kidneys or sigmoid kidney). Intraparenchymal tracer distribution of left ectopic kidney is mildly nonhomogeneous (decreased uptake in both poles), with no evidence of significant cortical defects

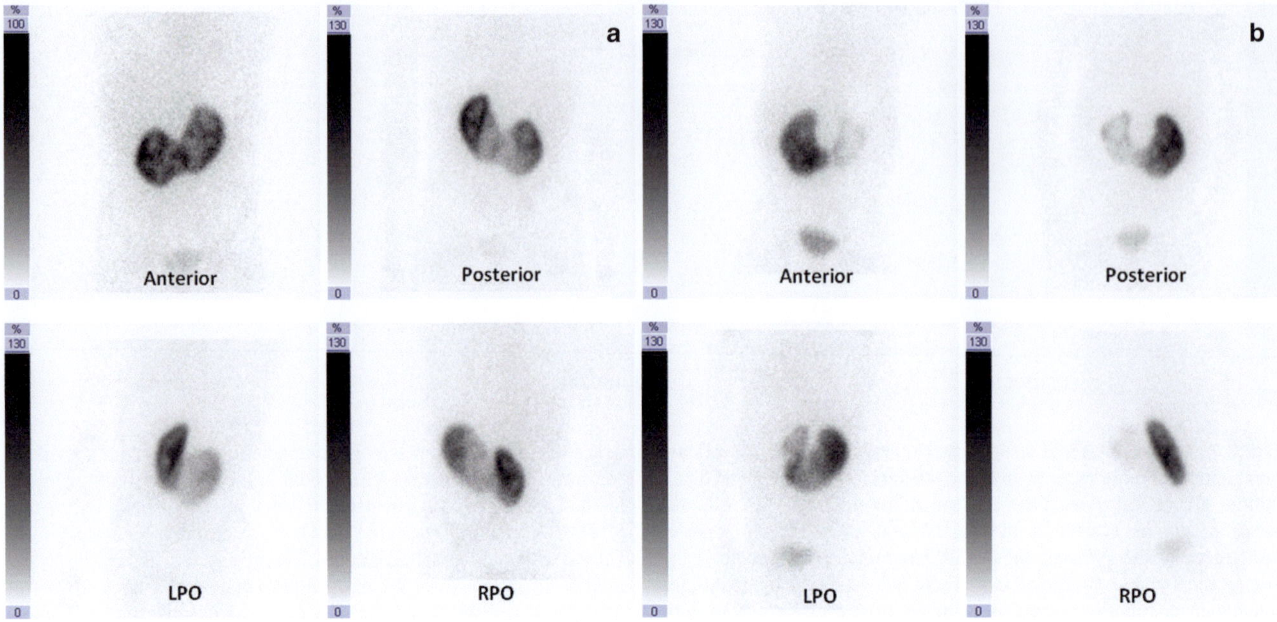

Fig. 8.9 (**a**) DMSA renal scan (posterior view, anterior view, *LPO* view, and *RPO* view): horseshoe kidney, with good uptake of radiotracer and homogeneous intraparenchymal distribution in both kidneys without cortical defects. (**b**) DMSA renal scan (posterior view, anterior view, *LPO* view, and *RPO* view) in horseshoe kidney. *Left kidney* shows reduction of radiotracer uptake and nonhomogeneous intraparenchymal distribution (due to an area devoid of tracer corresponding to dilated renal pelvis and collecting system) and multiple cortical defects. *Right kidney* shows good uptake of radiotracer, homogeneous intraparenchymal distribution, and no evidence of cortical defects

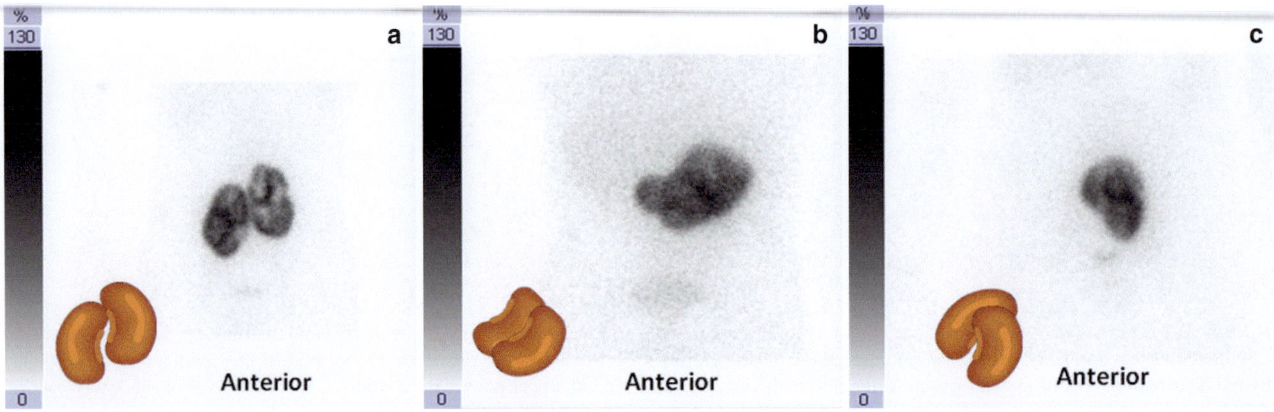

Fig. 8.10 (**a**) DMSA renal scan (anterior view) in ectopic pelvic kidneys fused on their medial border. *Left kidney* shows good and homogeneous uptake of radiotracer, with no evidence of cortical defects. *Right kidney* shows irregular shape, with nonhomogeneous radiotracer uptake; two small cortical defects are evident in the upper and middle two-thirds of the kidney, on the medial and lateral border. (**b**) DMSA renal scan (anterior view): as displayed by drawing, a single ectopic kidney is located in the abdomen on the left paramedian line, showing good and homogeneous uptake of radiotracer without evidence of cortical defects. (**c**) DMSA renal scan (anterior view): as displayed by drawing, a single ectopic pelvic kidney is evident, showing good uptake of radiotracer with two cortical defects in the upper and lower poles, respectively

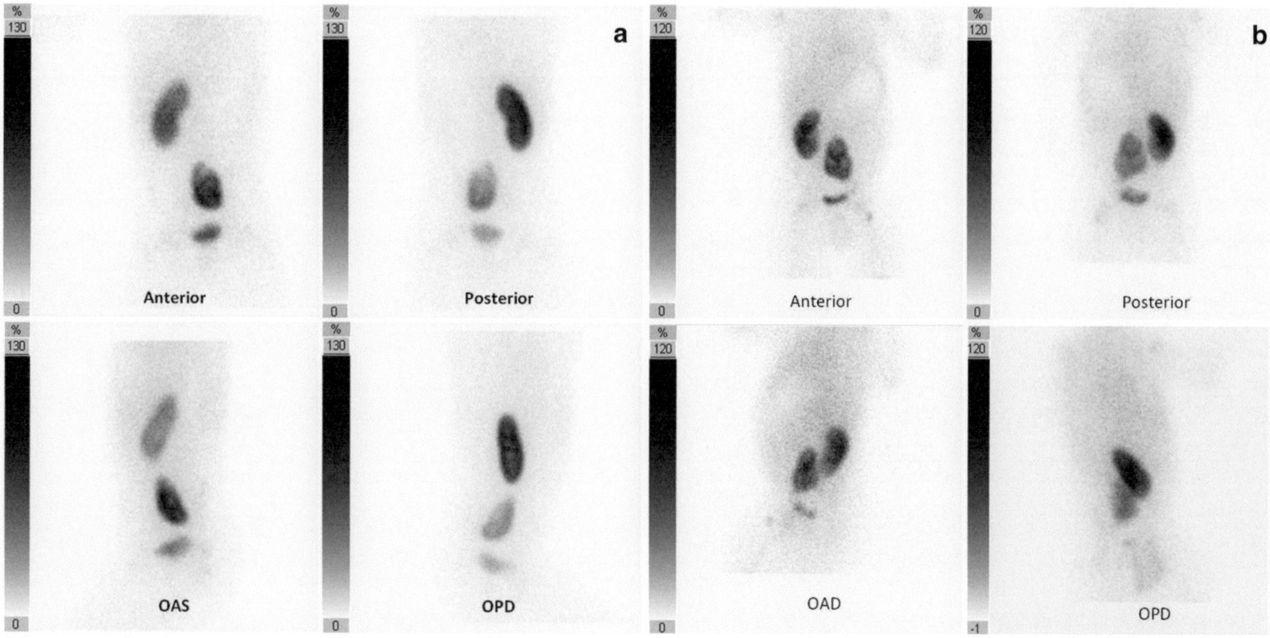

Fig. 8.11 (**a**) DMSA renal scan (posterior view, anterior view, *LAO* view, and *RPO* view) shows left ectopic kidney located in the pelvis, with irregular shape and mild reduction of radiotracer uptake; a cortical defect is evident in the upper pole. *Right kidney* is located in its own proper site and shows good uptake of radiotracer, homogeneous intraparenchymal distribution, and no evidence of cortical defects. (**b**) DMSA renal scan (posterior view, anterior view, *LAO* view, and *RPO* view) shows *left kidney* located in its own proper site with good uptake of radiotracer, homogeneous intraparenchymal distribution, and no evidence of cortical defects. Right ectopic kidney is located in the pelvis with irregular shape and mild reduction of radiotracer uptake. Intraparenchymal distribution is nonhomogeneous, with an area devoid of tracer corresponding to dilated renal pelvis and no cortical defects

Bibliography

Piepsz A, Colarinha P, et al.; Paediatric Committee of the European Association of Nuclear Medicine. Guidelines for ^{99m}Tc-DMSA scintigraphy in children. Eur J Nucl Med. 2001;28(3):BP37–41.

9 Nephrourology: Focus On Child with Bladder Dysfunctions and Urodynamics

Mario De Gennaro, Maria Luisa Capitanucci, and Giovanni Mosiello

9.1 Introduction

Bladder dysfunction is a broad term used to describe different dysfunctional conditions of the bladder-sphincter complex, due to nonneurogenic and neurogenic causes. The International Children's Continence Society (ICCS) provided guidelines on bladder dysfunctions which are better defined with the term *lower urinary tract dysfunctions* (LUTD) [3–6, 16, 17]. The ICCS classified two main groups of nonneurogenic conditions: nighttime (*enuresis*) and daytime (*overactive bladder – OAB*, *dysfunctional voiding* – DV, *underactive bladder* – UB, *bladder and bowel dysfunction – BBD*) conditions. They are more common problems in children and adolescents, leading to urinary incontinence (UI); LUTD seriously affect quality of life. *Neurogenic bladder (NB)* is the term applied to LUTD due to congenital or acquired neurological lesions. Depending on the site of neurological insult, urodynamic studies show pattern of detrusor overactivity or underactivity with or without sphincter dyssynergia. Due to pathophysiological reasons, urinary tract infection (UTI) and vesicoureteral reflux (VUR) are strong comorbid conditions in both nonneurogenic and neurogenic LUTD. This chapter focuses on definition, pathophysiology, and assessment of both nonneurogenic and neurogenic LUTD.

M. De Gennaro • G. Mosiello
Unit of Urology, Robotic Surgery and Urodynamic, "Bambino Gesù" Children Hospital, Rome, Italy

M.L. Capitanucci (✉)
Unit of Urology, Robotic Surgery and Urodynamic, "Bambino Gesù" Children Hospital, Rome, Italy
e-mail: mluisa.capitanucci@opbg.net

9.2 Nonneurogenic Lower Urinary Tract Dysfunctions [3, 5, 6, 16]

Since the final steps of lower urinary tract (LUT) control development are usually achieved at the age of 3 or 4 years, definitions of LUT symptoms and dysfunctions are relevant from the age of 5 years.

- *Lower urinary tract symptoms (LUTS)*: LUTS are classified according to their relation with the storage or voiding phase of bladder function.

  Storage Symptoms
  - *Increased or decreased voiding frequency*: The normal range is 3–7 voiding per day. *Voiding frequency* is *increased* in those children who void ≥8 times daily and *decreased* in the ones who void ≤3 times daily.
  - *Urinary incontinence (UI)*: It means involuntary leakage of urine. It can be continuous or intermittent. When UI is continuous, it is almost exclusively associated with congenital anomalies (ectopic ureter, posterior urethral valves, exstrophy-epispadias complex), iatrogenic damage (external sphincterotomy, vesicovaginal fistulas), and NB. Differently, intermittent UI is due to nonneurogenic LUTD. When associated with urgency, it is called urge UI.
  - *Urgency*: It means the sudden and unexpected experience of an immediate need to void.
  - *Nocturia*: The child must be awaken at night to void.

  Voiding Symptoms
  - *Hesitancy*: denotes difficulty in the initiation of micturition.
  - *Straining*: child applies abdominal pressure to initiate and maintain voiding.
  - *Weak stream*: observed ejection of urine with a weak force.
  - *Intermittency*: micturition occurs in several discrete spurts.
  - *Dysuria*: burning or discomfort during micturition.

© Springer International Publishing Switzerland 2017

M.C. Garganese, G.F.L. D'Errico (eds.), *Conventional Nuclear Medicine in Pediatrics*, DOI 10.1007/978-3-319-43181-9_9

Other Symptoms

- *Holding maneuvers*: they are observable strategies to postpone micturition as well as squatting, standing on tiptoe, forcefully crossing the legs.
- *Feeling of incomplete bladder emptying*.
- *Urinary retention*: sensation of the inability to void despite persistent effort in the presence of a fully, distended bladder.
- *Postmicturition dribble*: involuntary urine leakage which occurs immediately after voiding has finished.
- *Spraying (splitting) of the urinary stream*: urine passes as a spray or a split rather than a single discrete stream.

• *Lower urinary tract dysfunctions (LUTD)*: These include nighttime and daytime conditions:

Nighttime condition

- *Enuresis*: It is a form of *intermittent nocturnal UI* defined as involuntary voiding during sleep, at least three times a week, in nonneurologically impaired children over 5 years of age. Enuresis may be *monosymptomatic* (without daytime symptoms) or *nonmonosymptomatic* (with daytime symptoms) and *primary* (children who have never been free of bed-wetting for 6 months) or *secondary* (re-emergence of bed-wetting after a dry period of at least 6 months). The classification into mono- (MNE) and nonmono (NMNE) symptomatic enuresis is very important when we consider treatment strategies. MNE is an isolated phenomenon due to delayed maturation in one or more of the following systems: stability of bladder function, arginine–vasopressin release, or response and ability to wake from sleep to full bladder sensations. Combinations of all the three problems may be present in the same children. NMNE is not an isolated phenomenon but a part of symptom complex which is expression of LUTD. Therefore, children with NMNE are more appropriately managed in the context of LUTD.

Daytime Conditions

Classification of daytime LUTD is more complex due to heterogeneity of LUTS and considerable overlap between conditions. The main types of daytime LUTD have been reported:

- *Overactive Bladder (OAB)*: OAB is defined by urgency, usually accompanied by increased frequency and/or nocturia. UI may be concomitant with urgency (urge UI). The hallmark symptom of OAB, the urgency, arises from detrusor overactivity (DO): detrusor contractions are registered during the filling phase of invasive urodynamic study (UDS). During invasive UDS, DO is countered by voluntary contraction of the pelvic floor to postpone voiding and minimize urge UI. The predominant pathophysiological theory to explain OAB in children is that OAB is due to delayed maturation of reticulospinal pathways and inhibitory center in the midbrain and cerebral cortex [5]. Delay in bladder–sphincter coordination during voiding causes DO to be met with voluntary external sphincter contractions. Consequent increase in intravesical pressure is recognized by children as sense of urgency, and may lead to the development of VUR. Recurrent detrusor contraction against a closed or incompletely relaxed sphincter/pelvic floor can induce progressive detrusor hypertrophy, which may lead to decreased functional bladder capacity and increased DO; in this manner, a vicious circle is created in which OAB can only get worse [2].
- *Dysfunctional Voiding (DV)*: Children with DV are disabled to fully relax the sphincter or pelvic floor muscles during voiding. This condition can be defined only by means of flowmetry plus pelvic-floor electromyography showing staccato or interrupted pattern. Children with DV usually present with low voiding frequency, UI, and UTI, with or without VUR. Pathophysiology of DV remains unclear. It has been hypothesized that DO eventually leads to overactivity of the pelvic floor with subsequent insufficient relaxation during voiding [1]. Another theory suggests that poor relaxation of the pelvic floor muscles during voiding is a learned condition during the toilet training years, adopted following episodes of urinary tract infection or constipation or occurring after sexual abuse [10]. Moreover, toilet conditions and privacy issues can trigger or exacerbate voiding disturbances [8]. In some girls, DV may be associated with anatomical anomalies of the external urethral meatus: the urine stream may be deflected anteriorly and cause stimulation of the clitoris with reflex activity of the bulbocavernous muscle, causing intermittent voiding [14].
- *Underactive Bladder (UB)*: The term UB replaces the old entity of lazy bladder. This term is reserved for children with a need to increase abdominal pressure to initiate, maintain, or complete voiding. The children with UB show an inability to void using detrusor pressure alone; they often produce an interrupted or plateau flow pattern with relevant postvoiding residual urine (PVR). In these cases, UDS is mandatory to define the presence of detrusor underactivity during voiding. Long-standing overactivity of the pelvic floor may lead in some children to detrusor decompensation with detrusor hypocontractility and *UB*; however, no data are available to support this theory.

- *Bladder and Bowel dysfunction* (*BBD*): BBD is a combination of LUTD and bowel dysfunction in children with no identifiable or recognizable neurological abnormalities [3]. Children in the early stage of defecation disorders show an incomplete and infrequent bowel emptying. With the progression of the disorder, the rectum and descending colon are distended with a decrease in normal sensation; children develop constipation, which may be associated with fecal retentive incontinence [7]. Abnormal recruitment of the external anal sphincter during defecation may elicit concomitant urethral sphincter and pelvic floor co-contractions, leading to functional obstruction in both systems. Consequently, high pressure generated by detrusor to overcome functional obstruction can stimulate detrusor hypertrophy, DO, and lead to incompetence of the vesicoureteral junction with development of secondary VUR [2].

9.2.1 Assessment

Standardization documents for diagnostic evaluation of children with nonneurogenic daytime incontinence and LUTS have been recently published by the ICCS [5, 13]. A *noninvasive approach* is recommended with detailed history, questionnaires [9], physical examination, bladder diary, urinalysis, uroflowmetry, and pre- and postvoiding bladder ultrasound (Table 9.1). These tools enable to make differential diagnosis between different types of LUTD, to select patients who will need further evaluations (invasive urodynamic, micturition cystourethrography, and renal scintigraphy), and to identify children with NB or structural anomalies.

- *Bladder Diary*: Bladder diary records fluid intake, micturition frequency, voided volume, episode of urgency, and urine loss. For diagnostic purpose, it should cover at least 3 days of registration. A bowel movement chart and Bristol stool chart [12] are also important, either separate from or in conjunction with bladder diary.
- *Urinalysis*: It may provide information about urinary tract infection, possible associated diabetes and renal damage, or disease-causing proteinuria. Dipstick may be useful in clinical practice to achieve these information quickly [15].
  Uroflowmetry (*FLW*) [5]: It is the less invasive of all urodynamic studies and, therefore, is perfect for pediatric patients [11]. In children, more than one FLW recording should be obtained in the same session before drawing conclusions, and three evaluations are advised [3, 16]. Pelvic floor EMG and ultrasound PVR are recommended, increasing the value of FLW measurement. Results of FLW, combined with those of history, bladder diary, and PVR, seem to be more effective than UDS in detecting both OAB and DV. The shape of the flow curve is the most important factor to analyze in pediatric patients (Fig. 9.1) [5]. In normal voiding, the curve is bell-shaped. OAB may produce an explosive voiding contraction that appears as a

Table 9.1 First-line assessment in children with nonneurogenic lower urinary tract dysfunction

Diagnostic tools	Overactive bladder	Dysfunctional voiding
Medical history	Urgency Holding maneuvers to contrast urgency ± Increased void frequency[a] ± Urge incontinence ± Urinary tract infection ± Constipation	Holding maneuvers to postpone micturition Increased/decreased void frequency[a] ± Intermittent incontinence ± Urinary tract infection ± Constipation
Bladder diary	Episodes of urgency Increased number of voiding[a] Low voided volume[b] Episodes of incontinence + urge Amount of urine loss Bowel movements	Abnormal number of voiding[a] Normal/high voided volume[b] Episodes of incontinence without urge Amount of urine loss Bowel movements
Uroflowmetry	Tower-shaped curve	Staccato or interrupted curve
	Low voided volume[b]	Normal/high voided volume[b]
Pelvic floor EMG	Relaxed pelvic floor	Overactive pelvic floor
Pre-voiding US	Low bladder capacity[b]	Normal/increased bladder capacity[b]
	Bladder wall: normal or thickened	Bladder wall: normal or thickened
Postvoiding US	No postvoiding residuum	± Postvoiding residuum

[a]Normal voiding frequency in children: 5–7/day [3]
[b]Expected bladder capacity for age [30 + age in years × 30)] in ml [3]

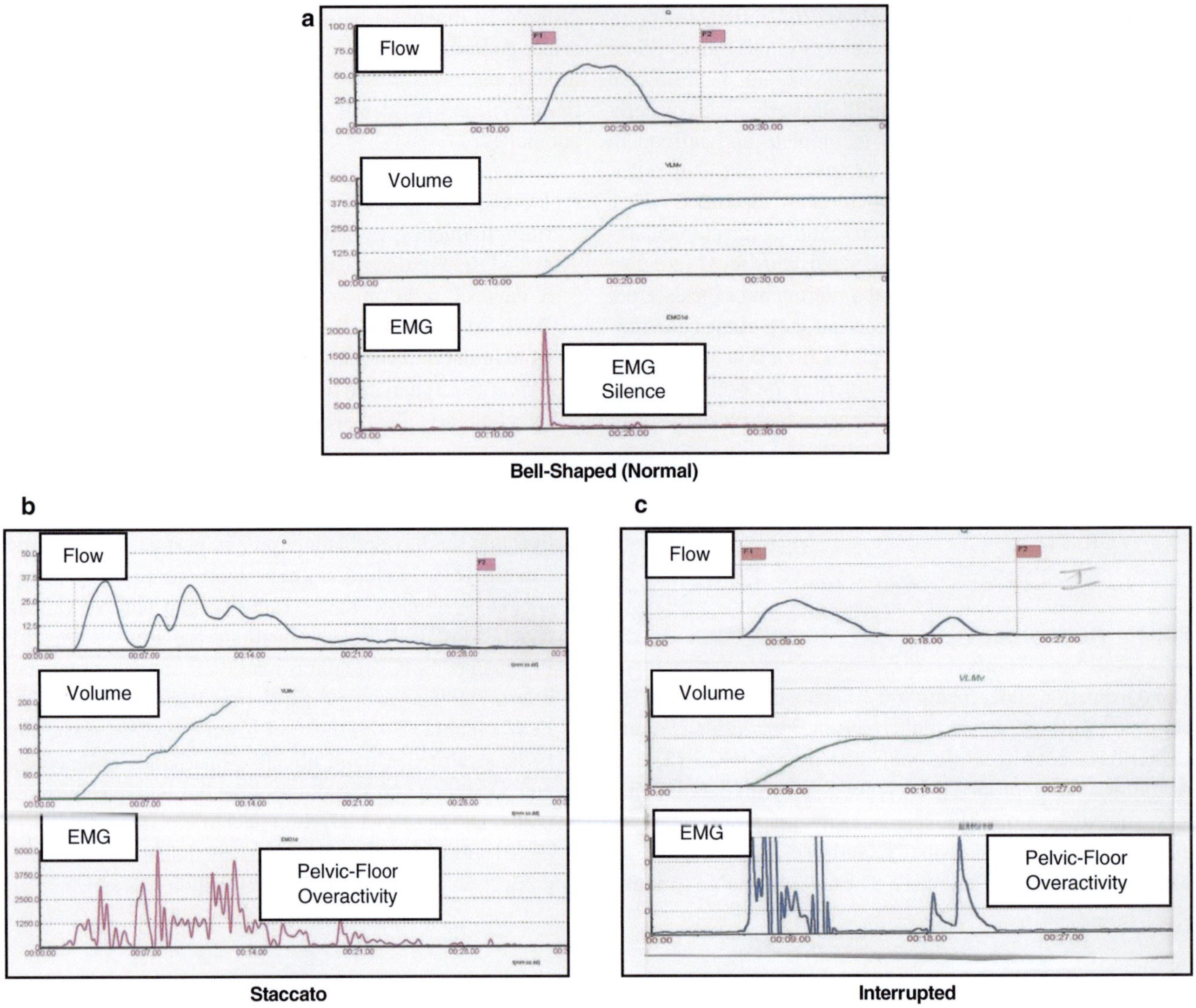

Fig. 9.1 Uroflowmetry pattern in children with nonneurogenic LUTD. (**a**) bell-shaped: normal flowmetric curve; (**b**) Staccato flow indicates dysfunctional voiding; (**c**) interrupted flow due to severe dysfunctional voiding or underactive bladder

high-amplitude flow curve of short duration, namely, a *tower-shaped curve*. In DV, sphincter overactivity during voiding produces a *staccato flow*, as a continuous urine flow with periodic reductions in flow rate precipitated by bursts of pelvic floor activity; voiding is commonly prolonged and incomplete. *Interrupted or fractionated flow* is micturition in separate fractions due to unsustained voiding contractions. Interrupted or fractionated flow can be seen in children with severe DV and UB. Functional and anatomical obstruction often has a low amplitude, and rather even flow curve, that is, a *plateau curve*. Generally, in children with OAB, voided volume (Vvol) is lower than the expected bladder capacity for age (EBC). On the contrary, in children with DV, Vvol can be higher than EBC. EBC for age is estimated by the formula: [30 + (age in years × 30)] in ml [16]. Evaluating FLW, EBC is of great importance, because it has been shown that uroflow curve changes when the voided volume is less than 50 % of EBC [5]. In children, poor correlation exists between Qmax and outflow resistance. Therefore, Qmax is of minor importance than in adult age.

- *Ultrasound*: In all children with proven LUTS, bladder ultrasound is indicated. It should be performed before and after voiding. Prevoid examination contributes to overall assessment of bladder capacity, bladder wall, lower ureteral dilatation, and bladder neck appearance. Since bladder wall thickness depends on the degree of bladder filling and age of children, it is of great variability

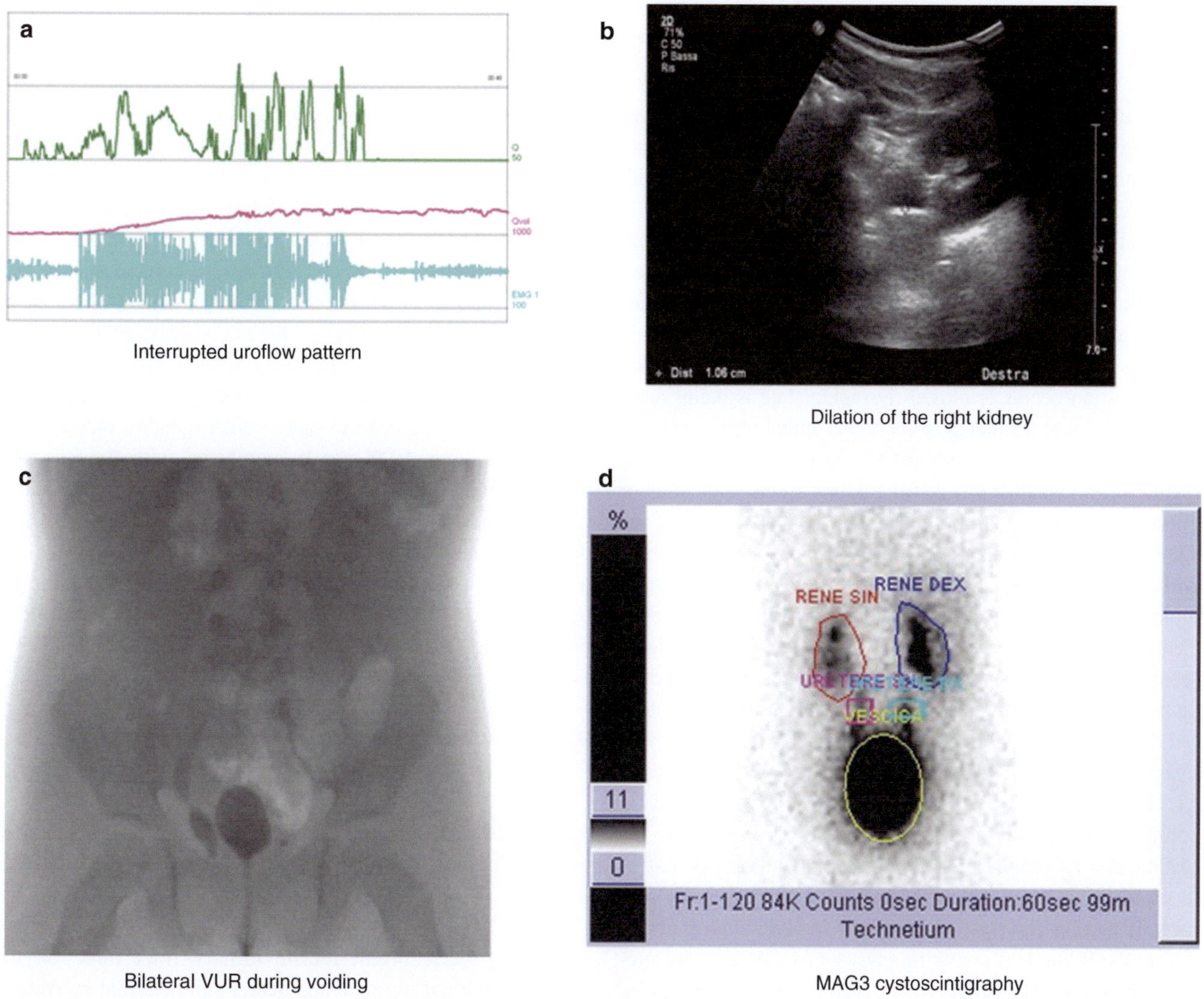

Fig. 9.2 Flowmetry and radiological findings of a 6-year-old girl with dysfunctional voiding, recurrent UTI, and VUR: (**a**) flowmetric pattern (interrupted) of severe dysfunctional voiding; (**b**) mild dilation of the right kidney at ultrasound evaluation of the urinary tract; (**c**) bilateral VUR during voiding at micturition cystourethrography; (**d**) appearance of VUR at MAG3 cystoscintigraphy

in pediatric age, and normal values are not disposable. However, correlations have been demonstrated in children with LUTD between bladder wall thickness, urodynamic pattern, and treatment outcome, with good specificity [18]. Therefore, a thickened bladder wall may alert clinicians on the presence of a long-standing LUTD, leading to detrusor hypertrophy. Ultrasound evaluation of bladder immediately after voiding can demonstrate PVR. A PVR ≥10% of EBC or ≥20 ml is considered significant [5].

Children with LUTD complicated by recurrent UTI and/or upper urinary tract dilation (Fig. 9.2), may need further investigations to detect:

- Secondary VUR and urethral anomalies (male), by means of micturition cystourethrography
- Renal parenchyma involvement, by means of renal scintigraphy

Technetium-99 m-dimercaptosuccinic acid (DMSA) is an excellent parenchymal imaging radiopharmaceutical, primarily used for detecting and defining pyelonephritis and renal cortical scars. Technetium-99 m mercaptoacetyl triglycine (MAG3) is rapidly extracted and secreted by tubular cells. It is used for evaluating obstructive uropathy. However, it may be useful in monitoring evolution of secondary VUR and in evaluating postvoiding residual urine.

9.3 Neurogenic Lower Urinary Tract Dysfunction [4, 17]

Neurogenic bladder dysfunction (NB) in children is an ever-evolving condition. In the mid-1950s, there were few insights and minimal alternatives to the children with NB. Starting with the development of adequate neurosurgical assessment and interventions and reliable urodynamic investigation, the advent of clean intermittent catheterization, various drug therapies, and urological surgical treatment modified long-term prognosis of children with NB. The most common cause of NB in children is neurospinal dysraphism, primarily an open back lesion, but an occult or closed dysraphic state is being diagnosed with more frequency, as neonatal spinal ultrasound and magnetic resonance imaging (MRI) are used with increasing regularity to visualize any lower midline spinal cutaneous or gluteal cleft malformation. Other causes of NB involving the spine include sacral agenesis, tethered spinal cord associated with imperforate anus, cloacal malformations, and spinal cord injuries from sporting injuries and motor vehicle accidents. Central nervous system abnormalities include spastic diplegia (cerebral palsy) and learning disabilities, that is, attention-deficit hyperactivity disorder (ADHD) or attention-deficit disorder (ADD). In 2012, ICCS defined indications and timing of investigations in children with NB (Fig. 9.3). The type of neurogenic LUTD is detected by UDS. UDS consists of the following components: transurethral double-lumen catheter to fill the bladder and record intravesical pressure; rectal balloon catheters which measure intra-abdominal pressure to identify artifacts of motion and monitor increases in abdominal pressure during the filling and emptying phases of UDS; external urethral sphincter electromyography (EMG), using a 24-gauge concentric needle electrode inserted perineally in boys or paraurethrally in girls and advanced into the skeletal muscle component of the sphincter until individual motor unit action potentials are seen or heard on a standard EMG recorder. Neurogenic DO is defined as any short-lived pressure rise of >15 cm H_2O from baseline before bladder capacity is reached. The examination findings are considered normal when there is an appropriate capacity, good compliant bladder, with no DO, and normal innervation of the sphincter with normal sacral reflexes, and an increase in sphincter activity during filling and complete silencing during emptying. An upper motor neuron lesion is present when there is DO and/or hyperactive EMG responses to sacral reflexes and/or a failure of the sphincter muscle, on EMG, to relax (either partially or completely) with a bladder contraction or leaking at capacity. A lower motor neuron lesion is noted when there are no contractions of the detrusor muscle (detrusor underactivity), and/or there is a degree of denervation, either partial or complete, in the sphincter muscle, with characteristic EMG changes in the motor units or no motor unit activity at all, respectively, and little or no response in the sphincter to sacral reflexes and/or bladder filling or emptying. UDS can be combined with fluoroscopic video-imaging (video-urodynamic study) using a dilute radio-opaque contrast agent to visualize the appearance of the bladder wall (Fig. 9.4) and bladder neck (Fig. 9.5) or to detect the presence of VUR (Fig. 9.6). In children with NB, evaluation of upper urinary tract is mandatory by means of ultrasonongraphy, voiding cystourethrography, and renoscintigraphy.

9.3.1 Renal Scintigraphy in Children with Lower Urinary Tract Dysfunction

In children with both neurogenic and nonneurogenic bladder dysfunction, the main indications of renal scintigraphy (RS) include:

1. History of recurrent febrile urinary tract infection to quantify renal function and detect parenchymal scarring
2. Secondary vesicoureteral reflux (VUR), to quantify renal function, detect parenchymal scarring, and monitor evolution of vesicoureteral reflux, avoiding micturition cystography
3. Symptomatic or relevant upper urinary tract dilatation without VUR to quantify renal function, detect parenchymal scarring, and evaluate obstruction

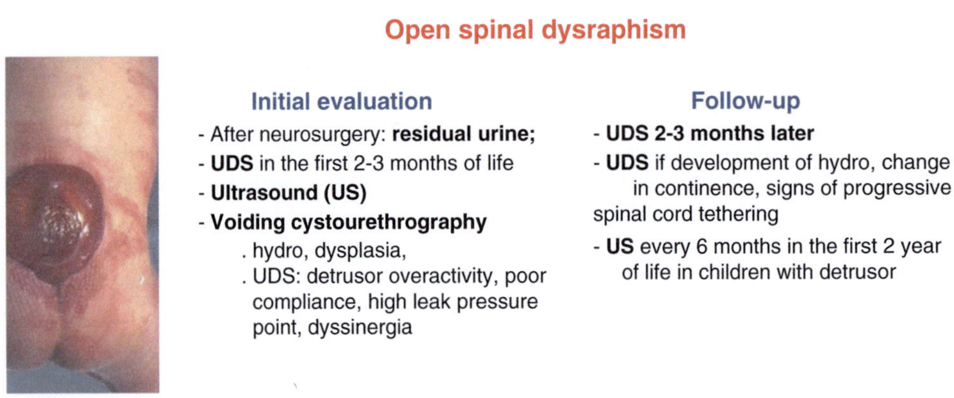

Fig. 9.3 ICCS recommendations for initial diagnostic evaluation and follow-up in congenital neuropathic bladder and bowel dysfunction in children

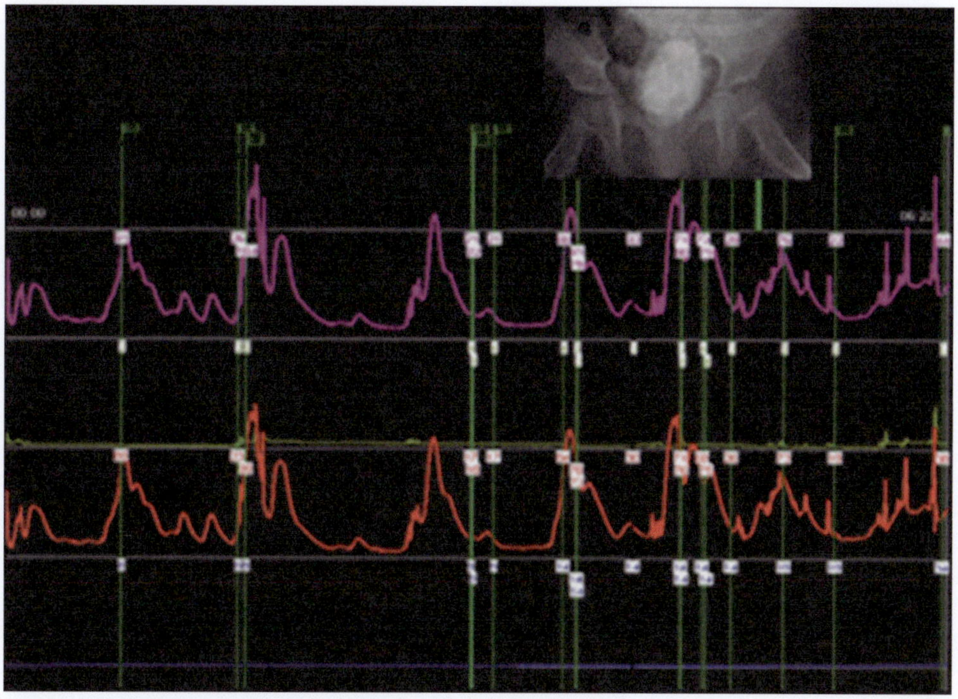

Fig. 9.4 Video-urodynamics in 2-year-old children with neuropathic bladder due to open spinal dysraphism: detrusor overactivity with bladder wall diverticula

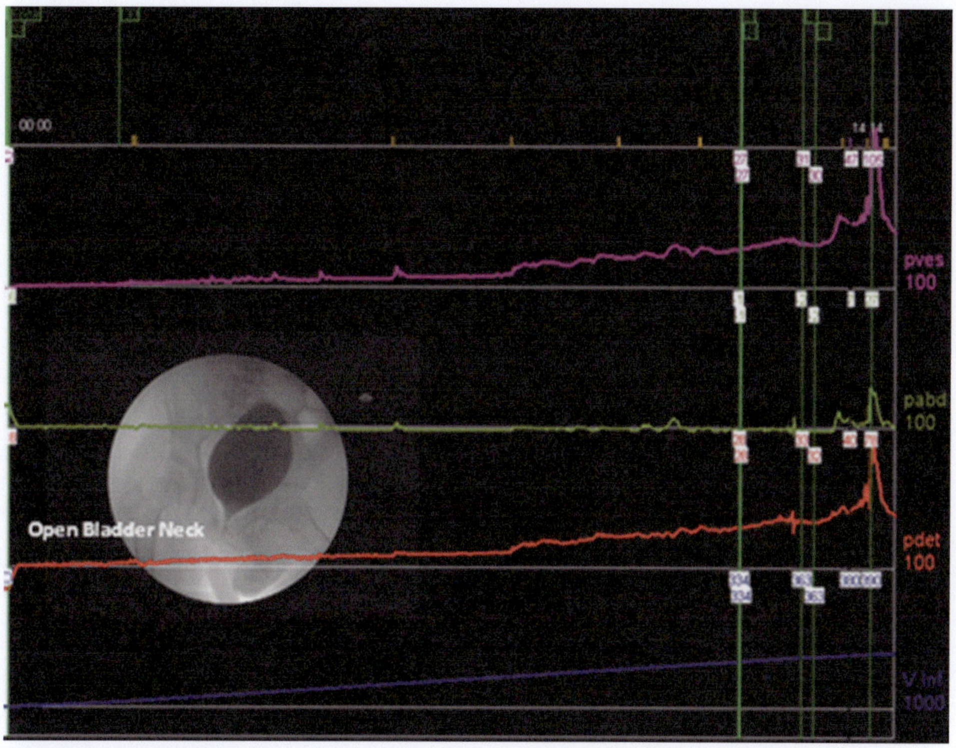

Fig. 9.5 Video-urodynamics in 14-year-old children with incontinence due to neurogenic bladder (NB) secondary to spinal cord injury: poor compliant and underactive NB with sphincter incompetence

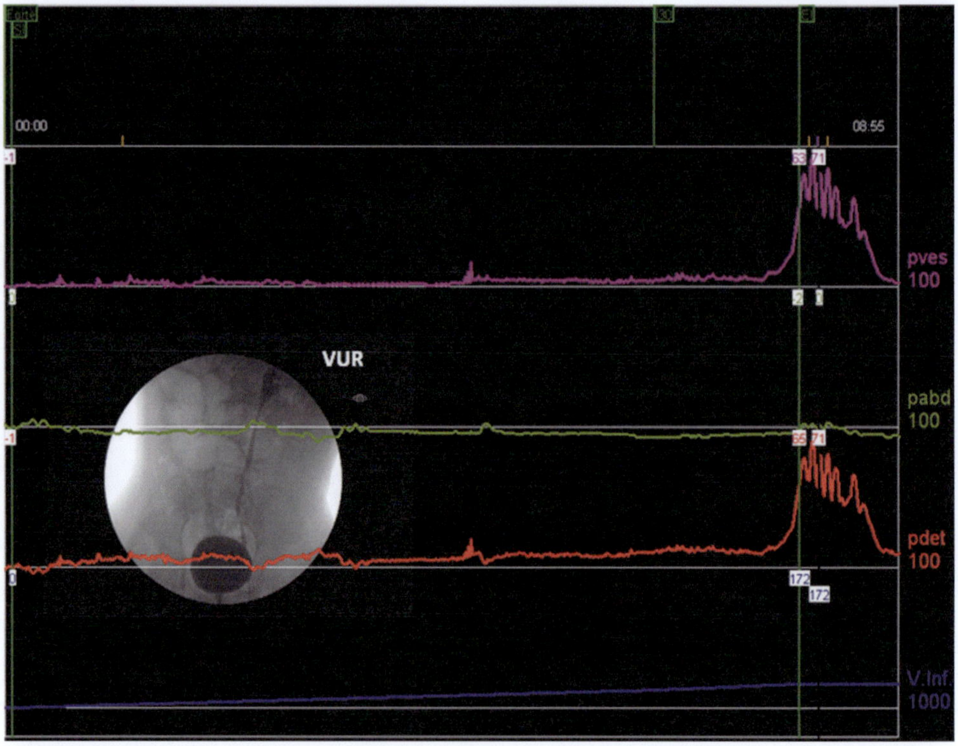

Fig. 9.6 Video-urodynamics in 10-year-old children with neuropathic bladder due to cerebral palsy: terminal detrusor overactivity with concomitant vesicoureteral reflux

Bibliography

1. Abidari JM, Shortliffe LM. Urinary incontinence in girls. Urol Clin North Am. 2002;29:661–75.
2. Abrams P, Cardozo L, Khoury S, Wein A. Incontinence. ICUD-EAU eds. 2013. Published by SMART-DOT, marketing & web consultants. Mtayleb - Lebanon
3. Austin PF, Bauer SB, Bower W, et al. The standardization of terminology of lower urinary tract function in children and adolescents: update report from the Standardization Committee of the International Children's Continence Society. Neurourol Urodyn. 2015;9999:1–11.
4. Bauer S, Austin F, Rawashdeh YF, et al. International Children's Continence Society's Recommendations for initial diagnostic evaluation and follow-up in congenital neuropathic bladder and bowel dysfunction in children. Neurourol Urodyn. 2012;31:610–4.
5. Bauer S, Nijman RJM, Drzewiecki BA, et al. International Children's Continence Society standardization report on urodynamic studies of the lower urinary tract in children. Neurourol Urodyn. 2015;34:640–7.
6. Chang SJ, Van Laecke E, Bauer S, et al. Treatment of daytime urinary incontinence: a standardization document from the International Children's Continence Society. Neurourol Urodyn. 2015. doi:10.1002/nau.22911.
7. Chase JW, et al. Functional constipation in children. J Urol. 2004;171:2641–3.
8. Cooper CS, et al. Do public school teach voiding dysfunction? Results of an elementary school teacher survey. J Urol. 2003;170:956–8.
9. De Gennaro M, Niero M, Capitanucci ML, et al. Validity of the international consultation on incontinence questionnaire-pediatric lower urinary tract symptoms: a screening questionnaire for children. J Urol. 2010;194:1662–7.
10. Ellsworth PI, Merguerian PA, Copening ME. Sexual abuse: another causative factor in dysfunctionl voiding. J Urol. 1995;153:773–6.
11. Griffiths DJ, Scholtmeijer RJ. Place of the free flow curve in the urodynamic investigation of children. Br J Urol. 1984;56:474–7.
12. Heaton KW, Radvan J, Cripps H, et al. Defecation frequency and timing and stool form in the general population: a prospective study. Gut. 1992;33:818–24.
13. Hoebeke P, Bower W, Combs A, De Jong T, Yang S. Diagnostic evaluation of children with daytime incontinence. J Urol. 2010;183:699–703.
14. Hoebeke P, et al. Anomalies of the external urethral meatus in girls with non-neurogenic bldder-sphincter dysfunction. BJU Int. 1999;83:294–8.
15. Mori R, Yonemoto N, Fitzgerald A, et al. Diagnostic performance of urine dipstick testing in children with suspected UTI: a systematic review of relationship with age and comparison with microscopy. Acta Paediatr. 2010;99(4):581–4.
16. Neveus T, von Gontard A, Hoebeke P, et al. The standardization of terminology of lower urinary tract function in children and adolescents: report from the Standardization Committee of the International Children's Continence Society. J Urol. 2006;176:314–24.
17. Rawashdeh YF, Austin P, Siggaard C, et al. International Children's Continence Society's recommendations for therapeutic intervention in congenital neuropathic bladder and bowel dysfunction in children. Neurourol Urodyn. 2012;31:615–20.
18. Sreedar B, Yeung CK, Leung VYF, Chu CW. Ultrasound bladder measurements in children with severe primary nocturnal enuresis: pretreatment and posttreatment evaluation and its correlation with treatment outcome. J Urol. 2008;179:1568–72.

10 Nephrourology: Bladder Dysfunctions

Maria Felicia Villani, Milena Pizzoferro, Mario De Gennaro, Maria Luisa Capitanucci, Giovanni Mosiello, and Maria Carmen Garganese

10.1 Study Technique and Interpretation

Study technique (dynamic renal scan, static renal scintigraphy and indirect radionuclide cystoscintigraphy) has been reported in the previous chapter.

10.2 Teaching Cases

10.2.1 Case 10.1 Incomplete Bladder Emptying in a Girl with Frequent UTI and Type 1 Glycogenosis

A 17-year-old girl, followed in our institution for type 1 glycogenosis and a prenatal diagnosis of renal hypoplasia, undergoes MAG3 dynamic renal scan and indirect radionuclide cystoscintigraphy (IRC) for frequent urinary tract infections (UTI) and dysuria without fever. Nuclear imaging is also required to determine differential renal function, in particular in hypoplastic kidney.

Renal scan shows a preserved function of right hypoplastic kidney, while IRC shows absence of vesicoureteral reflux (VUR), but detects incomplete bladder emptying. For this reason, the girl is scheduled for toilet and micturition training.

M.F. Villani • M. Pizzoferro
Nuclear Medicine Unit, Imaging Departement – "Bambino Gesù" Children Hospital, Rome, Italy

M. De Gennaro • G. Mosiello • M.L. Capitanucci (✉)
Unit of Urology, Robotic Surgery and Urodynamic, "Bambino Gesù" Children Hospital, Rome, Italy
e-mail: mluisa.capitanucci@opbg.net

M.C. Garganese
Diagnostic Imaging Department of Nuclear Medicine, IRCCS Bambino Gesù Paediatric Hospital, Rome, Italy

10.2.2 Case 10.2 Irregular Bladder Emptying in a Boy Previously Treated for VUR

A 4-year-old boy undergoes MAG3 dynamic renal scan and indirect radionuclide cystoscintigraphy (IRC) 1 year after endoscopic treatment of bilateral VUR in order to verify the efficacy of treatment. Renal scan confirms a known hypofunction of left kidney, and IRC shows absence of VUR and evidence of an irregular bladder emptying. Currently, the boy is still on follow-up, and he is asymptomatic.

10.2.3 Case 10.3 Difficult Micturition Without Evidence of VUR

A 13-year-old girl, treated at the age of 2 years for VUR, undergoes MAG3 dynamic renal scan and indirect radionuclide cystoscintigraphy (IRC) for recurrent fever and difficult and painful micturition. Renal scan shows hypofunction of right kidney while IRC confirms severe difficulty in micturition in the absence of vesicoureteral reflux (VUR). For this reason, the girl is scheduled for toilet and micturition training.

10.2.4 Case 10.4 Difficult Micturition with Evidence of VUR

A 3-year-old boy, previously treated for VUR, presents constipation, urinary retention habit, and recurrent episodes of pyelonephritis; therefore, a MAG3 scan with IRC is performed in order to evaluate renal function and to rule out the persistence of VUR. Renal scan shows bilateral scars with hypofunction of right kidney; IRC detects high-grade bilateral VUR and difficult micturition. Considering these findings, the boy undergoes bilateral ureteral reimplantation, and he is still on treatment for stipsis and on toilet training.

© Springer International Publishing Switzerland 2017
M.C. Garganese, G.F.L. D'Errico (eds.), *Conventional Nuclear Medicine in Pediatrics*, DOI 10.1007/978-3-319-43181-9_10

10.2.5 Case 10.5 Irregular Bladder Emptying with Scintigraphic Evidence of VUR

A 4-year-old girl is treated with toilet training for bilateral II grade VUR, probably due to detrusor sphincter dysynergia; during the treatment, a MAG3 renal scan with IRC is performed in order to evaluate renal function and to monitor training efficacy.

Renal scan shows normal function of both kidneys, while IRC shows a II grade right VUR and a possible low-grade left VUR; considering scintigraphic findings and the occurrence of further episodes of UTI although she is still on toilet training, the girl undergoes endoscopic correction of VUR.

10.2.6 Case 10.6 Evidence of VUR in Bladder Overfilling

IRC in a 6-year-old girl treated for left VUR at the age of 4. Frequent UTI and retentionist habit are referred during last year, despite toilet training program (Figs. 10.1, 10.2, 10.3, 10.4, 10.5, and 10.6).

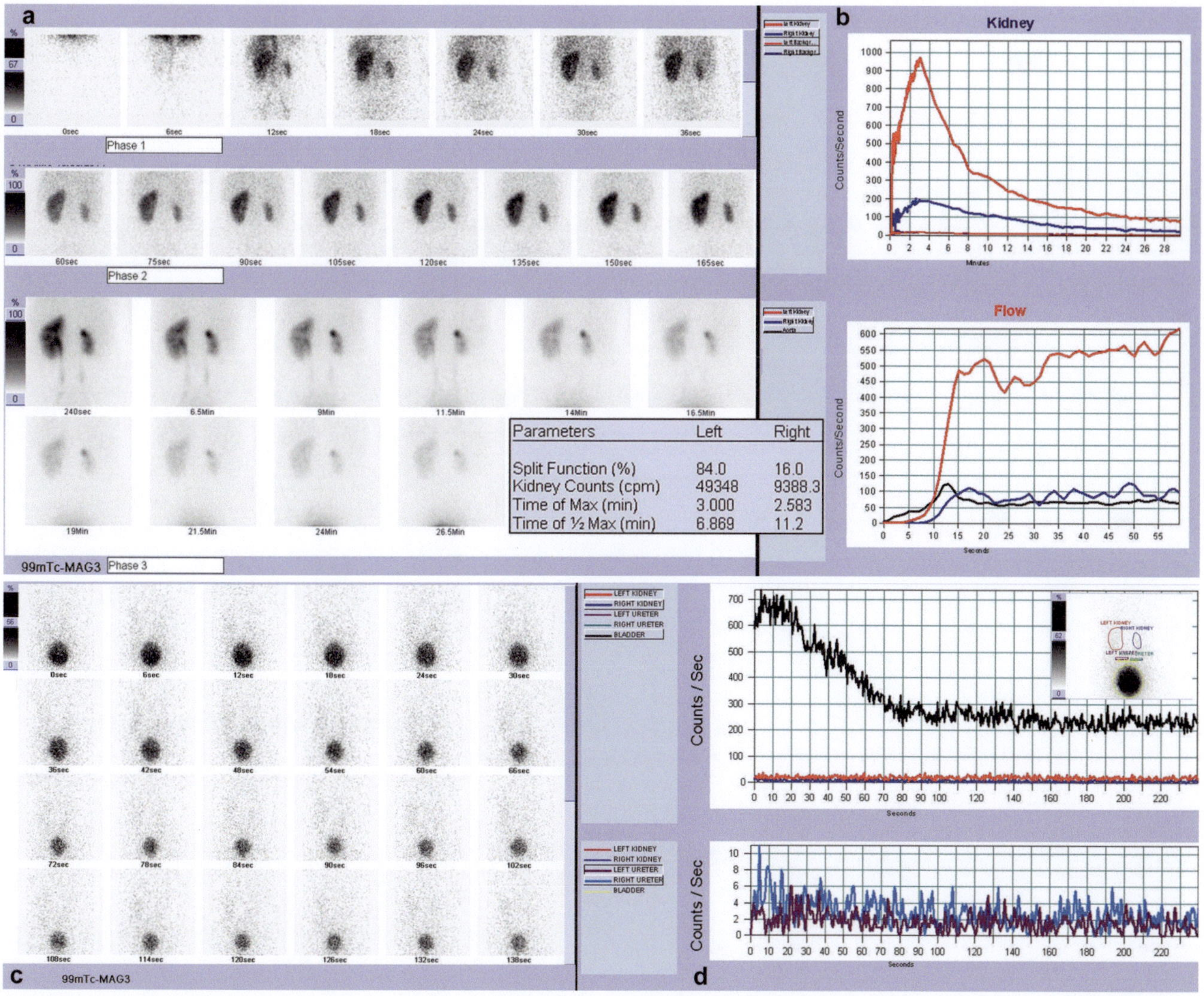

Fig. 10.1 MAG3 dynamic renal scan. Dynamic images (**a**) show good and homogeneous radiotracer uptake in *left* kidney. *Right* kidney is markedly smaller than the other one, with irregular shape and reduced uptake. Drainage is normal in both kidneys. *Left* renogram shows normal function and drainage; *right* renogram has low width, presents reduced slope of parenchymal phase and normal drainage. Flow T/A curves show synchronous but asymmetrical perfusion (reduced in *right* kidney) (**b**). IRC images (**c**) and time-activity curves (**d**) show regular but incomplete bladder emptying (30 % of residual radioactivity after voiding) and no evidence of VUR

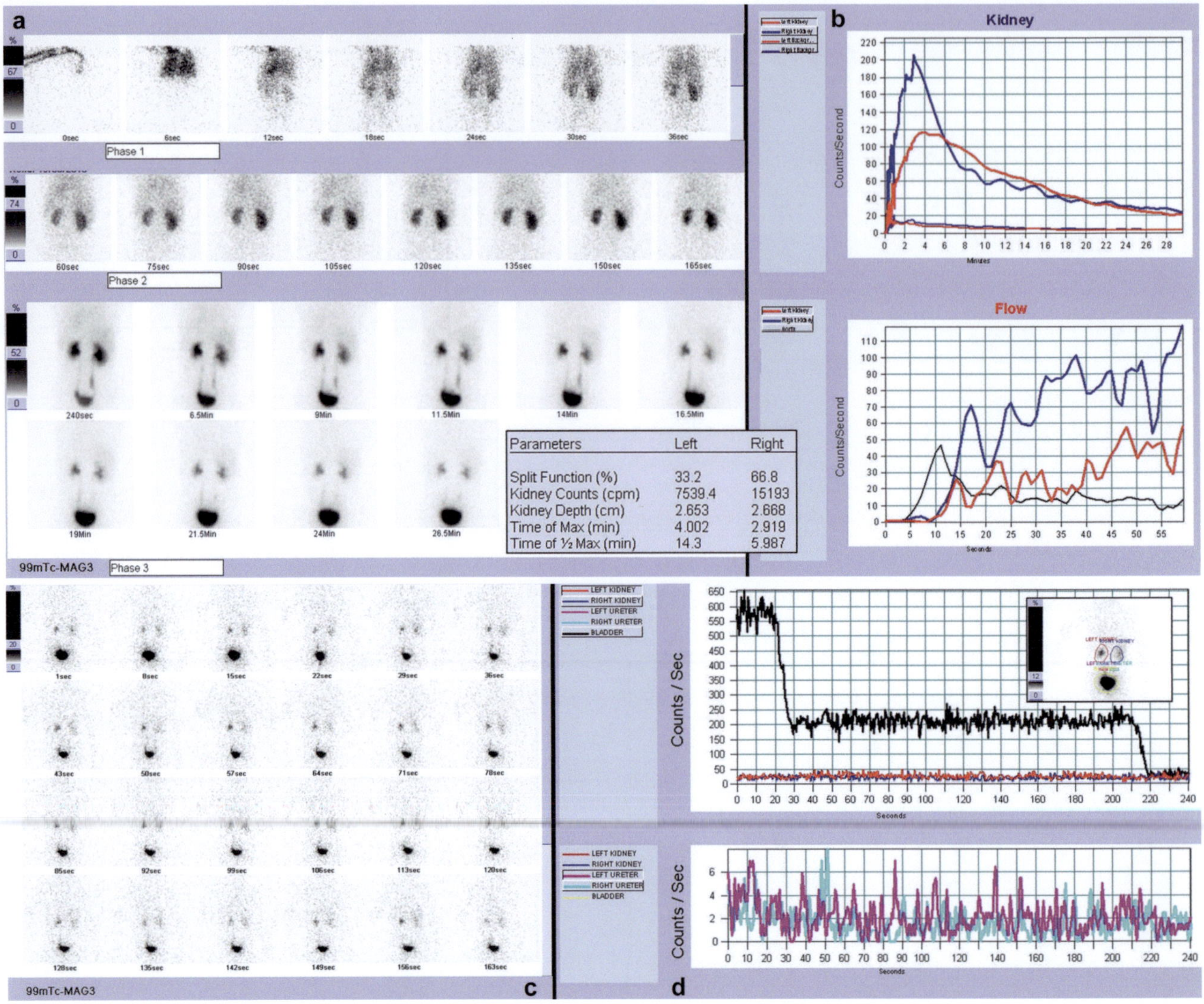

Fig. 10.2 MAG3 dynamic renal scan. Dynamic images (**a**) show reduction of uptake in left kidney, which is smaller than the other one, with irregular shape and normal drainage. *Right* kidney shows good and homogeneous radiotracer uptake and normal drainage. Renograms (**b**) confirm moderate hypofunction and normal drainage of *left* kidney and normal function and drainage of *right* kidney; flow T/A curves (**b**) show synchronous but asymmetrical perfusion (reduced in *left* kidney). IRC images (**c**) and time-activity curves (**d**) show complete but irregular bladder emptying and no evidence of VUR

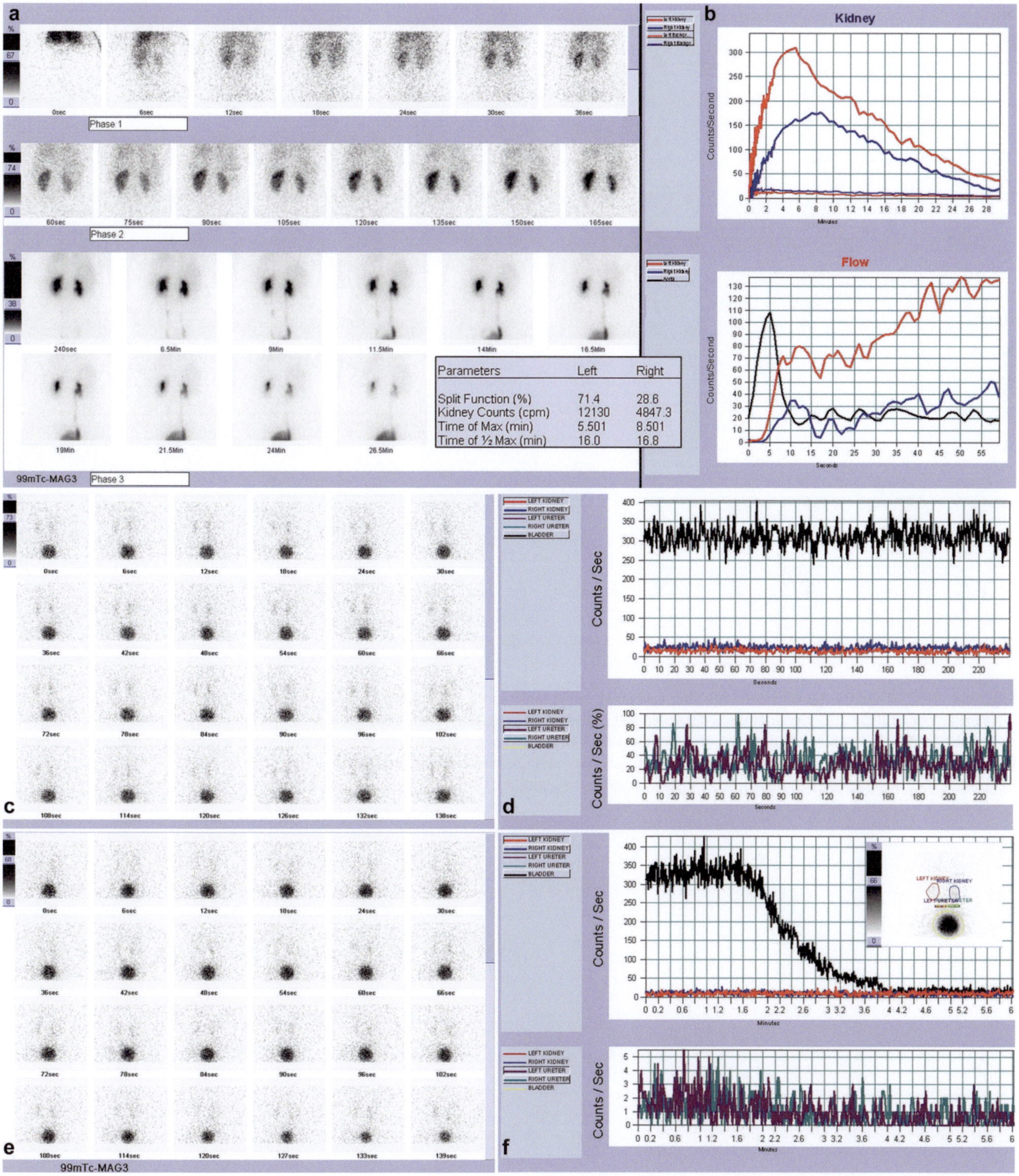

Fig. 10.3 MAG3 dynamic renal scan. Dynamic images (**a**) show good and homogeneous radiotracer uptake in *left* kidney. *Right* kidney is smaller than the other one, with irregular shape and reduction of uptake. Drainage is normal in both kidneys. *Left* renogram shows normal function and drainage; *right* kidney renogram has low width, reduced function, and normal drainage. Flow T/A curves (**b**) show synchronous but asymmetrical perfusion (reduced in *right* kidney). Micturition is obtained only after several attempts (all registered); one of these IRC registrations is displayed and shows no bladder emptying and no evidence of VUR (**c**, **d**); finally, voiding was obtained, and IRC images (**e**) and time-activity curves (**f**) show a complete and regular bladder emptying and no evidence of VUR

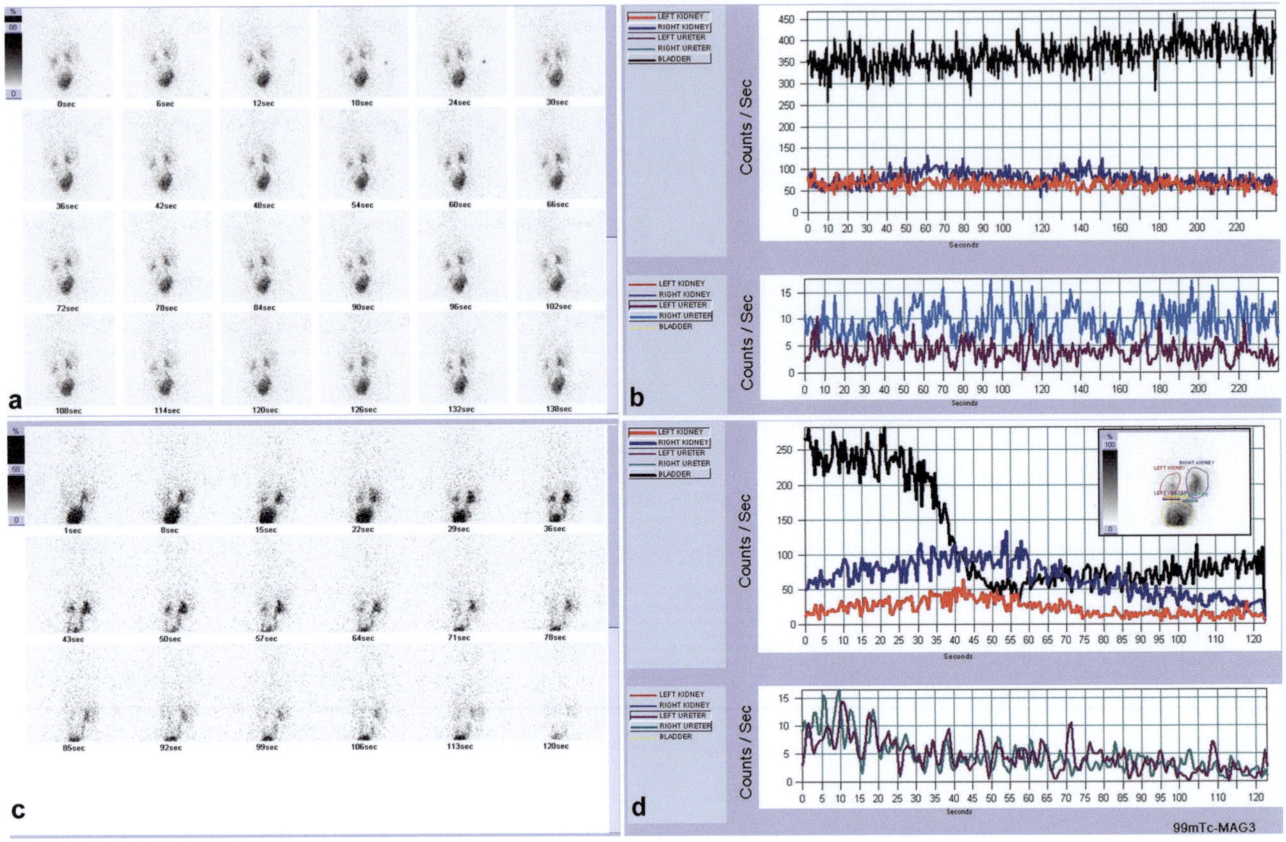

Fig. 10.4 IRC. Micturition is obtained only after several attempts (all registered); one of these IRC registrations is displayed and shows (**a**, **b**) no bladder emptying, but possible presence of radiourine reflux in right kidney that reaches the renal pelvis (interpretation of images and curves is difficult for the presence of urinary stasis in both renal pelvis and ureters). Finally, voiding is obtained, and IRC images (**c**) and time-activity curves (**d**) show a complete and regular bladder voiding with evidence of VUR in both kidneys that reaches the renal pelvis, which is bilaterally dilated (grade III)

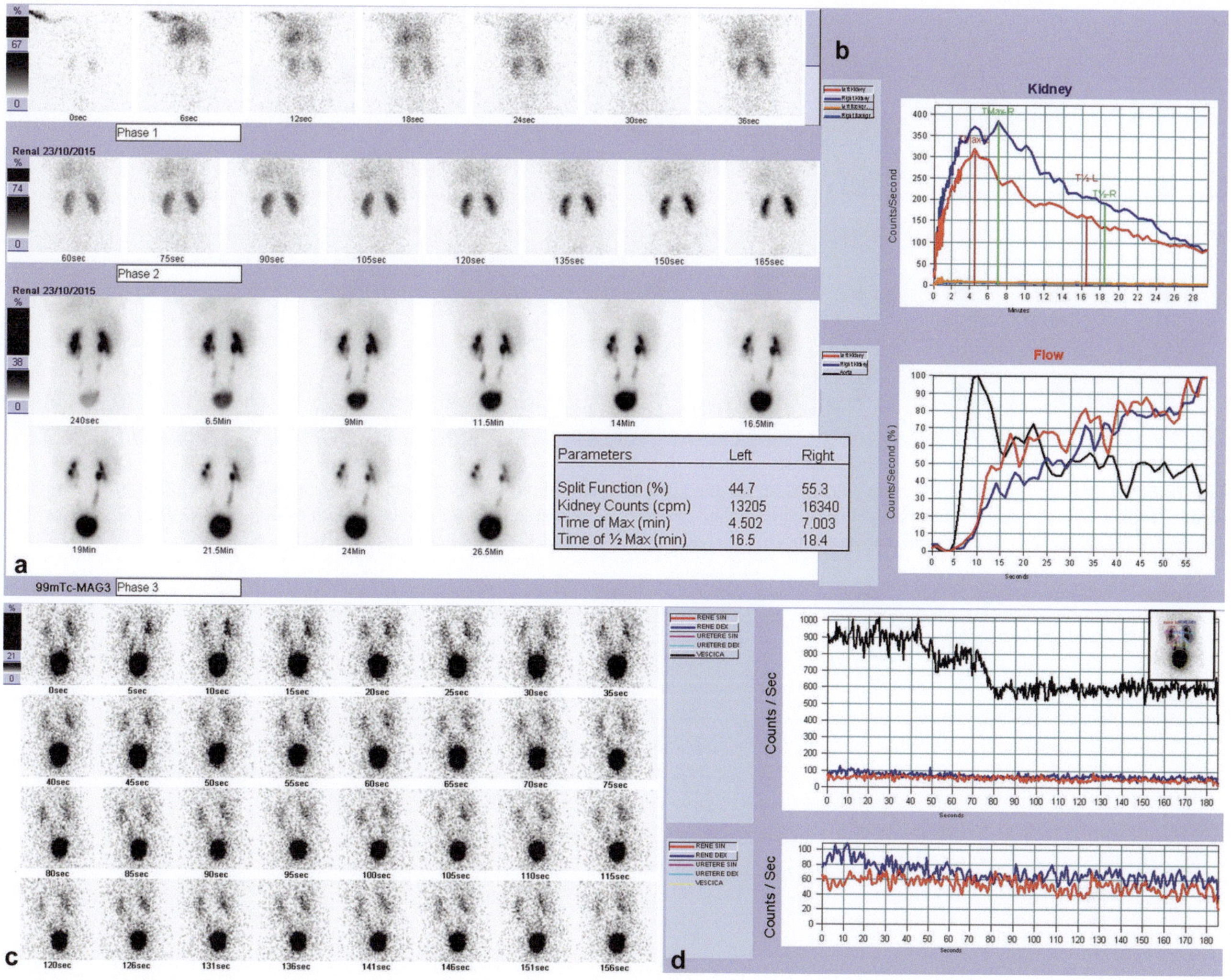

Fig. 10.5 MAG3 dynamic renal scan. Dynamic images (**a**) show good and homogeneous radiotracer uptake and normal drainage in both kidneys; renograms (**b**) confirm normal function and drainage of both kidneys. Flow T/A curves show synchronous and symmetrical perfusion. IRC images (**c**) and time-activity curves (**d**) show irregular and incomplete bladder emptying (60 % of postvoiding residual activity): for two times, a sudden interruption of urination is observed with evidence of VUR in *right* kidney that reaches the renal pelvis (grade II); a small amount of radiourine refluxed is also evident in *left* ureter

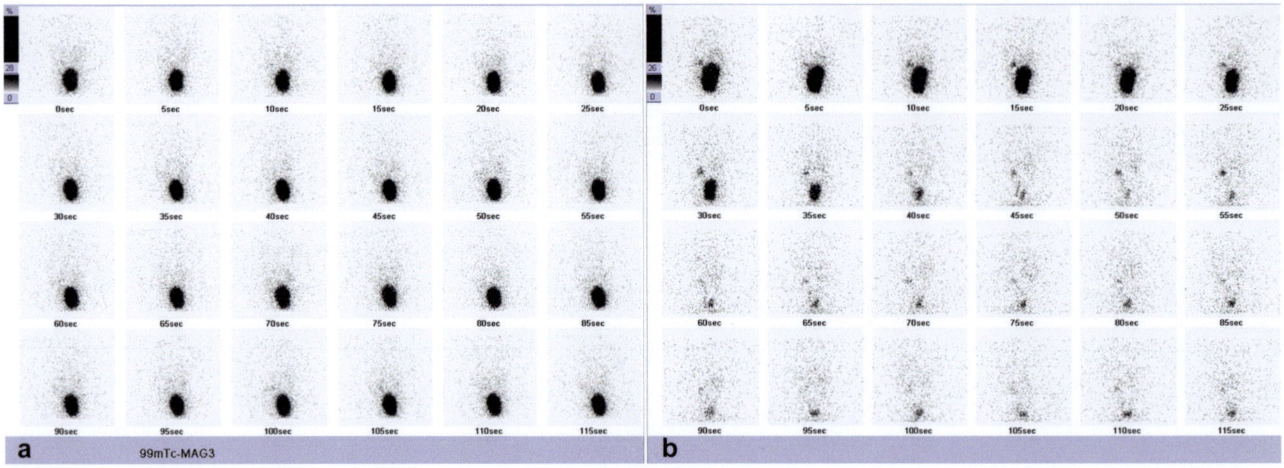

Fig. 10.6 At first attempt, the girl was not able to void, despite a good bladder filling; IRC images (**a**) show no bladder emptying and no evidence of VUR. After several hours and many attempts, the girl was able to void only when the bladder was overfilled. IRC (**b**) shows complete and regular bladder emptying with evidence of VUR in left kidney that reaches the renal pelvis (grade II–III)

10.2.7 Case 10.7 DMSA Renal Scan in Prune-Belly Syndrome

Prune-belly syndrome is a rare disorder characterized by poor development of the abdominal muscles (it causes wrinkles in the abdominal skin, which looks like a prune), cryptorchidism, and variable dilation of the lower urinary tract. In Fig. 10.7 is displayed a DMSA scan performed in a 1-year-old baby with prune-belly syndrome and bilateral VUR.

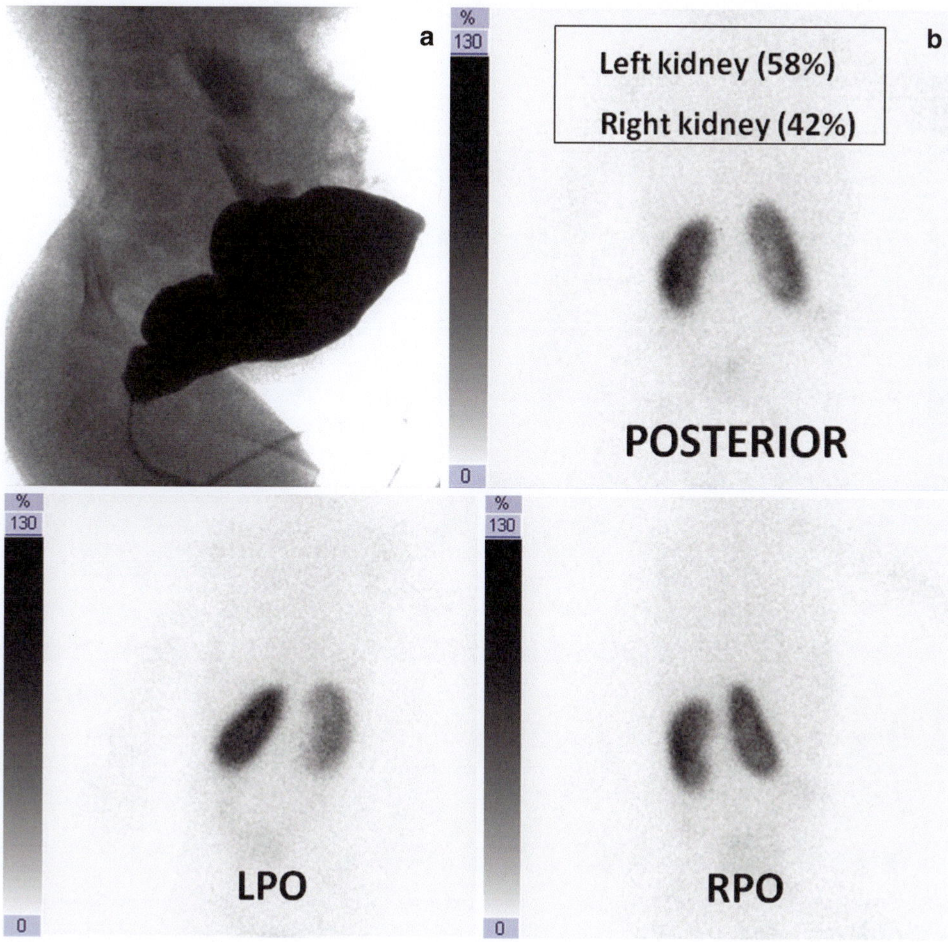

Fig. 10.7 (**a**) Cystography (lateral view) shows an abnormal, expanded bladder, and bilateral passive IV grade VUR with dilated ureters. (**b**) DMSA renal scan (posterior view, *LPO* view, and *RPO* view): *left* kidney shows good uptake of radiotracer and no evidence of cortical defects; *right* kidney is larger than the other one; it shows nonhomogeneous intraparenchymal distribution with multiple areas devoid of tracer corresponding to dilated renal pelvis and collecting system, without cortical defects

10.2.8 Case 10.8 Obstructive Uropathy in a Complicated Clinical Case

MAG3 renal scan in a 16-year-old girl with Down syndrome, previously treated for bilateral VUR, and neurogenic bladder due to ischemic event. During follow-up, bilateral hydronephrosis is observed, with progressive increase of dilatation. In this complicated case, renal scan is helpful in the evaluation of the whole urinary system (Fig. 10.8).

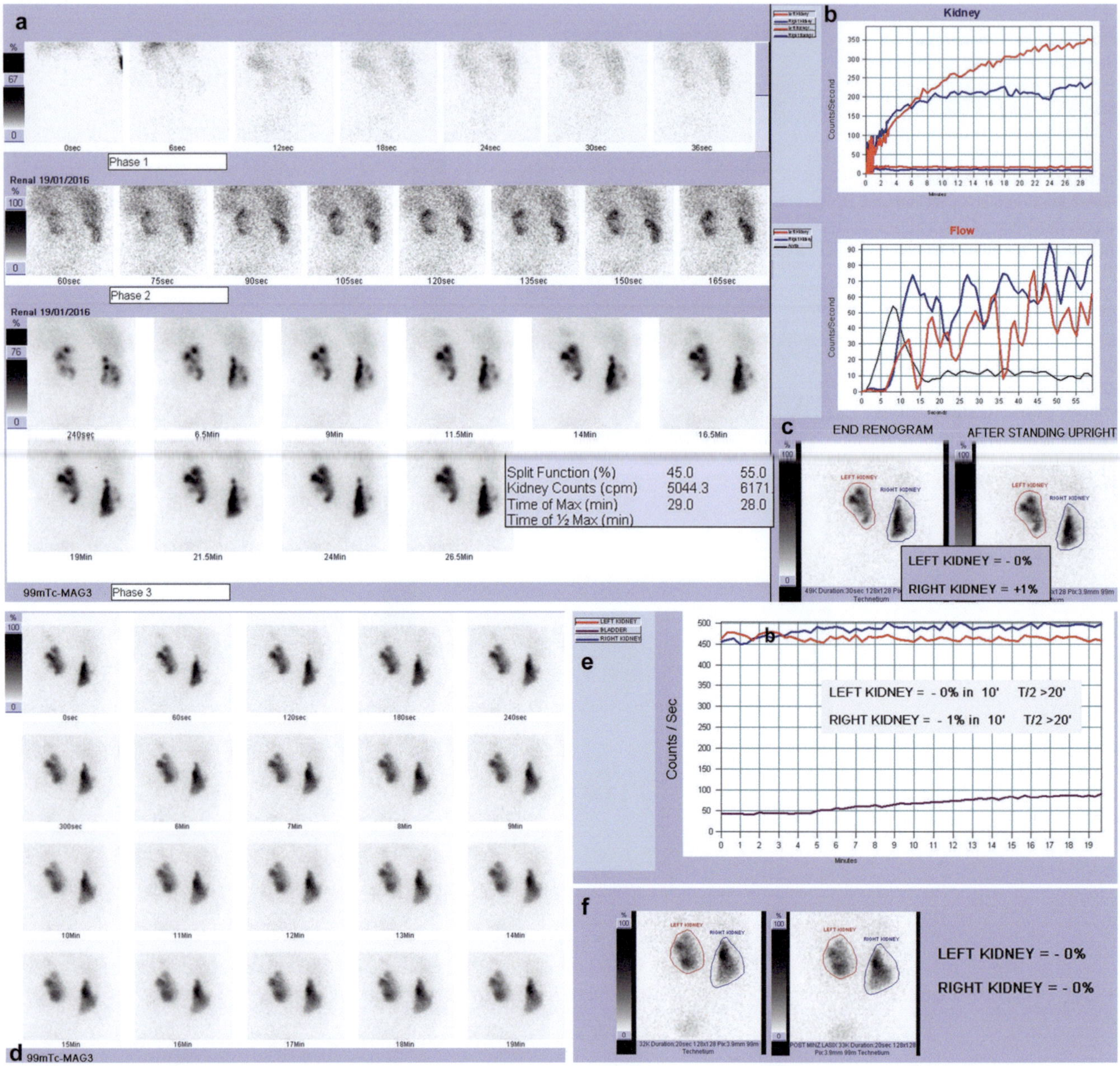

Fig. 10.8 MAG3 dynamic renal scan: dynamic images (**a**) show irregular shape of both kidneys, with evidence of multiple cortical defects and nonhomogeneous intraparenchymal radiotracer distribution with an area devoid of tracer corresponding to dilated renal pelvis; drainage is poor in both kidneys. A low target/background ratio is also evident. Renograms (**b**) show hypofunction and impaired drainage of both kidneys ("rising curves" in both kidneys); flow T/A curves (**b**) show synchronous and symmetrical perfusion. Gravity-assisted drainage-1 test (**c**) shows no significant improvement in drainage in both kidneys. Diuretic dynamic images (**d**) and diuretic renogram (**e**) show very slow response to furosemide and no significant improving in drainage in both kidneys. Drainage remains still poor even after gravity-assisted drainage-2 test (**f**)

Oncology

11

Luciana Vinti, Angela Mastronuzzi, Giuseppe Maria Milano,
Evelina Miele, Raffaele Cozza, and Franco Locatelli

11.1 Introduction

Although childhood cancer is rare, it is the second most common cause of death among children in Western countries, after accidents. Global incidence rate shows that there are 140–150 new cases for every million children aged 0–16. Childhood cancer rates have been rising slightly for the past few decades; increase in incidence has been attributed in part to improvements in diagnosis and changes in reporting patterns.

Thanks to investment in pediatric oncology, overall outlook for childhood cancer has improved greatly over the past 50 years. It is estimated that 65 % of children diagnosed with cancer can be successfully treated, so there is approximately 1 survivor of childhood cancer among 800–900 adults. Long-term survivors need follow-up care for the rest of their lives because of the risk of late effects (such as anthracycline-induced cardiotoxicity, higher breast cancer rates in women treated for Hodgkin's lymphoma with chest irradiation) that may occur many years after they complete treatment for cancer. This is the reason why a program that provides survivors of childhood cancer with lifelong health surveillance has to be planned and realized.

11.1.1 Acute Lymphoblastic Leukemia

Acute lymphoblastic leukemia (ALL) is the most common childhood cancer (accounting for 35 % of pediatric malignancies with 30–40 new cases for every million children aged 0–16) and represents a prototype of improvements in treatment and remarkable gains in survival. ALL accounts for about 80 % of leukemias and occurs at all ages, but the peak incidence is between 2 and 6 years of age.

L. Vinti • A. Mastronuzzi (✉) • G.M. Milano • E. Miele
R. Cozza • F. Locatelli
Pediatric Hematology and Oncology Department, "Bambino Gesù" Children Hospital, Rome, Italy
e-mail: angela.mastronuzzi@opbg.net

11.1.2 Non-Hodgkin's Lymphoma

Malignant lymphomas account for approximately 10 % of childhood cancers: in industrialized countries, they are the third most common neoplastic disease according to incidence rates. Lymphoma is a general term for a histologically heterogeneous group of neoplasms characterized by clonal proliferation of immunologically active cells (B, T, and NK lymphocytes). They are used to be divided into (HLs) and non-Hodgkin's lymphomas (NHLs).

NHL represents the most common lymphomatous neoplasm in children aged under 10 years, while HLs occur more frequently in adolescents. There are eight new cases of NHLs for every million children, and the peak incidence is between 7 and 10 years of age (extremely rare under 2 years).

Etiology of NHL remains unknown. Epstein Barr virus is associated with Burkitt lymphoma in equatorial Africa, but is observed only in 15 % of patients in Western countries. Unlike leukemias, NHLs arise from lymphoid tissues such as spleen, thymus, lymph nodes, and mucosa-associated lymphoid tissue (MALT). When neoplastic cells spread to the bone marrow (more than 25 %), malignant lymphoma turns into a leukemia.

Classification system for NHLs is very complex, but pediatric subtypes are basically four: Burkitt's lymphoma (T or B), lymphoblastic lymphoma, anaplastic large cells lymphoma (ALCL), and diffuse large B-cells lymphoma (DLBCL). Pediatric NHLs are highly aggressive with fast growing and dissemination, especially to extranodal sites.

Histological diagnosis of lymphoma is always required, and thus a biopsy is essential for the proper framing of the disease. Once NHL is diagnosed, tests are performed to determine the stage: whole body computer tomography (CT) scan can analyze primary site and any disseminations, while bone scintigraphy may reveal metastatic bone lesions. FDG-PET/CT scan detects metabolic activity both in primary localization and metastasis.

NHL staging system according to *St Jude Children's Research Hospital* criteria:

© Springer International Publishing Switzerland 2017
M.C. Garganese, G.F.L. D'Errico (eds.), *Conventional Nuclear Medicine in Pediatrics*, DOI 10.1007/978-3-319-43181-9_11

- Stage I: NHL is limited to one lymph node group (e.g., neck, underarm, groin, etc.) or tumor outside of the abdomen or mediastinum (middle chest)
- Stage II: NHL is limited to one tumor with local lymph node involvement, or NHL is limited to two or more tumors or lymph node groups on the same side of the diaphragm, or NHL is limited to a primary tumor of the gastrointestinal tract with/without involvement of the local lymph nodes.
- Stage III: NHL includes tumors or lymph node groups on both sides of the diaphragm, or any primary NHL tumor within the thorax (trunk) or extensive NHL within the abdomen, or any NHL around the spine or the outermost membrane of the brain and spinal cord (dura mater).
- Stage IV: NHL is in the bone marrow or central nervous system (CNS), with/without other sites of involvement. Bone marrow NHL is defined as 5 % malignant cells in an otherwise normal bone marrow with normal blood counts and smears. By contrast, lymphoblastic lymphoma that produces more than 25 % malignant cells in the bone marrow is defined as leukemia.

11.1.3 Hodgkin's Lymphoma

Hodgkin's lymphoma represents 6 % of childhood cancers and typically occurs in adolescents (more frequently in male), while it is extremely a rare entity in children under 6 years of age. Neoplastic cells (*Reed-Sternberg* or Hodgkin's cells) are usually derived from B lymphocytes in germinal center, and around 50 % of HL cases express EBV-encoded proteins.

HL is histologically classified into two groups: nodular lymphocyte-predominant and classic (subdivided into four pathological subtypes). Patients present painless enlargement of one or more lymph nodes (cervical and supraclavicular nodes are most frequently involved). Mediastinum is often affected and may be noticed on a chest radiograph. Definitive diagnosis is made by lymph node biopsy in order to accurately specify histological subtype. TC, bone scintigraphy, and PET/CT are also used during staging process.

The staging system for HL was initially developed by Ann Arbor, which was then revised in 1989:

- Stage I: single lymph node group
- Stage II: multiple lymph node groups on the same side of diaphragm
- Stage III: multiple lymph node groups on both sides of diaphragm
- Stage IV: multiple extranodal sites or lymph nodes and extranodal disease

X = bulky mass >10 cm. E = extranodal extension or single, isolated site of extranodal disease. A or B = B symptoms: weight loss >10 %, fever, drenching night sweats.

11.1.4 Langerhans Cell Histiocytosis

Langerhans cell histiocytosis (LCH) is a disorder with highly variable clinical presentation and biological behavior, characterized by proliferation and accumulation of cells phenotypically and functionally similar to the activated normal Langerhans cells (LCs) which move into tissues where they are not normally found, frequently involving bone and skin. Most cases of histiocytosis occur under the age of 15 years, and the incidence peak is in children aged 1–3 years.

A typical lesion consists of collections of LCs, interdigitating cells, and macrophages, accompanied by T lymphocytes with variable numbers of multinucleated giant histiocytes and eosinophils.

Staging is usually made by X-ray, CT scan, and scintigraphy. These disorders are often treated with chemotherapy and steroids; surgery may also be used for single or specific bone lesions.

Patients presenting with single bone LCH have a benign course and an excellent survival, while multifocal bone or multisystem LCH may have a risk of significant permanent sequelae. Multisystemic LCH (MS-LCH) with involvement/dysfunction of critical organs (e.g., liver, spleen, hematopoietic system) have a high risk of mortality.

MS-LCH patients initially responding well to treatment may experience disease reactivations that can lead to permanent consequences such as orthopedic problems, hormonal disorders, or neurological deficits.

11.1.5 Central Nervous System Tumors

Central nervous system (CNS) tumors are the second most common malignancies in children, after acute lymphoblastic leukemia, with a peak of incidence in the first decade. Today, CNS tumors represent the leading cause of death in children affected by any oncological diseases. They make up a very heterogeneous group, since tumors arise from different types of cells in the brain.

CNS tumors can be reported as sporadic case or linked to genetic predisposing syndrome, such as neurofibromatosis type I and II, Li-Fraumeni syndrome, Gorlin syndrome, and Turcot syndrome. Despite the classification of many different histotypes, all CNS tumors have biological characteristics in common: quite exclusively dissemination to cerebrospinal fluid (CSF), malignant features unless surgically resectable, and radiologically characteristic localization.

The most common types are medulloblastomas (25–30 %), low-grade (20–25 %), and high-grade (12–18 %) gliomas. Clinical presentation is variable as resulting from primary tumor localization, infiltration pattern, and patient's age. Subtentorial neoplasms may cause IV ventricle compression that leads to increased intracranial pressure and consequent manifestations (morning headache, vomiting, and visual problems). In supratentorial neoplasms, symptoms are only related to localization: seizure, severe headache, and focal neurological deficit.

Tests for brain tumors include neurological and ophthalmoscopic examination. Children presenting with focal symptoms or visual problems are required to undergo fundus photography. At present, magnetic resonance (MR) has replaced CT, which may be still the first scan to be used, especially in emergency.

Despite latest improvements in surgical procedures and radiochemotherapy combined treatment, survival in children affected by CNS tumors has slightly improved, and mortality has showed lesser decrease compared to other pediatric malignancies. Prognosis remains related to histological subtype (disease-free survival ranging from 5 % in Diffuse Intrinsic Pontine Gliomas (DIPGs) to 70–75 % in medulloblastoma).

11.1.6 Retinoblastoma

Retinoblastoma (RB) is the most relevant eye tumor in pediatric patients and accounts for approximately 3–4 % of all childhood cancers. About 60 % of affected individuals have unilateral RB with a mean age of 2 years, while the remaining 40 % have bilateral localization that develops earlier. In 40 % of cases, RB shows familial history, since RB gene mutations are germinal and inherited in an autosomal dominant pattern. Leukocoria represented the typical sign in large RB and, along with strabismus, may lead parents to refer child to ophthalmologists. Early diagnosis is essential for efficient treatment, which involves surgery and radiotherapy. At present, surgical removal (enucleation) is not needed for all retinoblastomas, especially for smaller and localized tumors.

11.1.7 Neuroblastoma

Neuroblastoma accounts for 8–10 % of all childhood tumors but shows the worst prognosis, especially for advanced stages. The incidence rate is about 1 new case per 7000 born children, and the average age is 19 months.

Neuroblastoma originates from in neural crest cells, often in the nerve tissue of the adrenal glands. There is a wide range in how neuroblastomas behave: it may grow slowly, while others spread quickly. In other cases, the cells sometimes mature on their own into normal ganglion cells and stop dividing (ganglioneuroma).

Children affected by neuroblastoma present with unspecific symptoms, usually related to primary or metastatic localization. Less frequently, it begins with spinal cord compression or *Claude-Bernard-Horner* syndrome, while opsoclonus-myoclonus syndrome is peculiar but rare.

In most cases, neuroblastoma cells secrete high levels of catecholamines detectable by blood or urine test; the two metabolites most often measured are homovanillic acid (HVA) and vanillylmandelic acid (VMA). Useful tests for diagnosis are ultrasonography, CT scan, and meta-iodobenzylguanidine (MIBG) scan, which are routinely used during diagnostic, staging, and monitoring processes.

For the neuroblastoma classification, see Chap. 12.

Prognosis in neuroblastoma patients is related to stage, age at diagnosis, presence of cytogenetic anomalies (e.g., n-Myc amplification), and histology. Advanced stages (III and IV) as well as Myc-amplified tumors show poor prognosis, while better survival rates are achieved in children under 1 year of age.

11.1.8 Other Abdominal Tumors

Nephroblastoma, or Wilm's tumor (WT), is the most common childhood abdominal malignancy. It represents a model of hereditary neoplastic disease, as WT is associated to WT1 or WT2 gene mutation, mapped on chromosome 11.

Diagnosis is often accidental or driven by the presence of abdominal mass. In only 20–30 % of WT cases, children present macroscopic hematuria and unspecific symptoms, while hypertension occurs in less than 25 % (due to renin production or renal artery compression). Nephrectomy defines conclusive histology, while ultrasonography and CT scan are required for tumor extension.

Thanks to combined treatments and multidisciplinary approach, at present, more than 90 % of children affected by localized WT and 60 % of metastatic patients can be cured.

Hepatoblastoma is a malignant hepatic tumor and is the most common pediatric liver cancer, followed by hepatocellular carcinoma. Liver tumors usually begin as asymptomatic abdominal mass, sometimes associated with anorexia, weight loss, and vomiting, while jaundice is rare at diagnosis. Alpha-fetoprotein (AFP) levels are commonly elevated (80–90 % of cases) and lead to ultrasonography and CT scan to define diagnosis, while liver biopsy allows final histological characterization.

Staging and prognosis classification are related to disease extension to hepatic sections (PRETEXT system):

- I: One section is involved, and three adjoining sections are free
- II: One or two sections are involved, but two adjoining sections are free
- III: Two or three sections are involved, and no two adjoining sections are free
- IV: All four sections are involved

11.1.9 Soft Tissue and Bone Tumors

Sarcoma is the general term for malignant neoplasms that start from mesenchymal cells. The most common soft tissue sarcoma is represented by rhabdomyosarcoma, where neoplastic cells are committed toward striated musculoskeletal differentiation, but may occur outside striated muscular tissue. Rhabdomyosarcoma accounts for half the sarcomas and 4–8 % of all childhood cancers. It belongs to small, blue, round-cell tumor group and is classified into histological subtypes:

- Embryonal
- Alveolar
- Botryoid
- Anaplastic
- Pleomorphic

Biopsy is required to define histology of soft tissue lesions that cannot be distinguished by clinical presentation. Radiological imaging (X-rays, CT, and RM) and bone scintigraphy are essential to determine tumor extensions, treatment, and prognosis. Rhabdomyosarcoma needs a multidisciplinary approach, but surgery still plays the main role.

On the contrary, osteosarcoma and Ewing's sarcoma are the most important bone tumors in children. The peak incidence is under 20 years, as fast bone growth is suspected to contribute to the development of osteosarcoma. Primary localizations are typically long bones, especially distal femur and proximal tibia. Usual clinical symptoms are mild pain for weeks, accompanied by swelling and limitation of motion, or fracture with minor trauma.

Several subtypes of osteosarcoma may be identified on X-rays (e.g., Codman's triangle) and biopsy above all; the biopsy of suspected bone tumor should be performed by a qualified orthopedic oncologist. A complete surgical resection of the tumor is the treatment of choice in osteosarcoma, while chemotherapy is usually administrered before surgery (neoadjuvant chemotherapy).

11.1.10 Germ Cell Tumors

Reproductive system cancers are rare in children and may originate from both germ (80 %) and stromal (10–20 %) cells. Germ cell tumors (GCTs) may develop not only ovary and testis, but extragonadal localization is typical in newborns and children under 3 years. GCTs can also involve the CNS. GCTs classification includes teratomas (mature and immature) and malignant GCTs. The latter are generally divided into the following:

- Germinomatous: dysgerminoma (ovary) and seminoma (testis)
- Nongerminomatous GCTs: yolk sac tumor, embryonal carcinoma, choriocarcinoma, and combined tumors

Genital tumors usually present with abdominal mass in girls and swelling testicles in boys, painless or accompanied by dull ache; ultrasonography is often the first test to be performed, followed by CT and MRI scan. Serum tumor markers, such as alpha-fetoprotein and human chorionic gonadotropin, may be detected in blood and guide clinicians in diagnosis, staging, and surveillance of patients.

Bibliography

1. Lanzkowsky P. Lanzkowsky's Manual of Pediatric Hematology and Oncology. 6th ed. ISBN: 978-0-12-801368-7. Elsevier Inc.
2. Pizzo PA, Poplack DG. Principles and practice of pediatric oncology. 7th ed. 2015. Wolters Kluwer- Philadelphia-Baltimore-New York- London- Buenos Aires- Hong Kong- Sidney-Tokyo. ISBN/ISSN :9781451194234.

Oncology: Solid Mass in Pediatrics and Malignant Bone Involvement

12

Maria Felicia Villani, Milena Pizzoferro, Luciana Vinti, Angela Mastronuzzi, Antonella Cacchione, Roberta Lombardi, Domenico Barbuti, Evelina Miele, and Maria Carmen Garganese

12.1 Study Technique and Interpretation

12.1.1 123I-MIBG Scintigraphy

Study technique has been reported in Chap. 13.

12.1.2 ^{99m}Tc-MDP Bone Scintigraphy

Whole-body bone scintigraphy is acquired 3 h after intravenous injection of Tc-99 m-MDP (methylene diphosphonate). The administered activity of radiotracer is adjusted to the patient's weight, according to EANM dosage card and to the national regulations.

Additional static scan and/or SPECT (single photon emission tomography) acquisition of interested skeletal segment are eventually performed, when required. SPECT images are also manually fused with CT and/or MRI when available.

In very young or uncooperative children, multiple static views of all skeletal segments can be performed, instead of whole-body acquisition.

M.F. Villani • M. Pizzoferro
Nuclear Medicine Unit, Imaging Departement – "Bambino Gesù" Children Hospital, Rome, Italy

L. Vinti (✉) • A. Mastronuzzi • A. Cacchione • E. Miele
Oncohematology Department, "Bambino Gesù" Children Hospital, Rome, Italy
e-mail: luciana.vinti@opbg.net

R. Lombardi • D. Barbuti
Imaging Department, "Bambino Gesù" Children Hospital, Rome, Italy

M.C. Garganese
Diagnostic Imaging Department of Nuclear Medicine, IRCCS Bambino Gesù Paediatric Hospital, Rome, Italy

12.2 Teaching Cases

12.2.1 Case 12.1 MIBG Scintigraphy in Diagnostic Workup of Abdominal Mass: MIBG-Avid Lesion

A 2-month-old baby underwent an ultrasonography for incidental finding of abdominal swelling; the study showed an abdominal mass, and following CT (Fig. 12.1a, b) defined the lesion as a retroperitoneal large tumor, suspected for neuroblastoma. During the hospitalization, arterial hypertension was diagnosed. A MIBG scintigraphy was then asked in order to verify if the lesion shows MIBG uptake and, in turn, to confirm the diagnostic hypothesis (Fig. 12.1c–e). Scintigraphy confirmed a MIBG-avid lesion, without secondary involvement. Diagnostic hypothesis was verified, and histological examination confirmed the diagnosis of poor neuroblastoma stroma. The genomic profile showed the presence of numerical chromosomal aberration, NMYC nonamplified.

The patient was enrolled in LINES protocol stage L2 <18 months NCA genomic profile with life-threatening symptoms (arterial hypertension).

The patient received chemotherapy according to the protocol, and because of the persistence of arterial hypertension, the chemotherapy was prolonged for a total two courses of carboplatin/etoposide plus two courses of cyclophosphamide/vincristine/doxorubicin. The patient underwent surgery at the end of chemotherapy.

© Springer International Publishing Switzerland 2017

M.C. Garganese, G.F.L. D'Errico (eds.), *Conventional Nuclear Medicine in Pediatrics*, DOI 10.1007/978-3-319-43181-9_12

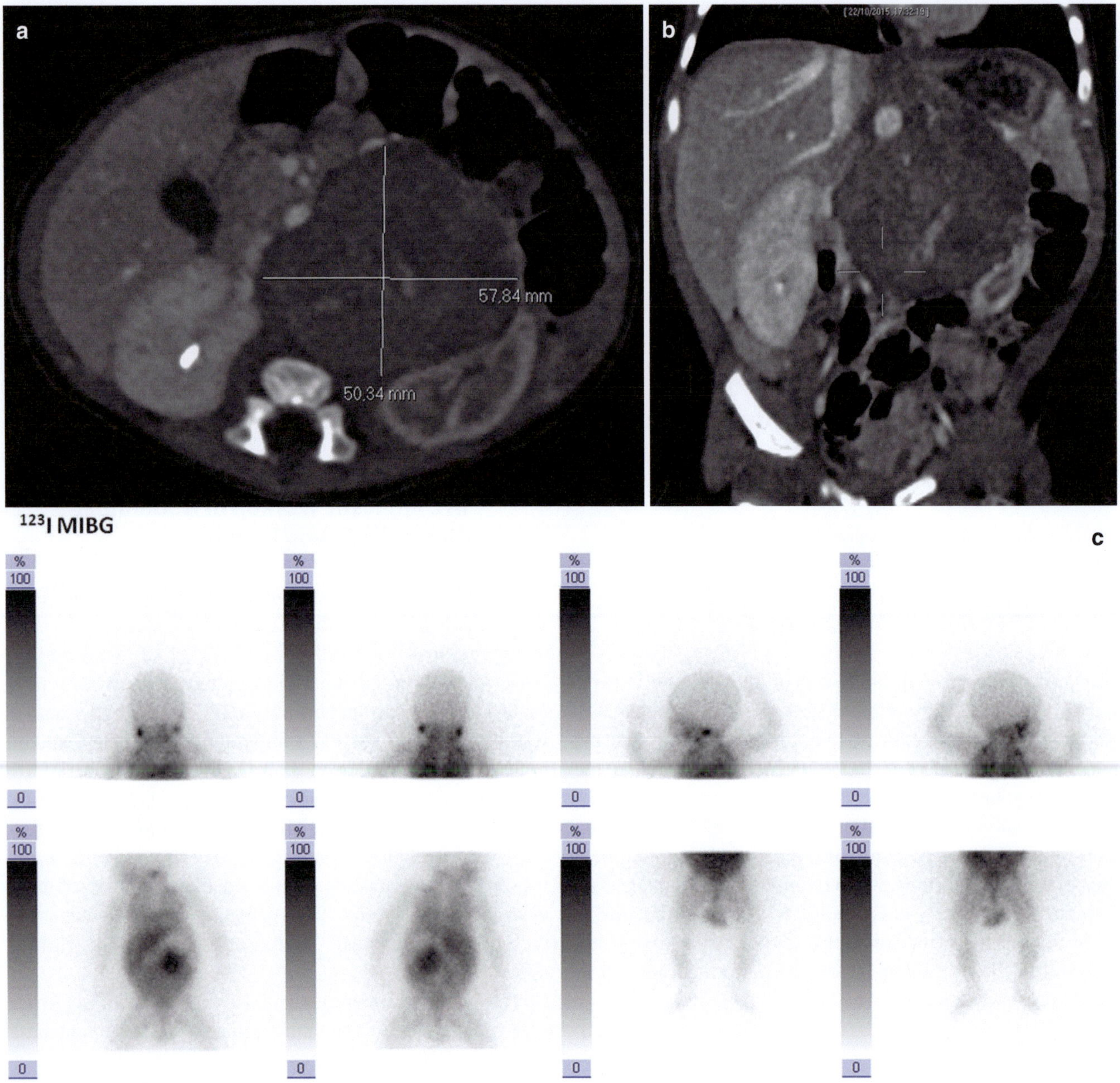

Fig. 12.1 (**a**, **b**) Contrast-enhanced CT. Axial (a) and MPR coronal (**b**) images showed a large retroperitoneal mass, appearing not homogeneously hypodense for the presence of multiple nonenhancing necrotic areas and tiny calcifications in the contest. The lesion, growing behind the aorta, encased left renal artery and displaced left adrenal gland and left kidney; abdominal aorta and inferior cava were pervious, although stretched, flattened, and displaced anteriorly, as well as the splenic vessels, pancreatic tail, and left renal vein. (**c**–**e**) MIBG scintigraphy (static views, **c**) showed an area of intense radiotracer uptake in the left abdomen, crossing the median line; no other areas of pathological uptake of radiotracer were evident. SPET-CT fused images (**d**, **e**) better defined that the area of uptake corresponded to the mass detected by CT

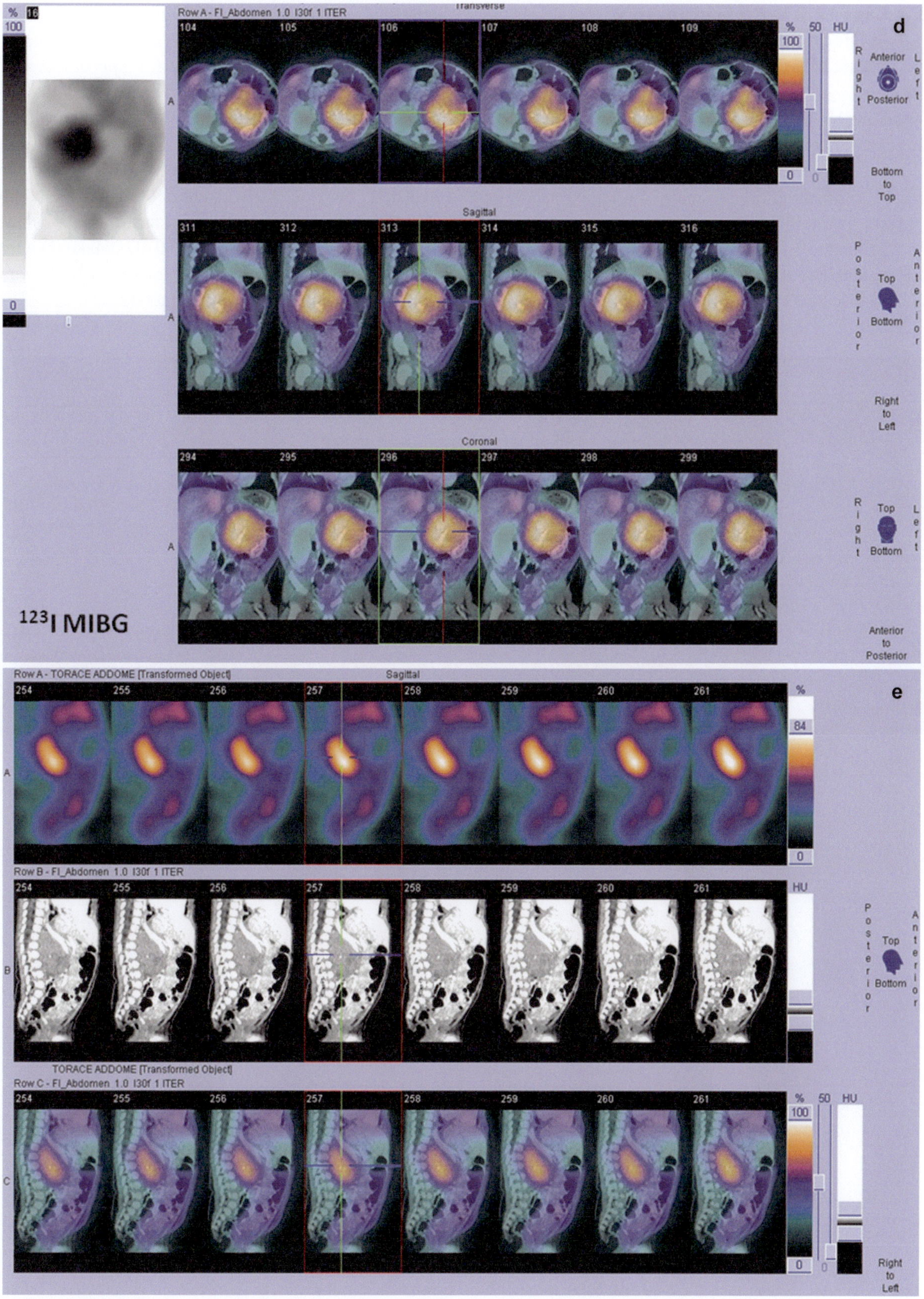

Fig. 12.1 (continued)

12.2.2 Case 12.2 MIBG Scintigraphy in Diagnostic Workup of Abdominal Mass: MIBG – Nonavid Lesion

A 2-year-old baby referred to our hospital for fever and limping; an ultrasonography revealed a median retroperitoneal lesion; therefore, a computed tomography (CT) was performed, confirming the presence of a large retroperitoneal mass, extending from celiac artery to mesenteric artery, suspected for neuroblastoma (Fig. 12.2a–c) Therefore, a MIBG scintigraphy was scheduled in order to verify if the lesion shows MIBG uptake, confirming the diagnosis. MIBG scintigraphy (Fig. 12.2d–e) did not show any area of pathological uptake of radiotracer; in particular, the abdominal lesion detected by CT appears as nonavid MIBG.

Subsequently, a biopsy of the lesion was performed, and histological examination showed a ganglioneuroma. As in this case, MIBG uptake and proliferative activity are strictly correlated, because MIBG reflects metabolic activity of tumor derived from neural crest; in fact, tumors with a high proliferative activity show higher MIBG uptake than lesions with lesser proliferation, such as ganglioneuromas or ganglioneuroblastoma, as reported in literature.

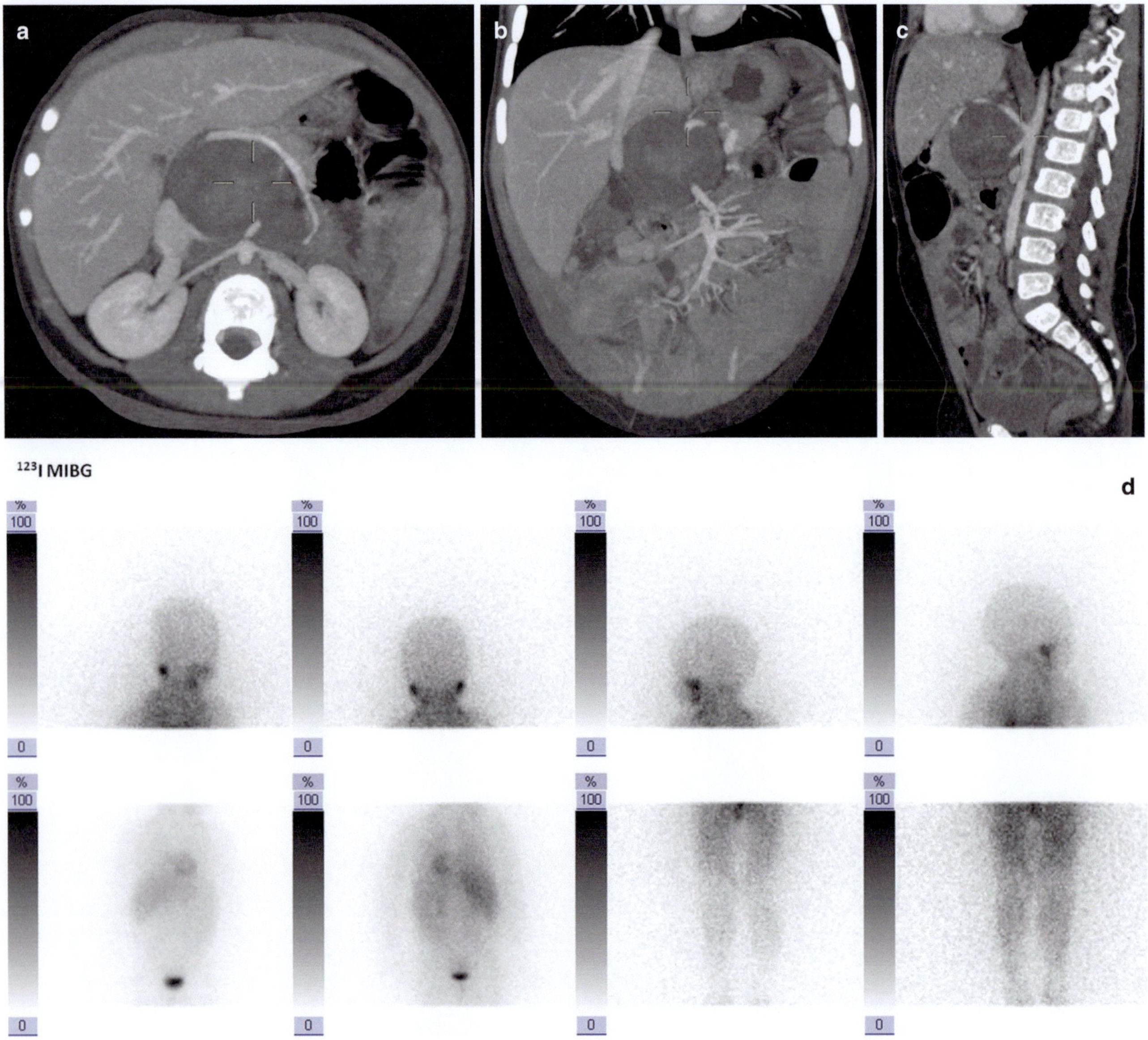

Fig. 12.2 (**a–c**) Contrast-enhanced CT axial (**a**), MPR coronal (**b**), and sagittal (**c**) images showed a large retroperitoneal mass, appearing polylobulated with well-defined borders, about 55 × 65 × 45 mm in size. The mass grew on the midline, between celiac artery and superior mesentery artery that were stretched and displaced, respectively, upper and lower in the abdomen. The lesion displaced inferior cava vein, pancreatic head and body, and portal vein, without signs of infiltration. There were also multiple enlarged nodes in mesenteric fat. (**d**, **e**) MIBG scintigraphy (static views, **d**) did not show any area of pathological uptake of radiotracer; in particular, the abdominal lesion detected by CT appeared as nonavid of MIBG. SPET-CT fused images (**e**) confirmed this finding

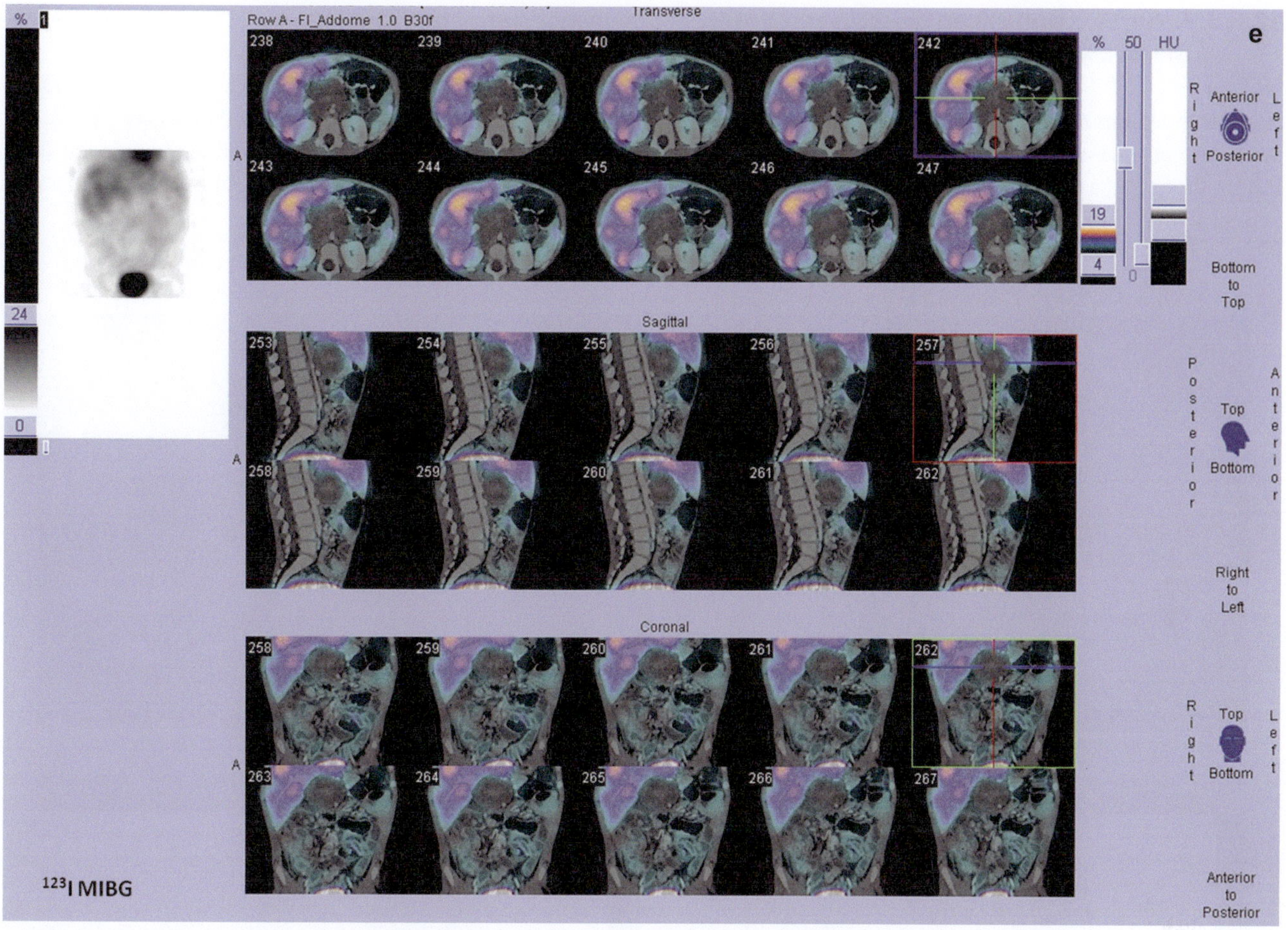

Fig. 12.2 (continued)

12.2.3 Case 12.3 Bone Scan in Paravertebral Mass: Ewing's Sarcoma

An 8-year-old girl referred to our hospital for dorsal pain and swelling; an ultrasonography revealed a right paravertebral lesion; therefore, a CT was performed, showing a large paravertebral mass, located above the right kidney, involving posterior segments of the ribs (Fig. 12.3a, b); histological examination indicated Ewing's sarcoma/PNET. The girl underwent a whole-body bone scan as part of diagnostic workup. Scintigraphy shows diffuse radiotracer uptake by right XII rib, without other pathological findings in the skeleton (Fig. 12.3c), and the girl was scheduled for therapy, adequate for tumor stage.

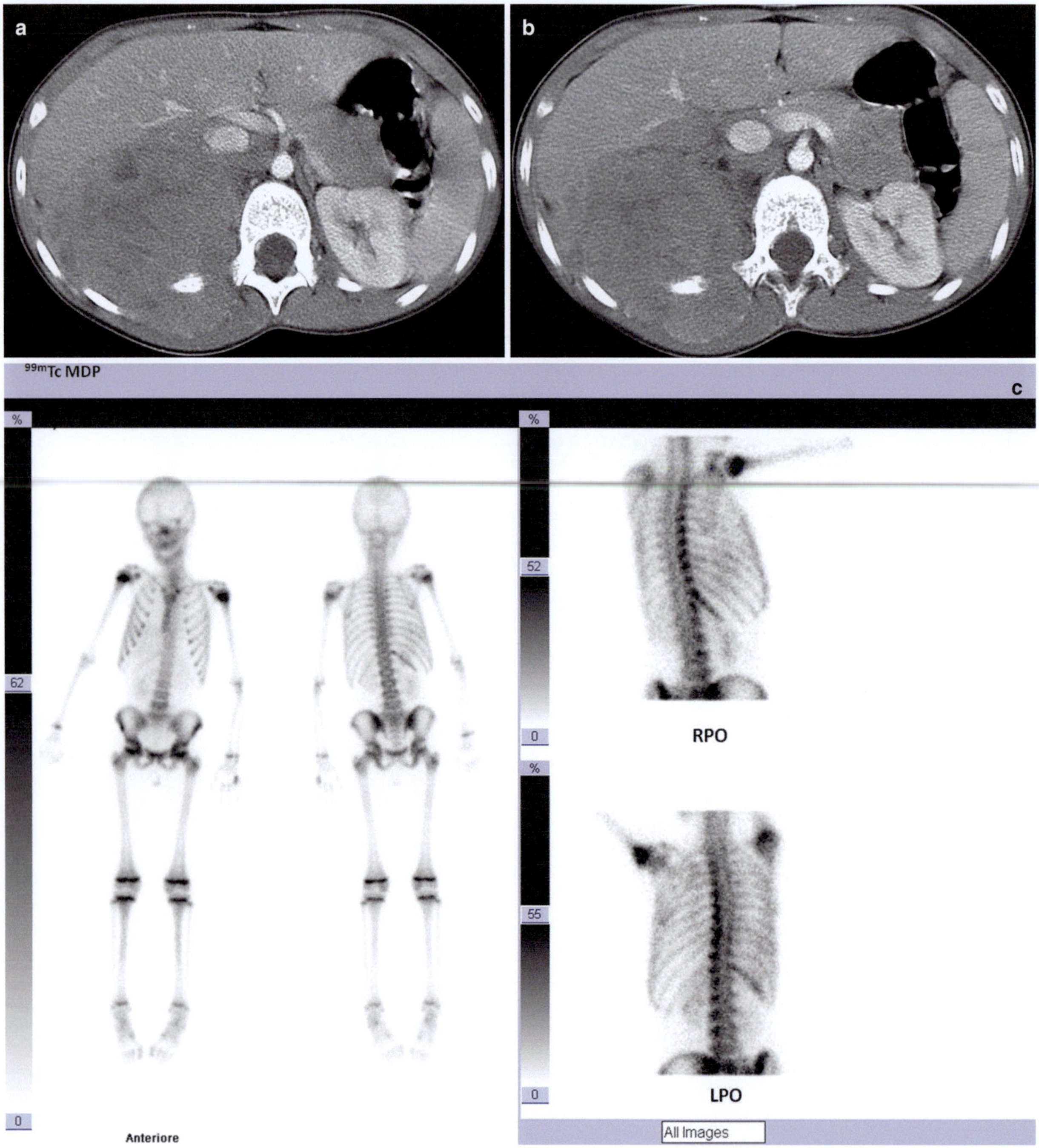

Fig. 12.3 (**a**, **b**) Contrast-enhanced CT axial (**a**, **b**) showed a large right suprarenal mass (about 8 × 8 × 15 cm in size), extending above and below the diaphragm with encasement of the back ribs and of the regional muscle tissue. The lesion, appearing nonhomogeneous after contrast agent administration, dislocated the right kidney inferiorly; liver and inferior cava vein were anteriorly compressed. (**c**) ^{99m}Tc-MDP whole-body scan; right posterior oblique (*RPO*) and left posterior oblique (*LPO*) views of thorax: a pathological, intense, and diffuse radiotracer uptake is evident in right XII rib; no other pathological findings are evident in the skeleton

12.2.4 Case 12.4 Bone Scan in Thoracic Wall Sarcoma: Evidence of Bone Metastases

A 15-year-old girl referred to our institution for swelling in correspondence to one of the last ribs of right hemithorax; during diagnostic workup, the girl underwent chest radiography, CT scan, and MRI, and a mass involving right X rib was detected (Fig. 12.4a–c). Histological examination revealed Ewing's sarcoma/PNET; therefore, a whole-body bone scan was performed for staging purpose (Fig. 12.4d, e). On the basis of scintigraphic results, a diagnosis of metastatic Ewing's sarcoma was made, and the girl began chemotherapeutic treatment.

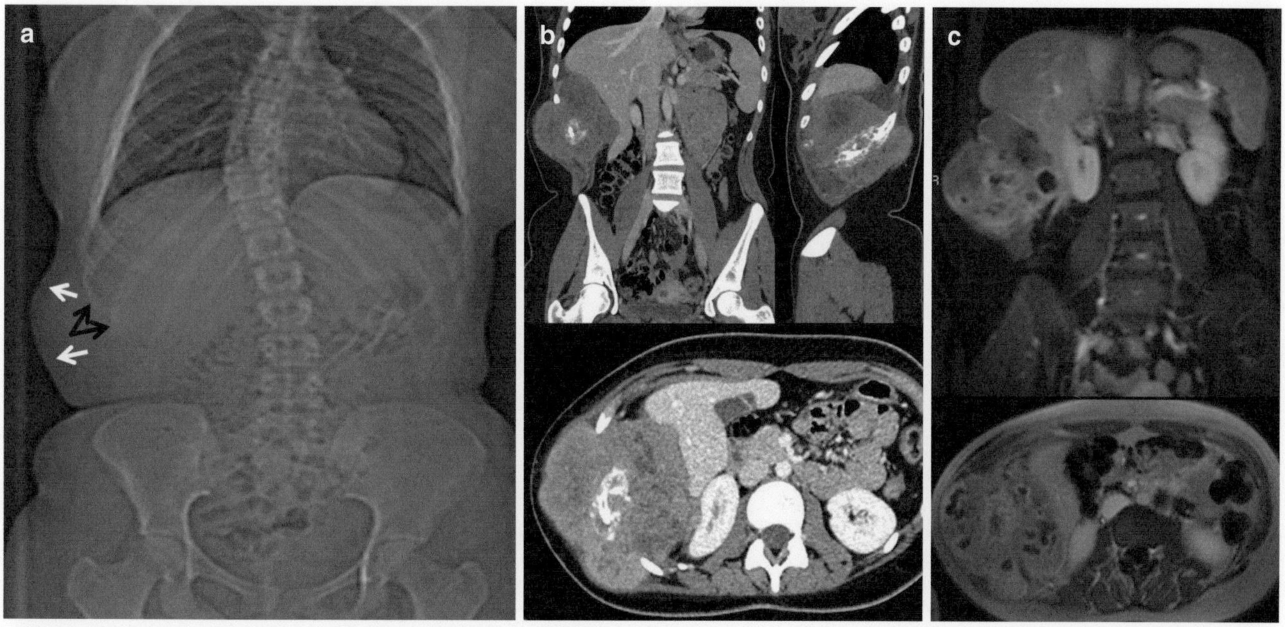

Fig. 12.4 (**a**): Anterior–posterior (AP) plain film of the chest and the abdomen: structural alteration of the IX and X right ribs (*black arrows*) with soft-tissue swelling (*white arrows*). (**b**): CT scan in the coronal, sagittal, and axial planes well highlights the costal osteolysis surrounded by inhomogeneous mass of soft tissue that displaces to the *left* of the liver and the *right* kidney. (**c**) MRI in the coronal and axial planes T1 fat/sat after contrast medium shows the mass of soft tissue with multiple hypointense areas in the context surrounded by peripheral ring enhancement related to necrotic areas. (**d**, **e**) ^{99m}Tc-MDP whole-body scan (**d**): a wide area of pathological, intense radiotracer uptake involving the anterolateral part of right X rib corresponding to the mass detected by CT; two small areas of pathological focal uptake are also evident in the posterior part of right XI rib and in the spinous process of one of the first cervical vertebrae (better defined in lateral views of skull, (**e**), respectively. A right posterior view of thorax (**e**) with arms up is also performed in order to define the focal uptake evident in inferior angle of right scapula, and it shows that it is due to an overlap of rib and scapula

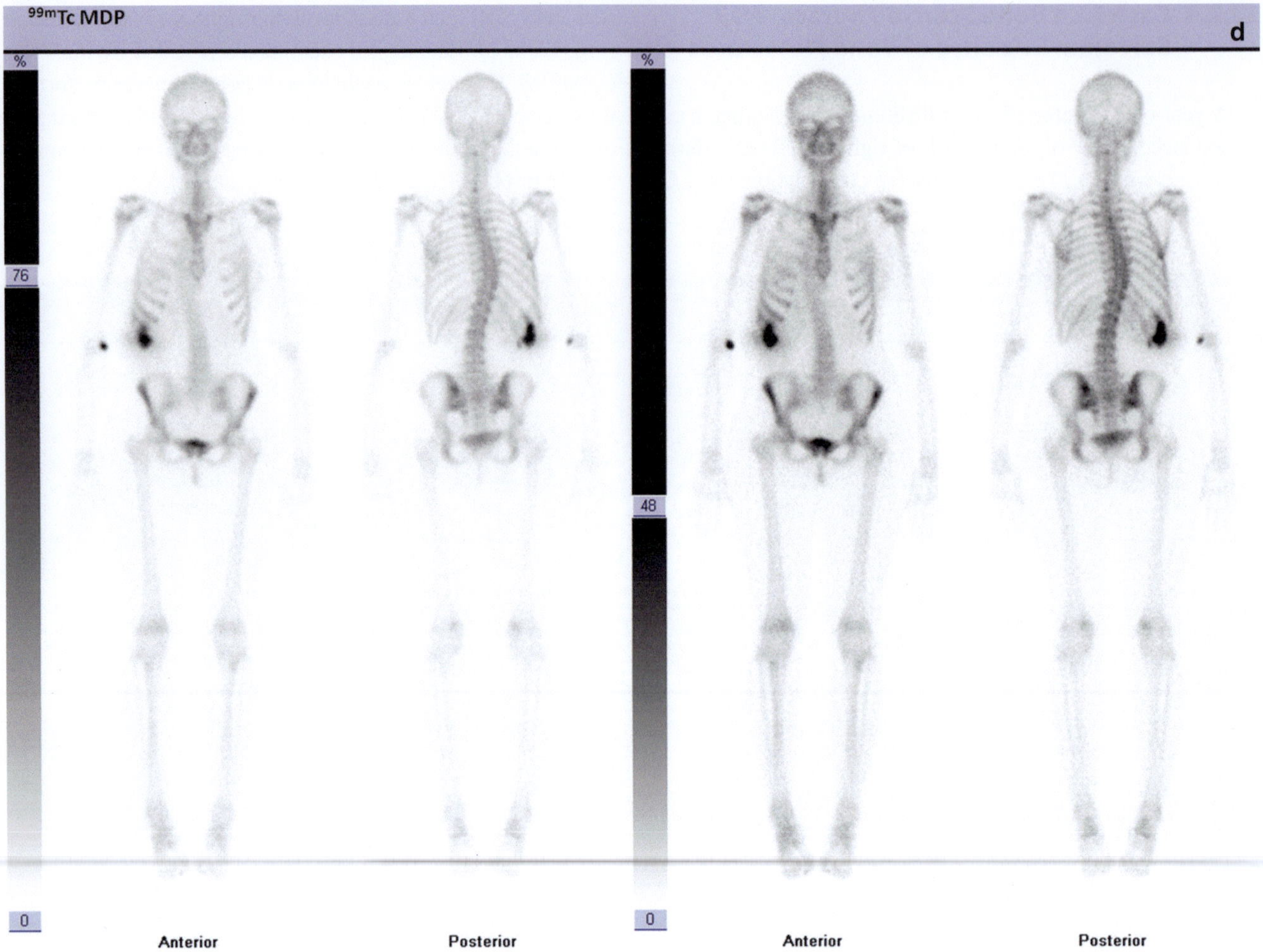

Fig. 12.4 (continued)

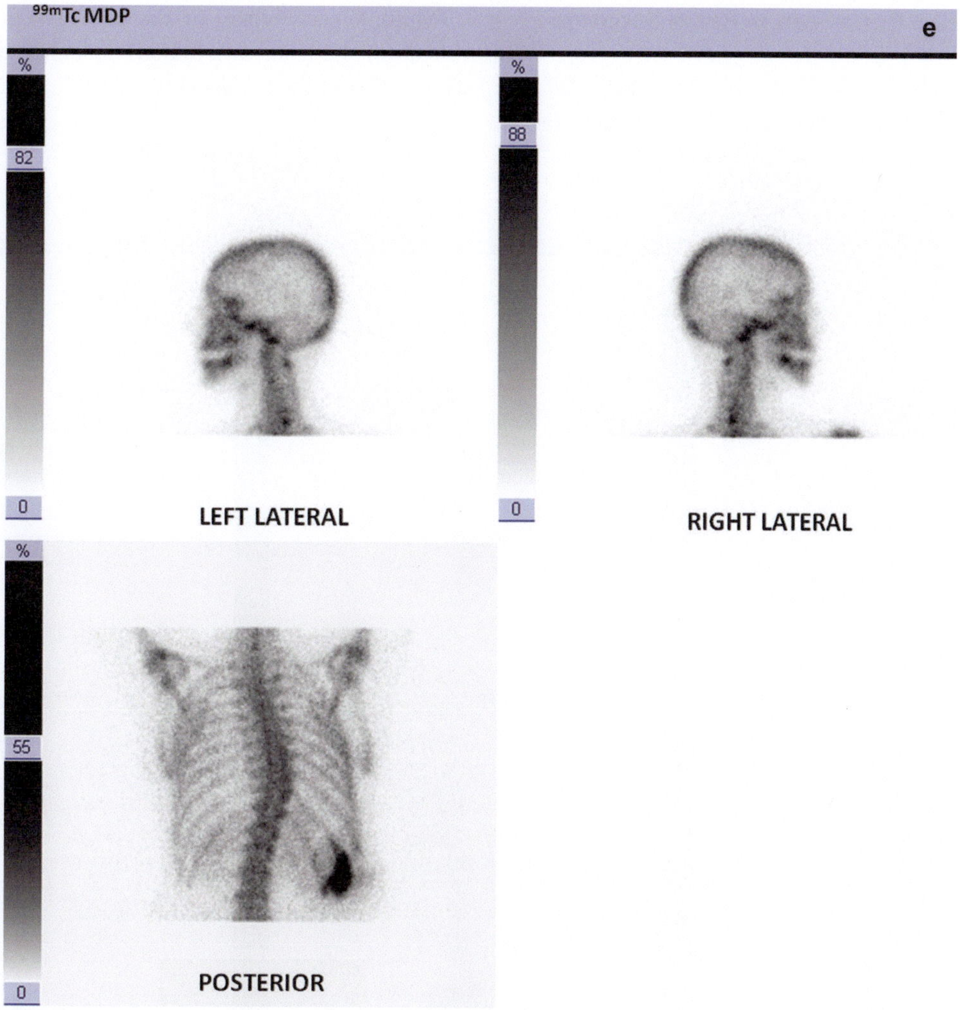

Fig. 12.4 (continued)

12.2.5 Case 12.5 Bone Scan in Renal Sarcoma

Staging bone scan in a 14-month-old baby with clear cell renal sarcoma, with lymph node and lung metastasis.

Multiple static views of skeletal segments are acquired, instead of the usual whole-body modality, due to the poor cooperation of the patient (Fig. 12.5).

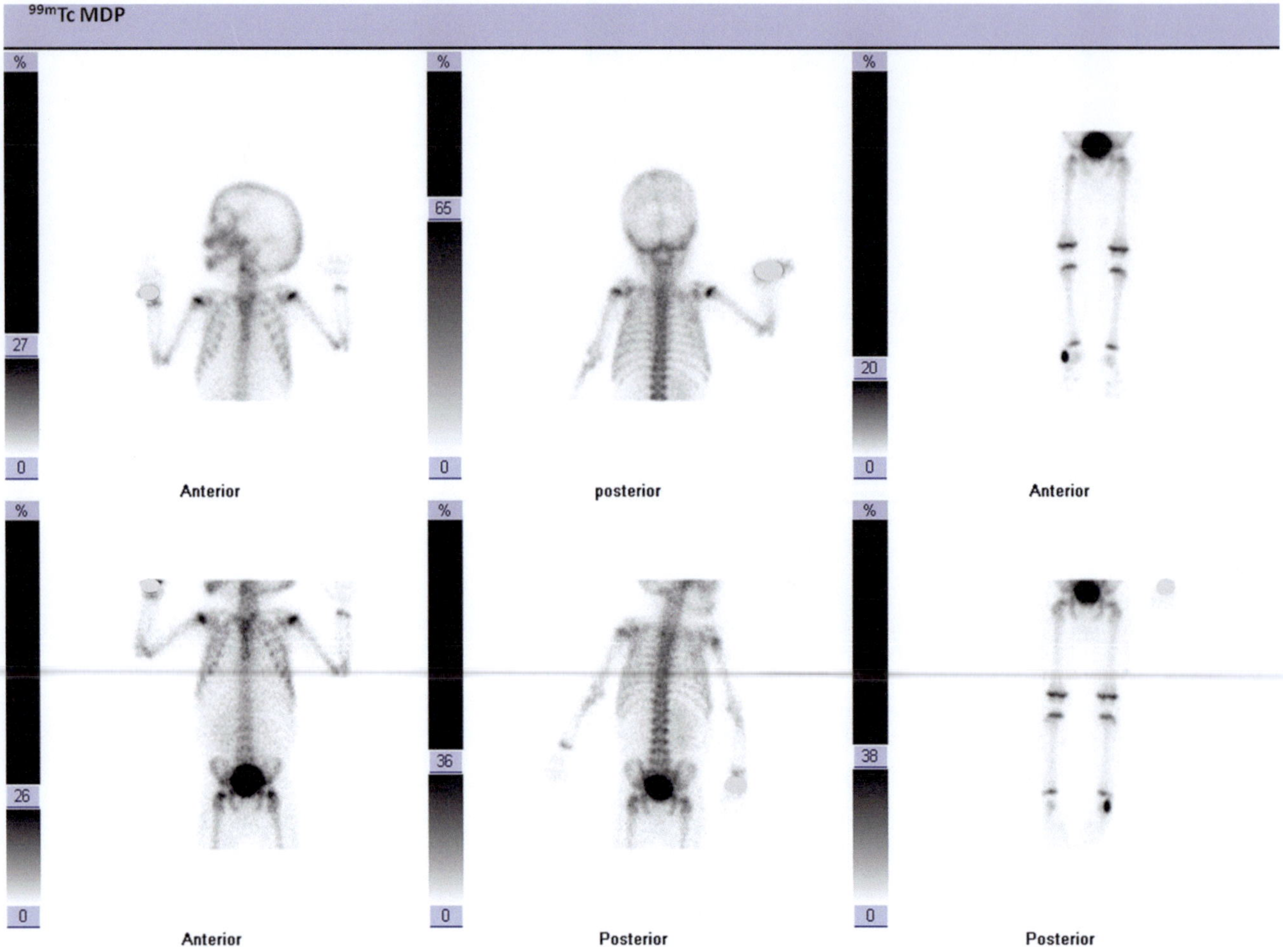

Fig. 12.5 ^{99m}Tc-MDP scintigraphy, multiple views of the skeleton: physiological distribution of radiotracer uptake and no evidence of pathological uptake in the skeleton

12.2.6 Case 12.6 Bone Scan in Pelvic Mass: Staging of Malignant Germinoma

A 9-year-old girl referred to our institution for vaginal bleeding; ultrasonography detected a pelvic mass; aFP and bHCG were very high; CT scan confirmed a large pelvic neoplasia involving right ovary and shows also a lung metastasis. Histological examination of the mass revealed a malignant germinoma, and a whole-body bone scan was performed to assess secondary bone involvement (Fig. 12.6).

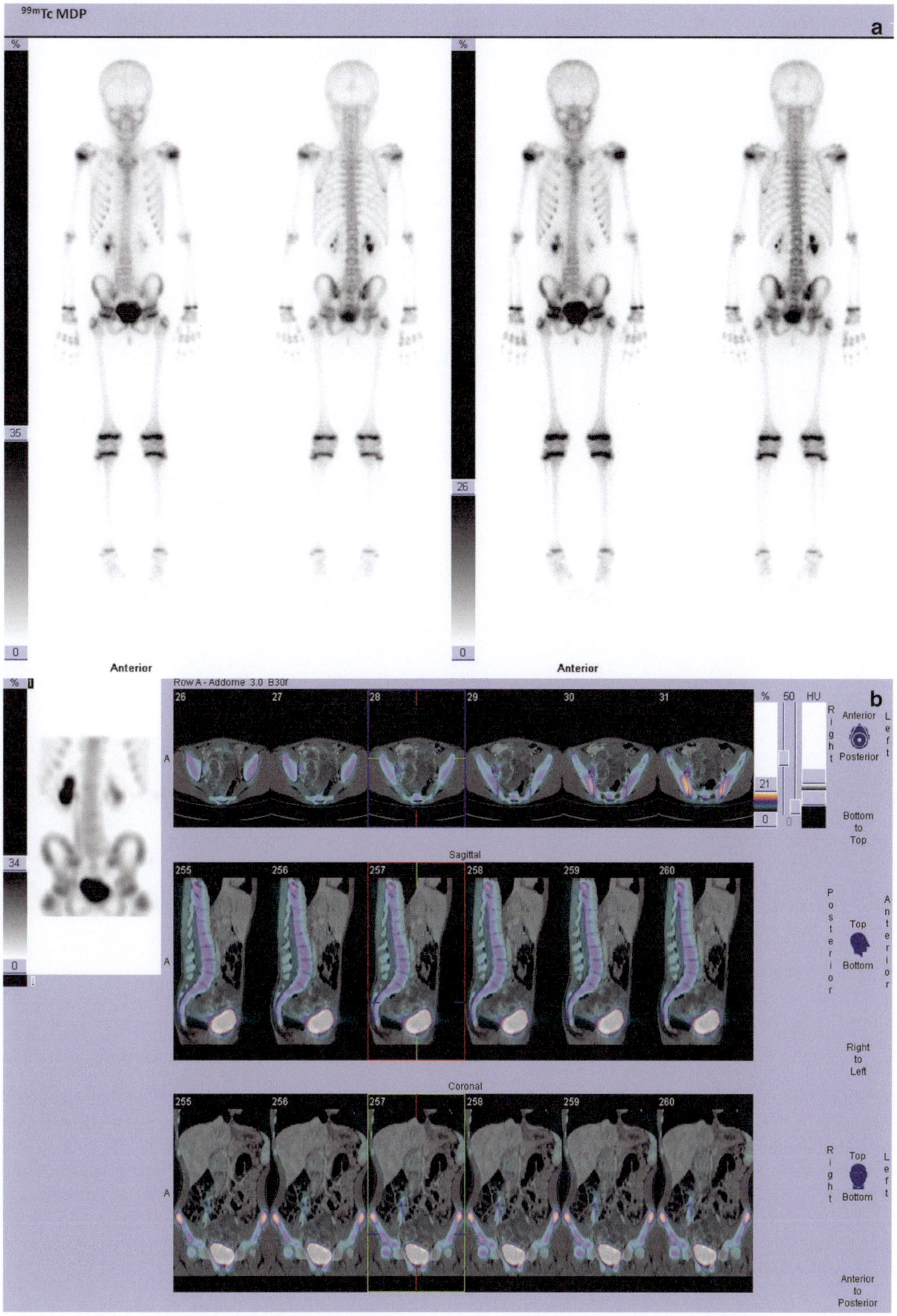

Fig. 12.6 ^{99m}Tc-MDP whole-body scan (**a**) shows physiological distribution of radiotracer uptake and no evidence of pathological uptake in the skeleton. Stasis of radioactive urine is evident in both kidneys and ureters (especially in *right* one), due to secondary hydroureteronephrosis. A SPECT of the pelvis is also performed, and SPECT-CT (**b**) manual fused image confirms the absence of pathological uptake in the pelvis and lumbar and sacral spine

12.2.7 Case 12.7 Bone Scan in Rhabdomyosarcoma

A 12-year-old boy referred to our hospital for swelling in right axilla; the boy underwent an ultrasonography and a CT scan, showing a neoplasia in pectoral muscles with involvement of axillary lymph nodes (histological examination: alveolar rhabdomyosarcoma). A whole-body bone scan was also performed for staging purpose (Fig. 12.7a, b); whole-body scan (a) showed a focal area of intense radiotracer uptake (better defined in lateral views of skull, (b) in superior part of left orbit; another small area of focal uptake is evident in the left posterior temporal bone. Furthermore, linear and diffuse radiotracer uptake is detectable in the right forearm, possibly due to the previous traumatic accident referred during clinical interview.

A CT scan (Fig. 12.7c, d) was performed, showing a hyperdense tissue, which extended to the left orbital cavity, starting from inferior border of the orbit roof.

Lesion was surgically removed, and histological examination revealed a lacrimal gland with MALT-tissue activation; after surgery, the boy went on with chemotherapeutic and radiotherapeutic treatment; ^{99m}Tc-MDP whole-body scan (Fig. 12.7e), after chemotherapy and radiotherapy, showed persistence of a faint focal area of radiotracer uptake in the superior part of left orbita (better defined in lateral views of skull (Fig. 12.7f). One year after stop therapy, the boy underwent a restaging workup for relapse of disease, including a ^{99m}Tc-MDP whole-body scan (Fig. 12.7g) that revealed multiple areas of pathological uptake of radiotracer in the whole skeleton.

Fig. 12.7 (**a**, **b**) Whole-body bone scan (**a**) shows a focal area of intense radiotracer uptake (better defined in lateral views of skull, (**b**) in superior part of left orbit; another small area of focal uptake is evident in left posterior temporal bone. Furthermore, linear and diffuse radiotracer uptake is detectable in right forearm, possibly due to the previous traumatic accident referred during clinical interview. (**c**, **d**) CT scan in axial, coronal, and sagittal planes with a soft tissue "window" (**c**); CT scan in axial, coronal, and sagittal planes with "bone window"(**d**). Small lenticular mass just less dense than the bone starting from the left orbital roof which protrudes inside the orbit contacting the eyeball and the other intraorbital structures. (**e**, **f**) Whole-body bone scan (**e**), after chemotherapy and radiotherapy, shows persistence of a faint focal area of radiotracer uptake in superior part of left orbita (better defined in lateral views of skull, **f**). (**g**) Whole-body scan (**g**) reveals multiple areas of pathological uptake of radiotracer in the whole skeleton

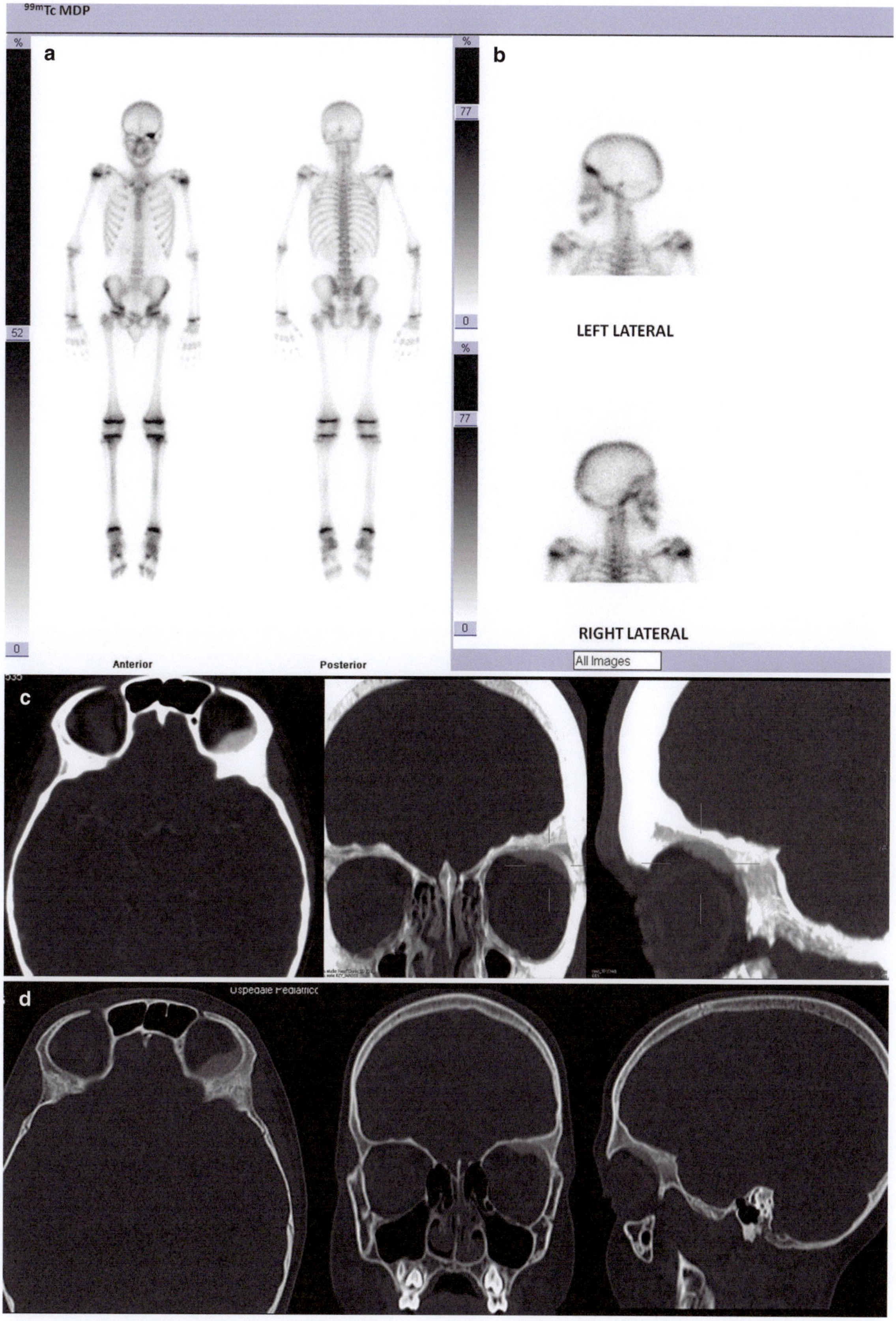
99mTc MDP
a
b
Anterior
Posterior
LEFT LATERAL
RIGHT LATERAL
All Images
c
d

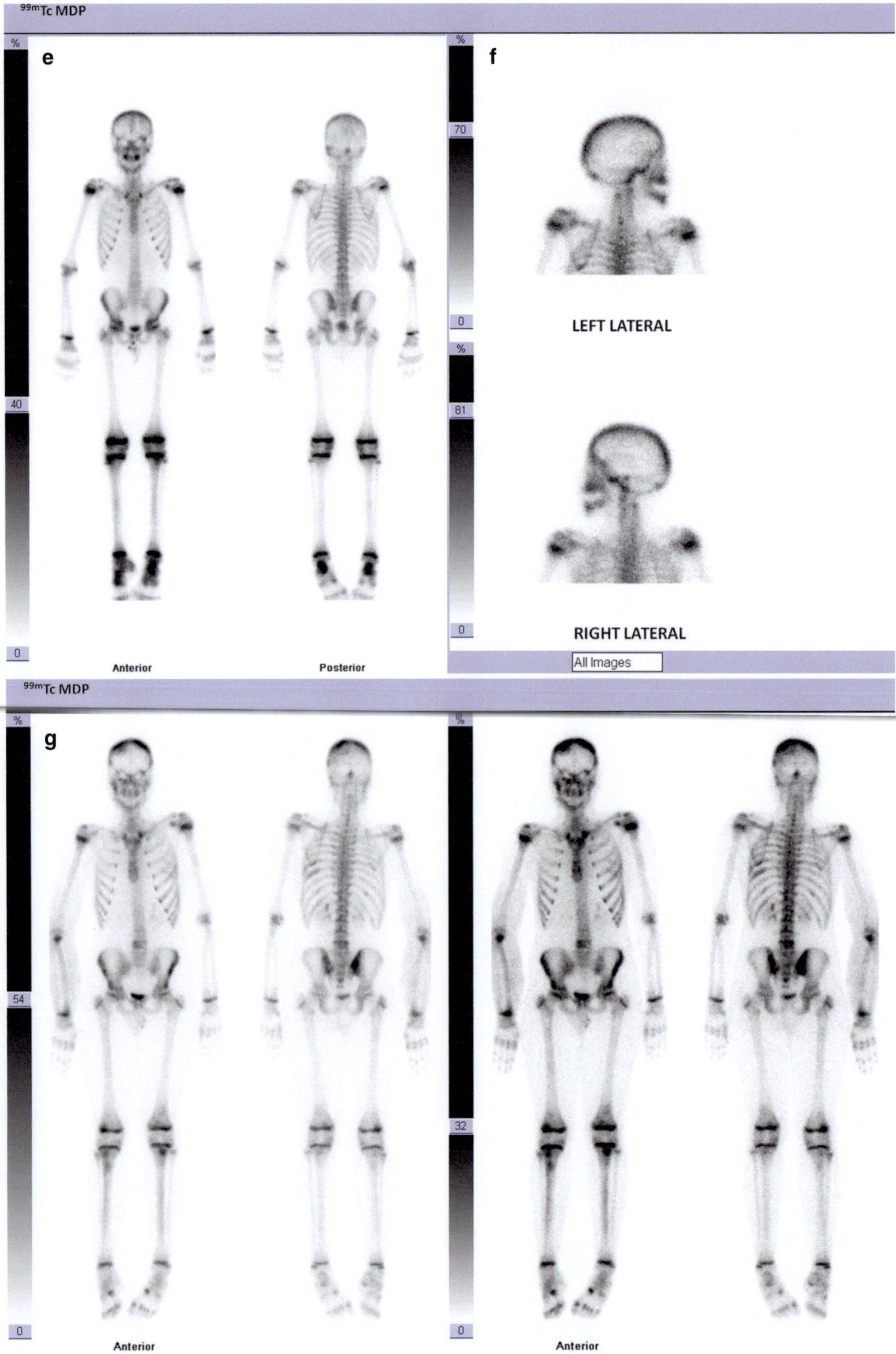

Fig. 12.7 (continued)

12.2.8 Case 12.8 Bone Scan in Large Chest Mass with Limited Bone Involvement

A 15-year-old girl referred to our hospital for diagnostic assessment of a thoracic mass, previously investigated in another center. Chest radiography (Fig. 12.8a) detected a diffuse opacity of the whole left lung field, and subsequent CT scan (Fig. 12.8b) showed a left lung mass eroding a rib, with pleural effusion. Histological examination of the mass showed Ewing's sarcoma, and a bone scintigraphy was scheduled for staging purpose. ^{99m}Tc-MDP whole-body scan (Fig. 12.8c, d) shows a pathological radiotracer uptake in the anterolateral part of a rib of the left hemithorax (probably IV rib) and no other pathological findings.

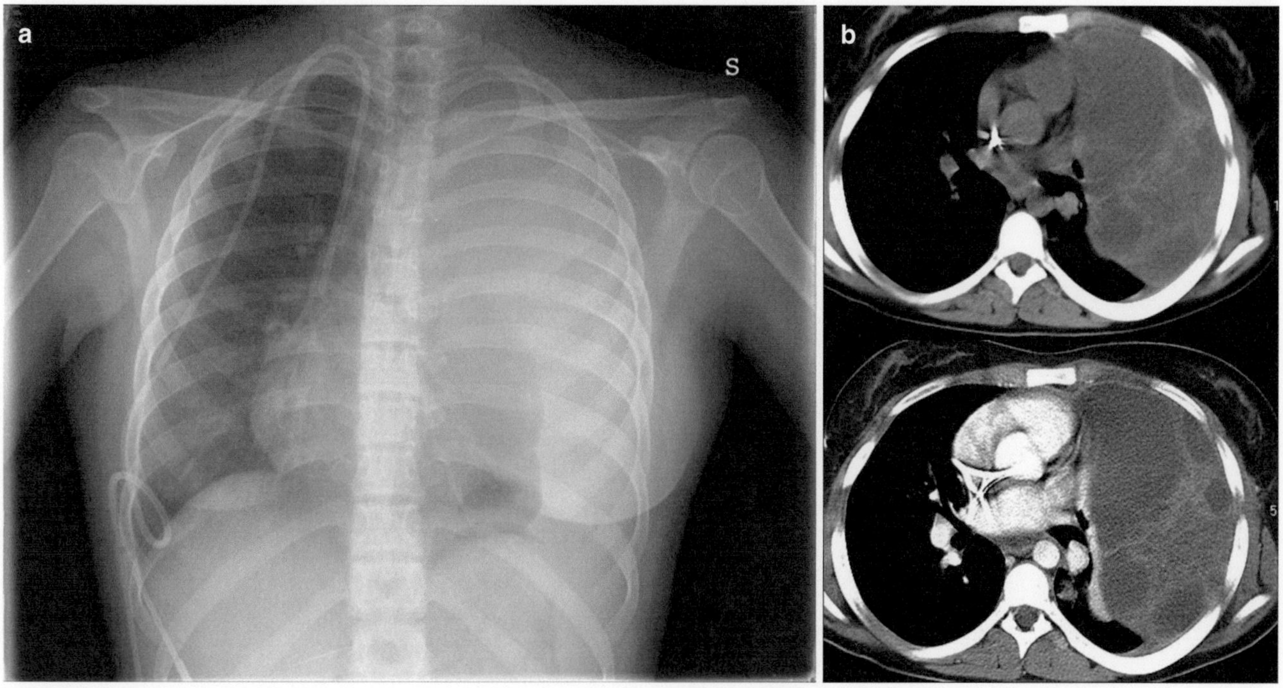

Fig. 12.8 (**a**) Frontal chest X-ray. Complete opacification of the left hemithorax with moderate displacement of the trachea, mediastinal structures, and the central venous catheter to the right. (**b**) CT scan before and after contrast medium. A big mass with multiple hypodense areas with small peripheral enhancement after contrast medium for prevalence of necrotic areas. Dislocation of the mediastinal structures toward the *right side*. (**c**, **d**) ^{99m}Tc-MDP whole-body scan (**c**) shows a pathological radiotracer uptake in anterolateral part of a rib of left hemithorax (probably IV rib), better defined in RAO and LAO views (**d**); no other pathological findings were evident in the skeleton. Moreover, radiotracer distribution in left VII and VIII ribs is not homogeneous. In this patient, despite the presence of a very large mass, bone scintigraphy detected a bone involvement, limited at ribs contiguous to the tumor

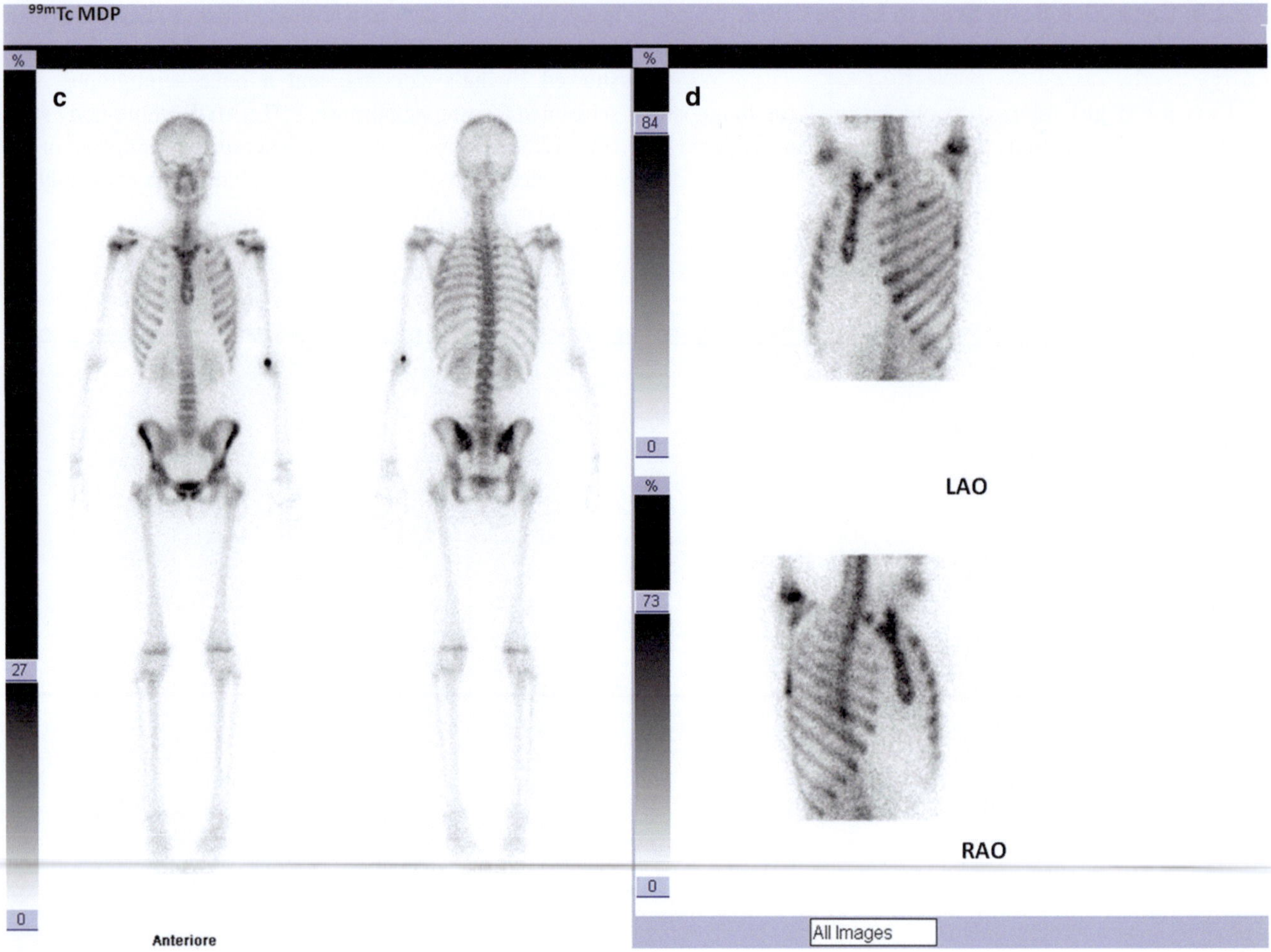

Fig. 12.8 (continued)

12.2.9 Case 12.9 Scintigraphic Diagnosis of Oncogenic Osteomalacia, Secondary to Phosphaturic Mesenchymal Tumor

An 8-year-old boy presented difficulty in running and jumping; he also referred myalgia and migrating arthralgia. Biochemical investigations showed hypophosphatemia, increased serum alkaline phosphatase, and hyperphosphaturia, with normal levels of calcium, PTH, creatinine, beta-2-microglobulin, and vitamin D3, thus excluding both primary and secondary hyperparathyroidism. Hand and ankle radiographies (Fig. 12.9a, b) showed diffuse decreases in radiodensity, and growth plates were widened. Bone MRI was inconclusive. Bone marrow biopsy was negative for malignancy. Therefore, a whole-body bone scintigraphy with ^{99m}Tc-MDP was performed in order to exclude a systemic bone involvement secondary to a skeletal inflammatory disease. The scan (Fig. 12.9c) showed the coexistence of multiple "hot spots" (suggestive for "pseudofractures"), and of scintigraphic signs of a metabolic disorder, suggesting a diagnosis for osteomalacia. Suspecting a paraneoplastic syndrome, a chest CT was performed which revealed a soft-tissue tumor of the posterior chest wall, which was surgically excised; histopathological examination revealed a phosphaturic mesenchymal tumor of mixed connective tissue type with signs of malignancy. Resection of the mass resulted in resolution of symptoms and in a complete biochemical response within 2 weeks.

In this case, bone scintigraphy was useful in making the diagnosis of osteomalacia and addressed subsequent management of the patient.

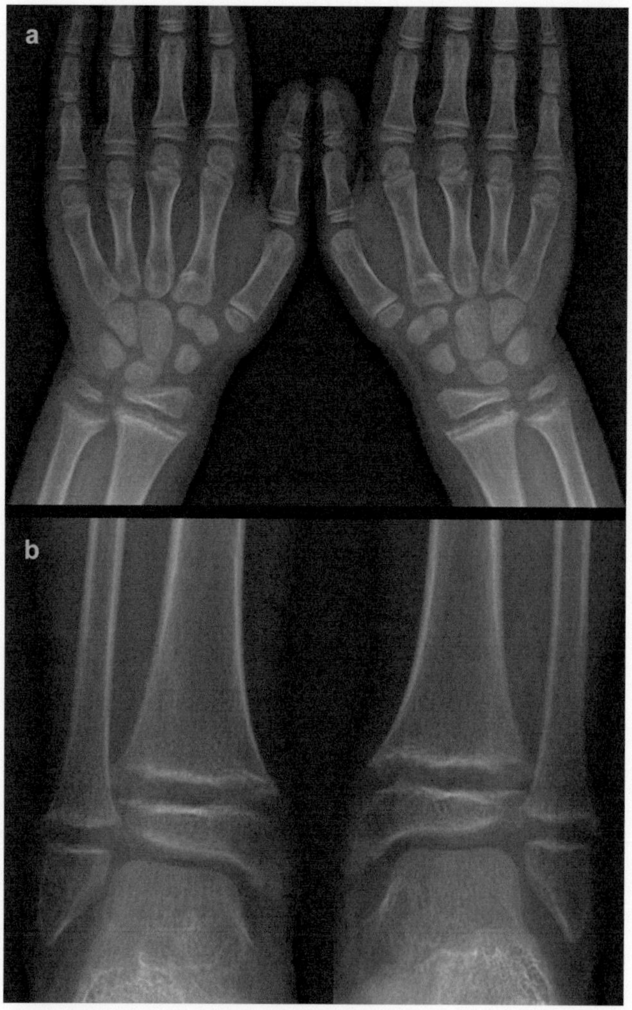

Fig. 12.9 (**a**, **b**) PA plain film of the hands (**a**); AP plain film of the ankles (**b**). Enlargement of radioulnar, tibial, and fibular physes with frayed aspect of the distal metaphyseal margins: findings compatible with rickets. (**c**) ^{99m}Tc-MDP whole-body scan: multiple areas of both focal and diffuse increased uptake in the ribs, in left scapula, both humeri, both sacroiliac joints, in right femur, and tibiae; increased uptake throughout the sternum and in the costochondral junctions and very faint radiotracer uptake in the kidneys with increased uptake in the axial skeleton. The coexistence of multiple "hot spots" (suggestive for "pseudofractures") and of scintigraphic signs of a metabolic disorder suggests a diagnosis of osteomalacia

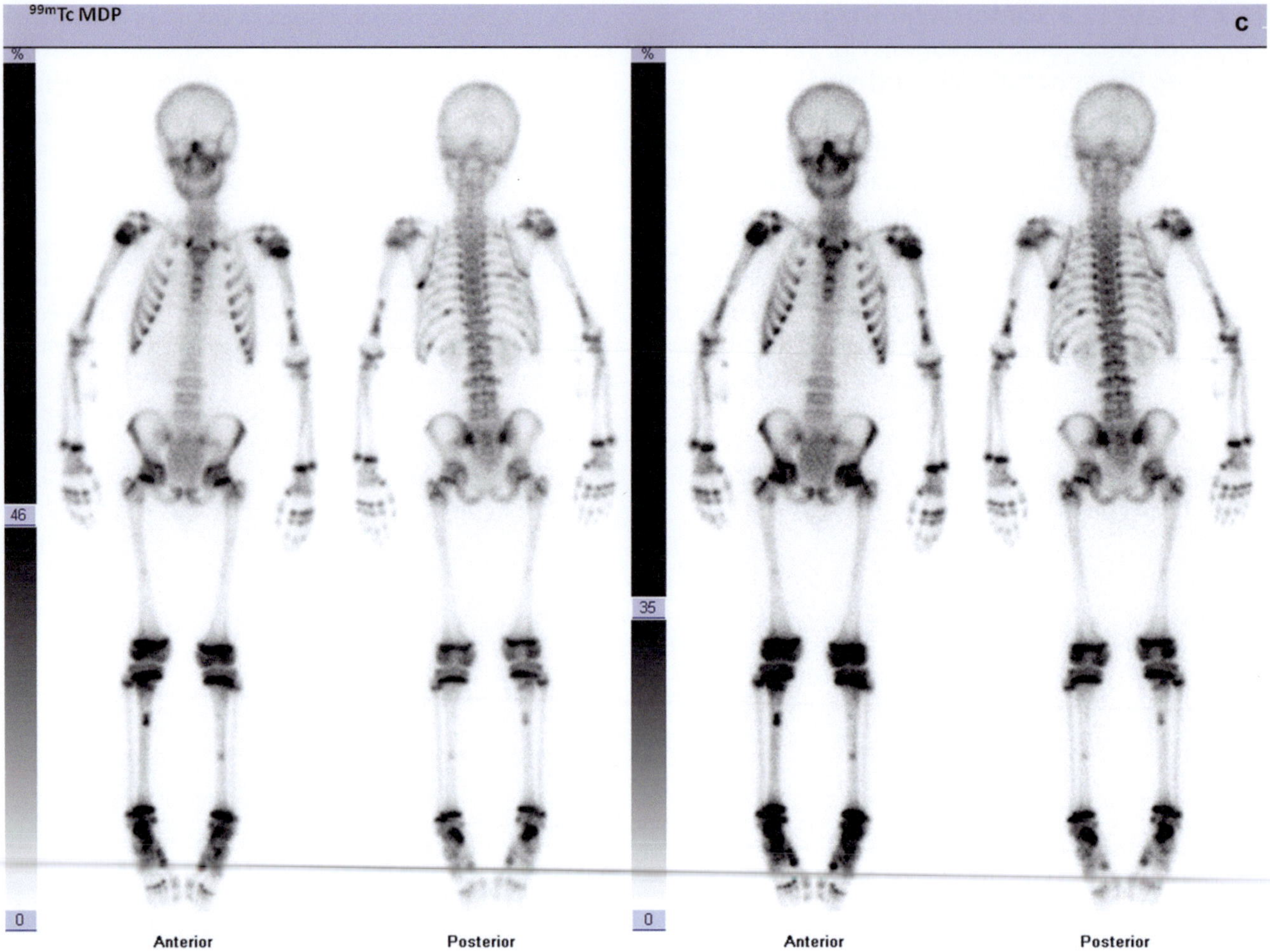

Fig. 12.9 (continued)

12.2.10 Case 12.10 (Fig. 12.10) Warning

Similar scintigraphic patterns, characterized by intense radiotracer uptake, can be present in different diseases as shown in the following pictures. Indeed, histological examination revealed a different disease in each case.

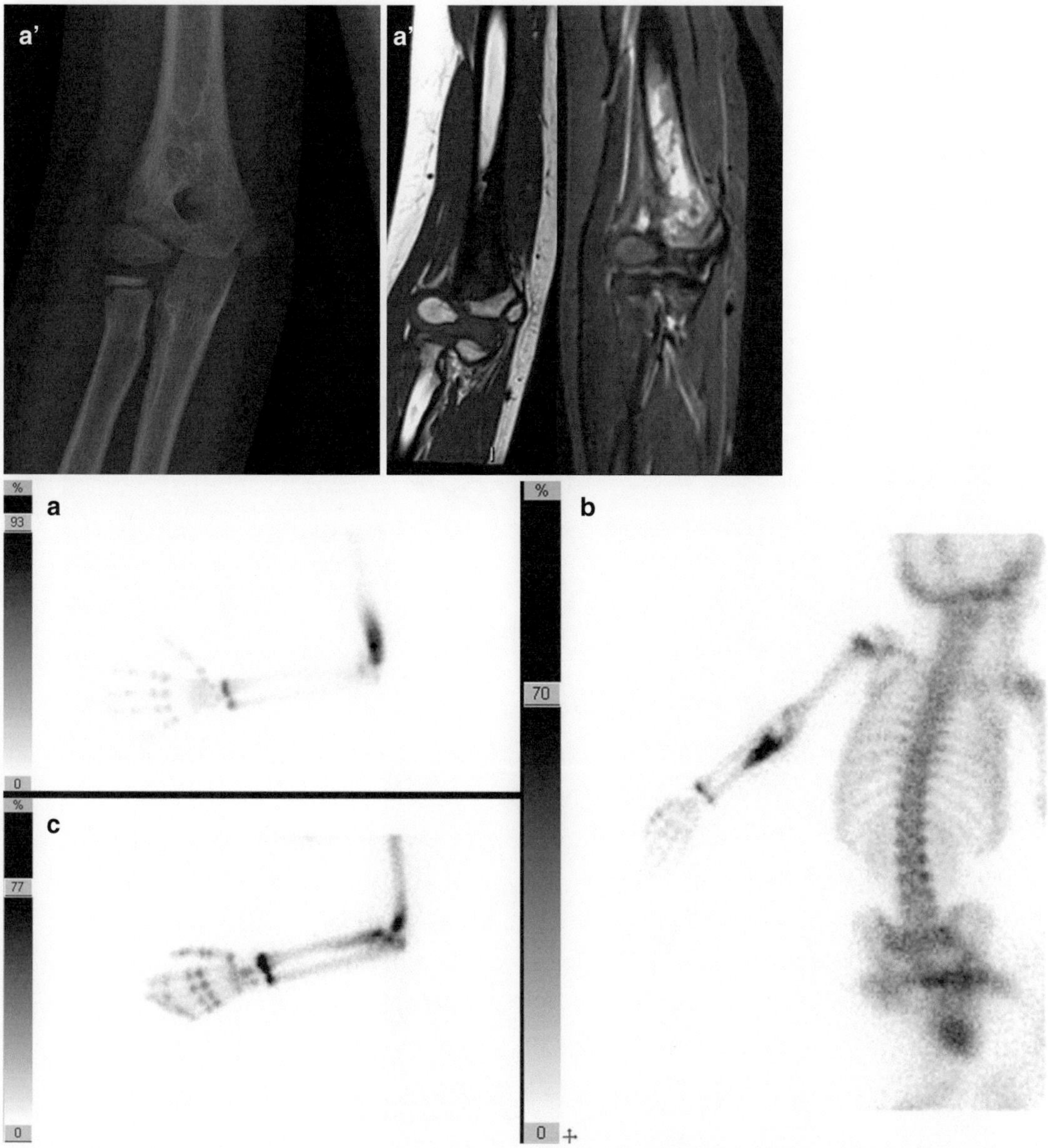

Fig. 12.10 (**a**–**c**) In this figure are displayed scintigraphic patterns that look very similar to each other, that is, intense radiotracer uptake in upper limb (distal humerus in image (a), proximal radius in image (b), and proximal ulna in image (**c**), respectively), though histological examination detects a different disease in each case: Ewing's sarcoma in patient in image (a), osteoid osteoma in patient in image (b), and Langerhans' cell histiocytosis in image (c), respectively. Radiological findings of each patient are reported in Figure (**a'**, **a''**) (Ewing's sarcoma), Figure (**b'**, **b''**) (osteoid osteoma), and in Figure (**c'**) (Langerhans' cell histiocytosis), respectively. (**a'**, **a''**) AP elbow plain film: distal humerus, moth-eaten appearance (**a'**); RM coronal T1 and T2 fat/sat: reduced signal in T1 and increased in T2 fat/sat except epitrochlea, a small distal portion of the humeral palette, and capitulum humeri for replacement of normal bone marrow by tumor tissue (Ewing's sarcoma) (**a''**). (**b'**, **b''**). AP and LL plain film: a small radiolucent area in the radial neck (*black arrow*) surrounded by continuous and regular periosteal apposition (**b'**, *white arrows*). RM coronal T1 and axial T1 fat/sat after contrast medium: small area of reduced signal in the radial neck (*black arrow*) corresponding to the nidus of an osteoid osteoma, surrounded by bone marrow edema and edema of the extra-bone soft tissue with enhancement after contrast medium (**b''**, *white arrows*). (**c'**): AP and LL elbow plain film : osteolytic area with polycyclic margins with partial destruction of the olecranon articular surface. Dense and continuous periosteal apposition extended until the middle diaphysis (*black arrows*). It is necessary, in fact, to integrate scintigraphic findings with clinical presentation, laboratory test, and other imaging methods; moreover, it is mandatory in children to ever choose an imaging tool that investigates all skeletal segments, to identify multifocal disease, and consequently to support the diagnosis

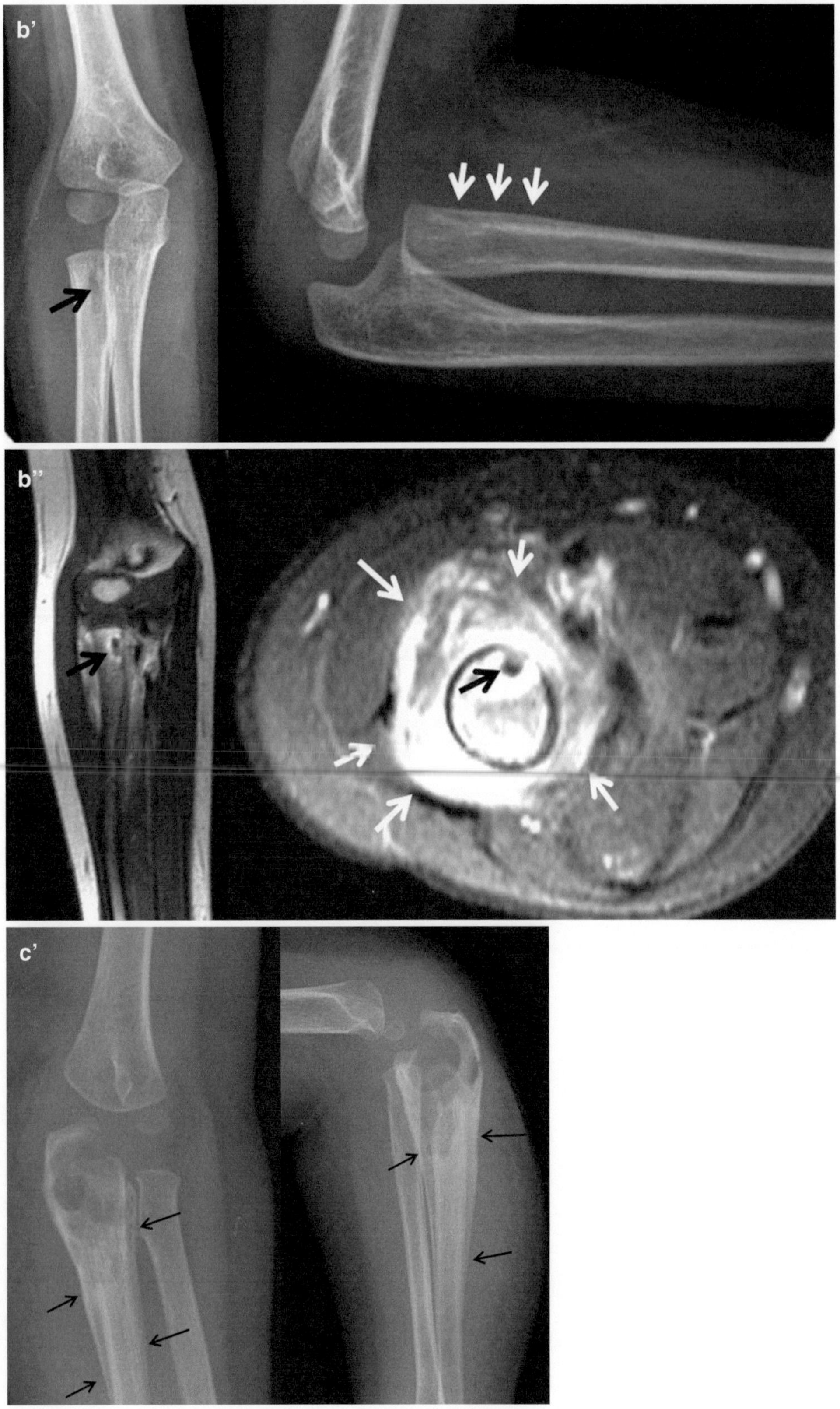

Fig. 12.10 (continued)

12.2.11 Case 12.11 Bone Involvement in Non-Hodgkin's Lymphoma

A 17-year old boy with a diagnosis of B-cell lymphoblastic lymphoma of appendix referred to our hospital for staging and therapeutic management.

A whole-body bone scan (Fig. 12.11a) was performed which showed a large lytic lesion in diaphysis of left femur and small lytic lesion in a vertebra in middle cervical spine.

Femoral lesion was confirmed by plain radiography (Fig. 12.11b).

Standard investigations performed at the beginning of diagnostic workup (CT and FDG-PET/CT) did not detect femoral lesion, because they did not include lower limbs.

The boy underwent chemotherapeutic treatment, and the ^{99m}Tc-MDP whole-body scan after therapy (Fig. 12.11c) showed a mild, linear, radiotracer uptake in the proximal diaphysis of left femur; the photopenic areas in the femur and in the cervical vertebra were no longer evident, such that indicating an almost complete response to therapy in the skeleton.

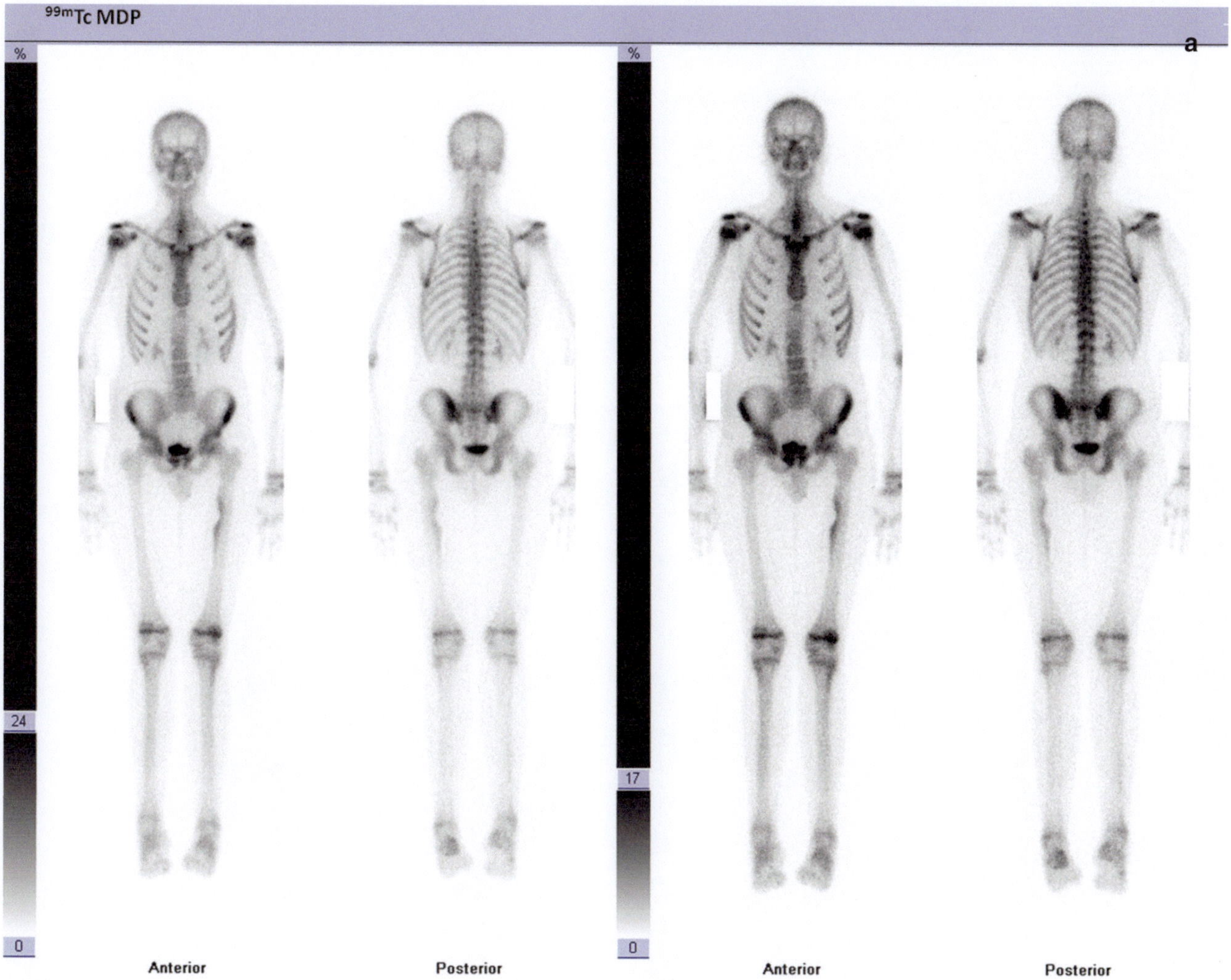

Fig. 12.11 (**a**) Whole-body bone scan shows a large photopenic area, surrounded by a rim of intense radiotracer uptake, in medial border of the proximal diaphysis of left femur; radiotracer distribution is not homogeneous in left femur, especially in both proximal and distal epiphyses; a small focal photopenic area surrounded by a rim of radiotracer uptake is also evident in a vertebra in middle cervical spine. (**b**): AP and LL plain films of the left femur. Extended thickening of the inner cortex of the femoral shaft (*black arrows*) interrupted by a large semilunar defect of the medial diaphyseal bone profile (*white arrow*). (**c**) Whole-body bone scan shows a mild, linear, radiotracer uptake in the proximal diaphysis of left femur; the photopenic areas in the femur and in cervical vertebra were no longer evident, indicating an almost complete response to therapy in the skeleton

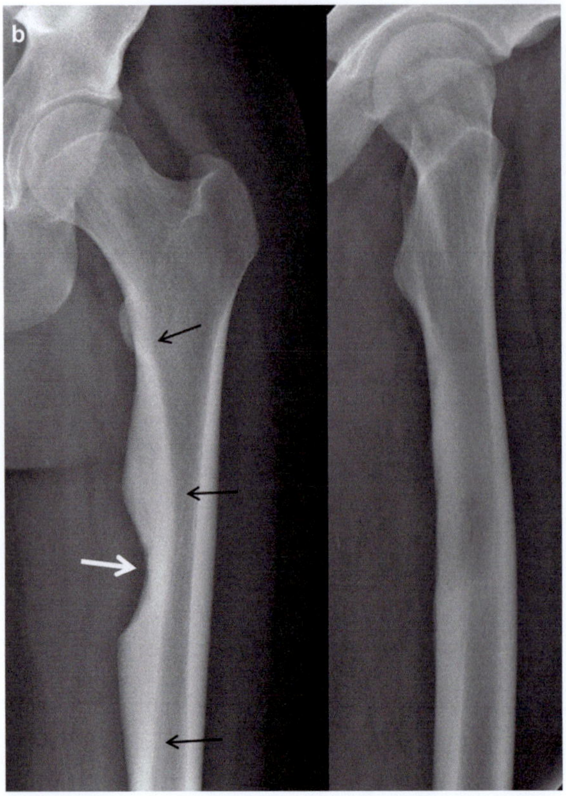

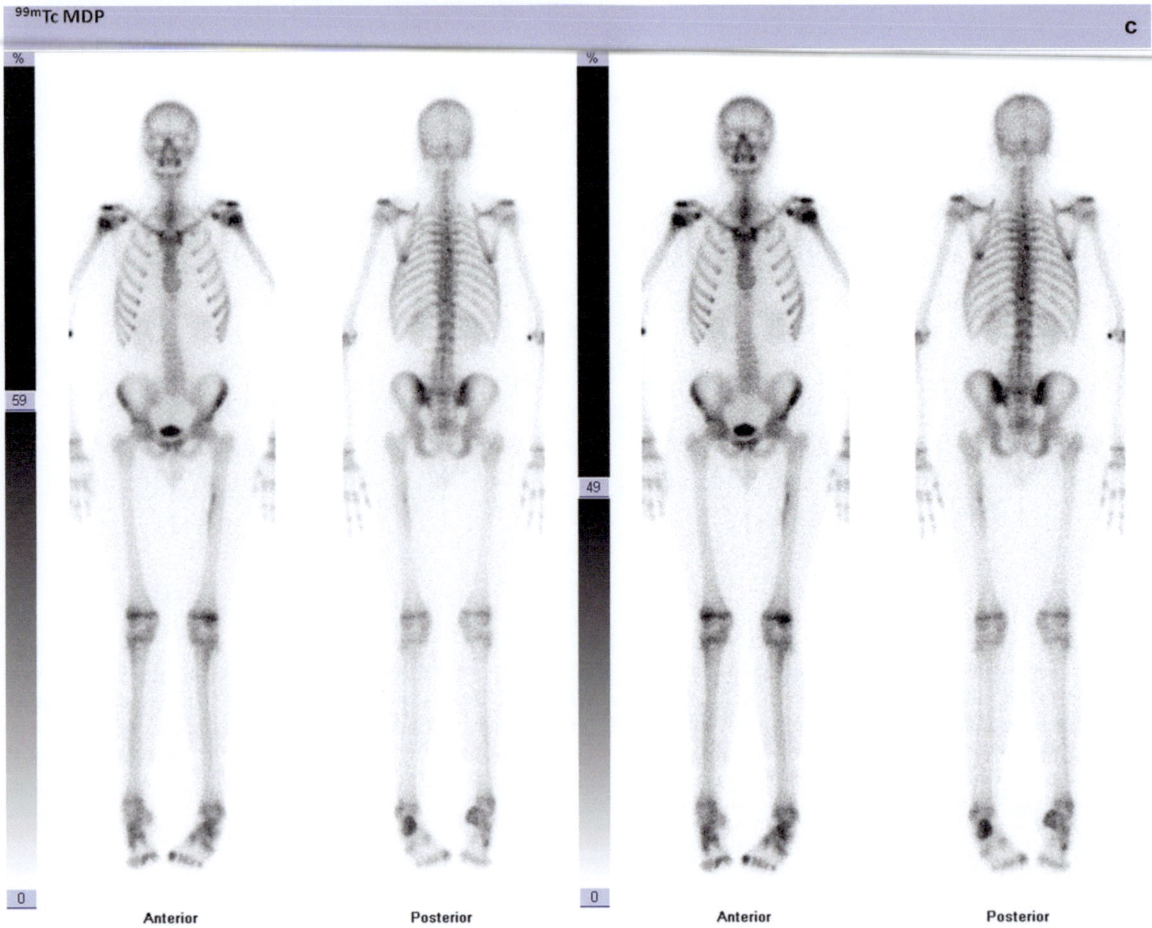

Fig. 12.11 (continued)

12.2.12 Case 12.12 Bone Scan in Osteosarcoma with Secondary Lung Involvement: No Evidence of Bone Metastases

A 12-year old girl with a recent diagnosis of osteosarcoma of left femur (plain radiography, Fig. 12.12a; MRI, Fig. 12.12b) with lung involvement referred to our hospital for staging and therapeutic management. A whole-body bone scan (Fig. 12.12c) was performed that showed a large area of intense and nonhomogeneous uptake of radiotracer, involving middle and distal diaphysis of left femur, reaching distal metaphysis; no other pathological findings were evident in the skeleton. Therefore, the girl underwent chemotherapy and surgical resection of neoplasia with a prosthetic implant (Fig. 12.12d); ^{99m}Tc-MDP whole-body scan performed after treatment (Fig. 12.12e) showed small areas of radiotracer uptake in middle-proximal left femur and in middle-distal left tibia, near the prosthesis, due to previous surgical treatment and no pathological findings in the skeleton.

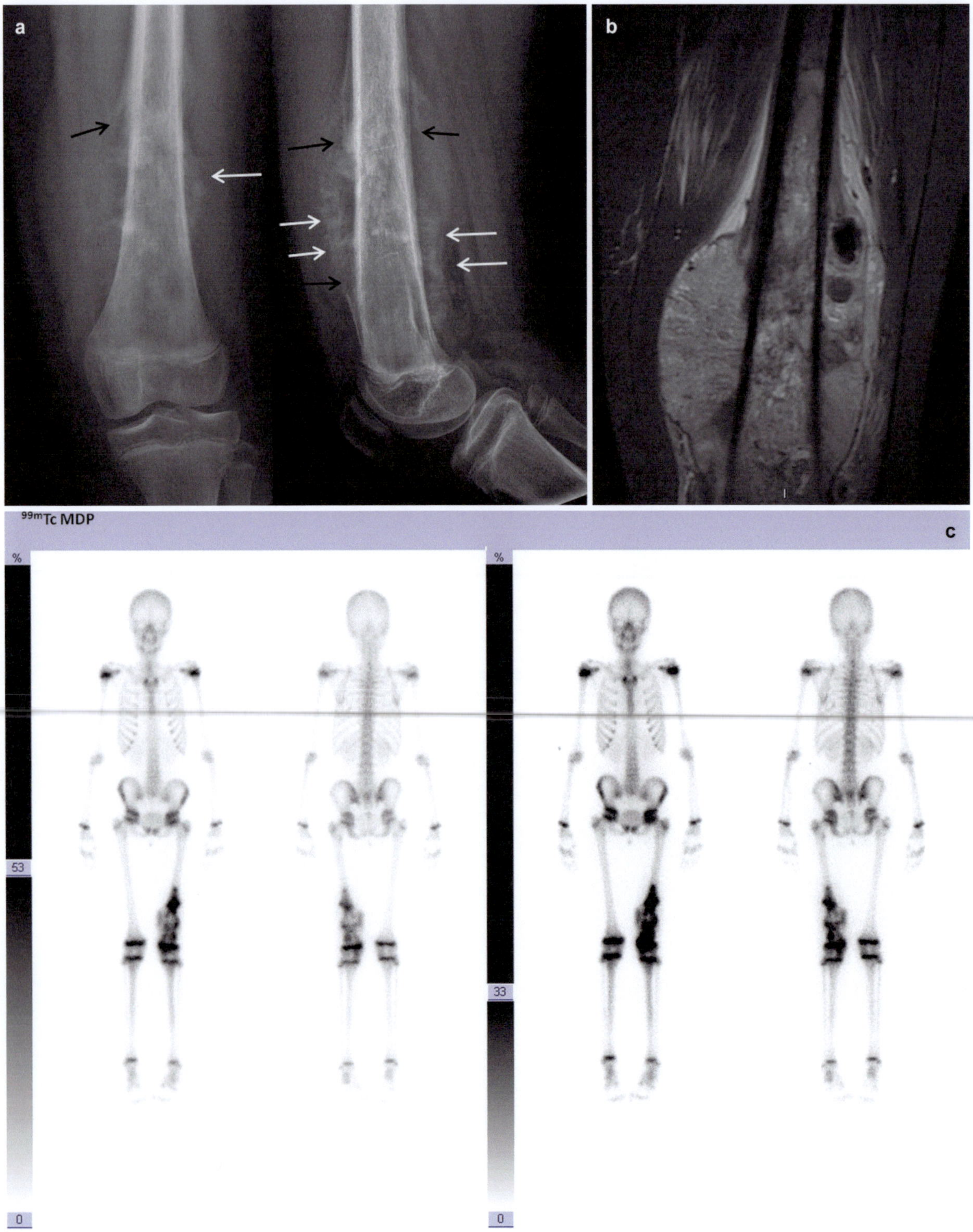

Fig. 12.12 (**a**) AP and LL plain film of the left femur. Extensive alteration of bone structure with multiple osteolytic areas in the diaphysis and distal metaphysis of the femur. Thinning of the internal cortical. Coarse and irregular periosteal apposition in the central part of the lesion (*white arrows*); peripherally, the periosteal apposition is interrupted with Codman triangle (*black arrows*). (**b**) MRI coronal T1 fat/sat after contrast medium: extensive alteration of the diaphyseal bone marrow signal. Cortical distally thinned. Extra-osseous mass with inhomogeneous enhancement and small hypointense areas due to necrosis. (**c**) Staging whole-body bone scan shows a large area of intense and nonhomogeneous uptake of radiotracer involving middle and distal diaphysis of left femur, reaching distal metaphysis; no other pathological findings were evident in the skeleton. (**d**): radiographic examination after joint prosthetic replacement. (**e**) Whole-body bone scan of small areas of radiotracer uptake in middle-proximal left femur and in middle-distal left tibia, near the prosthesis, due to previous surgical treatment and no pathological findings in the skeleton

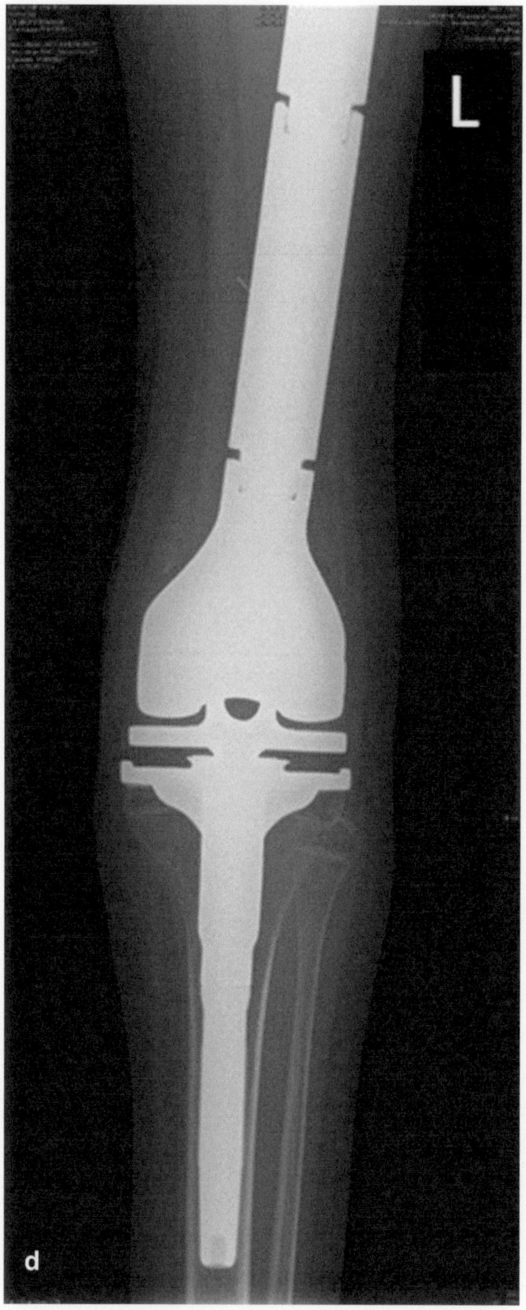

Fig. 12.12 (continued)

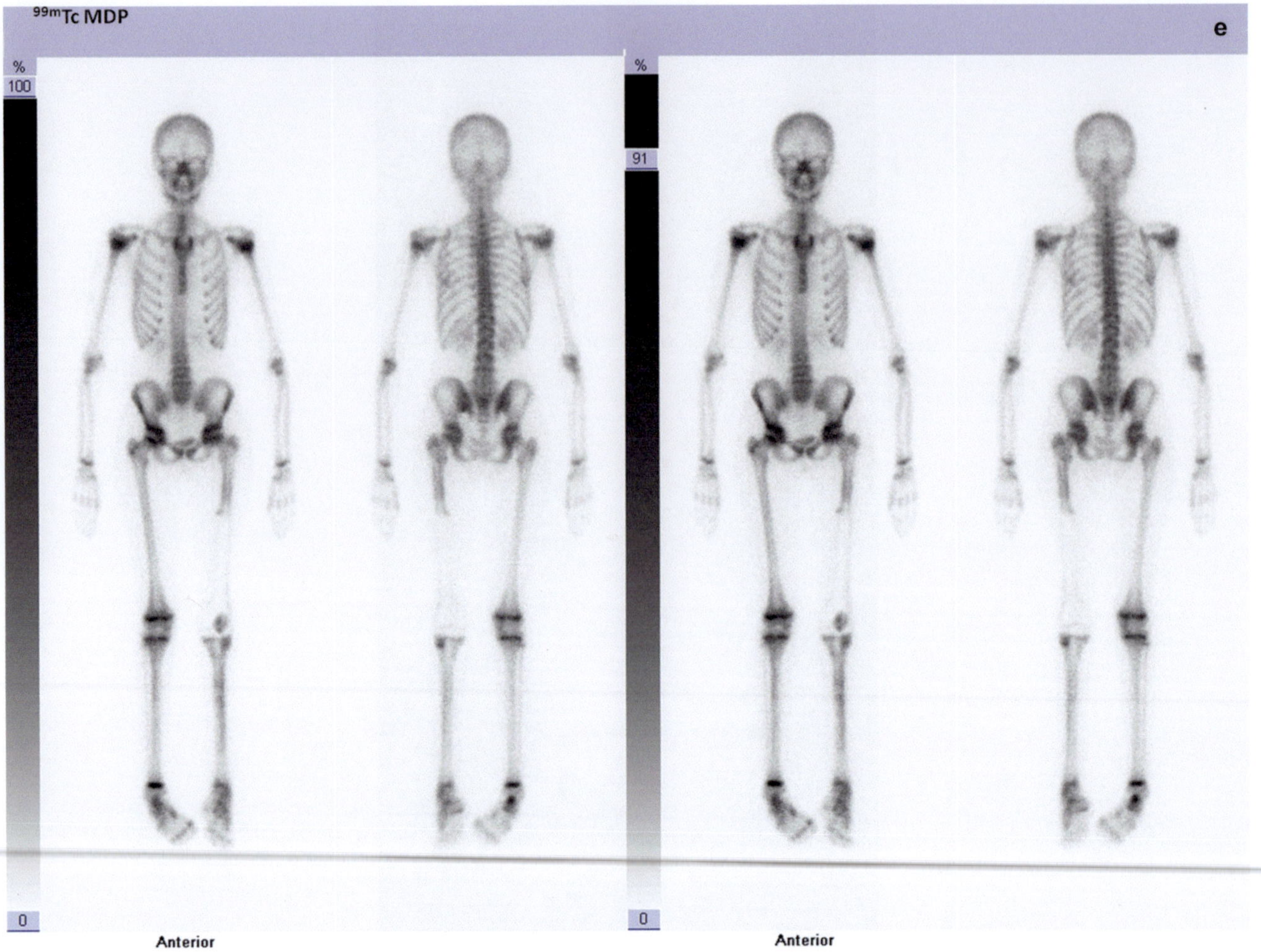

Fig. 12.12 (continued)

12.2.13 Case 12.13 Bone Scan in Osteosarcoma: Evidence of Bone Metastases

An 8-year old girl with a diagnosis of osteosarcoma of right femur with "skip lesion" (MRI, Fig. 12.13a) referred to our hospital for disease staging. ^{99m}Tc-MDP whole-body scan (Fig. 12.13b) showed a large area of intense and non-homogeneous uptake of radiotracer involving distal diaphysis of right femur; furthermore, a focal area of intense radiotracer uptake in proximal femur ("skip lesion") and a diffuse and intense uptake in XII thoracic vertebra are evident, respectively, such that indicating a metastatic osteosarcoma.

Therefore, the girl underwent chemotherapy and a complete surgical resection of right femur with a prosthetic implant (Fig. 12.13c). CT scan after chemotherapy detected a disease progression, with lung involvement; ^{99m}Tc-MDP whole-body scan (Fig. 12.13d) revealed multiple areas of pathological uptake of radiotracer in several skeletal segments; focal areas of intense uptake of radiotracer were also evident in left hemithorax, corresponding to lung metastasis detected by CT; moreover, three focal areas of uptake were present in the soft tissue of right thigh, which can be attributed to metastases.

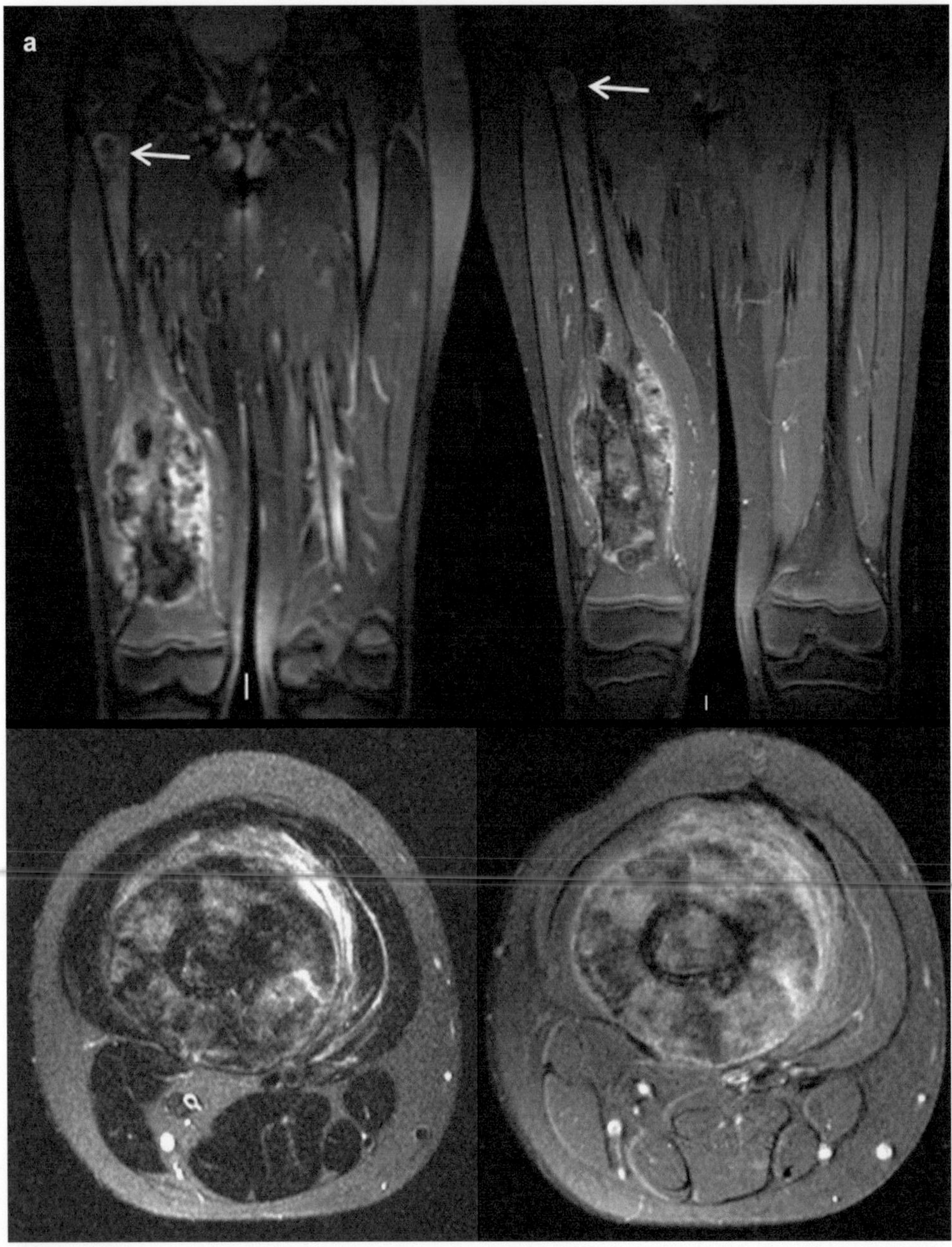

Fig. 12.13 (**a**)Above: RM coronal T1 fat/sat after contrast medium; below: MRI axial T2 fat/sat and T1 fat/sat after contrast medium; extended bone marrow signal alteration in the distal femur. Cortical is thinned and interrupted. Extra-osseous mass with inhomogeneous enhancement and small hypointense areas due to necrosis. Skip metastasis in the subtrochanteric area (*white arrow*). (**b**) ^{99m}Tc-MDP whole-body scan shows a large area of intense and nonhomogeneous uptake of radiotracer involving distal diaphysis of right femur; furthermore, a focal area of intense radiotracer uptake in proximal femur ("skip lesion") and a diffuse and intense uptake in XII thoracic vertebra are evident, respectively, indicating a metastatic osteosarcoma. (**c**) Radiographic examination after prosthetic replacement. (**d**) ^{99m}Tc-MDP whole-body scan reveals multiple areas of pathological uptake of radiotracer in several skeletal segments; focal areas of intense uptake of radiotracer are also evident in left hemithorax, corresponding to lung metastasis detected by CT; moreover, three focal areas of uptake are present in soft tissue of right thigh, which can be attributed to metastases. In this case, bone scintigraphy played a significant role both in diagnostic and in restaging phase; at diagnosis, in fact, the whole-body modality allows to detect skip lesion and distant metastasis, changing disease stage; restaging showed disease progression. Moreover, restaging scan shows a peculiarity of osteosarcoma metastases, that is, the ability to produce bone matrix and to fix ^{99m}Tc-MDP

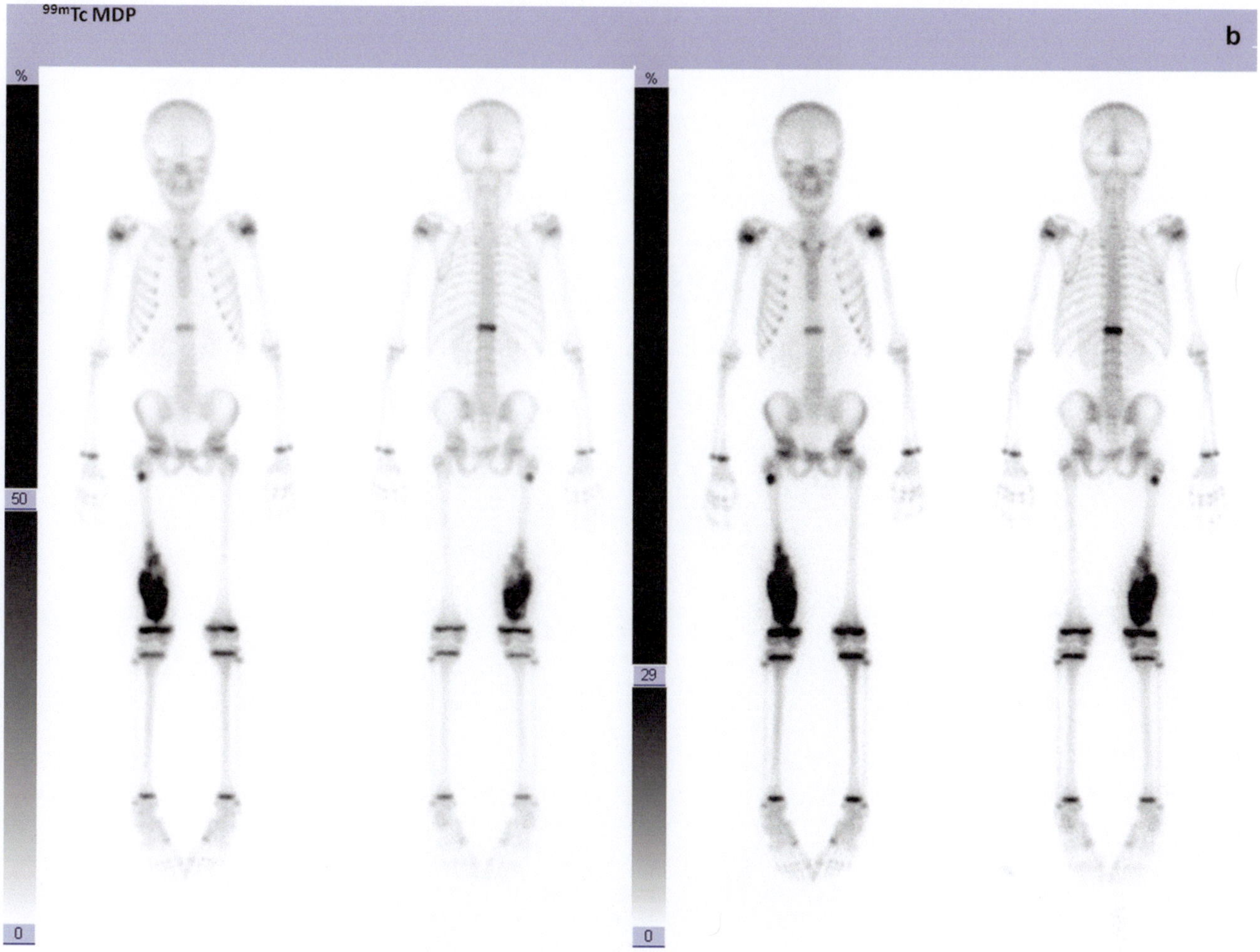

Fig. 12.13 (continued)

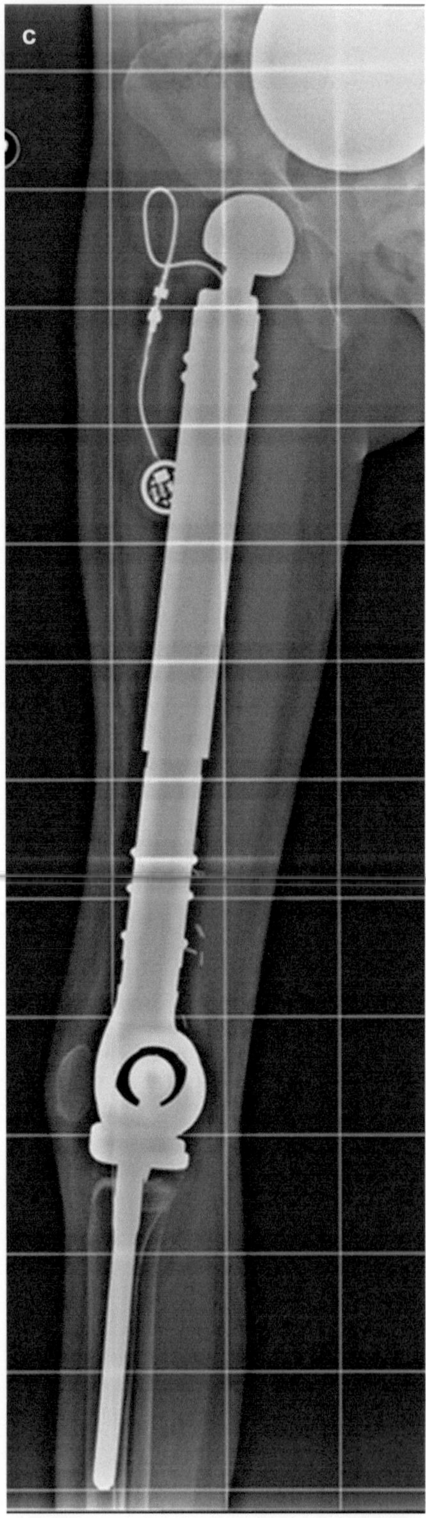

Fig. 12.13 (continued)

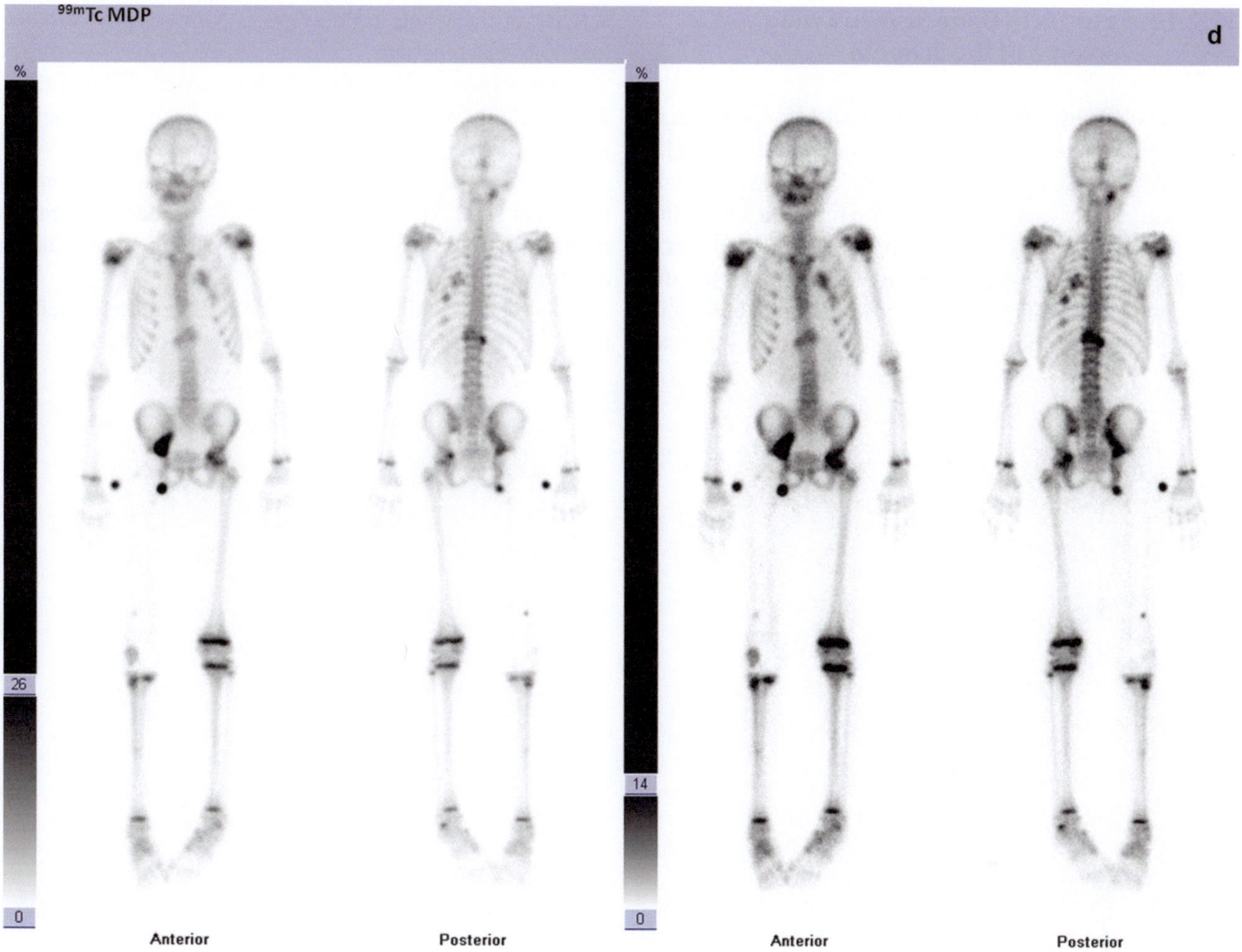

Fig. 12.13 (continued)

12.2.14 Case 12.14 Bone Scan in Ewing's Sarcoma of the Scapula

A 2-year-old baby referred to our institution for pain in right scapula and underwent plain radiography, CT, and MRI (Fig. 12.14a) that evidenced a lesion in the right scapula, strong suspect for malignancy, with no further relevant findings. A biopsy of the lesion was performed and diagnosis of Ewing's sarcoma was made. In order to complete the disease staging, the baby underwent a whole-body bone scintigraphy (Fig. 12.14b), showing a pathological increased activity in the whole right scapula. No evidence of other locations was reported.

A neoadjuvant chemotherapy was started. Then, a right scapulectomy was performed and a good pathological response was assessed. Adjuvant chemotherapy was administered according to the good-responders arm of treatment (ISG AIEOP EW1-Protocol). To date, the girl is in the fifth year of disease-free follow-up in good clinical conditions.

Total body scintigraphy was useful to definitely exclude metastatic disease, orienting the therapeutic approach.

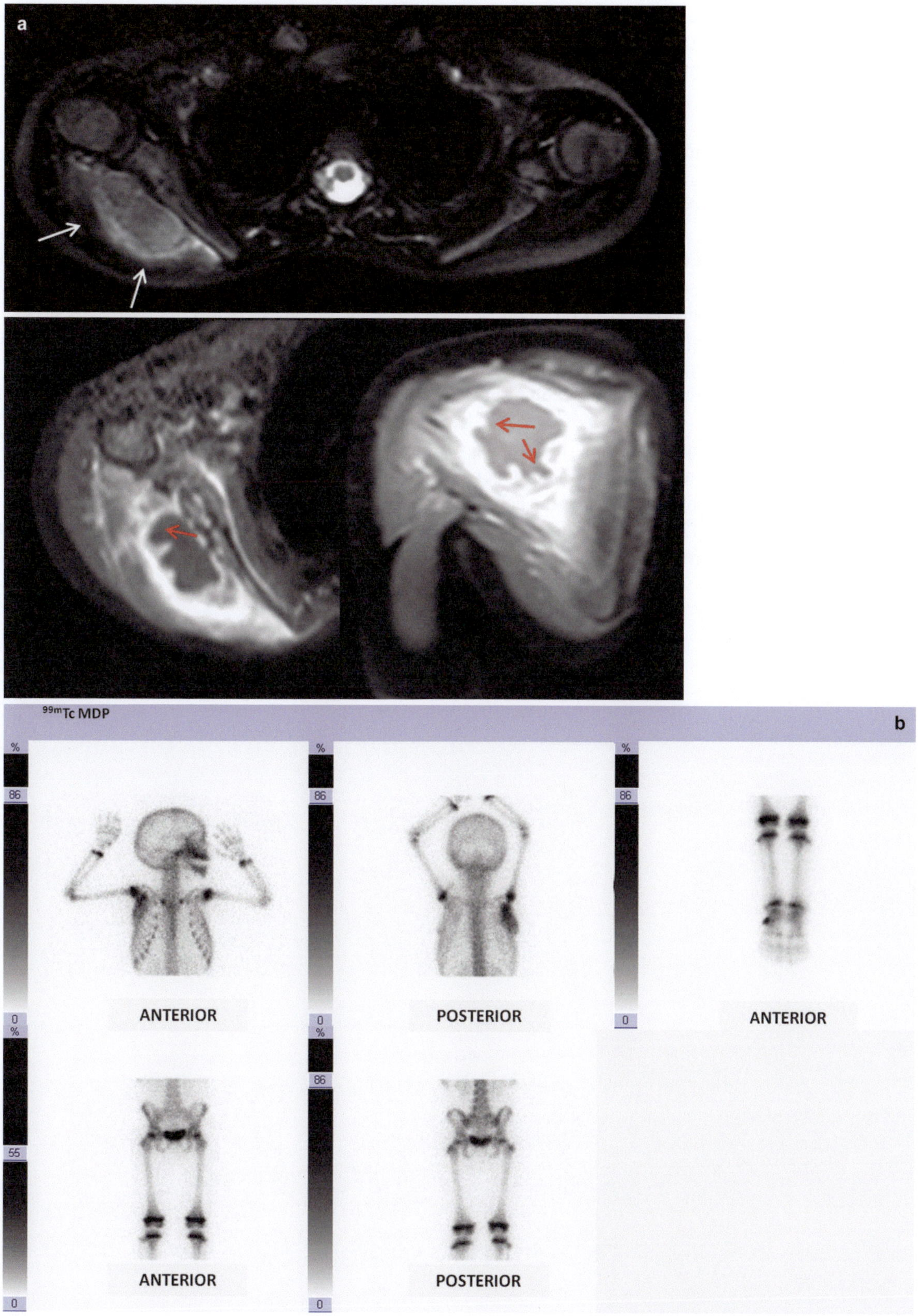

Fig. 12.14 (**a**) Above: Axial MRI T2 fat/sat; below: RM axial and coronal T1 fat/sat after contrast medium; swelling of the posterior margin of the scapula (*white arrows*) with a large extraosseous mass with contrast enhancement, but with wide central hypointense area due to necrosis (*red arrows*). (**b**) ^{99m}Tc-MDP scintigraphy: multiple static views of skeletal segments are acquired, instead of the usual whole-body modality, due to the poor cooperation of the baby; scintigraphy showed intense and diffuse radiotracer uptake in almost all right scapula and no other pathological findings in the skeleton. An accumulation of radiophosphate in skeletal growth plates was also observed that was judged physiological for age

12.2.15 Case 12.15 Bone Scan in Paraneoplastic Cushing's Syndrome, Secondary to Ewing's Sarcoma

A 10-year-old boy presented with history of progressive weight increase, hypertrichosis, and weakness. At physical examination, he presented the classical facial and body habitus of Cushing's syndrome.

Blood tests documented high levels of ACTH and plasma cortisol that suppressed with high-dose dexamethasone test; therefore, the boy underwent brain MRI for evaluation of pituitary gland that appeared normal. Ultrasonography and abdominal MRI revealed bilateral adrenalic hyperplasia with pseudonodular appearance of the cranial portion of the left adrenal gland.

A paraneoplastic Cushing's syndrome was diagnosed, and the patient underwent thorax and abdomen CT in order to identify primary neoplasia. Plain radiography of the pelvis (Fig. 12.15a) and CT scan (Fig. 12.15b, c) identified a diffuse alteration of the bone structure with predominant osteoblastic aspects of the right ischiopubic and ileopubic branches.

CT findings were strongly suggestive for a bone neoformation, suspected for osteosarcoma.

^{99m}Tc-MDP scintigraphy (Fig. 12.15d, e) showed intense uptake of radiotracer in right ischiopubic and ileopubic branches (better defined in pelvis static views) corresponding to the lesion detected by CT. Multiple areas of radiotracer uptake are also evident in skull (more evident in the lateral views of the skull,) spine, several ribs of both hemithorax, sternum, left scapula, both femurs (in particular, the left one), and in right proximal tibia.

Scintigraphic findings were confirmed by radiological examination, as shown in Fig. 12.15f–h.

The final diagnosis of metastatic Ewing's sarcoma with paraneoplastic Cushing's syndrome was made by core biopsy of the left ischiopubic branch lesion.

In this case, bone scan allowed to identify the metastatic nature of the disease, not evident at the CT scan evaluation, thus changing the therapeutical approach toward a metastatic disease protocol.

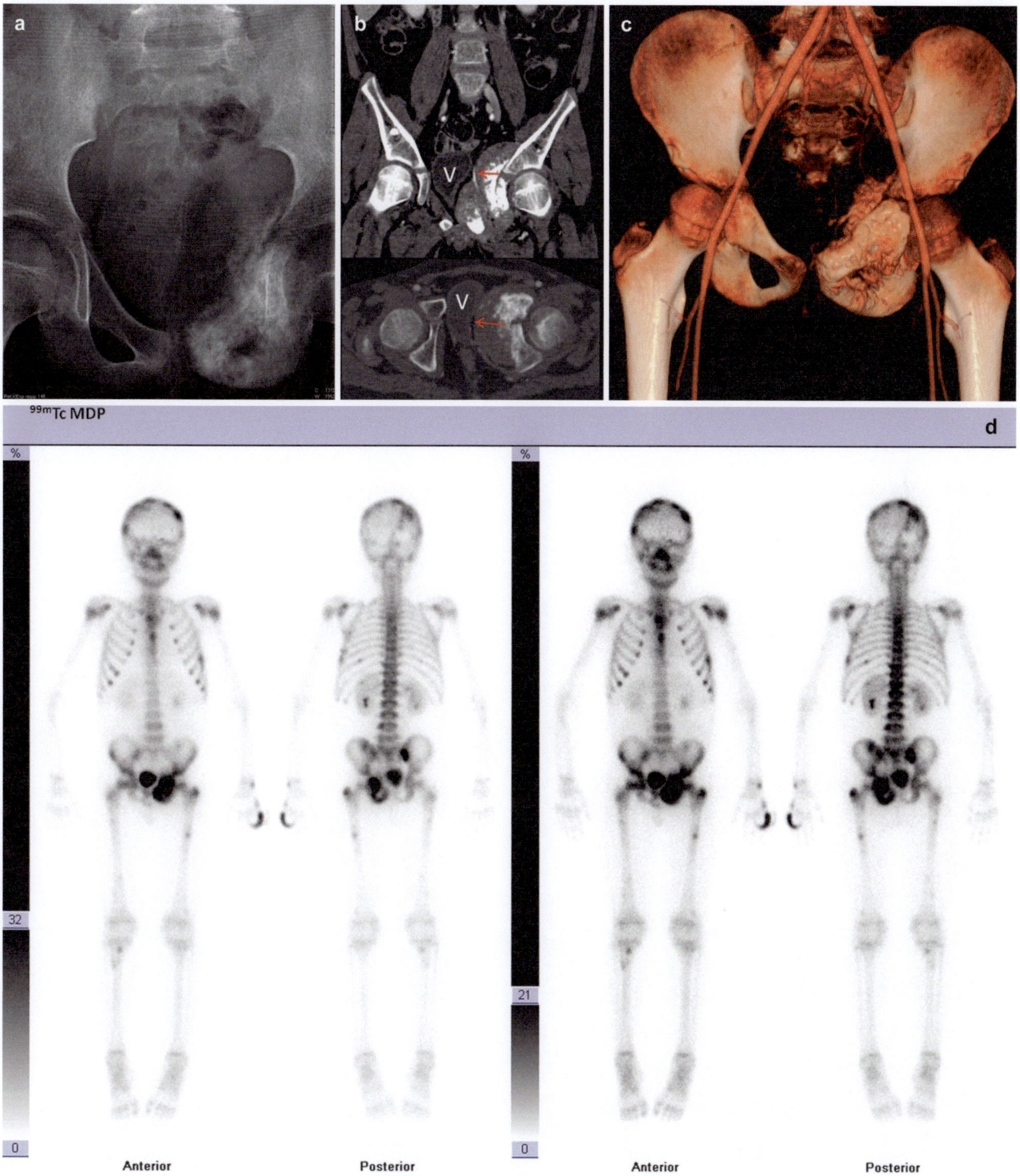

Fig. 12.15 (**a**) AP pelvic plain film: swelling with predominantly sclerotic appearance of left ischiopubic area. (**b**) Coronal and axial CT after contrast medium: bone alteration mainly hyperdense of left ischiopubic area with extraosseous endopelvic mass that displaces the bladder (V) toward the right (*red arrows*). (**c**) Three-dimensional CT shows bone alterations. Notice the integrity of iliac vessels with some newly formed vessels from external and internal iliac arteries that supply the tumor area. (**d**, **e**) ^{99m}Tc-MDP scintigraphy shows intense uptake of radiotracer in right ischiopubic and ileopubic branches (better defined in pelvic static views. (**e**) Corresponding lesion detected by CT. Multiple areas of radiotracer uptake are also evident in skull (more evident in lateral views of the skull, (e) spine, several ribs of both hemithorax, sternum, left scapula, both femurs (in particular in left one), and in right proximal tibia. (**f**–**h**) Cerebral MRI scans sagittal and coronal T1-weighted after contrast medium and axial FLAIR: (**f**) repetitive alteration with right parietal bone bulging, and extracranial and intracranial mass (*red arrow*); CT chest; (**g**) metastatic pulmonary nodules (*red arrow*); T2 sagittal MRI of the spine; (**h**) somatic collapse with hypointense signal in T3 and osteolysis of the anterior half of the L1 body (*white arrow*). Partial somatic collapse of T5–T6 without signal alteration due to osteoporosis (*red arrow*)

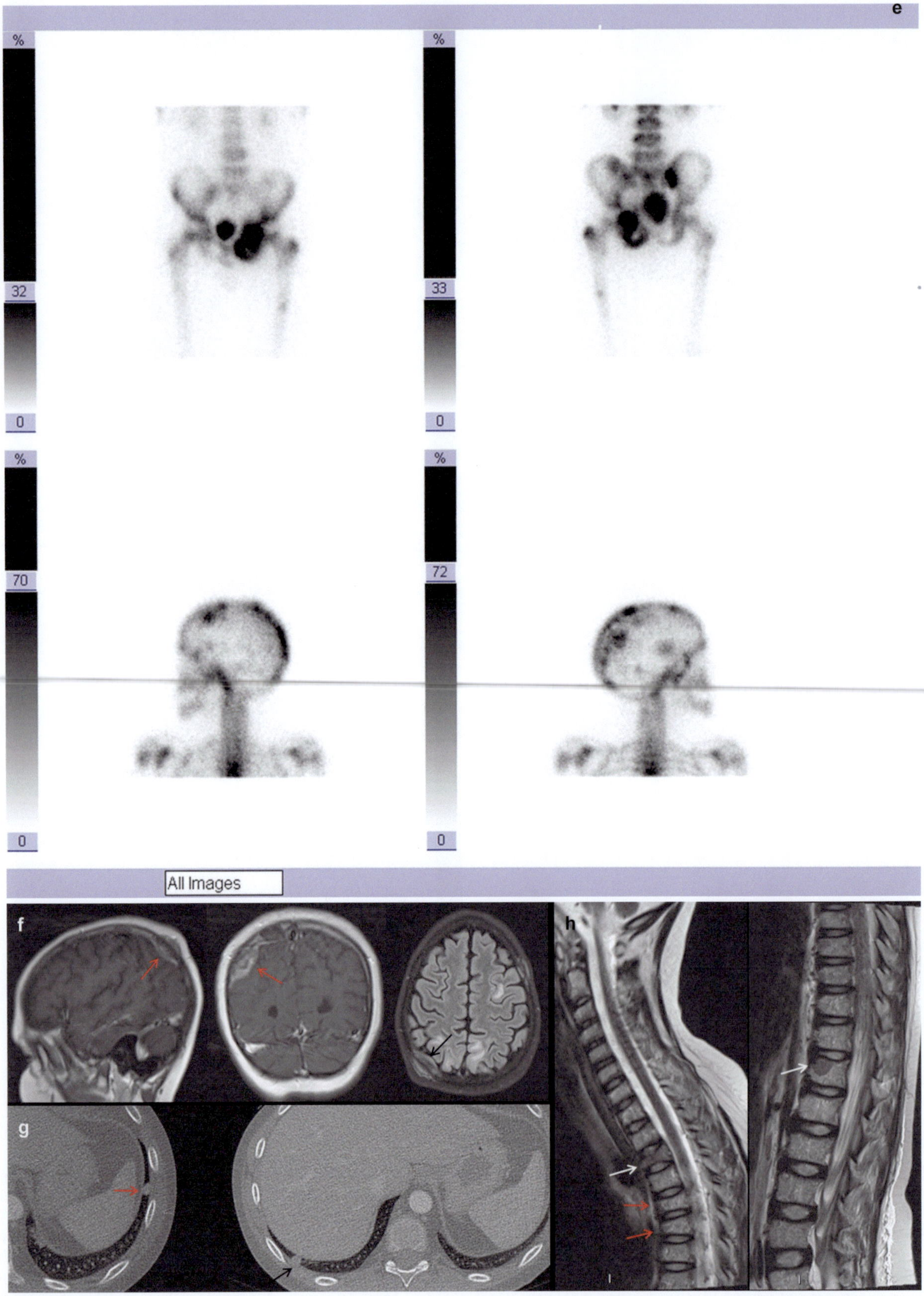

Fig. 12.15 (continued)

12.2.16 Case 12.16 Langerhans' Cell Histiocytosis: Utility of Bone Scan in the Choice of Lesion Eligible for Diagnostic Biopsy

A 15-year old boy presenting cervical pain, asthenia, and weight loss referred to our hospital for diagnostic workup of a vertebral collapse, diagnosed in another center; a CT and spine MRI previously performed detected a preparavertebral lesion extending from C7 to T5, involving intervertebral foramina and spinal canal; a complete vertebral collapse of T1 and lytic lesions in C7–T5 soma and in T1 were also evident, respectively. A biopsy of the lesion was not conclusive. In our hospital, the boy underwent plain radiography, further CT, and spine MRI (Fig. 12.16 a, b, b', c and c'), confirming vertebral lesion, and a brain MRI for evaluation of pituitary gland showed pituitary gland hyperplasia and pituitary gland stalk thickening, thus suggesting a Langerhans' cell histiocytosis.

Therefore, a ^{99m}Tc-MDP whole-body scan was performed in order to detect active lesions and in particular to identify a site eligible for biopsy.

Whole-body bone scintigraphy (Fig. 12.16d–f) showed increased radiotracer uptake in left mastoid process, several vertebrae of cervical and dorsal spine, left sacroiliac joint, and both iliac wings.

Considering scintigraphic finding, a CT-guided biopsy of lesion located in left iliac wing (appearing as lytic in CT) was performed, and histological examination confirmed Langherans' cell histiocytosis.

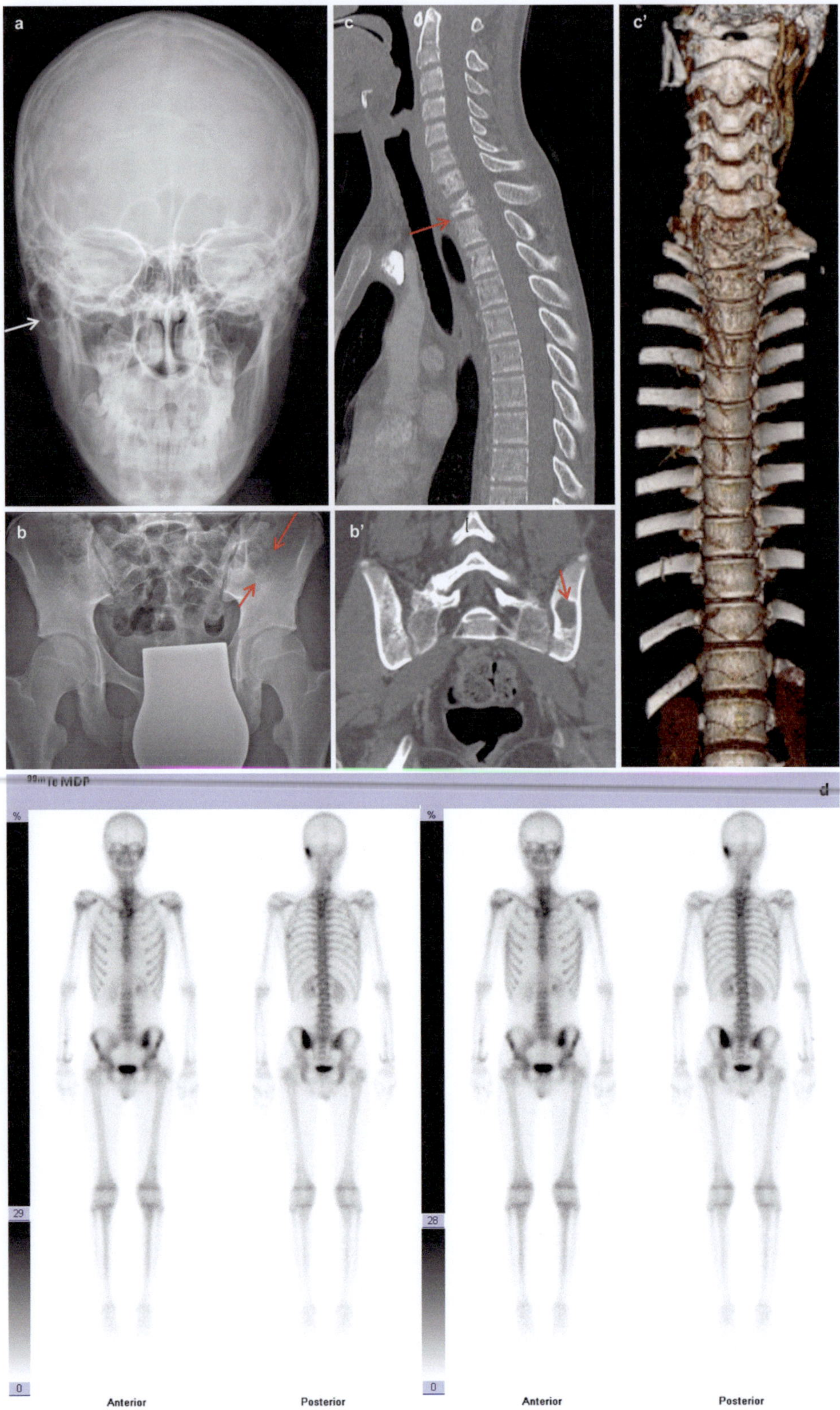

Fig. 12.16 (**a**, **b**, **b'**, **c**, and **c'**) AP Skull plain film. (**a**) Osteolytic area of the right mastoid (*white arrow*). X-ray (b) and coronal CT of the pelvis (**b'**): osteolysis in the left iliac wing (*red arrow*) sagittal CT (**c**). Three-dimensional CT of the spine (**c'**). Multiple somatic alterations from C7 to T4 with partial collapse of T1 (*black arrow*). (**d–f**) Whole-body bone scintigraphy shows increased radiotracer uptake in left mastoid process, several vertebrae of cervical and dorsal spine, left sacroiliac joint, and both iliac wings. Nonhomogeneous radiotracer uptake is also evident in proximal-middle two-third of right humerus and in right scapulohumeral joint. SPECT of the skull and of cervical and dorsal spine are also acquired; SPECT-CT manual fused images (**e**) allows to better localize radiotracer uptake in left mastoid process, while SPECT-MRI manual fused images (**f**) give a better definition of vertebral involvement

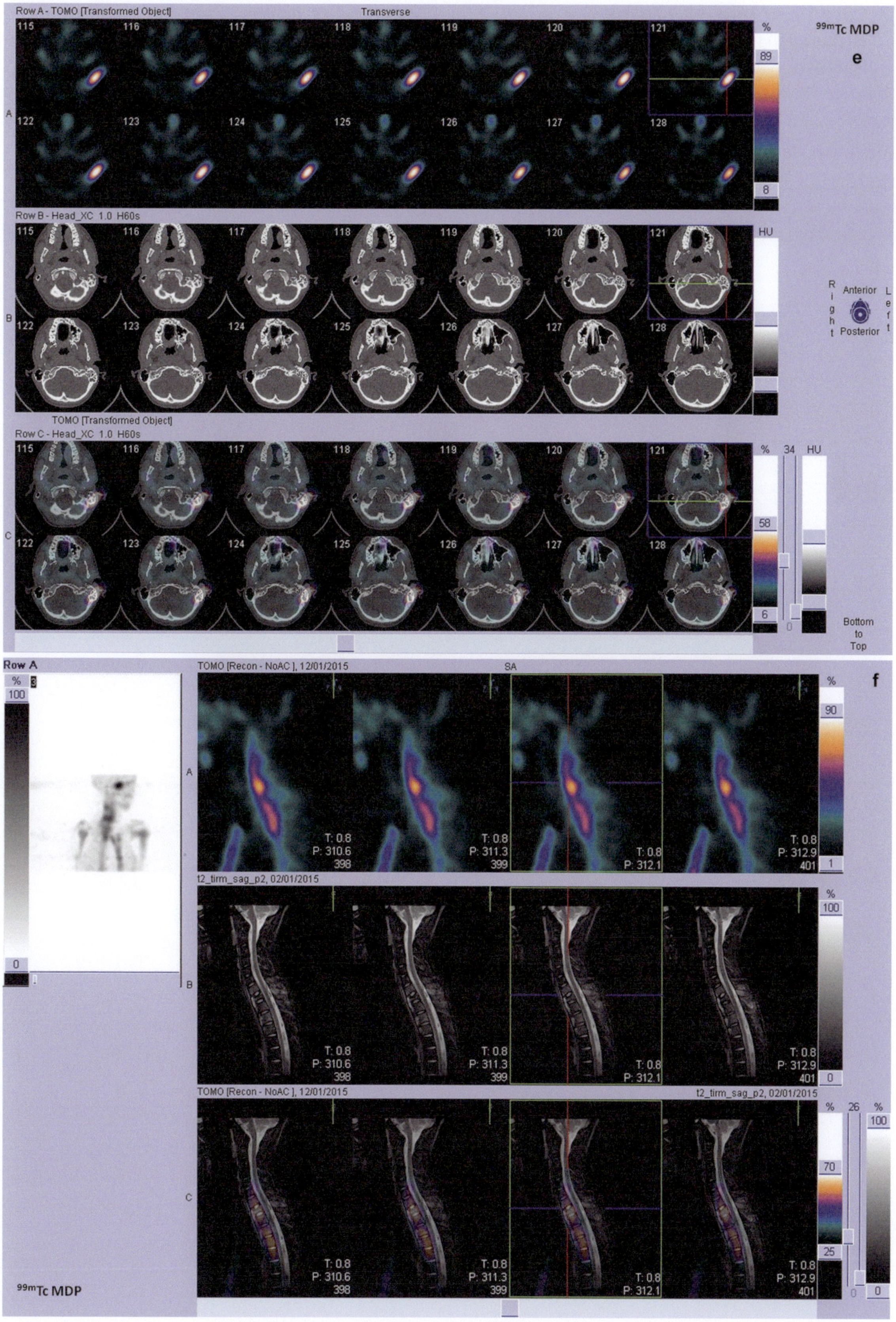

Fig. 12.16 (continued)

12.2.17 Case 12.17 (Fig. 12.17a, b) Histiocytosis: Typical Scintigraphic Pattern

A 3 year old boy was admitted to our department with a history of vomiting, diarrhea, delayed growth and weight loss. A diagnosis of diabetes insipidus was performed. X-ray showed a large osteolytic lesion. Scintigraphy demonstrated a typical pattern of histiocytosis.

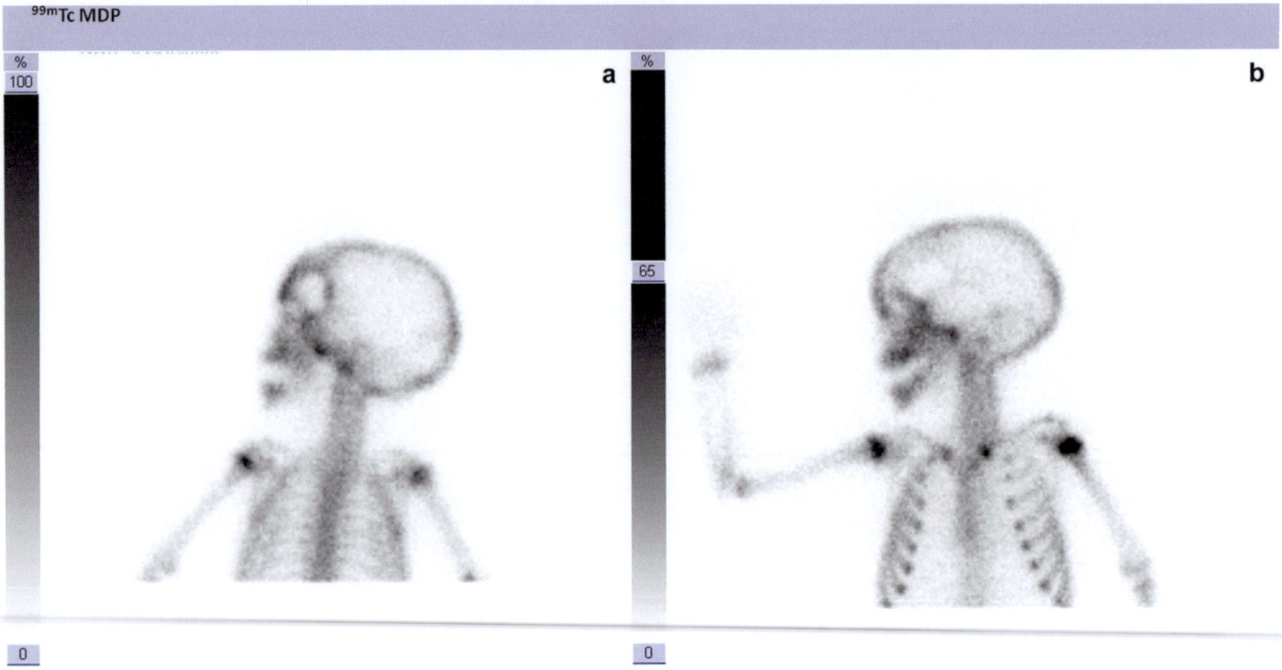

Fig. 12.17 In (**a**) is displayed a typical scintigraphic pattern of histiocytosis: a large photopenic area, surrounded by a rim of intense radiotracer uptake, expression of osteoblastic reaction, in left frontal bone; in (**b**) is showed bone scintigraphy of the same patient, after treatment: a photopenic area is still evident, without rim of uptake (absence of osteoblastic activity)

12.2.18 Case 12.18 (Fig. 12.18a, b) Scintigraphic Features and Typical Sites of Histiocytosis

LCH most commonly affects the skin and bones, but it can involve any organ in the body including lymph nodes, lungs, liver, spleen, bone marrow or brain. Following pictures show typical sites of histiocytosis.

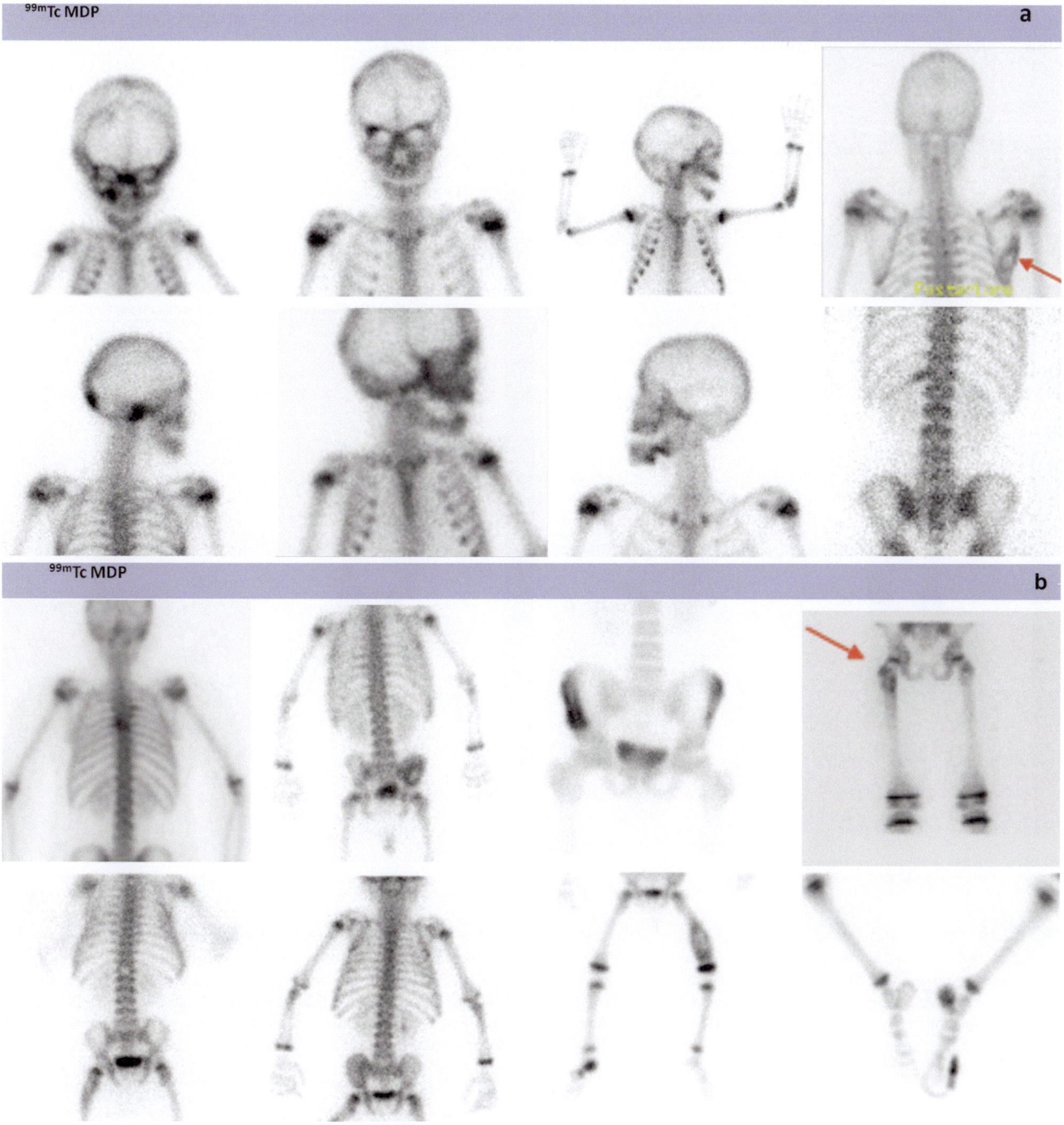

Fig. 12.18 (**a**, **b**) Scintigraphic features and typical sites of histiocytosis

12.2.19 Case 12.19 Bone Scan in Erdheim–Chester Syndrome

Erdheim–Chester disease (ECD) is a rare non-Langerhans' histiocytosis, involving multiple tissues and organs (i.e., skin, lungs, brain, pituitary gland). Bone involvement is characteristic of ECD and typically affects diaphyses and metaphyses of long bones, in particular of lower limbs.

In this figure is displayed a bone scintigraphy of a 16-year-old girl followed in our hospital for ECD.

^{99m}Tc-MDP whole-body bone scintigraphy (Fig. 12.19a) shows bilateral intense and diffuse increased radiotracer uptake in lower limbs, in particular, in metaphyses of distal femurs (extending to region above the metaphyses), proximal tibiae (extending to region below the metaphyses), and distal tibiae (extending to region above the metaphyses), respectively.

Multiple areas of increased radiotracer uptake in skull, proximal right clavicula, sternum, both humeral diaphyses, and left elbow are also evident.

This scintigraphic pattern, especially in lower limbs, is characteristic of skeletal involvement in ECD; corresponding radiological images are reported in Fig. 12.19b–e.

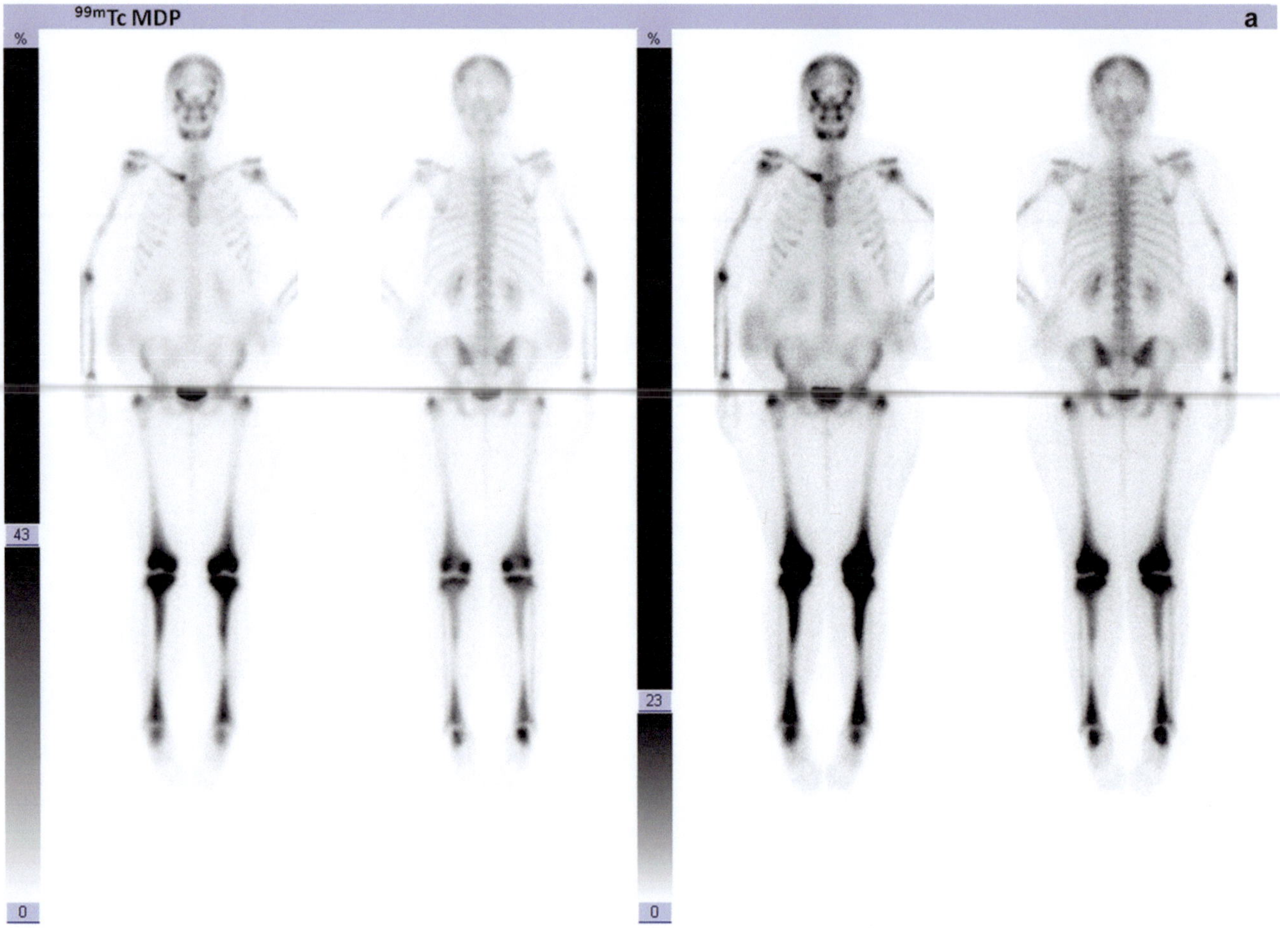

Fig. 12.19 (**a**) Bilateral intense and diffuse increased radiotracer uptake in lower limbs, in particular, in metaphyses of distal femurs (extending to region above the metaphyses), proximal tibiae (extending to region below the metaphyses) and distal tibiae (extending to region above the metaphyses), respectively. (**b–e**): AP skull plain film (**b**) Multiple osteolytic areas in the vault and skull base and in half right jaw (*black arrows*). AP radiograph of the upper chest (**c**) enlargement of right medial clavicle extremity with cortical thinning (*white arrows*). AP plain film of the elbow (**d**) shows flexion contracture and slight inhomogeneous osteosclerosis of articular bones. AP plain film of the legs (**e**): osteosclerotic tibias with thickening of the inner cortex and reduced size of the medullary channel (*black arrows*)

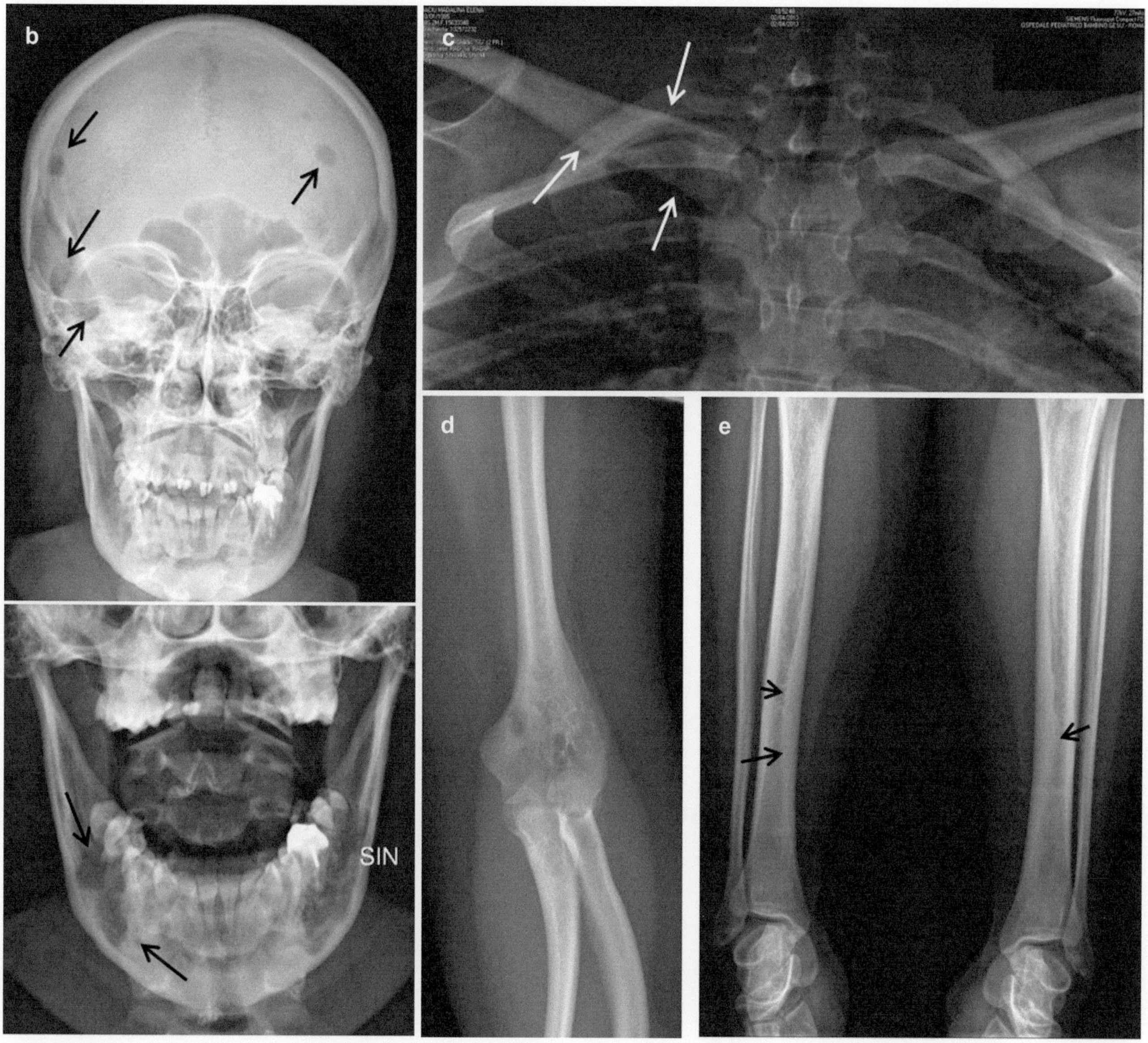

Fig. 12.19 (continued)

Bibliography

1. Fendler WP, Melzer HI, Walz C, von Schweinitz D, Coppenrath E, Schmid I, Bartenstein P, Pfluger T. High 123I-MIBG uptake in neuroblastic tumours indicates unfavourable histopathology. Eur J Nucl Med Mol Imaging. 2013;40(11):1701–10.

Oncology: Neuroblastoma

13

Maria Felicia Villani, Milena Pizzoferro, Aurora Castellano, Roberta Lombardi, Annalisa Serra, Maria Carmen Garganese, and Franco Locatelli

13.1 Introduction

Neuroblastoma is the most common solid extracranial tumor of childhood. It originates from the cell of the neural crest intended to form sympathetic nervous system. It accounts for 7 % of all childhood cancers and for approximately 15 % of cancer deaths in children. Most frequently neuroblastoma arises from the adrenal gland (65 %) but it could originate along the ganglia of sympathetic nervous system. Other common sites are the ganglia in the retroperitoneum followed by the ganglia localized in the chest, neck, and pelvis. The median age at diagnosis is 17 months, but it can occur in children from the prenatal age to young adult age. Around 50 % of patients present with disseminated disease at the time of diagnosis. Dissemination occurs through lymphatic and hematogenous routes, with the involvement of bone, bone marrow, and liver.

Neuroblastoma is staged according to the International Neuroblastoma Staging System (INSS). Stage 1 or 2 neuroblastoma is localized, stage 3 neuroblastoma consists of locoregional extended disease, and stage 4 neuroblastoma is marked by distant metastases. A unique pattern of dissemination, limited to the liver, skin, and less than 10 % of bone marrow in children younger than 18 months old, is defined as stage 4S, which has a potential for spontaneous regression.

M.F. Villani • M. Pizzoferro
Nuclear Medicine Unit, Imaging Departement – "Bambino Gesù" Children Hospital, Rome, Italy

A. Castellano (✉) • A. Serra • F. Locatelli
Oncohematology Department, "Bambino Gesù" Children Hospital, Rome, Italy
e-mail: aurora.castellano@opbg.net

R. Lombardi
Imaging Department, "Bambino Gesù" Children Hospital, Rome, Italy

M.C. Garganese
Diagnostic Imaging Department of Nuclear Medicine, IRCCS Bambino Gesù Paediatric Hospital, Rome, Italy

During the last two decades, there have been major advances in understanding the genetics of NB. Although the unfavorable prognostic factor MYCN amplification is used by all cooperative groups for risk-group stratification and therapeutic decisions, other prognostically significant genetic features have been incorporated into risk classification schemas. For these reasons, the International Neuroblastoma Risk Group (INRG) published a new clinical staging system in 2008: the INRG classification was designed to stratify patients at the time of diagnosis; before any treatment, in the International Neuroblastoma Risk Group Staging System (INRGSS), extent of locoregional disease is determined by the absence or presence of image-defined risk factors (IDRFs) (L1 and L2, respectively). Stage M will be used for widely disseminated disease, and MS describes metastatic NB limited to skin, liver, and bone marrow, without cortical bone involvement in children aged 0–18 months with L1 or L2 primary tumors. This new stratification takes into account histology, age, stage at diagnosis, and chromosomal aberrations.

Children with metastatic disease are quite ill at presentation. As the tumor disseminates to the bone, patients often present with nonspecific symptoms such as fever, bone pain, limping, or all of these. Metastasis in the orbits can cause periorbital ecchymosis (raccoon eyes), sometimes accompanied by proptosis, caused by metastases in the orbital bone.

Particular clinical presentation of disease are the tumor arising from paraspinal site that may cause spinal cord compression resulting in neurological symptoms, such as motor weakness, pain, and sensory loss, which can be medical emergencies. In these cases, multidisciplinary competences are required.

Clinical presentation of patients affected by localized disease depends on the site of tumor; so, the abdominal localization presented with abdominal pain, while thoracic localization often presented with cough or as an incidental finding.

The treatment of metastatic neuroblastoma generally consists of induction chemotherapy, surgery, myeloablative

© Springer International Publishing Switzerland 2017

M.C. Garganese, G.F.L. D'Errico (eds.), *Conventional Nuclear Medicine in Pediatrics*, DOI 10.1007/978-3-319-43181-9_13

chemotherapy with stem cell rescue, radiotherapy, and immunotherapy. The treatment of localized neuroblastoma ranges from observation to chemotherapy, surgery, radiotherapy, and differentiating therapy. The clinical course in patients affected by metastatic neuroblastoma varies enormously, ranging from spontaneous regression to rapid and fatal tumor progression, despite extensive treatment.

The outcome of the patient affected by neuroblastoma is extremely variable in the case series and strongly depends on the presence of metastatic disease.

Improvement in the knowledge about tumor genome, more refined pathological definition, and more sophisticated diagnostic techniques allow to better characterize neuroblastoma in all its features, in order to tailor the treatment to the patients and to improve their prognosis.

13.2 Study Technique and Interpretation: 123I-MIBG Scintigraphy

123I-MIBG is administered by slow intravenous injection (administered activity adjusted to the patient's weight, according to EANM dosage card and to the Italian regulations), and scintigraphic images are acquired 24 h after the injection.

Anterior and posterior static spot images of chest, abdomen, pelvis, upper and lower extremities, and anterior, posterior, left lateral, and right lateral spot images of the skull are acquired; the study is single proton emission tomography (SPECT) of interested segments; SPECT images are also manually fused with CT and/or MRI when available.

123I MIBG scan represents the gold standard for disease staging and treatment response evaluation in NB patients. MIBG labeled with 123I has superior imaging characteristics than 131I-MIBG due to its physical properties (159 keV photon energy, 13 h half-life, and paucity of 123I particulate emission) and to the high activity that can be administered. 123I characteristics and its favorable dosimetry, even at high administered doses, make its use preferable in children. Moreover, the SPECT and SPECT/CT overcome the limitation of planar 123I MIBG scan imaging and can distinguish false-positive uptake, thus improving the detection rate and accuracy. A better anatomical localization of the lesions is achieved by the three-dimensional reconstruction of CT images, while imaging definition is improved by the lesion contrast evident at the CT scan.

Overall, MIBG scintigraphy alone is a sensitive (88–93 %) and specific (83–92 %) tool in detecting NB cells. False-positive MIBG findings are due to misinterpretation of physiological uptake, as in normal adrenal gland, bowel, muscle, heart, and liver. Instead, MIBG uptake in bone or bone marrow is always abnormal and has to be considered as a sign of focal bone involvement and/or diffuse bone marrow infiltration.

There are many drugs that can interfere with MIBG uptake, in particular, cardiovascular and sympathomimetic drugs (such as amiodarone, combined alpha and beta-blockers, adrenergic neurone blockers, alpha-blockers, calcium channel blockers), systemic and local nasal decongestants, and several neurological drugs. A full list of interfering drugs is reported in EANM Guidelines on MIBG Scintigraphy.

However, in pediatric clinical practice, most used medications are cardiovascular drugs, in particular, antihypertensives, because hypertension is often present in NB patients.

13.2.1 Case 13.1 MIBG Scan in Prenatal Diagnosis of Adrenal Mass: MIBG-Avid Lesion

A newborn with prenatal diagnosis of right adrenal mass, confirmed by ultrasonography (US, 1) at birth and with elevated urinary catecholamines, undergoes 123I-MIBG scintigraphy (Fig. 13.1c, d) to confirm the suspicion of neuroblastoma (NB). MIBG scan shows a MIBG avid lesion, without evidence of metastases. According to European guidelines, the baby is enrolled in observational protocol for neonatal adrenal mass.

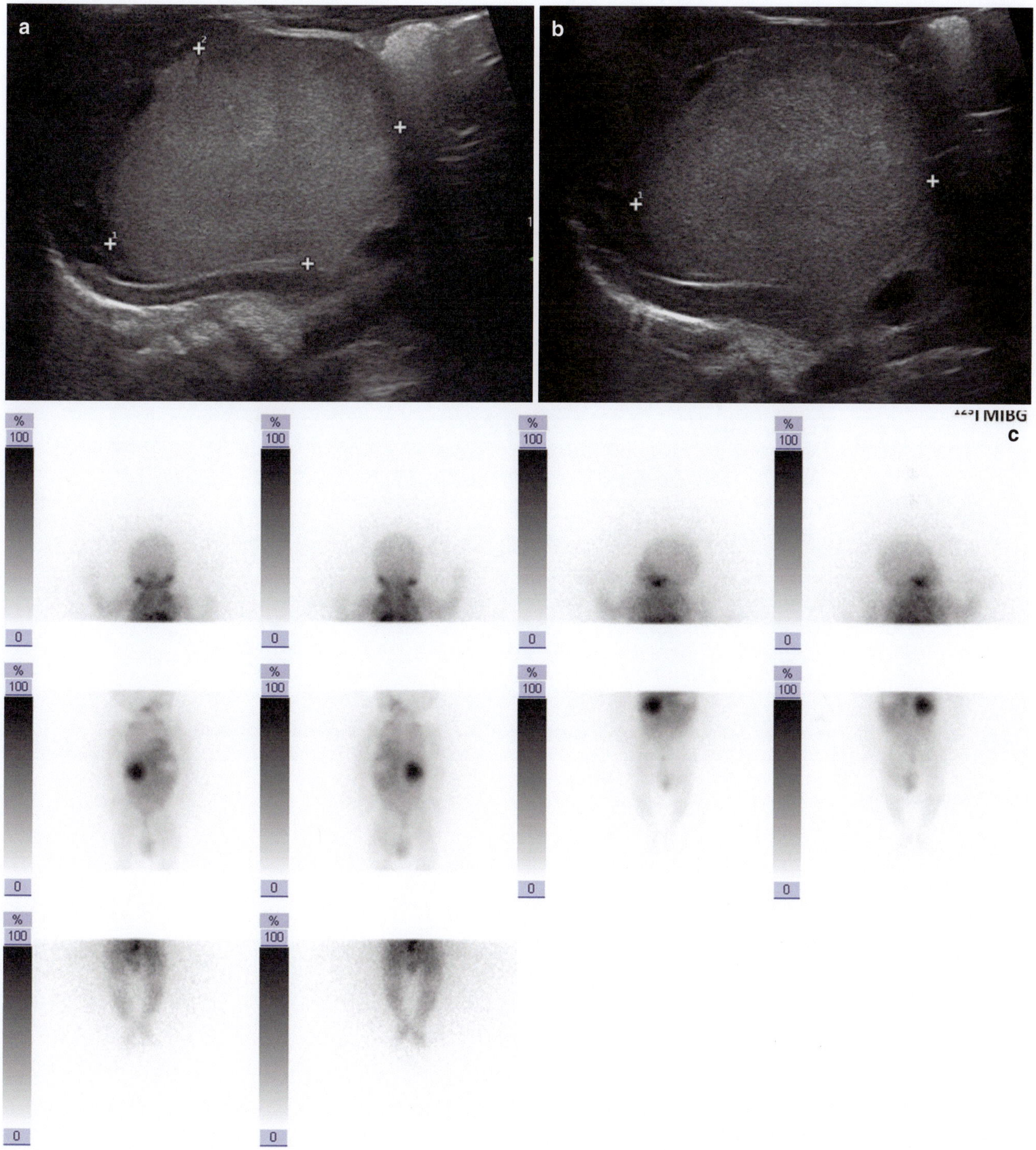

Fig. 13.1 (**a**, **b**) Ultrasonographic images detect a large, oval, "comma"-shaped suprarenal mass showing an echoic fine nonhomogeneous pattern; neither calcifications nor necrotic areas are seen within the lesion. Diameters are about 40 × 27.5 × 34.5 mm. Right kidney is displaced and distorted, but not infiltrated by the tumor, and adrenal flaps are opened wide; a "contact" is present between the mass and the inferior vena cava that appears "flattened," reduced in diameter in retro-hepatic tract, but with partially visible lumen. Color-Doppler ultrasound (CDUS) evaluation shows some flow signal peripherally and within the lesion. (**c**, **d**) MIBG scintigraphy (static views (**c**) show an area of intense and nonhomogeneous radiotracer uptake in the abdomen, corresponding to the mass detected by ultrasonography; no other areas of pathological uptake of radiotracer are evident. SPECT images (**d**) help to better identify the site of the uptake (right adrenal region)

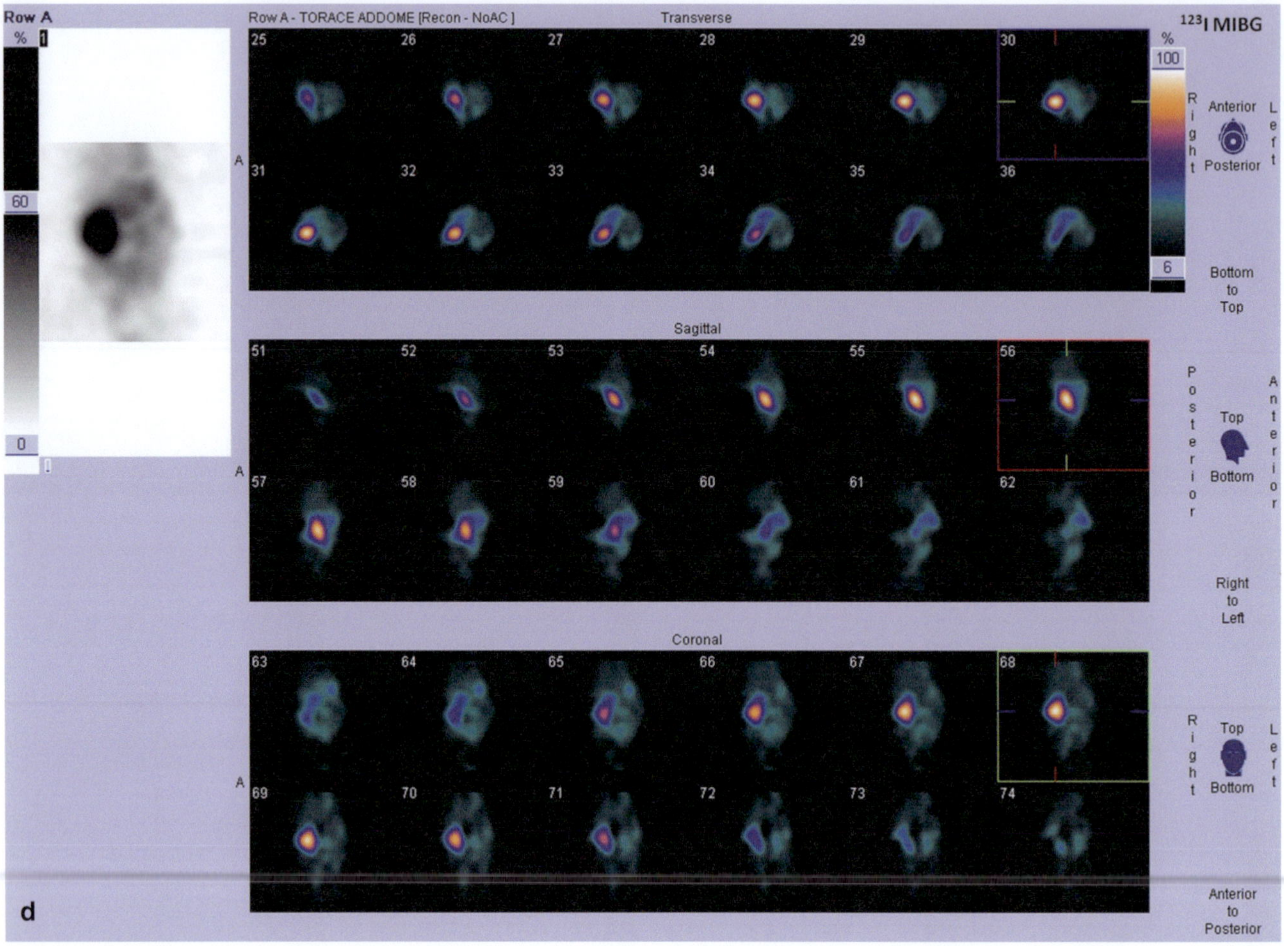

Fig. 13.1 (continued)

13.2.2 Case 13.2 Prenatal Diagnosis of Adrenal Mass: Nonavid Lesion at MIBG Scan

A newborn with prenatal diagnosis of left adrenal mass undergoes at birth an ultrasonography (Fig. 13.2a–d), which shows a reduction of diameters of the lesion; therefore, 123I-MIBG scintigraphy is performed in order to exclude a NB (Fig. 13.2e, f). The lesion appears as nonavid of MIBG, and the baby is enrolled in observational protocol for neonatal adrenal mass.

Lesion was no longer detectable at ultrasonography performed at 1 year of age.

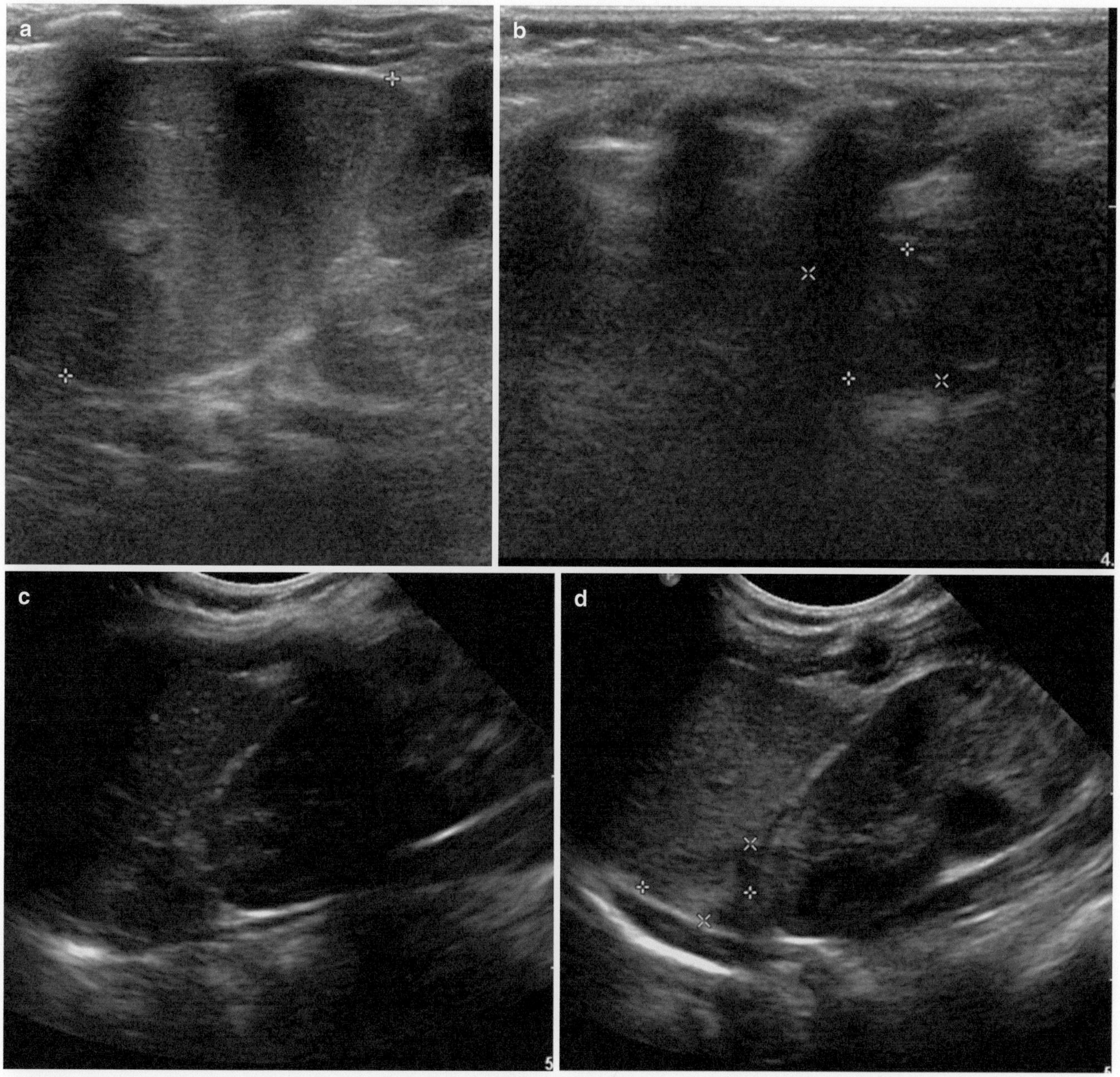

Fig. 13.2 (**a–d**) Ultrasonographic images of the left hypochondrium shows a lesion with size reduced compared to the previous ultrasound examination performed in gestational age (now measuring about 14 × 12 × 10 mm). This lesion presents another homogeneous pattern, mainly hypoechoic with tiny hyperechoic spots in the central part, probably due to small calcifications. At CDUS, no flow signals are detected within the adrenal mass. Spleen and left kidney are separated from the lesion by a fatty layer. (**e, f**) MIBG scintigraphy (static views, **c**) does not show any areas of pathological uptake of radiotracer; in particular, the lesion detected by ultrasonography appears as nonavid of MIBG. SPECT images (**f**) confirm this finding

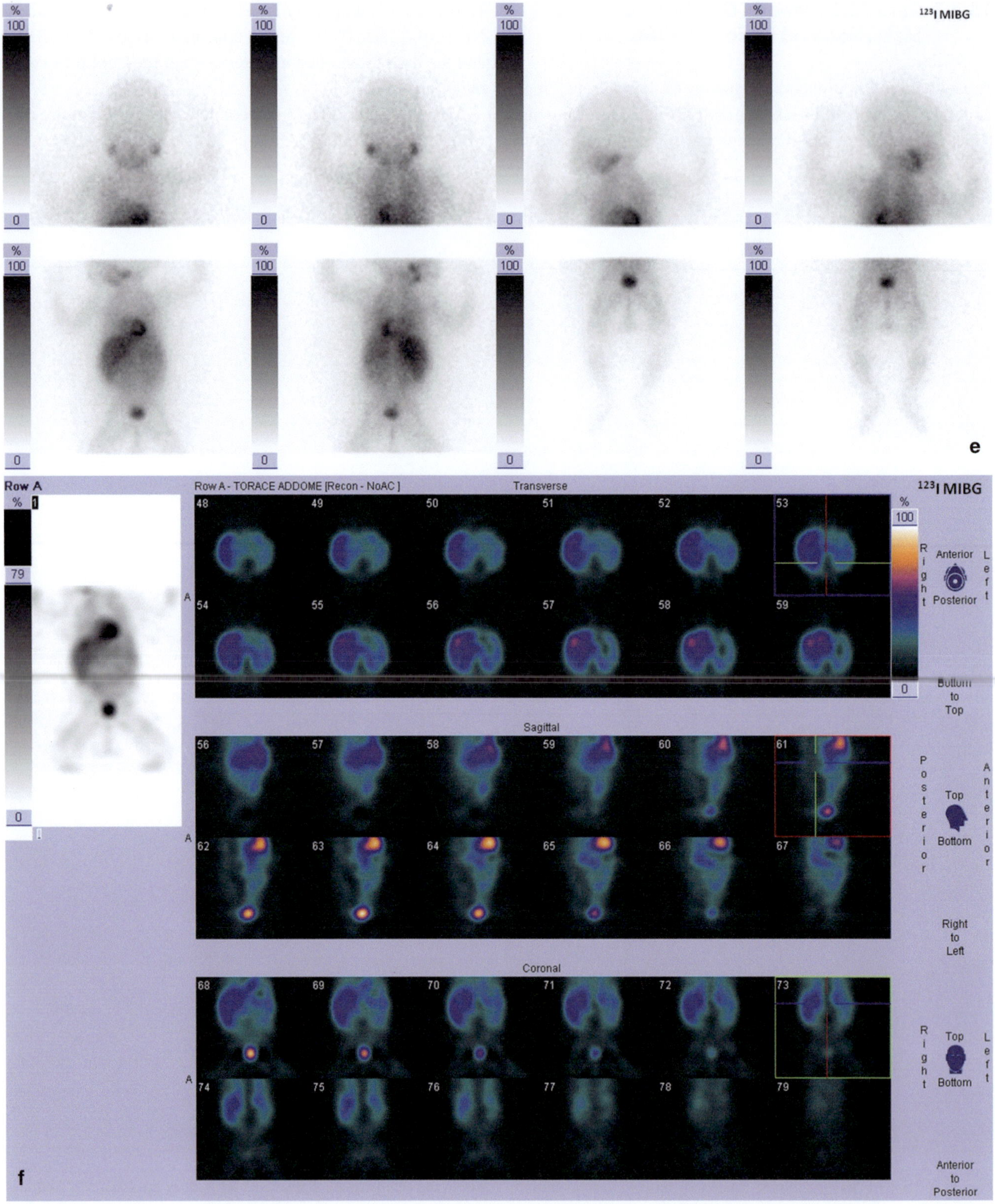

Fig. 13.2 (continued)

13.2.3 Case 13.3: MIBG Scintigraphy in Localized Thoracic Neuroblastoma Infiltrating Spinal Canal

An 11-month-old baby presents sudden hypotonia and difficulty in crawling; physical examination confirms hypotonia of the lower limbs. Suspecting a spinal cord compression, a brain and spine magnetic resonance (MR) (Fig. 13.3a–d) and a chest and abdomen computed tomography (CT) (Fig. 13.3e,f) are performed, and a left mediastinal mass is detected localized at the costovertebral junction between the T1 and T6 spinal levels, with foraminal and intraspinal extension. Histological examination shows a stroma-poor NB, and, subsequently, a MIBG scintigraphy for staging purpose is scheduled and confirms the presence of the mass without metastases (Fig. 13.3g, h). Genomic profile shows absence of numerical chromosomal aberration, and so the case is defined as L2 neuroblastoma <12 months of age at diagnosis with IDRFs – NCA genomic profile with life-threatening symptoms. Patient is enrolled in LINES protocol – Group 2, and underwent chemotherapy. After receiving two courses of chemotherapy with carboplatin and etoposide, a complete resolution of symptoms is observed. A re-evaluation of disease shows the persistence of IDRFs; so, patient undergoes follow-up.

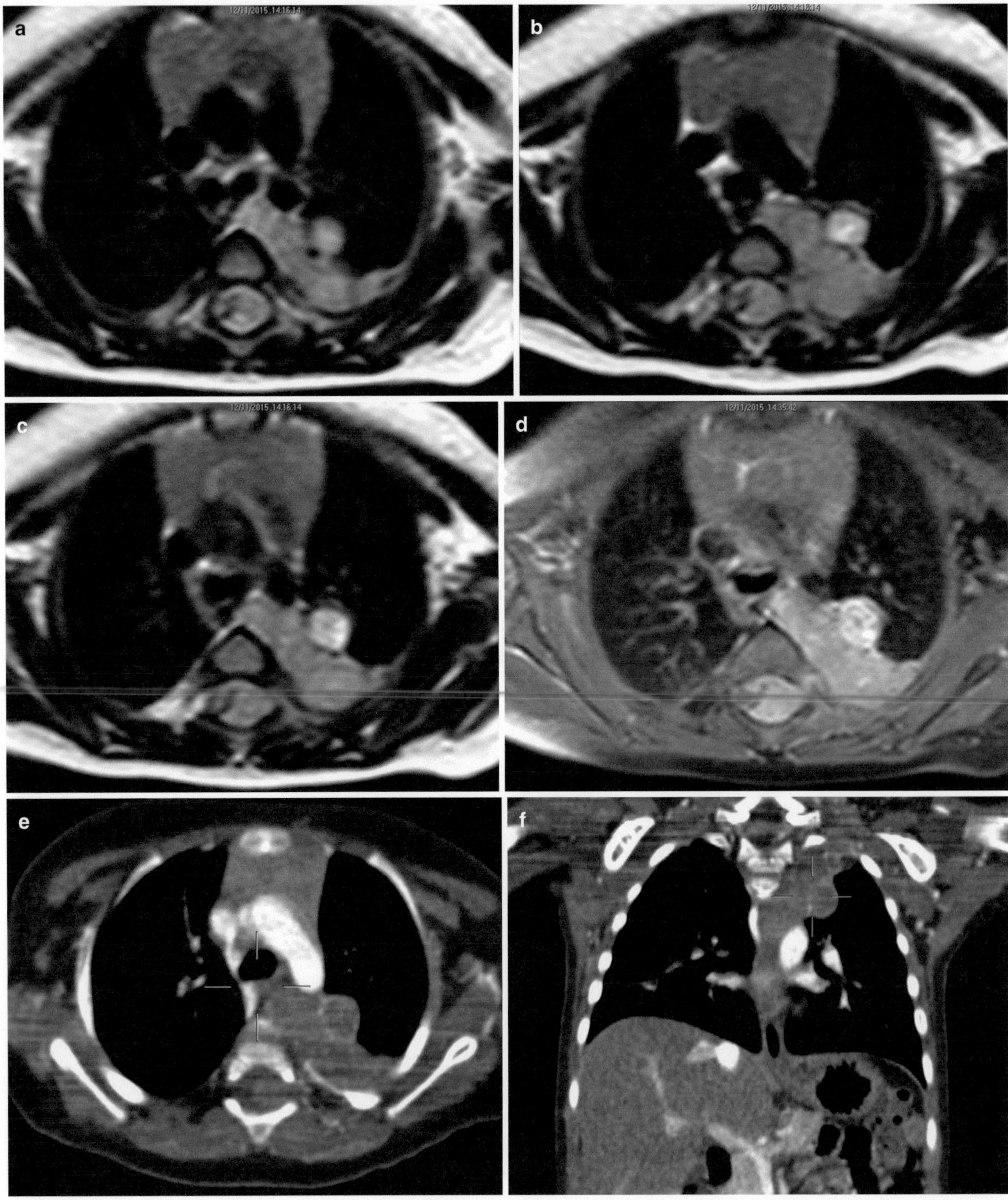

Fig. 13.3 (**a**–**f**) Transverse nonenhanced T2-weighted MR image and postcontrast T1-weighted image (**a**–**d**), and transverse and MPR coronal contrast-enhanced CT (**e**, **f**) imaging show left mediastinal mass localized at the costovertebral junction between T1 and T6 spinal levels, with foraminal and intraspinal extension (dumbbell tumor). A "contact" is present between the lesion and the aorta (aortic arch and descending aorta), the left subclavian vein, and the azygous vein, respectively. In postcontrast imaging (both CT and MRI), more than one-third of the spinal canal in the transverse plane is invaded, and the leptomeningeal spaces are not visible; the spinal cord MR signal intensity appears altered, as for marrow infiltration. (**g**, **h**) MIBG scintigraphy (static views, **g**) shows an area of intense and nonhomogeneous radiotracer uptake in the posterior chest; SPECT-CT fused images (**h**) confirm that the area of uptake corresponds to the mass detected by CT; no other areas of pathological uptake of radiotracer are evident

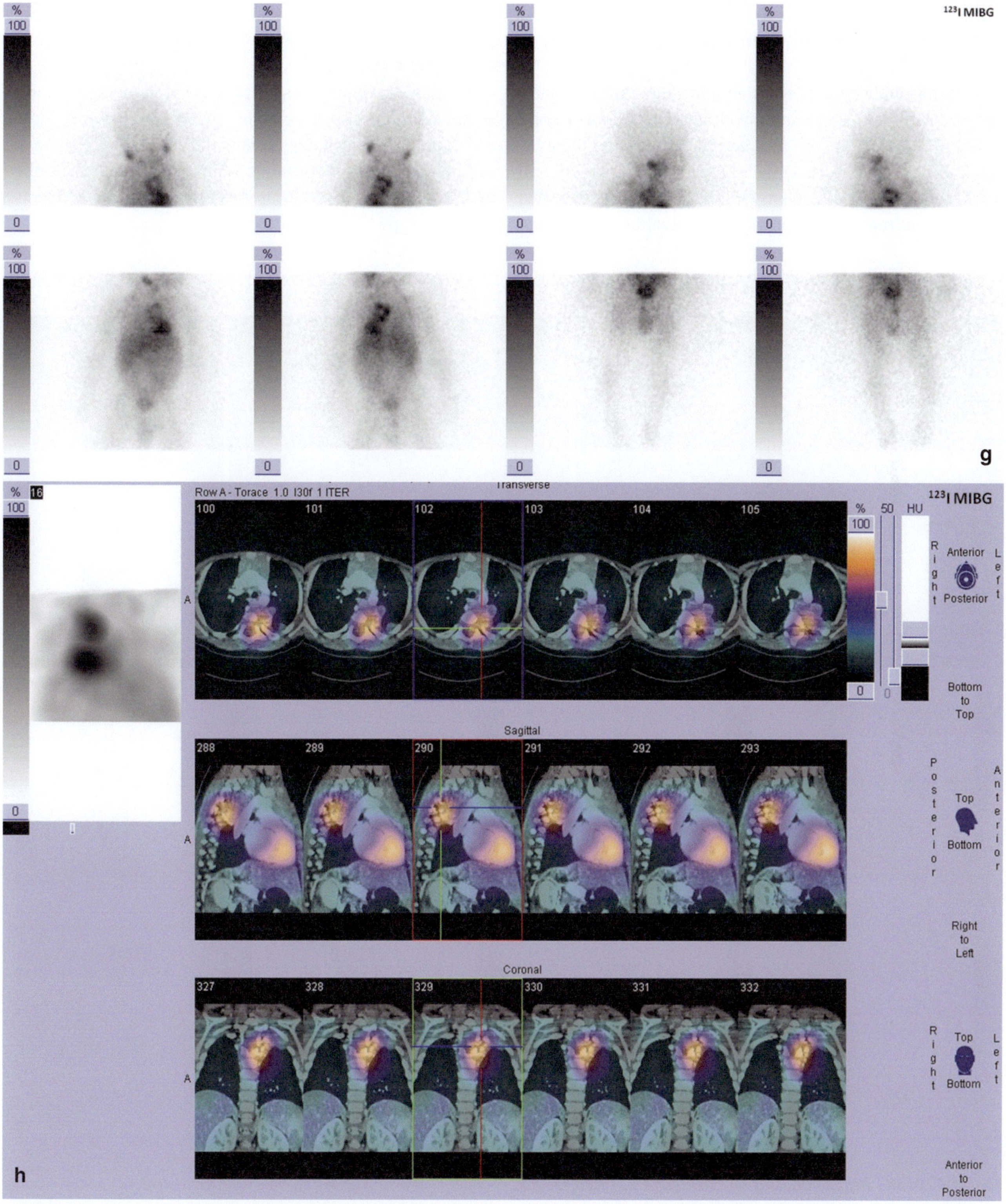

Fig. 13.3 (continued)

13.2.4 Case 13.4: MIBG Scintigraphy in Localized Abdominal Neuroblastoma

A 5-month-old baby undergoes an ultrasonography for incidental finding of abdominal swelling; US shows a solid lesion localized in the left retroperitoneal space on the middle line. CT detected a large retroperitoneal, prevertebral mass, with some calcifications (Fig. 13.4a–c), and suspected for NB, confirmed by histological examination (NB stroma poor). Subsequently, MIBG scan is scheduled for staging purpose and detects the presence of the mass without metastases (Fig. 13.4d, e).

Genomic profile shows the absence of numerical chromosomal aberration; so, the case is defined as L2 neuroblastoma <12 months of age at diagnosis with IDRFs – NCA genomic profile without life-threatening symptoms. Patient is enrolled in LINES protocol – Group 1 and randomized to receive chemotherapy.

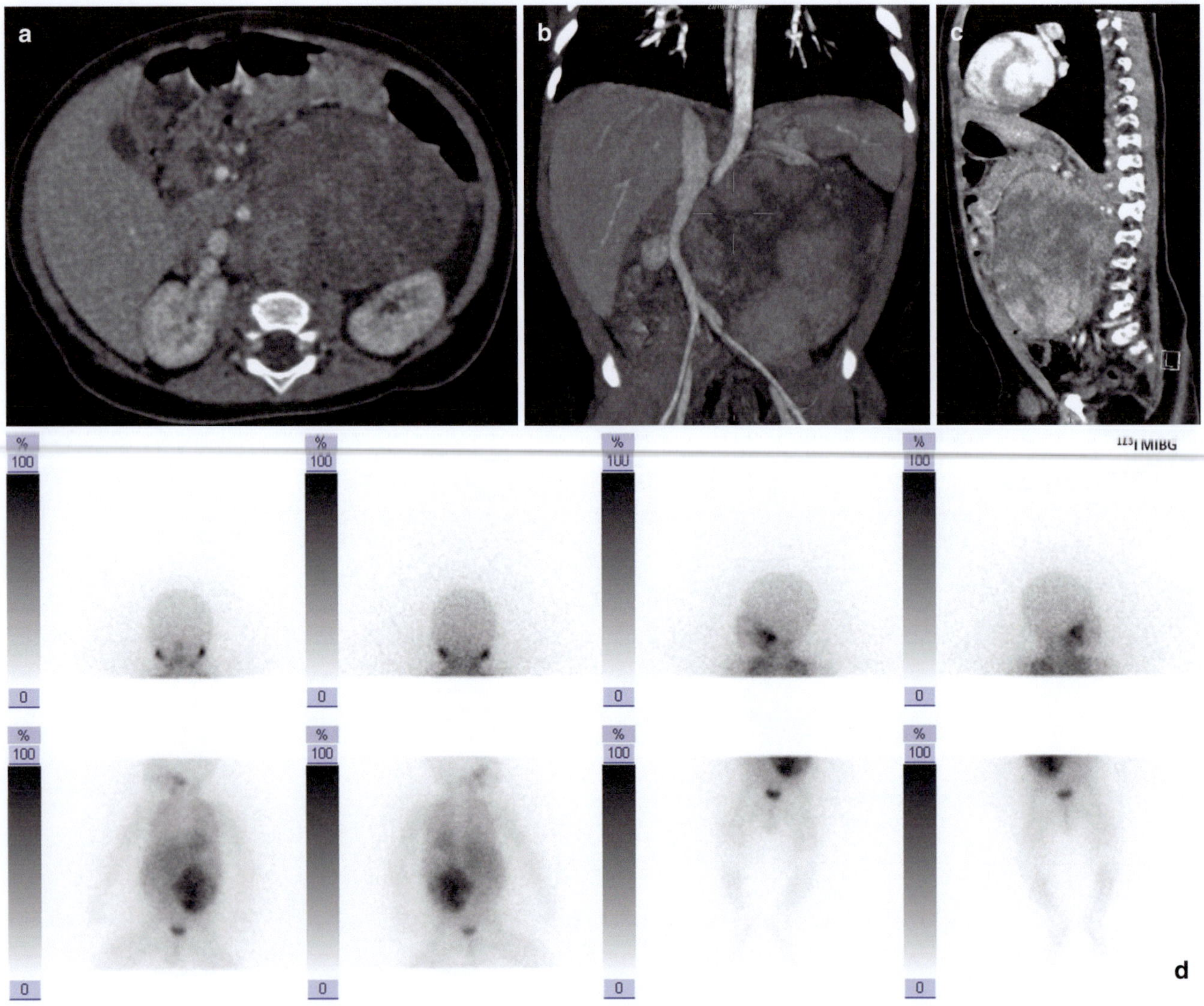

Fig. 13.4 (**a**–**c**) Contrast-enhanced CT. Transverse (**a**), MPR coronal (**b**), and sagittal (**c**) images show a large tumor in left abdomen, crossing the midline, containing large areas of amorphous calcifications, with nonhomogeneous enhancement after contrast media administration. Left kidney is displaced and distorted by the tumor but not infiltrated, as the normal cortex is still visible; aorta and inferior cava are pervious, although stretched, flattened, and displaced anteriorly, such as celiac artery, hepatic artery, and superior mesenteric vessels. Tumor infiltrates the iliolumbar fossa, without foraminal and intraspinal extensions. (**d**, **e**) MIBG scintigraphy (static views, **d**) detects a large area of intense and nonhomogeneous radiotracer uptake in abdomen-pelvis, crossing the middle line; SPECT-CT fused images (**e**) confirm that the area of uptake corresponds to the mass detected by CT; no other areas of pathological uptake of radiotracer are evident

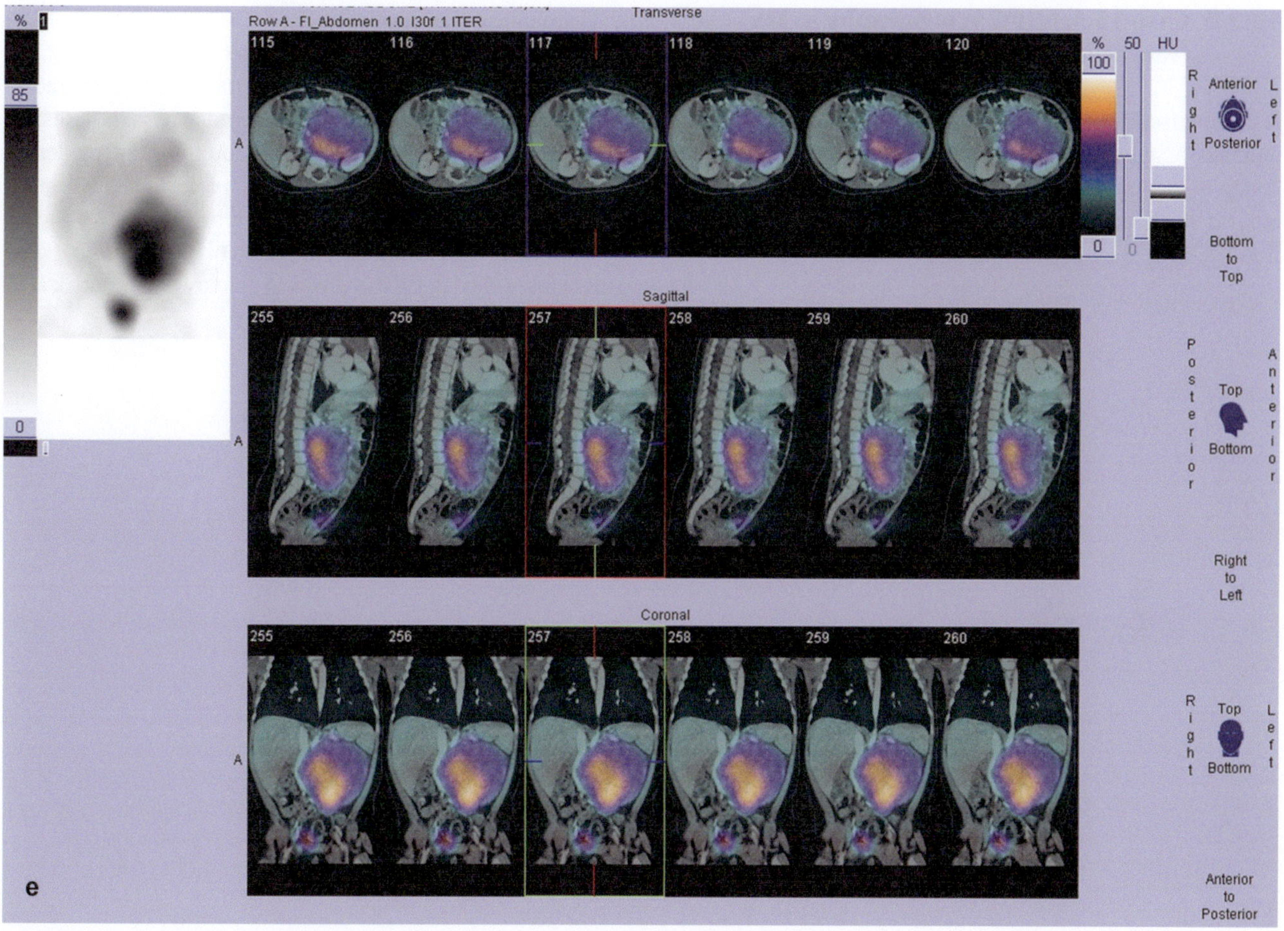

Fig. 13.4 (continued)

13.2.5 Case 13.5: MIBG Scintigraphy in MS Neuroblastoma

A 2-month-old baby refers to our institution for vomiting and lack of appetite; an ultrasonography shows a left adrenal lesion that compresses left kidney and multiple hyperechoic areas in the liver, respectively. CT confirms ultrasonographic findings (Fig. 13.5a–f).

Histological examination reveals a NB; therefore, the baby undergoes a MIBG scan for staging purpose (Fig. 13.5g, h); scintigraphy detects the mass and a nonhomogeneous radiotracer uptake in the liver, due to the presence of metastases; no other areas of pathological uptake of radiotracer are evident.

Genomic profile shows the absence of segmental chromosomal aberration; so, the case is defined as MS neuroblastoma without SCA and without life-threatening symptoms. The patient is enrolled in LINES protocol – Study arm low-risk MS.

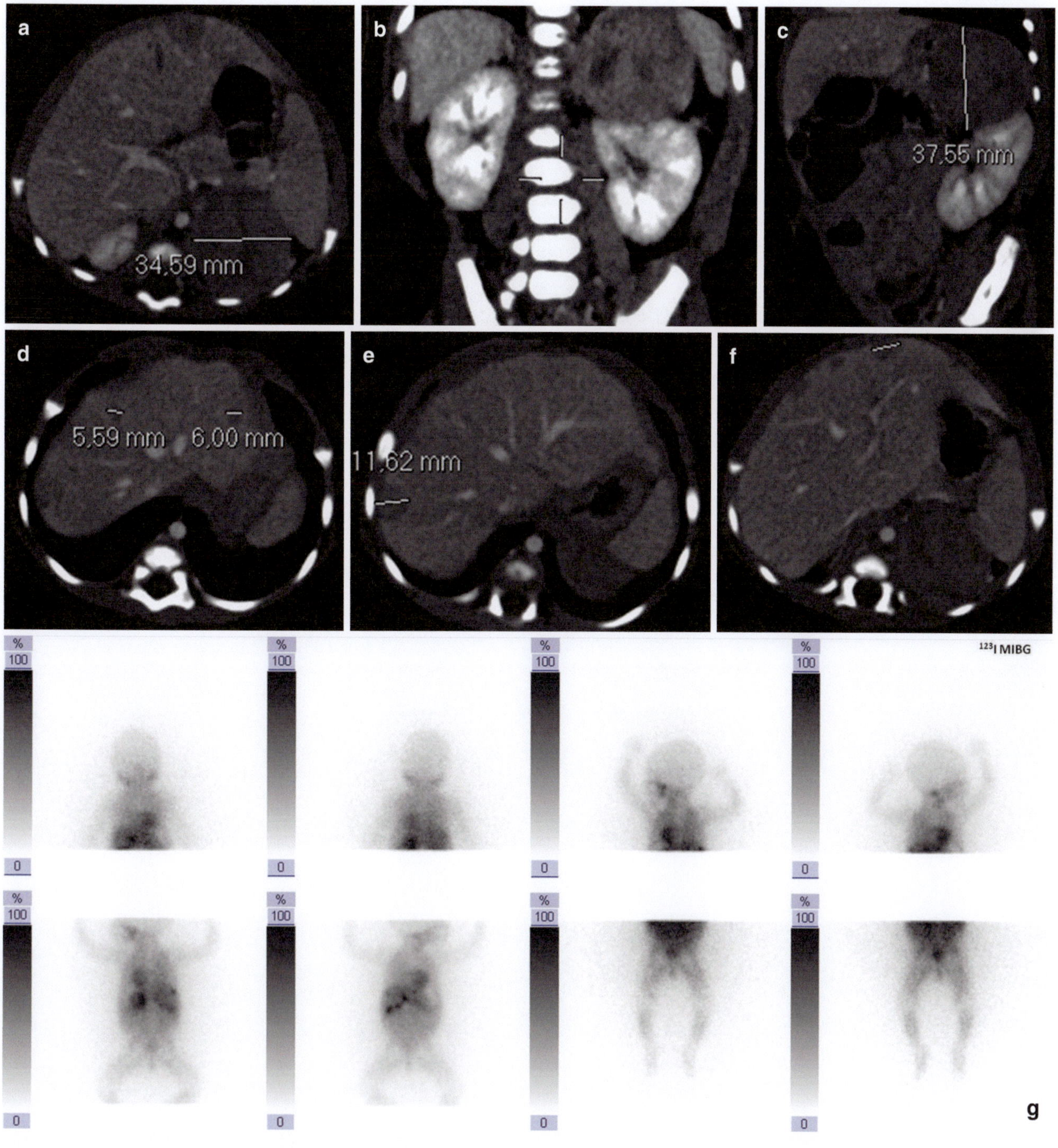

Fig. 13.5 (**a–f**) Contrast-enhanced CT. Transverse (**a**), MPR coronal (**b**), and sagittal (**c**) images show a mass in left adrenal lodge (with diameters about 41 × 35 × 38 mm); tumor appears round-shaped and well-circumscribed; it displaces and compresses left kidney, separated from the tumor by a fatty layer. The mass has a wide contact with aorta, celiac artery, and splenic vessels, stretched and flattened; a part of the left vein is completely encased by the tumor. CT scan shows also multiple peripherally enhancing lesions throughout the liver, consistent with the metastases (transverse images, **d–f**). (**g**, **h**) MIBG scintigraphy (static views, **g**) detects a large area of intense and nonhomogeneous radiotracer uptake in abdomen, in left paravertebral region; SPECT-CT fused images (**h**) confirm that the area of uptake corresponds to the adrenal lesion detected by CT; the liver shows nonhomogeneous radiotracer uptake, due to multiple secondary nodules evident at CT (**g**, **h**); no other areas of pathological uptake of radiotracer are evident

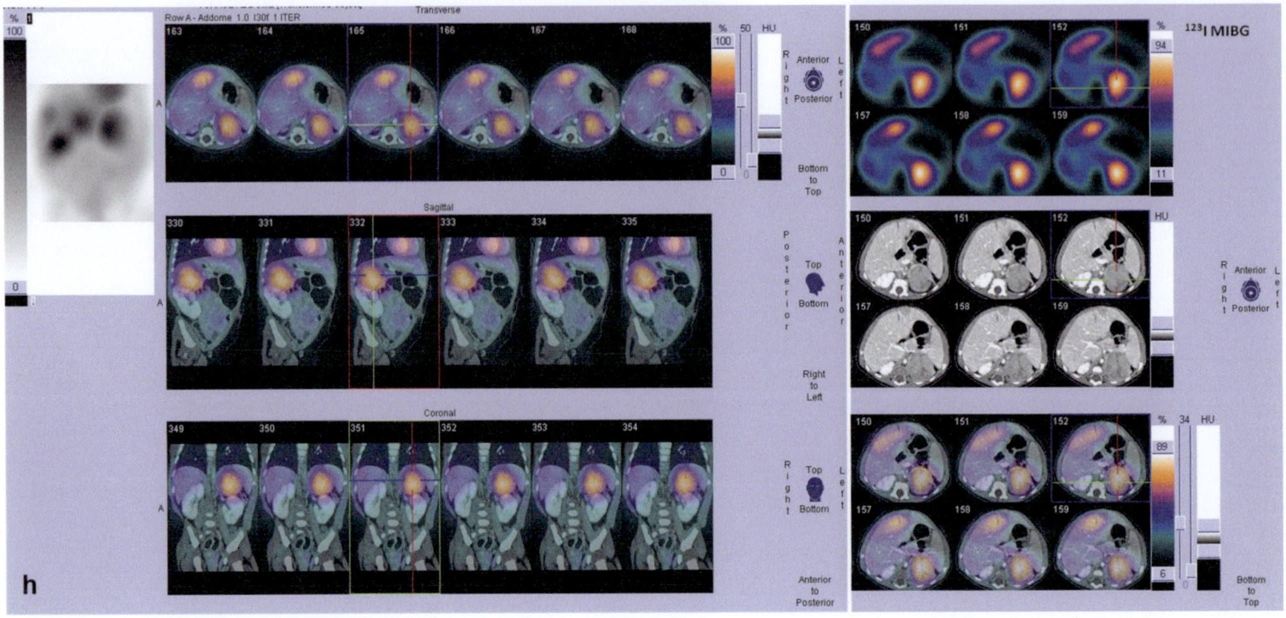

Fig. 13.5 (continued)

13.2.6 Case 13.6: Infant Stage IV Neuroblastoma: MIBG and Bone Scan Imaging Integration

A 2-month-old baby refers to our institution for appearance of multiple blue nodules on the skin; an ultrasonography shows a left adrenal mass that compresses left kidney and multiple hyperechoic areas in the liver. CT detects a prevertebral mass located in the left adrenal lodge with multiple calcification and multiple hypodense areas in the liver, respectively; several nodules are also evident in subcutaneous fat tissue of chest, abdomen, and pelvis; no lesions are evident in the skeleton (Fig. 13.6a–f). Histological examination of one of this nodules reveals a metastasis of NB; therefore, the baby undergoes a MIBG scan for staging purpose (Fig. 13.6g); scintigraphy shows a MIBG-avid mass and a nonhomogeneous radiotracer uptake in the liver, due to the presence of metastases; multiple areas of focal radiotracer uptake are evident in the abdomen, in the pelvis, and in the lower limbs (corresponding to known skin lesions).

Moreover, two focal areas of MIBG uptake are evident in the right orbital region and in the left proximal humerus, respectively; it has been considered that these two foci of uptake are probably due to bone metastasis.

For this reason, the child undergoes 99Tc-MDP bone scan (Fig. 13.6h) that shows uptake of radiotracer in the right orbital region, corresponding to MIBG uptake.

Chemotherapeutic treatment is carried out, and MIBG scintigraphy after chemotherapy (Fig. 13.6i) shows persistence of MIBG uptake in the primitive lesion and known skin lesions; nonhomogeneous radiotracer uptake in the liver is still present. Uptake in bone is no longer evident, such that indicating response to chemotherapy of the bone lesions.

The girl then undergoes surgery on primary NB, and is followed up with laboratory examination and periodic CT and MIBG scan.

At last follow-up, MIBG scintigraphy (Fig. 13.6j shows a single, very small area of faint MIBG uptake in one of the known skin lesions and nonhomogeneous uptake in the liver.

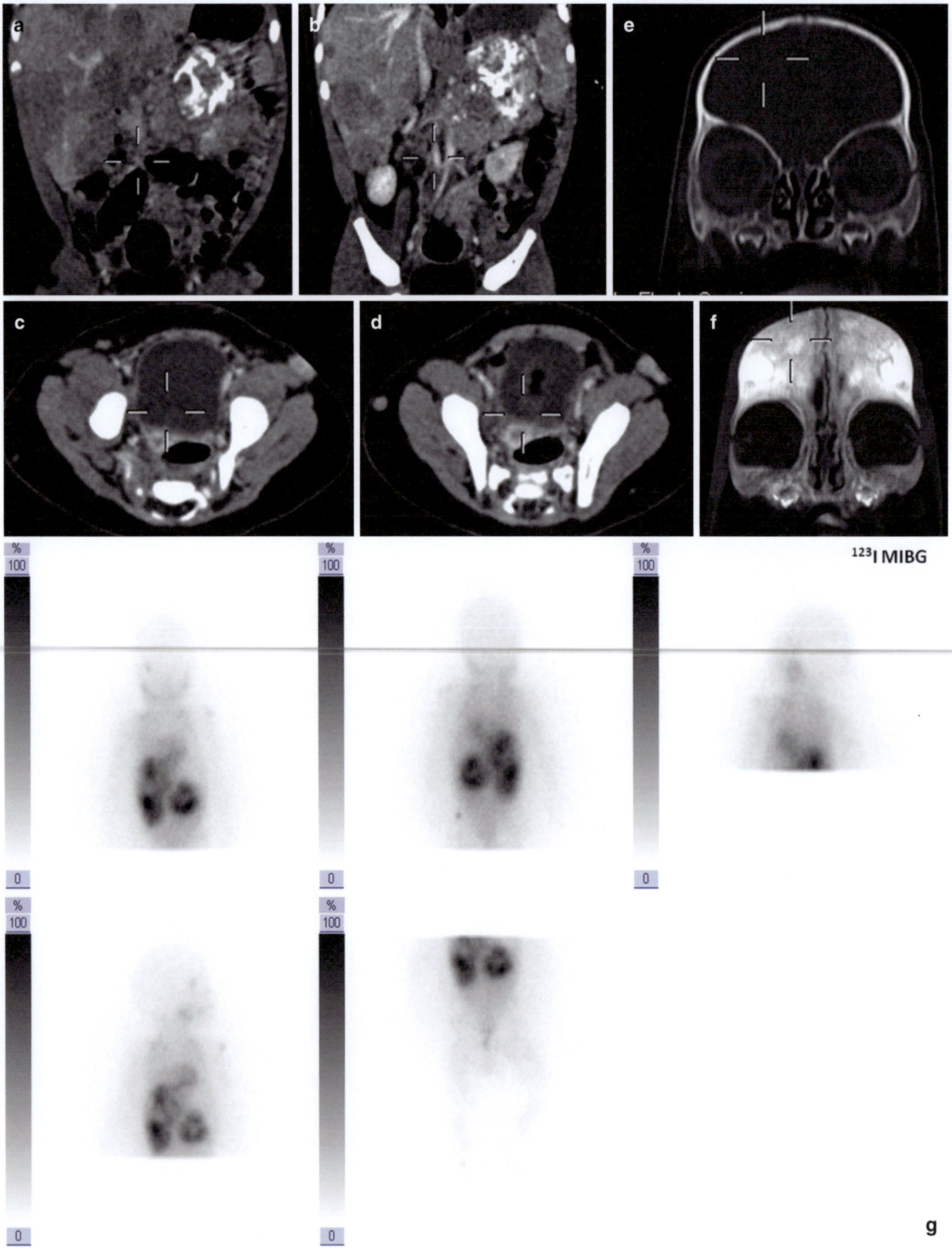
a
b
e
c
d
f
^{123}I MIBG
%
100
0
g

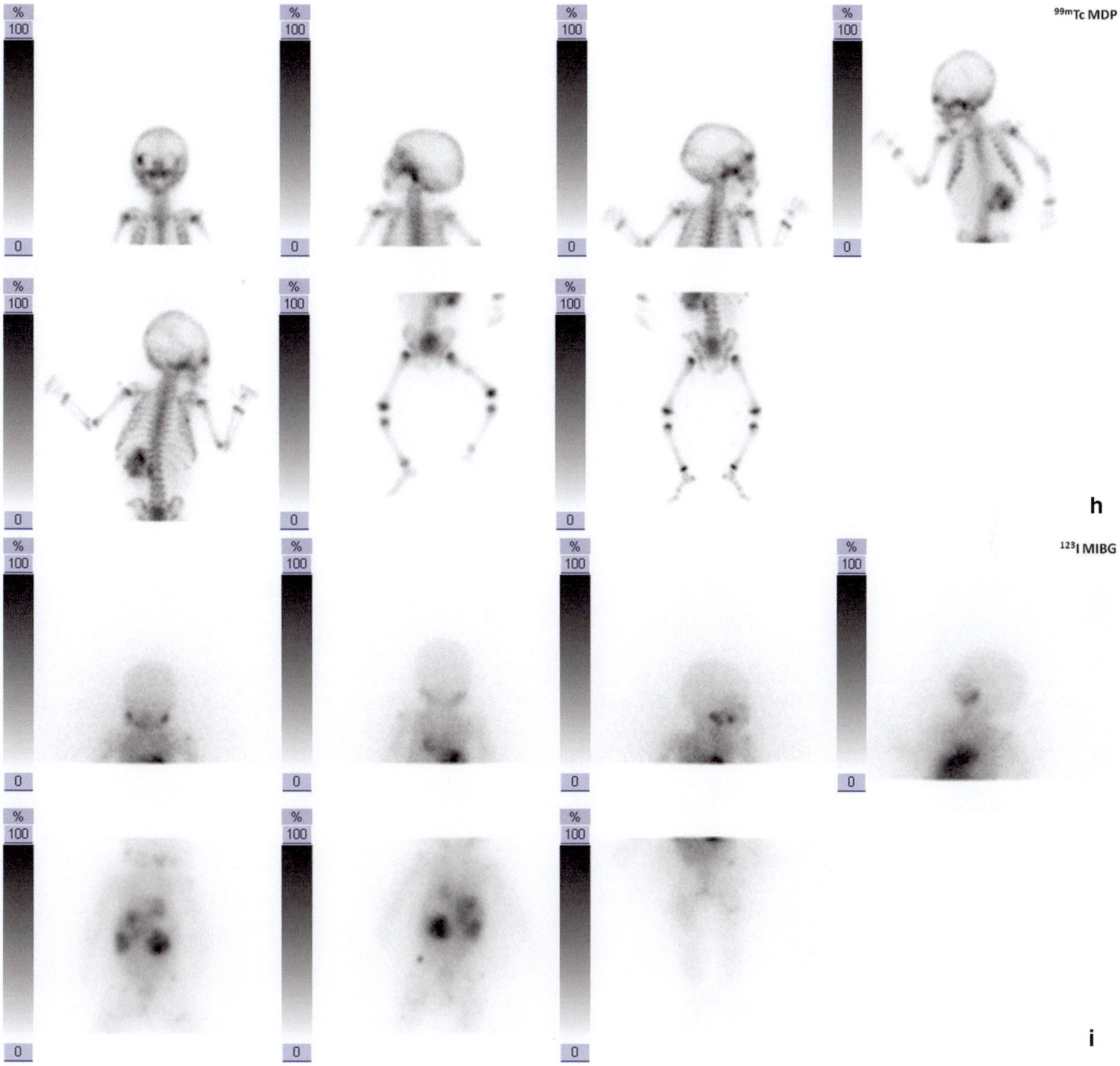

Fig. 13.6 (continued)

Fig. 13.6 (**a–f**) Contrast-enhanced CT. MPR coronal (**a**, **b**) and transverse (**c**, **d**) images show a nonhomogeneous and aggressive retroperitoneal mass containing many amorphous calcifications and located in the area of the left adrenal gland; the mass does not infiltrate the kidney and was about 40 × 35 × 48 mm in size. Many lymph node metastases, multiple subcutaneous nodules, and liver enhancing lesions are also seen. Head CT scan (**e**, **f**) does not show images consistent with metastases. (**g**) Staging MIBG scintigraphy (static views) detects a large area of intense and nonhomogeneous radiotracer uptake in abdomen, in left paravertebral region, corresponding to the lesion showed by CT that does not cross the middle line; the liver shows nonhomogeneous radiotracer uptake, due to multiple secondary nodules evident at CT; multiple areas of focal radiotracer uptake are evident in proximal region of left humerus, in abdomen, in the pelvis, and in lower limbs (corresponding to known skin lesions). A focal area of radiotracer uptake is evident in the right orbital region, suspected for bone metastases. (**h**) 99Tc-MDP bone scan (static views) shows focal uptake of radiotracer in the right orbital region, corresponding to MIBG uptake. Faint uptake is evident in known skin lesions; intense uptake of radiotracer is also evident in abdominal mass (frequent in NB, due to the presence of calcifications). (**i**) MIBG scintigraphy after chemotherapy (static views) shows persistence of intense radiotracer uptake in abdomen, in the primitive lesion, and of nonhomogeneous radiotracer uptake in the liver, respectively; focal uptake in known skin lesions is still present, while radiotracer uptake in right orbital region and in left proximal humerus is no longer evident, such indicating response to chemotherapy of the bone lesions. (**j**) MIBG scintigraphy during follow-up (static views) shows a single, very small area of faint extraskeletal radiotracer uptake in soft tissue of left iliac region (corresponding to known skin lesion) and nonhomogeneous uptake in the liver

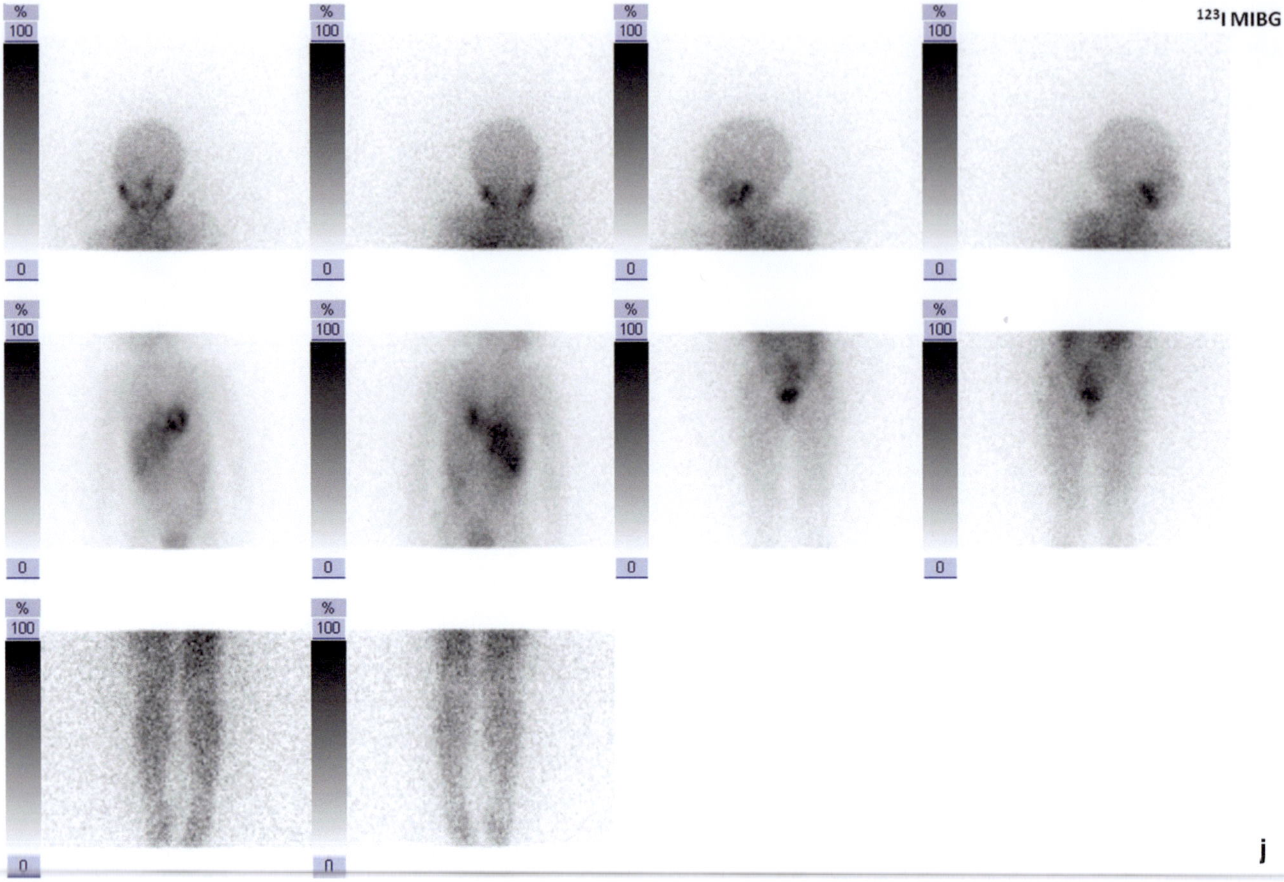

Fig. 13.6 (continued)

13.2.7 Case 13.7 MIBG Scintigraphy in Localized Abdominal Ganglioneuroma/Ganglioneuroblastoma

A 7-year-old girl refers to our institution for abdominal pain; an ultrasonography shows a left adrenal mass that dislocates left kidney; CT confirms a solid mass with calcifications that impresses the upper pole of the left kidney, suspected for NB (Fig. 13.7a–c). The girl undergoes 123I-MIBG scintigraphy to confirm the suspicion (Fig. 13.7d, e), and the lesion appears as nonavid of MIBG. Subsequently, a biopsy of the lesion is performed, and histological examination shows a peripheral neuroblastic tumor, borderline between ganglioneuroma "maturing" and intermixed ganglioneuroblastoma, such that explaining the absence of MIBG uptake.

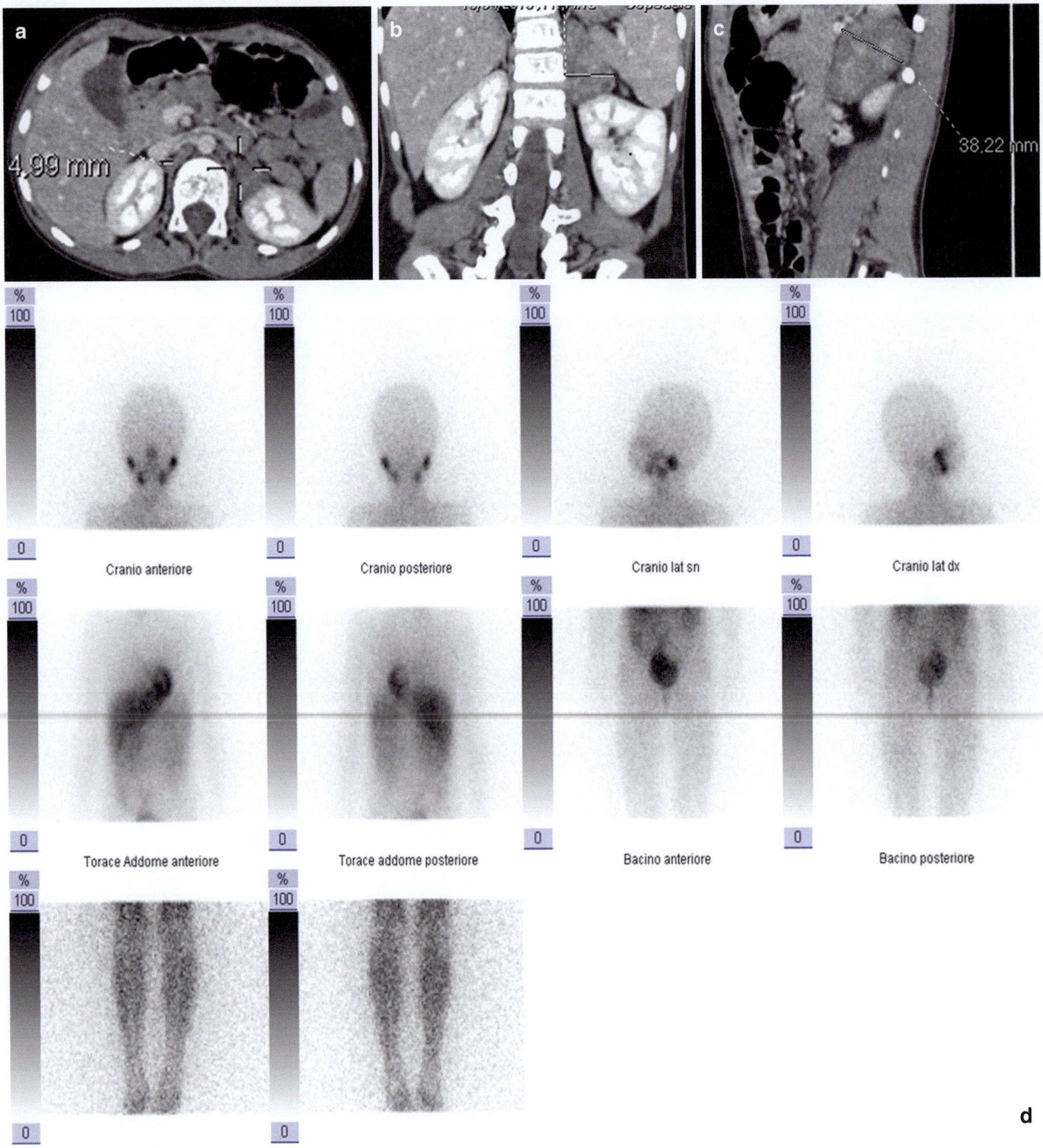

Fig. 13.7 (**a–c**) Contrast-enhanced CT. Transverse (**a**), MPR coronal (**b**), and sagittal (**c**) images show a large mass in the left suprarenal region (about 58 × 28 × 39 mm in diameter). The lesion, containing tiny dystrophic calcifications, is oval-shaped and shows nonhomogeneous enhancement after contrast agent administration. Left kidney is inferiorly displaced; left adrenal gland, pancreatic tail, and medial border of the spleen are also displaced, although separated from the tumor by a fatty layer. (**d**, **e**) MIBG scintigraphy (static views, **d**) does not show any area of uptake of radiotracer; in particular, the lesion detected by CT appears as nonavid of MIBG. SPECT-CT fused images (**e**) confirm this finding

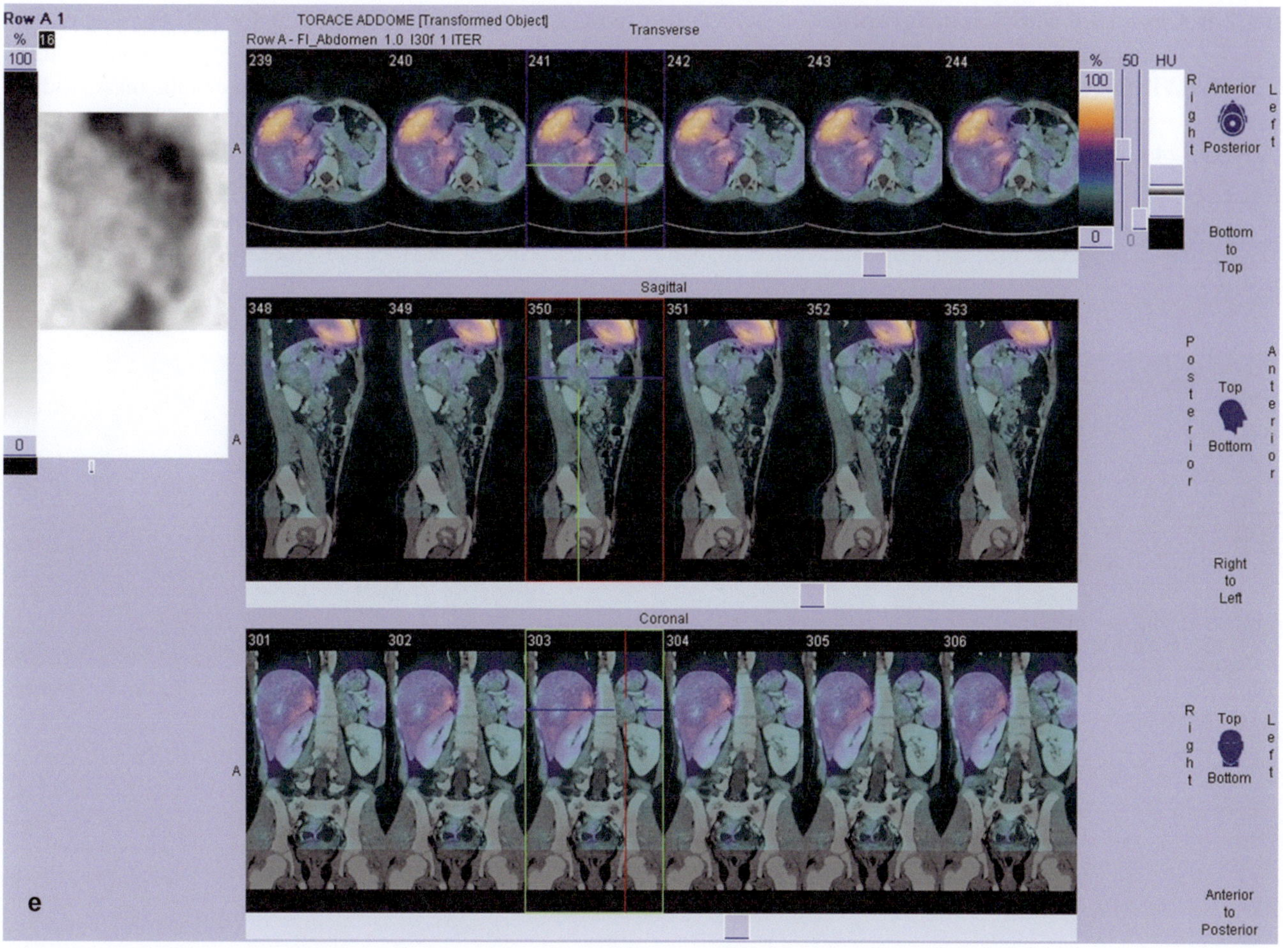

Fig. 13.7 (continued)

13.2.8 Case 13.8 MIBG Scintigraphy in Localized Thoracic Neuroblastoma Without Involvement of Spinal Canal

A 3-year-old girl presents persistent cough since 1 month; she received specific therapy, but because of the persistence of symptom, a chest radiography, a CT scan, and a MR (Fig. 13.8a–c) are performed, and neoplasia is detected in the posterior mediastinum, suspected for NB. For this reason, the girl undergoes 123I-MIBG scintigraphy (Fig. 13.8d, e), which shows intense radiotracer uptake in the mass, without evidence of metastases.

To better characterize the neoplasia, a biopsy was performed, and diagnosis of differentiating ganglioneuroblastoma nodular performed. Patient was treated according to LINES protocol, and then the tumor was completely resected.

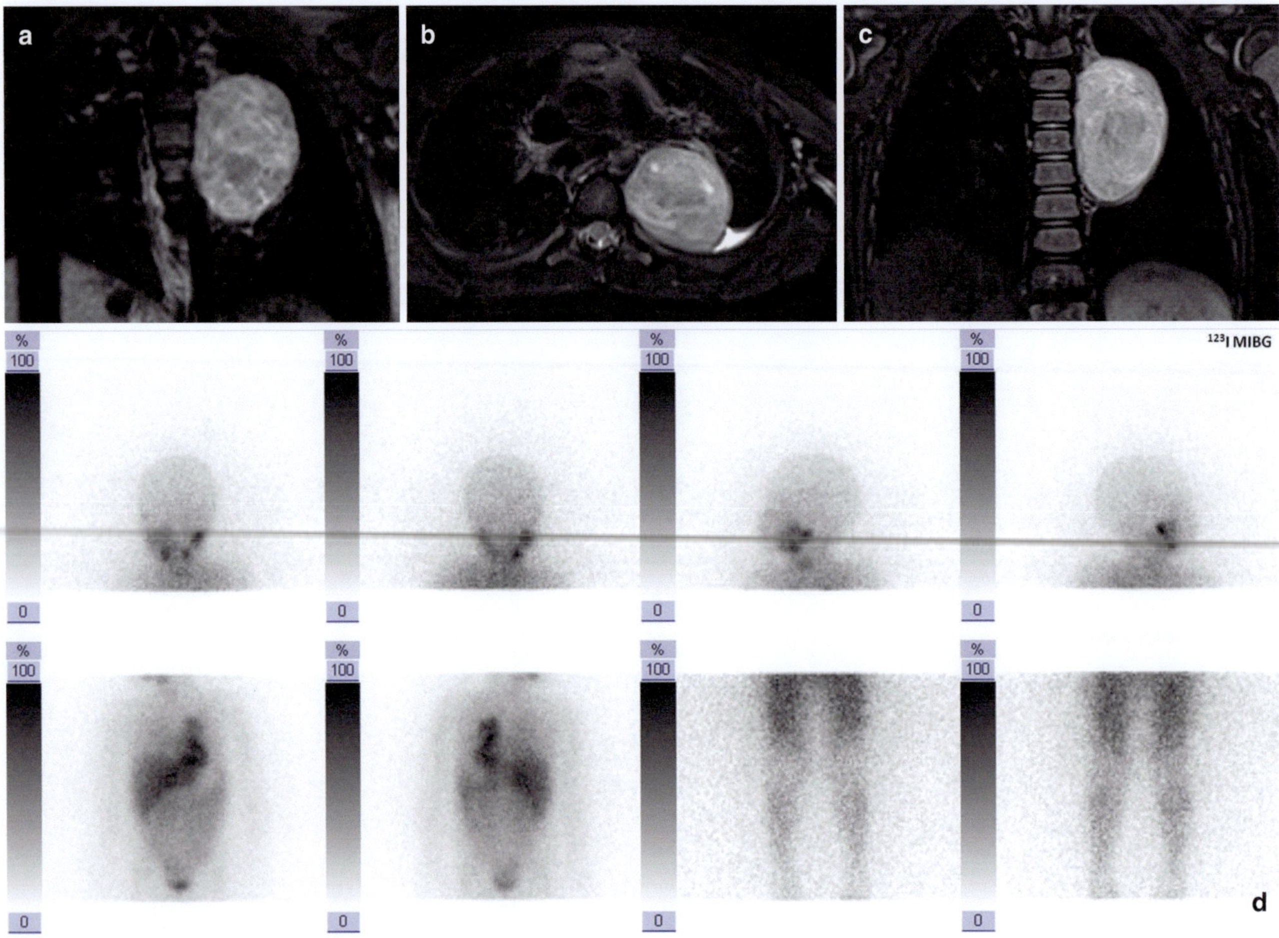

Fig. 13.8 (**a–c**) TransverseT2-weighted fat-sat (**a**), coronal T2-weighted TIRM (**b**), and postcontrast transverse T1-weighted MR images show a large, left upper posterior mediastinal mass; it is localized between T3 and T8 spinal levels, and it does not show foraminal and intraspinal extensions. A "contact" is present between the lesion and the descending aorta, without signs of infiltration of the nearest anatomical structures. (**d**, **e**) MIBG scintigraphy (static views (**d**) detects a large area of intense radiotracer uptake in the chest, corresponding to large mass in posterior mediastinum, in paravertebral region, corresponding to the lesion showed by MRI, as better evident on SPECT-MRI fused images (**e**)

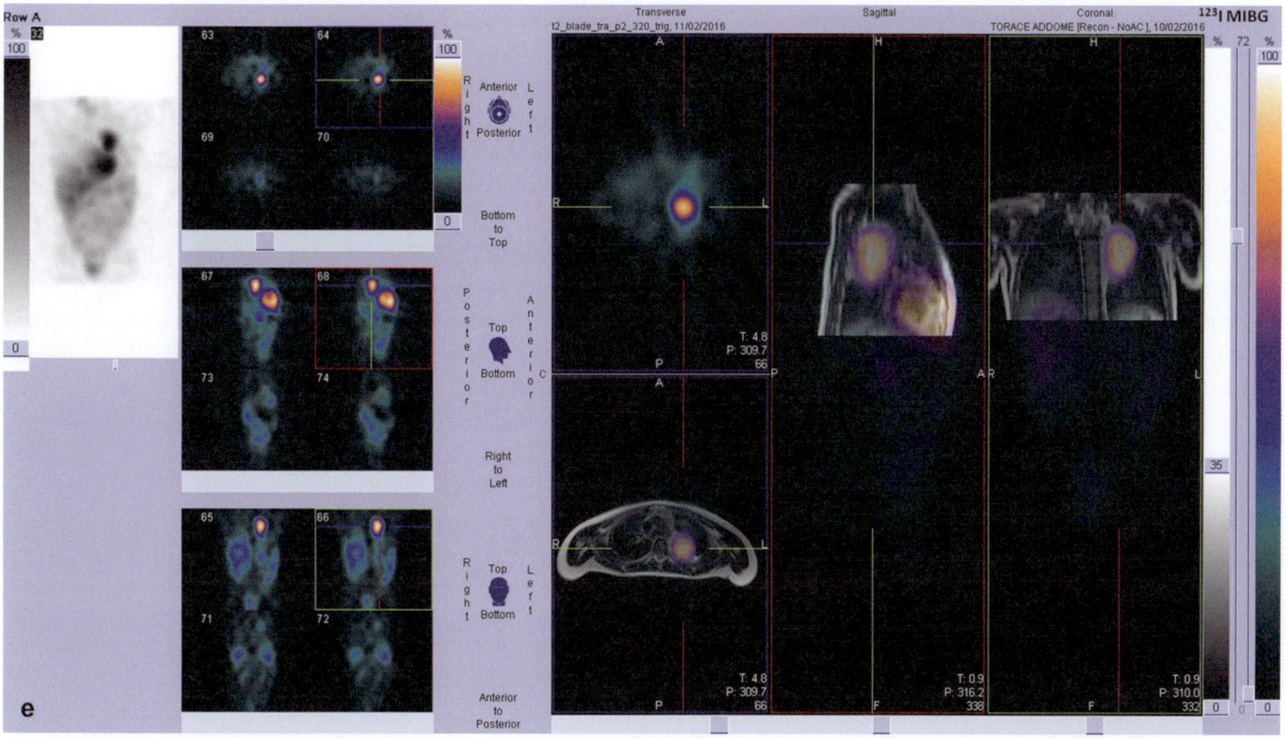

Fig. 13.8 (continued)

13.2.9 Case 13.9 Stage IV NB: Scintigraphic Evidence of Complete Response to Induction Chemotherapy in Metastatic Sites

A 5-year-old girl refers to our institution for pain in pelvis and lower limbs; at clinical evaluation, the girl presents a hard swelling in abdomen. Therefore, an abdominal US and a subsequent CT are performed, and a large mass in the abdomen is detected (Fig. 13.9a, b), suspected for NB; histological examination confirms the diagnosis (NB stroma poor), and a MIBG scintigraphy is scheduled as part of diagnostic workup; the scan detects spread of disease in the bone and bone marrow, as well as the mass (Fig. 13.9c). Genomic profile shows NMYC not amplified. Patient is treated according to NBHR01 European protocol and patient randomized to N7 arm.

At the end of induction treatment, a new balance of disease by CT scan, bone and bone marrow biopsy, and MIBG scan is performed. The CT scan showed a partial response of primary tumor (Fig. 13.9d, e); bone and bone marrow biopsy are negative for infiltration of disease; MIBG scintigraphy shows disappearance of metastatic disease (Fig. 13.9f).

Fig. 13.9 (**a**, **b**) MPR coronal contrast-enhanced computed CT shows large retroperitoneal mass (**a**), with nonhomogeneous density after contrast agent administration and tiny peripheral calcifications. The lesion, oval-shaped, with irregular borders, displaces anteriorly the pancreatic gland and the superior mesenteric artery. There are also multiple metastatic nodes with inner coarse calcifications located in retroperitoneal fatty space and extending along iliac vessels both on the right and on the left. CT scan does not show images consistent with bone metastases (**b**). (**c**) Staging MIBG scintigraphy (static views, **c**) shows nonhomogeneous uptake in large tumor in abdomen; multiple areas of uptake are evident in skull, skull base, both orbits, sternum, many ribs in both hemithorax, in all spine, both humeri, right radius, pelvis, femurs, tibiae, and left foot, indicating bone-bone marrow involvement. (**d**, **e**) MPR coronal (**d**) and transverse (**e**) and contrast-enhanced computed tomography (CT) after chemotherapy show no significant reduction in size of the primary mass (about 52 × 82 × 45 mm), neither of the previous reported lymphadenopathies. At MIBG scintigraphy after treatment (**f**), metastatic lesions are no longer evident, while radiotracer uptake in right adrenal lodge (corresponding to residual mass) is still detectable, indicating a complete metabolic response to chemotherapy of bone and bone marrow metastasis

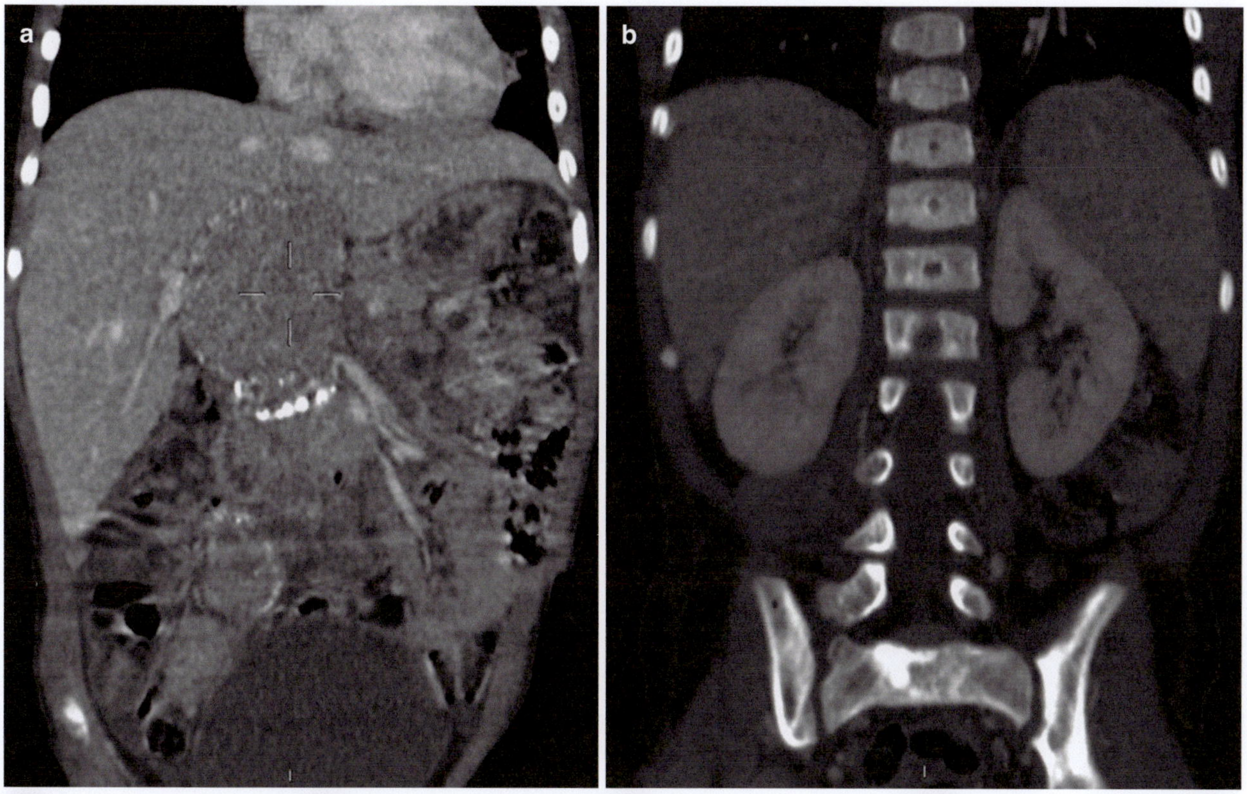
a
b

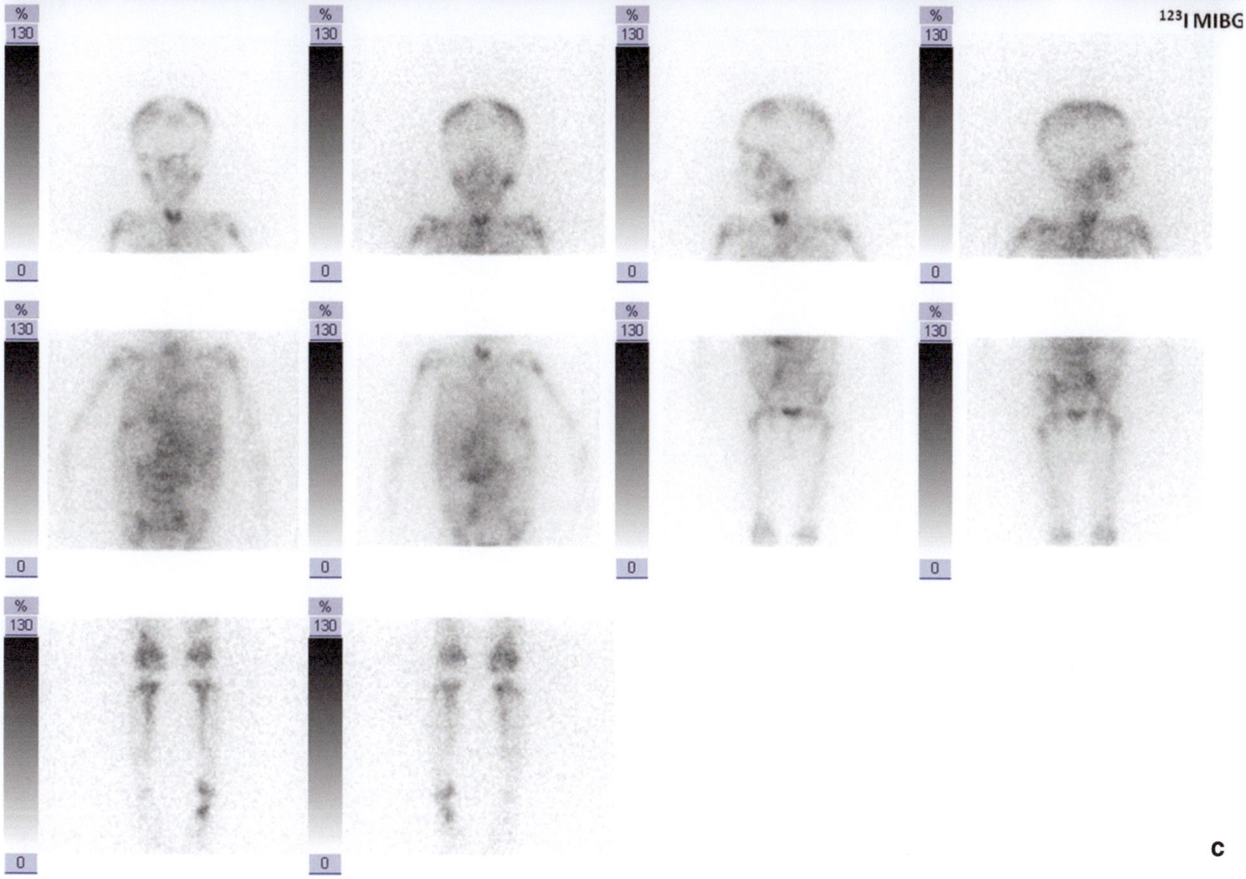
123I MIBG
%
130
0
c

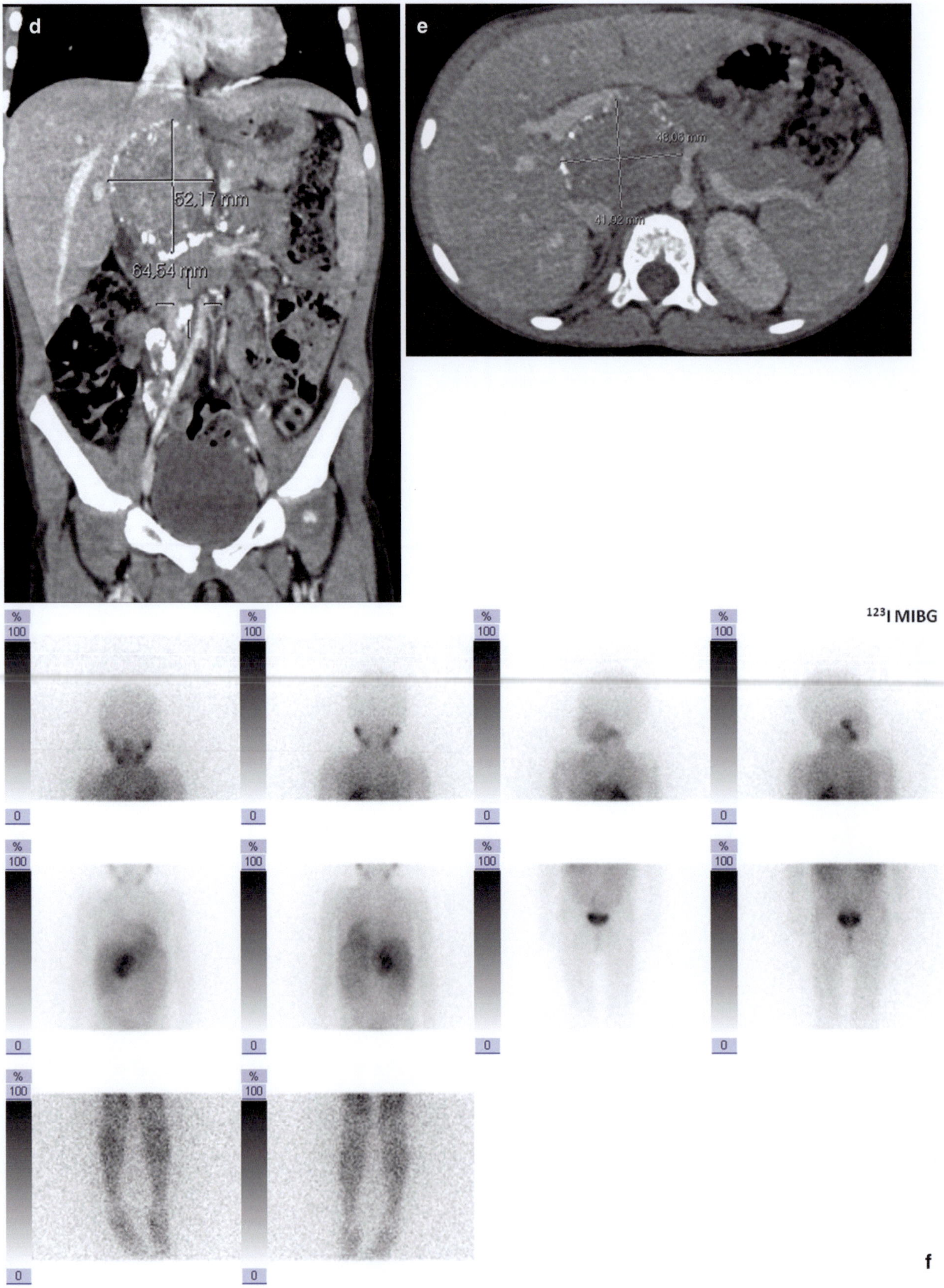

Fig. 13.9 (continued)

13.2.10 Case 13.10 Stage IV Neuroblastoma: Scintigraphic Evidence of Partial Response to Induction Chemotherapy in Metastatic Sites

A 2-year-old boy presenting limping since 1 month refers to our institution with a previous diagnosis of hip synovitis, treated with NSAI and steroid therapy; because of the persistence of symptoms, blood and biochemistry tests are performed. Blood test is normal, while biochemistry shows high level of LDH. An US is performed to check the hip synovitis, and it is extended to the abdomen, such that allowing to detect a lesion in the left adrenal gland; the next CT confirms a large tumor arising from left adrenal lodge and reaching in its distal part lumbar and sacral vertebrae; a portion of this tissue, extending from L5 to S2–S3, presents foraminal and intraspinal extension (Fig. 13.10a–c). Histological examination shows a NB stroma-poor, and MIBG scintigraphy is performed in order to complete disease staging. Scan detects spread of disease in the bone and bone marrow, as well as the mass (Fig. 13.10d). Genomic profile shows NMYC amplification.

Patient is treated according to NBHR01 European protocol and randomized to N7 arm.

At the end of induction treatment, a new balance of disease by CT scan, bone and bone marrow biopsy, and MIBG scan is performed. The CT scan shows a partial response of primary tumor (Fig. 13.10e–g); bone and bone marrow biopsy are negative for infiltration of disease; MIBG scintigraphy shows the persistence of disease in the lower limbs (Fig. 13.10h–k). For these reasons, patient receives TVD (topotecan-vincristine-doxorubicin) intensification chemotherapy regimen according to the protocol NBHR01.

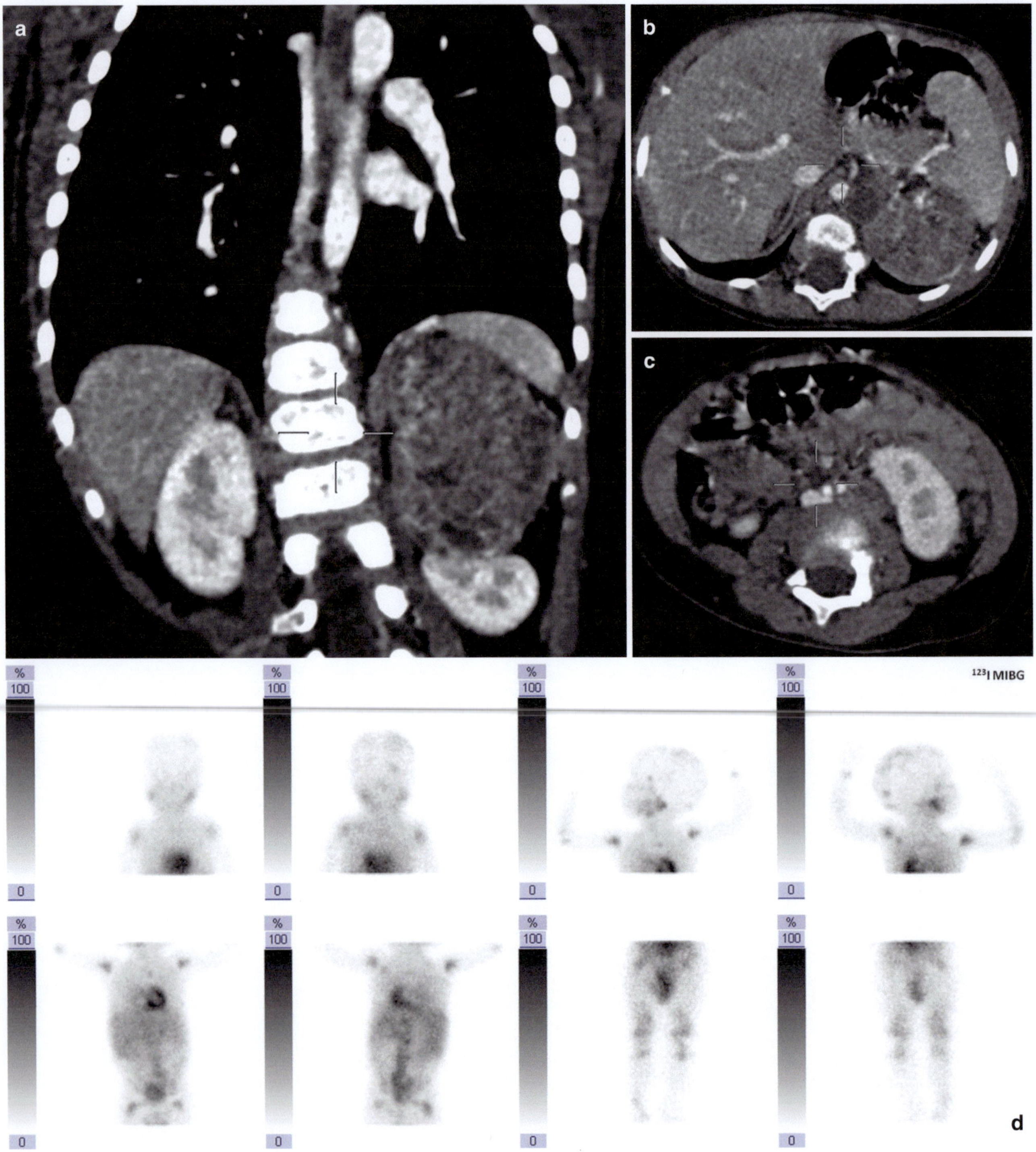

Fig. 13.10 (**a–c**) MPR coronal (**a**) and transverse (**b**) contrast-enhanced CT image show a large left adrenal mass, appearing at nonhomogeneously hypodense because of multiple inner nonenhancing areas after contrast agent administration. The lesion, oval-shaped, with well-defined borders, is about 51 × 43 × 62 mm in size; the left kidney is displaced and distorted but not infiltrated, as well as the spleen and the pancreatic tail. The tumor, extending in the iliolumbar fossa, invaded the spinal canal at the level between L5 and S3 via the neuroforamina (**c**). There are also multiple enlarged, metastatic retroperitoneal nodes. (**d**) Staging MIBG scintigraphy (static views) shows nonhomogeneous radiotracer uptake in the abdomen, probably corresponding to tumor evident on CT. Multiple areas of uptake are evident in skull, skull base, both orbits, sternum, left scapula, both humeri, both radii, pelvis, femurs, tibiae, and diffuse uptake in the spine, indicating bone and bone marrow involvement. (**e–g**) MPR (**e**) coronal and transverse (**f**) contrast-enhanced CT after treatment shows a partial response to therapy supported by a marked reduction in size of the primary mass (actually 22 × 26 × 24 mm) showing large inner calcifications. There is also a significant regression both in nodal involvement and in foraminal and intraspinal component (**g**). (**h**, **k**) MIBG scintigraphy after treatment (static views, **h**, **i**): radiotracer uptake is still evident only in distal femurs, proximal tibiae, and in right distal tibia; SPECT-CT fused images show absence of radiotracer uptake in primary tumor (**j**, **k**) and in tissue-infiltrating spinal canal. This pattern indicates a partial response to chemotherapy of bone and bone marrow lesions.

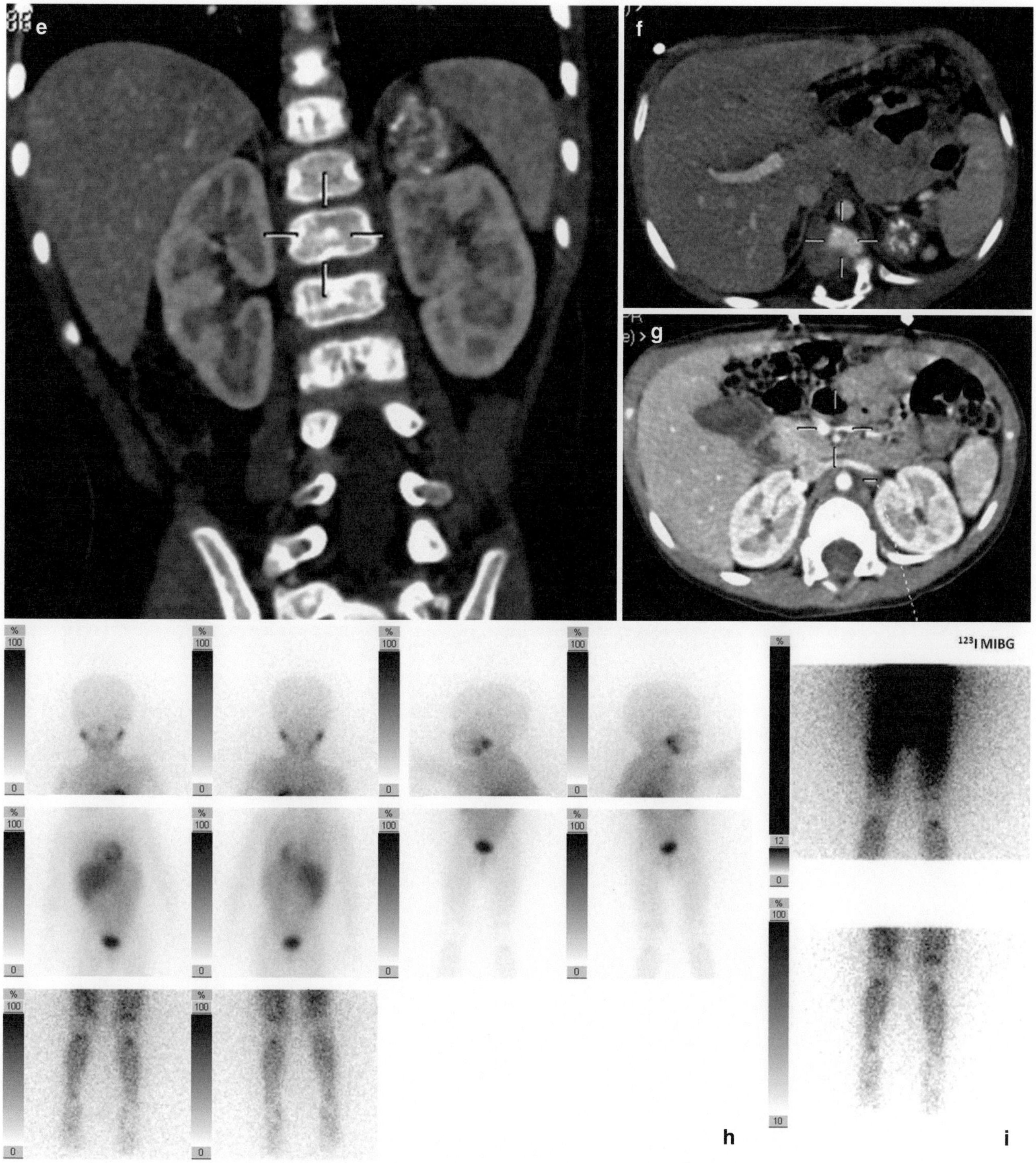

Fig. 13.10 (continued)

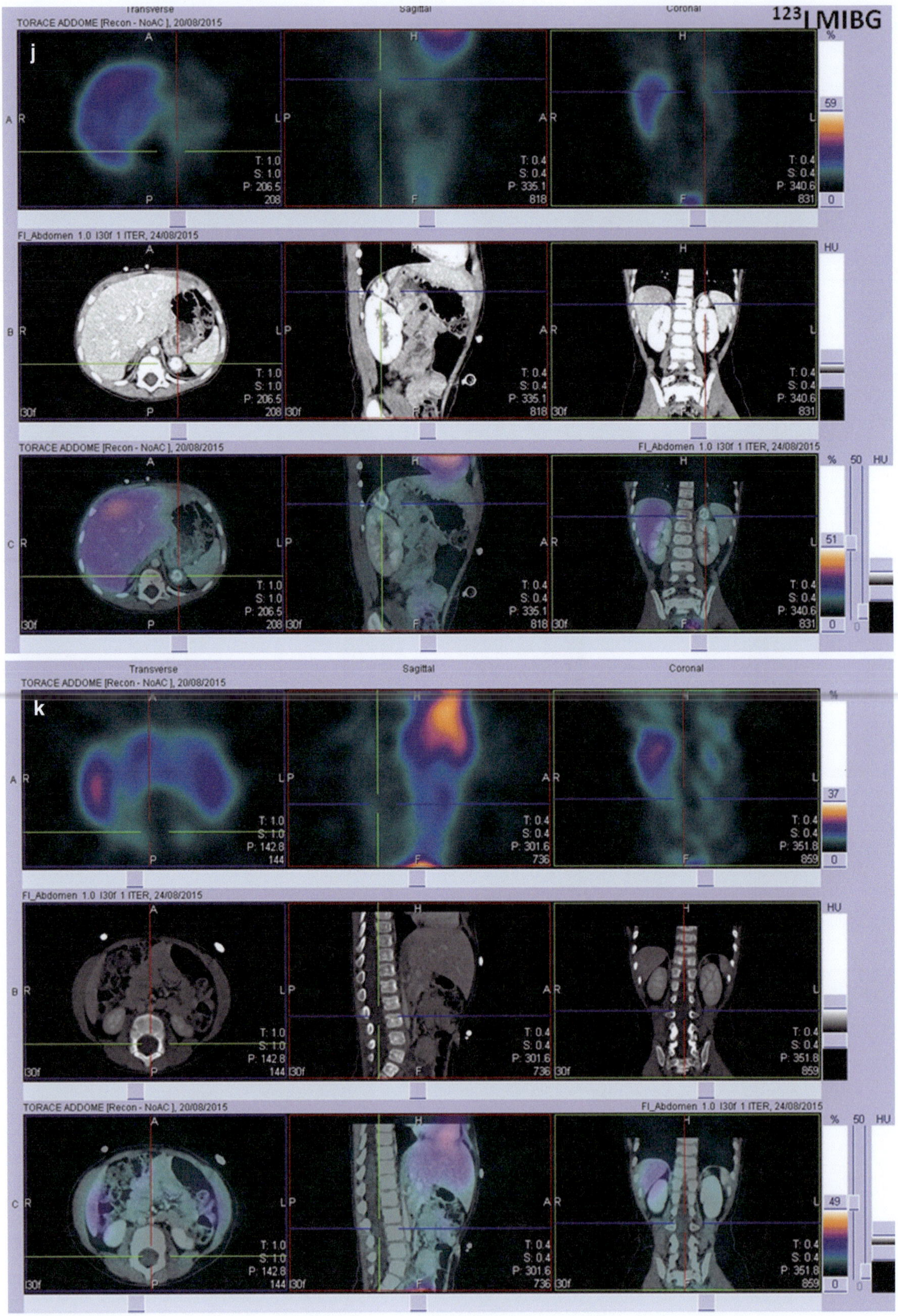

Fig. 13.10 (continued)

13.2.11 Case 13.11 Stage IV Neuroblastoma: Scintigraphic Evidence of Persistent Disease

A 15-month-old baby refers to our emergency for left orbital swelling and exophthalmos; suspecting a periorbital cellulitis, a brain CT scan is performed, which shows a pathological tissue starting from left temporofrontosphenoidal region and infiltrating the left wing of sphenoid bone and lateral wall of the orbit (Fig. 13.11a–d). To complete the study, a whole-body CT (Fig. 13.11e, f) is performed, and a neoplasia in the left adrenal gland is identified. For the characterization of the neoplasia, a biopsy of the adrenal mass is performed, and the suspected diagnosis of neuroblastoma is confirmed. Consequently, a MIBG scintigraphy is scheduled for staging and shows radiotracer uptake in the mass and bone and bone marrow involvement (in particular, in skull base) (Fig. 13.11g). Genomic profile shows NMYC amplification.

Patient is treated according to NBHR European protocol – N7 arm

At the end of the induction treatment, a new balance of disease by CT scan, bone and bone marrow biopsy, and MIBG scan is performed. CT scan shows a partial response of primary tumor and stable disease in the left orbit. One of two bone marrow biopsies was positive for infiltration of disease; MIBG scintigraphy shows persistence of disease compared with the staging (Fig. 13.11h). For this reason, patient receives TVD (topotecan-vincristine-doxorubicin) intensification chemotherapy regimen according to the protocol NBHR01.

Then, the girl undergoes surgery on primary tumor and further chemotherapeutic treatment.

At last follow-up, MIBG scintigraphy shows persistence of disease in skull and orbits, with no other areas of metastatic involvement (Fig. 13.11i, j.)

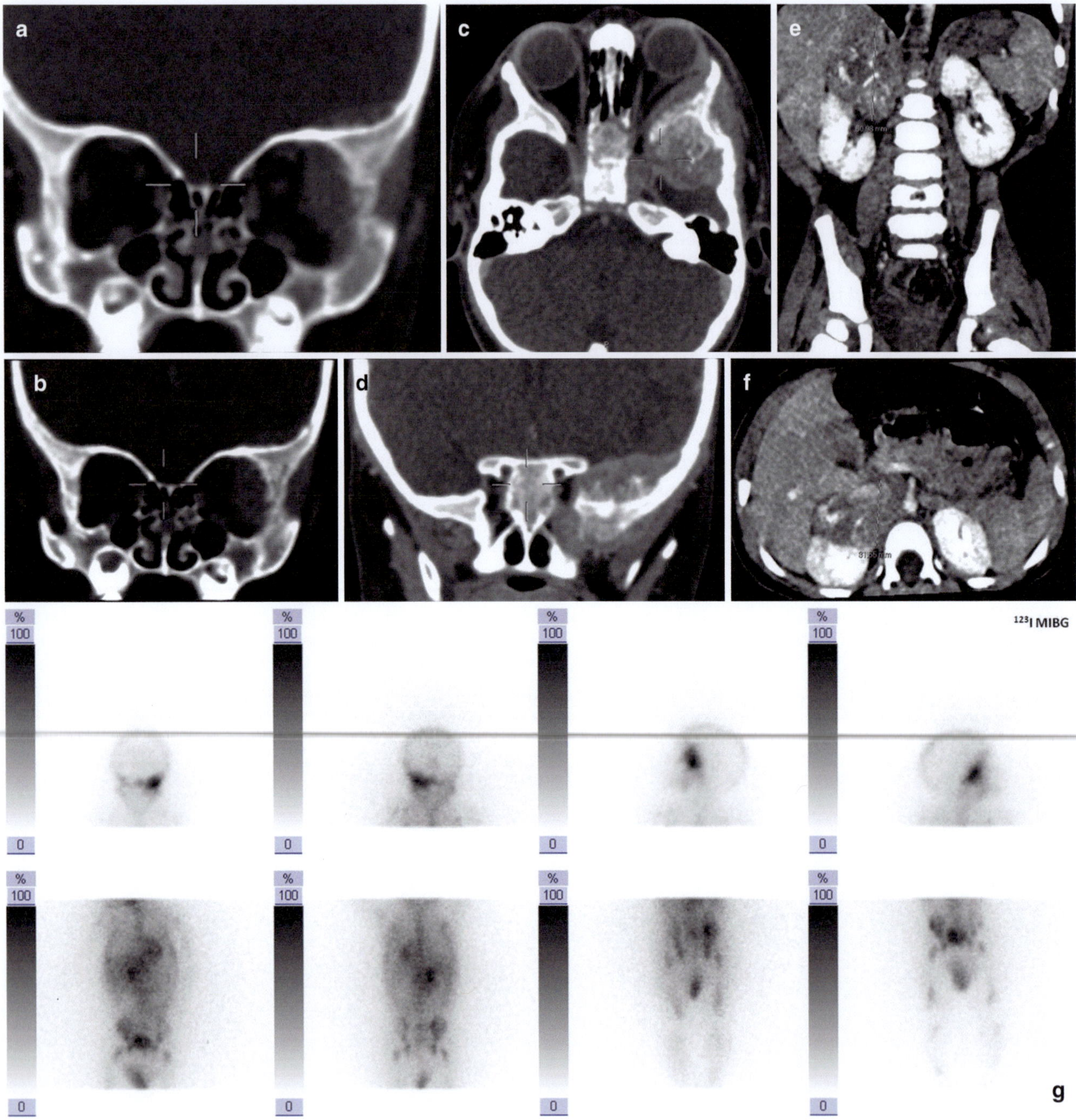

Fig. 13.11 (**a–f**) Contrast-enhanced CT: MPR coronal image of the head shows a large lesion originating in the bone marrow, as evidenced by bone destruction on bone windows (**a**, **b**), and then extending to paraosseous soft tissues, causing intraorbital or extratransverse intracranial soft tissue masses with an inhomogeneous enhancement after contrast media administration, better seen on soft tissue windows (transverse and MPR coronal images. (**c**, **d**) Abdomen CT scan shows a large, infiltrating neuroblastoma arising from right adrenal gland, appearing nonhomogeneous after contrast agent administration (MPR coronal and transverse images (**e**, **f**), with large, amorphous calcifications in the contest. The lesion completely encases right renal vessels; the "contact" between the tumor and the aorta and the inferior cava vein is wide. The margins between the tumor and the kidney are ill defined as well as the one between the mass and the liver. Multiple enlarged and nonhomogeneous retroperitoneal node metastases are also evident. (**g**) Staging MIBG scintigraphy (static views) shows nonhomogeneous radiotracer uptake in the abdomen, corresponding to tumor evident on CT. Multiple areas of uptake are evident in skull, skull base, both orbits, sternum, left scapula, ribs, both humeri, both radii, pelvis, femurs, and tibiae, and diffuse uptake in the spine, indicating bone and bone marrow involvement. (**h**) MIBG scintigraphy after treatment (static views): radiotracer uptake still evident shows the tumor in right adrenal lodge (evident on CT scan) and in quite all the sites evident in staging scan, even if intensity of uptake is mildly reduced. This pattern indicates a persistence of disease despite the chemotherapy. (**i**, **j**) MIBG scintigraphy during follow-up (static views, **i**) shows persistent radiotracer uptake in the skull, skull base, and in both orbits, better defined in SPECT-CT fused images (**j**). N other areas of pathological uptake are evident

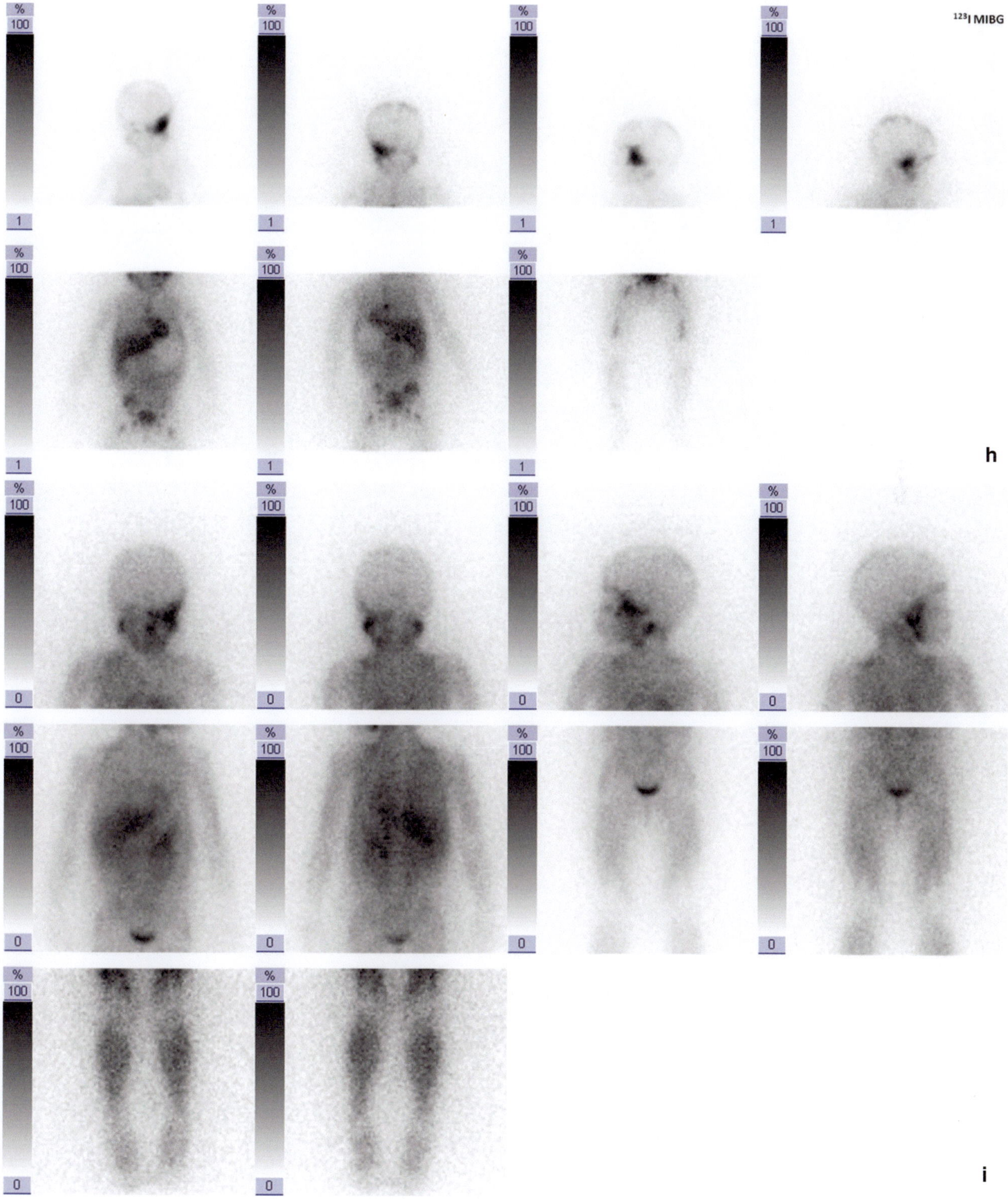

Fig. 13.11 (continued)

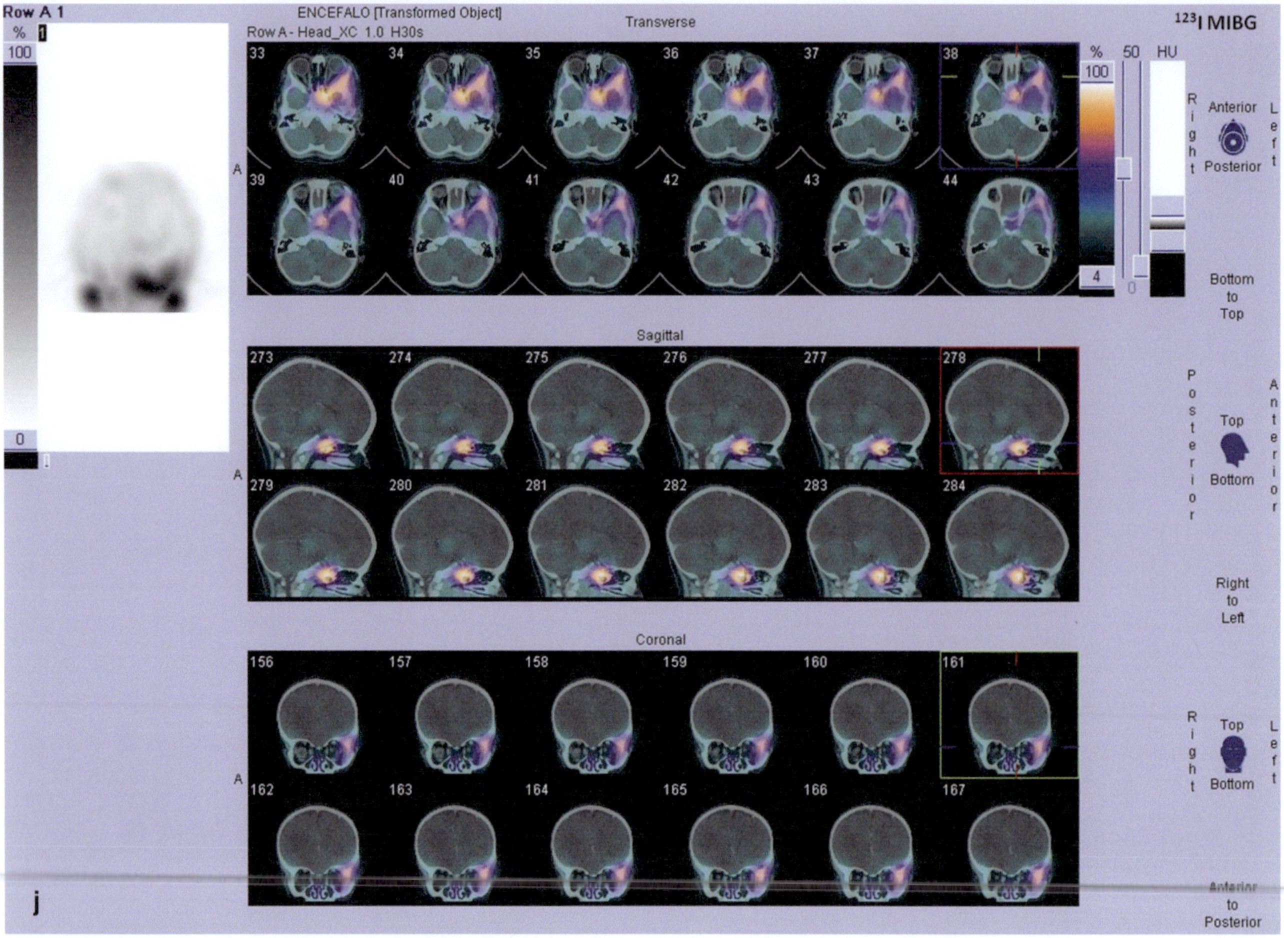

Fig. 13.11 (continued)

13.2.12 Case 13.12: Stage IV Neuroblastoma: Scintigraphic Evidence of Relapse

A 3-year-old child refers to our institution for fever and hard swelling in abdomen at clinical evaluation. Ultrasonography shows evidence of an abdominal mass; a CT detects a large abdominal mass with pleural metastases (Fig. 13.12a–d). MIBG scintigraphy is performed which shows nonhomogeneous radiotracer uptake in the mass and metastases in pleura, and in bone and bone marrow (Fig. 13.12e–g).

Therefore, the girl undergoes chemotherapy, surgery, and radiotherapy; MIBG scintigraphy at the end of treatment shows absence of areas of pathological radiotracer uptake (Fig. 13.12h, i).

During follow-up, a relapse is suspected for increase of LDH value, and a CT scan is scheduled. CT detects a large mass extending above and below the diaphragm, in pre- and paravertebral regions on the midline and on the right paramedian line (Fig. 13.12j–m), and then the girl undergoes a MIBG scintigraphy to restage the disease. The scan shows intense radiotracer uptake in the mass, without other areas of pathological uptake (Fig. 13.12n, o)

Currently, the girl is following chemotherapeutic treatment.

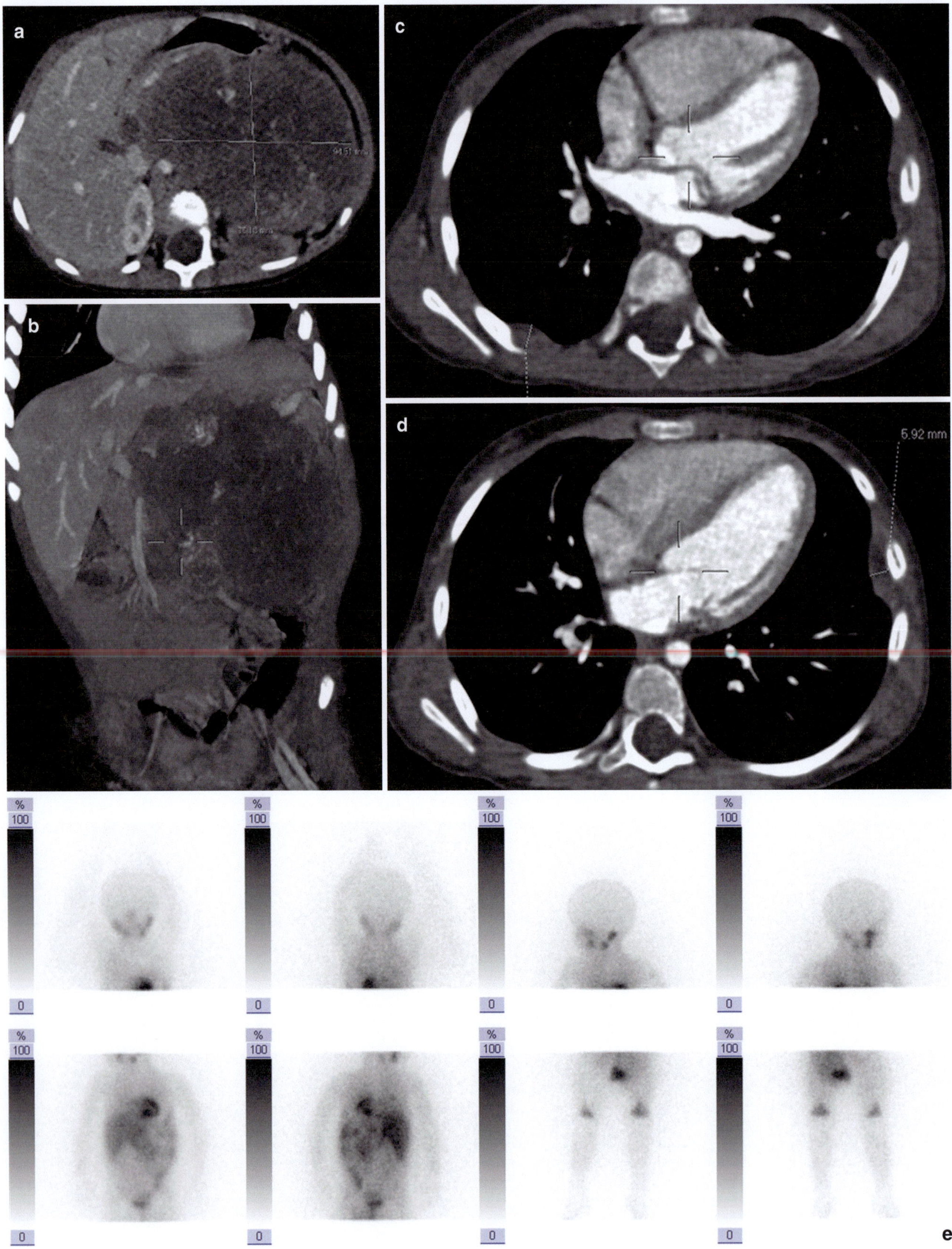
a
b
c
d
5.92 mm
%
100
0
e

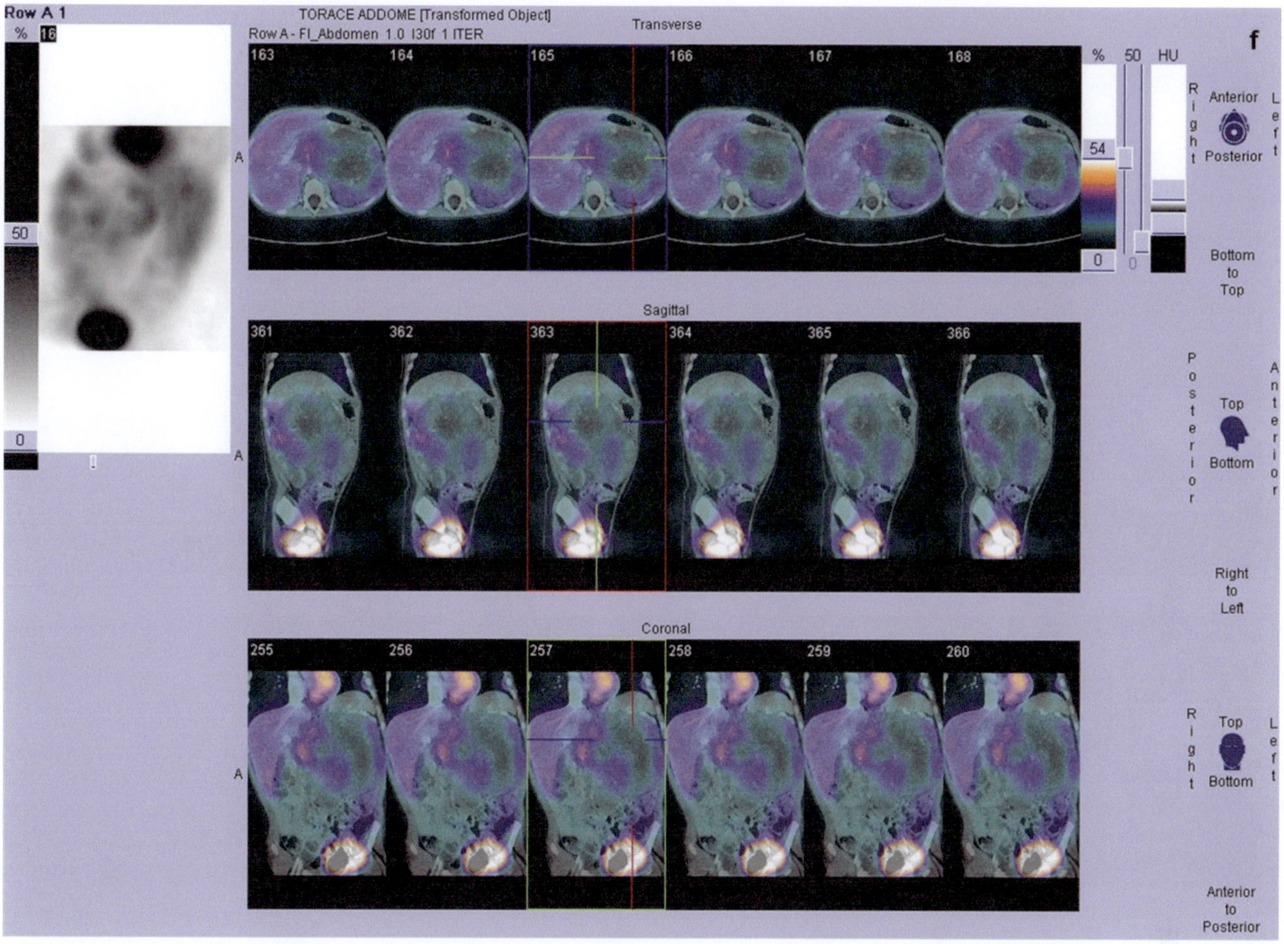

Fig. 13.12 (continued)

Fig. 13.12 (**a–d**) Contrast-enhanced CT: left adrenal infiltrating mass with wide retroperitoneal spread (MPR coronal and transverse images, **a**, **b**) and pleural metastases (transverse images, **c**, **d**). (**e–g**) MIBG scintigraphy (static views, **e**) shows nonhomogeneous radiotracer uptake in the large mass evident on CT, located in left abdomen, and crossing the midline; it presents wide hypoactive areas, as for colliquative necrosis (often seen in NB). Focal areas of intense radiotracer uptake are evident in distal femurs. SPECT-CT fused images confirm nonhomogeneous radiotracer uptake in the mass (**f**) and show uptake in the pleural lesions evident on CT (**g**). (**h**, **i**) MIBG scintigraphy after treatment (static views, **h**): no evidence of areas of pathological radiotracer uptake; SPECT images confirm this finding (**i**). (**j–m**) Contrast-enhanced CT. MPR coronal (**j**), sagittal (**k**), and transverse (**l**, **m**) images show a large mass extending above and below the diaphragm, in pre- and paravertebral region on the midline and on right paramedian line. The lesion is not homogeneous, hypodense after contrast agent administration, without inner calcified areas. It is oval-shaped with ill-defined borders and is about 58 × 55 × 53 mm in size. (**n**, **o**) Restaging MIBG scintigraphy shows intense radiotracer uptake in upper abdomen, above and below the diaphragm, in paravertebral region, corresponding to the mass evident on CT. No other areas of pathological uptake of radiotracer are present. In this case, SPECT-CT fused images (**o**) are mandatory for accurate evaluations of the lesion and its metabolic pattern

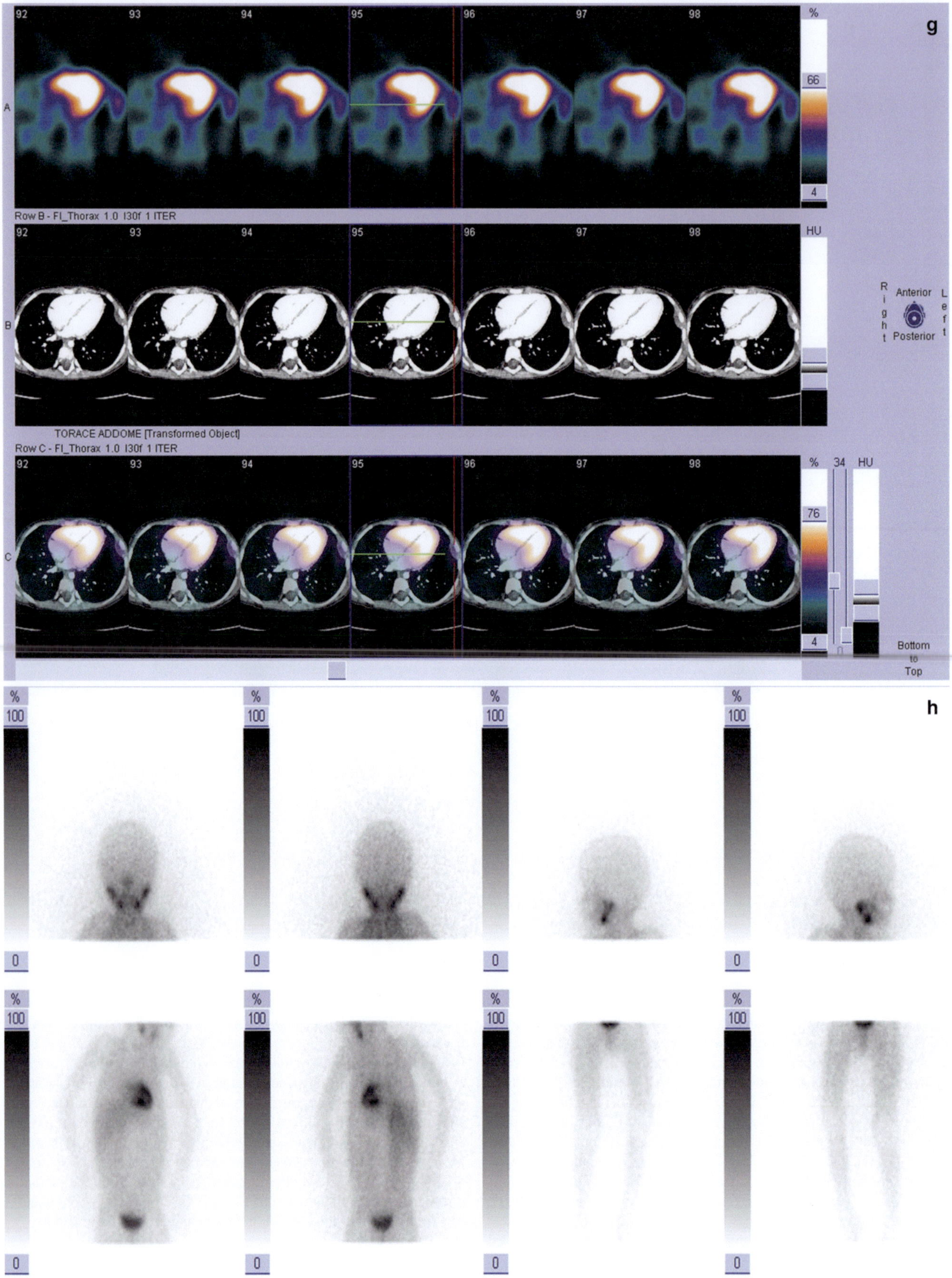

Fig. 13.12 (continued)

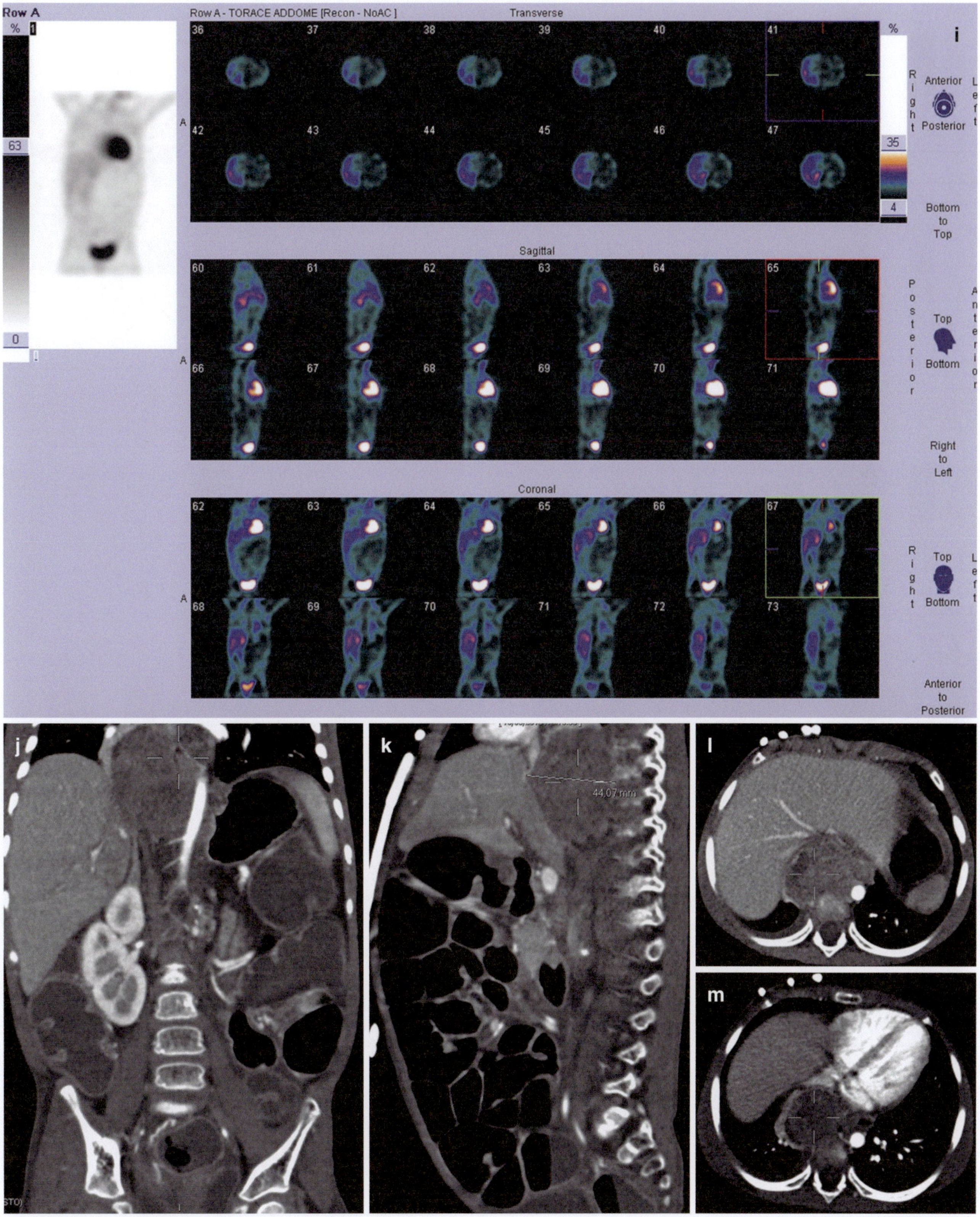

Fig. 13.12 (continued)

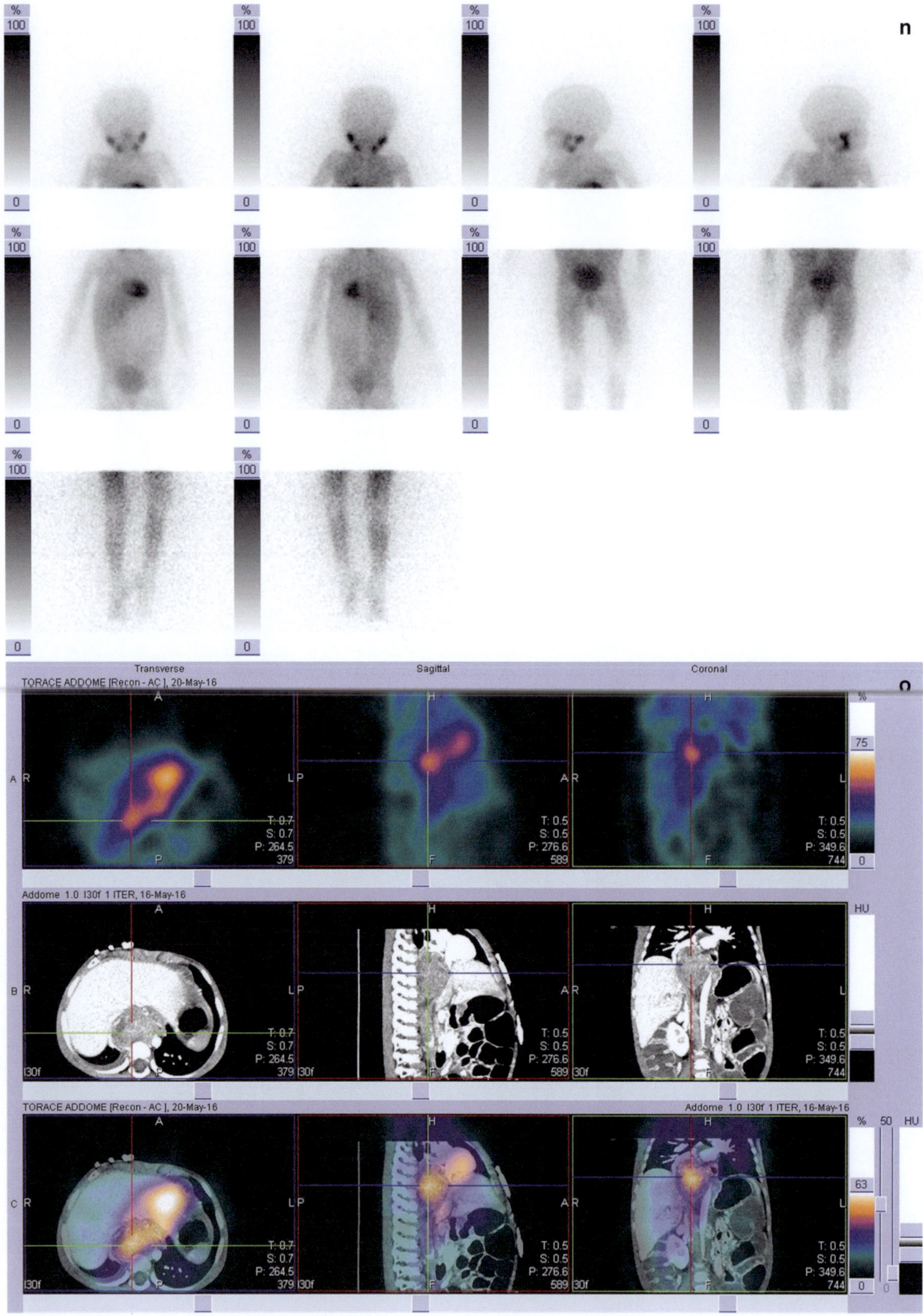

Fig. 13.12 (continued)

13.2.13 Case 13.13 123I-MIBG Scintigraphy in the Evaluation of Patients Eligible for 131-MIBG Therapy

A 13-year-old girl affected by relapsed NB. She had surgery at 5 years of age for an abdominal paravertebral NB Stage I with unfavorable histology, NMYC-negative and multiple further therapy for local recurrence. After 2 years of wellness, the girl experienced an ascend relapse of disease localized in the pleura.

In Fig. 13.13 are displayed restaged 123I-MIBG scintigraphy (a-b) and CT scan (Fig. 13.13c–g). The girl was treated with a course of chemotherapy, and the evaluation of disease at the end of treatment showed stable disease. For this reason, a radiometabolic therapy with I131- MIBG was scheduled (Fig. 13.13l, m), and she received 15 mcg/kg+Melphalan followed by PB stem cells rescue, before therapy.

Although there was a good clinical response to therapy with wellness, at last follow-up, the girl experienced a relapse in lung.

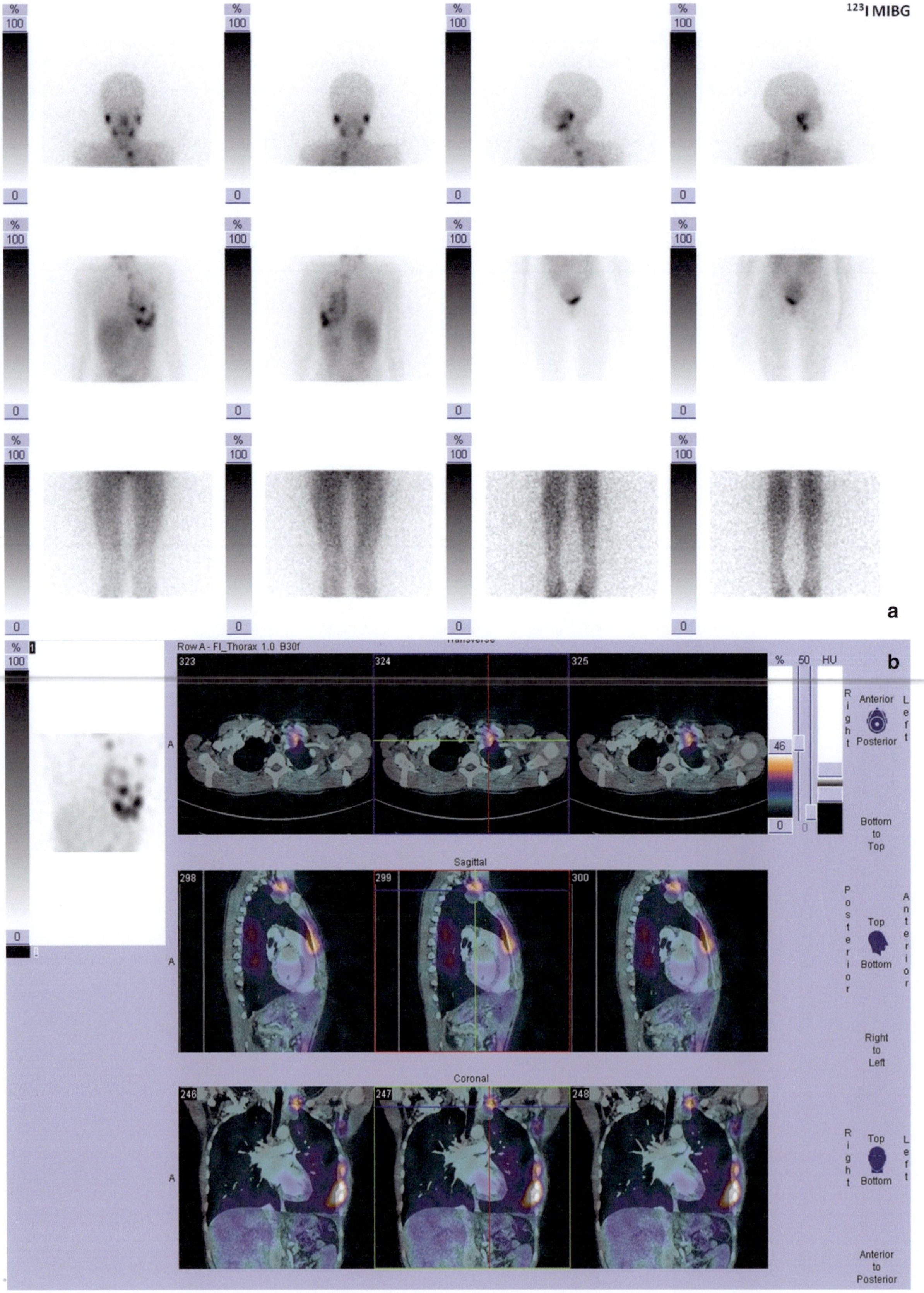

123I MIBG
a
b
Row A - FI_Thorax 1.0 B30f
Sagittal
Coronal
Anterior
Posterior
Bottom to Top
Top
Bottom
Right to Left
Anterior to Posterior
Right
Left
HU

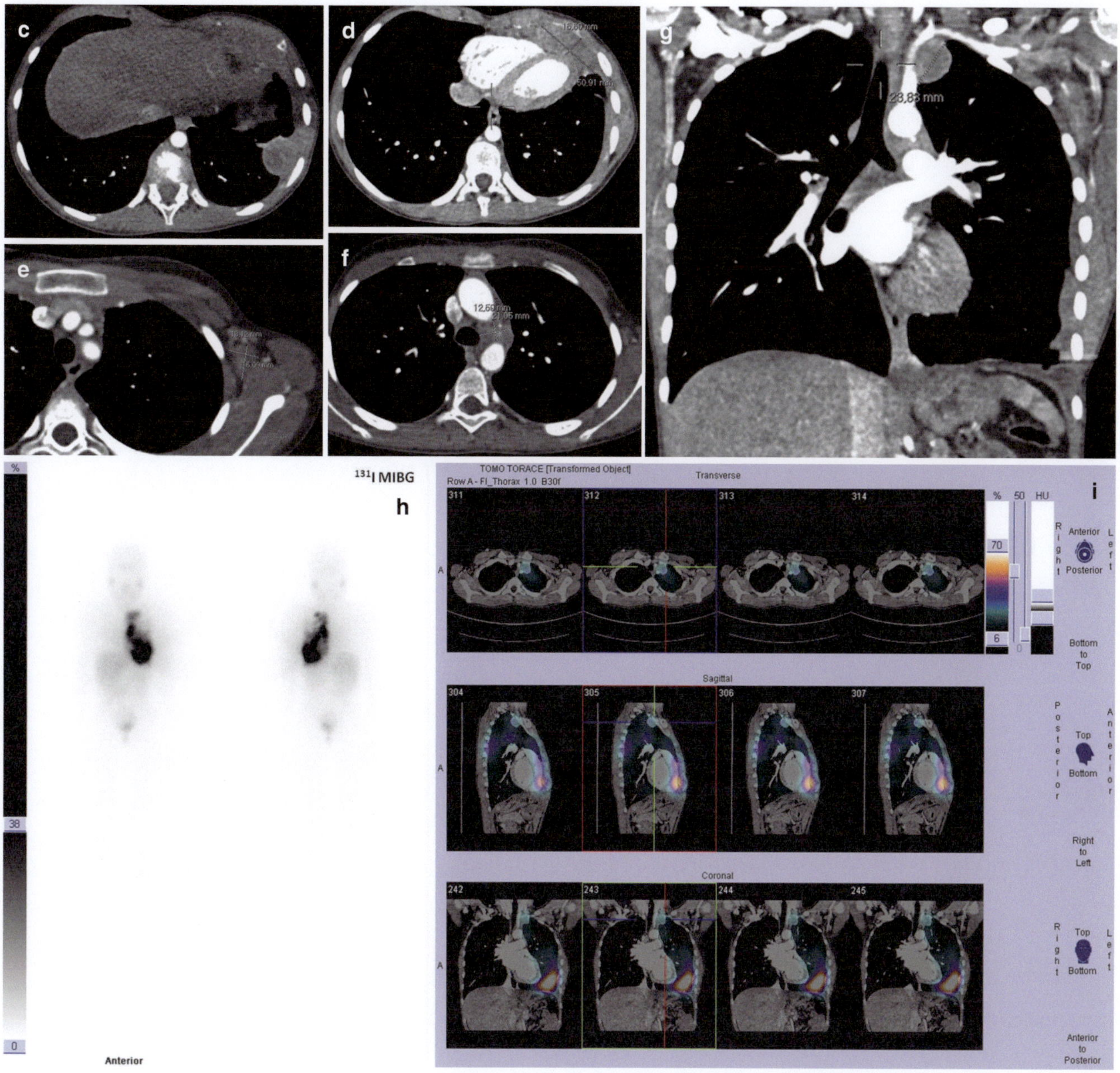

Fig. 13.13 (continued)

Fig. 13.13 (**a**, **b**) 123I-MIBG scintigraphy (static views, **a**) shows multiple focal areas of intense uptake in left hemithorax; SPECT-CT fused images (**b**) localize these areas in correspondence of nodular lesions detected by CT scan in upper left mediastinum and in quite all parietal pleural membranes of left hemithorax; radiotracer uptake is also evident in a tissue in cardiophrenic angle. MIBG uptake is also evident in a pathological tissue in left axilla. (**c–g**) Contrast-enhanced CT shows multiple solid and nonhomogeneous nodules located in the superior mediastinum (MPR coronal image, **g**), at the left pulmonary hilum and along the chest wall in subpleural region (transverse image, **c**); the presence of a soft tissue mass in the middle mediastinum, in the aortopulmonary window (transverse image, **f**), and in the left axilla fatty space (transverse image, **e**), respectively, is also observed. (**i–h**) 131I-MIBG scintigraphy after administration of therapeutic activity (whole-body, **h**, and SPECT-CT fused images, **i**) confirms the finding of diagnostic 123I-MIBG scintigraphy

Bibliography

1. Giammarile F, Chiti A, et al.; EANM. EANM procedure guidelines for 131I-meta-iodobenzylguanidine (131I-mIBG) therapy. Eur J Nucl Med Mol Imaging. 2008;35(5):1039–47.
2. Monclair T, Brodeur GM, Ambros PF, Brisse HJ, Cecchetto G, Holmes K, Kaneko M, London WB, Matthay KK, Nuchtern JG, von Schweinitz D, Simon T, Cohn SL, Pearson AD, INRG Task Force. The International Neuroblastoma Risk Group (INRG) staging system: an INRG Task Force report. J Clin Oncol. 2009;27(2): 298–303.
3. Olivier P, Colarinha P, et al. Guidelines for radioiodinated MIBG scintigraphy in children. Eur J Nucl Med Mol Imaging. 2003;30(5): B45–50. Epub 2003 Mar 26.

Gastroenterology: Focus on Children with Gastrointestinal Problems

14

Luigi Dall'Oglio and Renato Tambucci

Gastrointestinal imaging tests are a cornerstone of the gastroenterologist's diagnostic armamentarium. Over the last decades, nuclear medicine has gained increasing importance for the assessment of the digestive system disorders.

Since the first description of a radiolabeled meal administration in 1966, scintigraphy has become the standard test to measure the gastric emptying; however, despite promising results, no other significant progress in clinical practice has been made for studying gastrointestinal motility [10].

By definition, gastroparesis is a gastric motility disorder characterized by delayed gastric emptying without evidence of mechanical obstruction [3]. In adults, diabetic, postsurgical, and idiopathic etiologies account for approximately one third each of cases. In children, the majority of cases are idiopathic [15].

Classically, symptoms of gastroparesis include abdominal pain, nausea, vomiting, abdominal fullness, and early satiety. These are complaints commonly seen in pediatric clinical practice and may be found in other etiologies. Therefore, the diagnostic workup should include an upper gastrointestinal contrast study or an esophagogastroduodenoscopy in order to rule out mechanical obstruction or other organic underlying disorders (e.g., esophagitis and peptic ulcer disease). Once anatomical or organic diseases are excluded, gastroparesis and functional dyspepsia (defined by the Rome III criteria) can be considered; indeed, there is a significant clinical overlap between them. Moreover, it has been shown that a subset of children with clinical diagnosis of functional dyspepsia has a delayed gastric emptying [4].

Gastric emptying scintigraphy is the most reliable method to make a diagnosis of gastroparesis. It provides a noninvasive, physiological, quantitative measurement of gastric emptying. Especially in infants and in neurologically impaired children, a gastric emptying study may also be indicated for patients with refractory symptoms of gastroesophageal reflux disease, since gastroparesis may contribute or aggravate gastroesophageal reflux symptoms [11].

Identifying patients with delayed gastric emptying is important in treatment decision-making.

According to the symptoms' severity and based on scintigraphy results, the management may include dietary modification, pharmacological therapy, and endoscopic or surgical approaches [2, 15].

A field of very useful scintigraphic application is the assessment of the oropharyngeal and esophageal motor function. A complex coordination of sequences, controlled by multiple levels of the nervous system, is required for a safe and efficient swallowing. The phases of the swallowing process allow the normal bolus propulsion from the mouth to the stomach, avoiding the passage of food through the larynx into the respiratory tree. Oropharyngeal dysphagia can be caused by disorders of the central nervous system (e.g., cerebral palsy) and by neuromuscular diseases. Pulmonary aspiration during feeding is an important cause of acute, recurrent, and chronic pulmonary disease in children [18]. Moreover, during gastroesophageal reflux episodes, when the refluxate does enter the pharynx, the airway is protected by reflexive glottal closure and a pharyngoglottal closure reflex; impairment in this mechanism may result in aspiration. Infants who are born preterm, those that are small for gestational age, and those with cerebral palsy are at greatest risk of developing pharyngeal and/or esophageal motility disorders [16].

After an accurate patient's history and clinical assessment, instrumental testing is necessary for definitive diagnosis of swallowing dysfunction and aspiration. Videofluoroscopic swallow study and fiber-optic endoscopic evaluation of swallowing are the most commonly used tools, but nuclear scintigraphy may play an important role in aspiration assessment. As previously stated, aspiration can occur either during swallowing (antegrade) or as retrograde aspiration of gastric or esophageal contents [14]. The radionuclide salivagram primarily detects aspiration during swallowing (antegrade events), and the gastroesophageal reflux scintigraphy ("milk

L. Dall'Oglio • R. Tambucci (✉)
Unit of Endoscopic Surgery, "Bambino Gesù" Children Hospital, Rome, Italy
e-mail: renato.tambucci@gmail.com

© Springer International Publishing Switzerland 2017

M.C. Garganese, G.F.L. D'Errico (eds.), *Conventional Nuclear Medicine in Pediatrics*, DOI 10.1007/978-3-319-43181-9_14

scan") is more likely to detect events related to gastroesophageal reflux (retrograde events). During both tests, aspiration diagnosis is made when radiopharmaceutical activity is detectable within the lung fields [1]. Gastroesophageal scintigraphy scanning can detect reflux episodes occurring during meals administration and/or during study registration (at least 1 h) independently of the gastric pH; consequently, late postprandial acid exposure and occurrence of reflux episodes are missed with scintigraphy. The number of reflux episodes, level reached within the esophagus, and the clearance rate of reflux episodes may then be determined by scintigraphy. However, a lack of standardized techniques and the absence of age-specific norms are important limits of the test in the assessment of the gastroesophageal reflux disease [19].

Although not as well standardized as gastric emptying scintigraphy, esophageal transit scintigraphy may provide a quantitative and qualitative analysis of single- and multiple-swallow studies. Esophageal manometry is the standard test in assessing esophageal motility; however, when it is not available or results are equivocal, esophageal scintigraphy can be clinically useful. The transit time and/or retention in the esophagus can be assessed by scintigraphy. Scintigraphy studies of esophageal transit have shown a high sensitivity for detecting a wide range of esophageal disorders (e.g., achalasia, diffuse esophageal spasm, scleroderma), but a lower sensitivity, especially for disorders with intact peristalsis but high-amplitude contractions or isolated elevated pressures in the lower esophageal sphincter. Despite specific criteria for diagnosing the primary esophageal motility disorders have been proposed (in adults), its clinical utility in clinical practice is not well defined, and its widespread use is still limited [11].

As far as gastrointestinal motility is concerned, nuclear medicine efforts are channeled toward the standardization of small bowel and colon transit studies. Scintigraphy is a safe and noninvasive method for the quantitative evaluation of overall and regional intestinal transit. Scintigraphic test also allows the possibility to study gastric emptying and whole bowel transit as part of the same study. Indications for small bowel and colon transit scintigraphy include dyspepsia, irritable bowel syndrome, chronic constipation, chronic diarrhea, and chronic idiopathic intestinal pseudo-obstruction [12]. A partial, but encouraging, success in advancing gastrointestinal scintigraphy was achieved through the development of methods for the study of the colonic transit [13]. Compared to traditional tests (e.g., radiopaque markers), disadvantages of the colonic scintigraphy are related to the lack of standardization, especially in children, and its limited availability due to high costs and need for specialized equipment. However, radiolabeled meal allows a more physiological radioisotope incorporation into the gut content compared with the indigestible solid pellet. In 2005, a task force committee on gastrointestinal transit studies has stated that "the scintigraphic method is the only one that reliably allows the determination of both total and regional transit times" [9].

Scintigraphy studies are classically employed in the localization of active and obscure overt gastrointestinal bleeding and are the methods of choice for identifying ectopic gastric mucosa in a Meckel's diverticulum.

Although most bleeding ultimately resolves spontaneously, sometimes it might lead to hemodynamic instability resulting in potential life-threatening event that may require prompt surgical intervention.

Bleeding may originate from the upper or lower gastrointestinal tract, by convention defined as bleeding occurring respectively proximally and distally to the ligament of Treitz at the duodenal flexure. Upper and lower gastrointestinal bleeding require different clinical approaches. Although clinical signs may guide the localization – hematemesis and melena for upper bleeding, and hematochezia for lower bleeding – sometimes, the source of bleeding can be difficult to distinguish clinically. Endoscopic assessment is the first-line choice for the diagnosis and treatment of acute GI bleeding. Clinical guidelines for management of patients with acute lower gastrointestinal bleeding suggest that radiographic interventions (tagged red blood cell scintigraphy, computed tomographic angiography, and angiography) should be considered in high-risk patients with ongoing bleeding who do not respond adequately to resuscitation and who are unlikely to tolerate bowel preparation and colonoscopy [17]. Moreover, after performance of a normal upper and lower endoscopic examination, a source of small bowel bleeding should be considered. Video capsule endoscopy should be considered a first-line procedure for small bowel investigation followed by deep enteroscopy when endoscopic evaluation and therapy are required. In acute overt massive bleeding, conventional angiography should be performed for hemodynamically unstable patients, while in hemodynamically stable patients, multiphasic computer tomography can be performed to identify the site of bleeding and guide further management. However, in patients with acute overt gastrointestinal bleeding and slower rates of bleeding (0.1–0.2 mL/min), red blood cell scintigraphy should be performed if deep enteroscopy or video capsule endoscopy are not performed to guide timing of angiography [6].

Tagged red blood cell scintigraphy is a noninvasive test that detects active bleeding that is occurring at a slow rate (0.1–0.5 mL/min), and it is a very sensitive radiographic test for gastrointestinal bleeding [5]. Advantages of scintigraphy include the ability to detect lower rates of bleeding and the ability to perform delayed imaging that can improve detection of intermittent or delayed bleeding [17]. A major disadvantage of radionuclide imaging is that it can only localize bleeding to a general area of the abdomen. Poor localization occurs because blood can move in either a peristaltic or antiperistaltic direction. In addition, localization to an area of the abdomen is not equivalent to identifying a specific site [8]. It has been indicated that the optimal time for red blood cell-labeled scintigraphy is less than 24 h after the patient has received a minimum of 500 mL of red blood cell transfusion. A negative red blood cell scintigraphy study has been shown to be predictive of a good outcome [17].

Especially in children with ongoing overt bleeding and negative evaluation with video capsule endoscopy, or other testing modalities, consideration should be made for testing with a ^{99m}Tc pertechnetate scan for detection of Meckel's diverticulum. Approximately 10–60 % of these diverticula contain ectopic gastric mucosa, gastric acid, and pepsin production may result in mucosal damage and bleeding. Scintigraphic imaging is based on the fact that ^{99m}Tc pertechnetate is actively secreted by the mucous cells found within the gastric mucosa. A Meckel scan is performed in order to localize the abnormal tissue in preparation for surgical removal. On imaging, a Meckel's diverticulum is identified as a focus of activity in the lower abdomen or upper pelvis that generally appears at the time of stomach visualization and increases as stomach activity increases. Diagnostic accuracy of 90 % has been reported [7].

Bibliography

1. Baikie G, South MJ, Reddihough DS, et al. Agreement of aspiration tests using barium videofluoroscopy, salivagram, and milk scan in children with cerebral palsy. Dev Med Child Neurol. 2005;47:86–93.
2. Caldaro T, Garganese MC, Torroni F, et al. Delayed gastric emptying and typical scintigraphic gastric curves in children with gastroesophageal reflux disease: could pyloromyotomy improve this condition? J Pediatr Surg. 2011;46:863–9.
3. Camilleri M, Parkman HP, Shafi MA, et al. Clinical guideline: management of gastroparesis. Am J Gastroenterol. 2013;108:18–37.
4. Chitkara DK, Camilleri M, Zinsmeister AR, et al. Gastric sensory and motor dysfunction in adolescents with functional dyspepsia. J Pediatr. 2005;146:500–5.
5. Dusold R, Burke K, Carpentier W, et al. The accuracy of technetium-99m-labeled red cell scintigraphy in localizing gastrointestinal bleeding. Am J Gastroenterol. 1994;89:345–8.
6. Gerson LB, Fidler JL, Cave DR, et al. ACG clinical guideline: diagnosis and management of small bowel bleeding. Am J Gastroenterol. 2015;110:1265–87.
7. Howarth DM. The role of nuclear medicine in the detection of acute gastrointestinal bleeding. Semin Nucl Med. 2006;36:133–46.
8. Hunter JM, Pezim ME. Limited value of technetium 99m-labeled red cell scintigraphy in localization of lower gastrointestinal bleeding. Am J Surg. 1990;159:504–6.
9. Lin HC, Prather C, Fisher RS, et al. Measurement of gastrointestinal transit. Dig Dis Sci. 2005;50:989–1004.
10. Maurer AH. Guest editorial: gastrointestinal nuclear medicine: are we making progress? Semin Nucl Med. 2012;42:74–5.
11. Maurer AH. Gastrointestinal motility, part 1: esophageal transit and gastric emptying. J Nucl Med Technol. 2016;44:1–11.
12. Maurer AH. Gastrointestinal motility, part 2: small-bowel and colon transit. J Nucl Med Technol. 2016;44:12–8.
13. Maurer AH, Camilleri M, Donohoe K, et al. The SNMMI and EANM practice guideline for small-bowel and colon transit 1.0. J Nucl Med. 2013;54:2004–13.
14. Middleton ML, Strober MD. Planar scintigraphic imaging of the gastrointestinal tract in clinical practice. Semin Nucl Med. 2012;42:33–40.
15. Saliakellis E, Fotoulaki M. Gastroparesis in children. Ann Gastroenterol. 2013;26:204–11.
16. Singendonk MM, Rommel N, Omari T, et al. Upper gastrointestinal motility: prenatal development and problems in infancy. Nat Rev Gastroenterol Hepatol. 2014;11:545–55.
17. Strate LL, Gralnek IM. ACG clinical guideline: management of patients with acute lower gastrointestinal bleeding. Am J Gastroenterol. 2016;111(4):459–74.
18. Tutor JD, Gosa MM. Dysphagia and aspiration in children. Pediatr Pulmonol. 2012;47:321–37.
19. Vandenplas Y, Rudolph CD, Di Lorenzo C, et al. Pediatric gastroesophageal reflux clinical practice guidelines: joint recommendations of the North American Society for Pediatric Gastroenterology, Hepatology, and Nutrition (NASPGHAN) and the European Society for Pediatric Gastroenterology, Hepatology, and Nutrition (ESPGHAN). J Pediatr Gastroenterol Nutr. 2009; 49:498–547.

Gastroenterology: Gastric Emptying – Gastroesophageal Reflux

15

Tamara Caldaro, Paola De Angelis, Filippo Torroni, Francesca Rea, Giulia Angelino, Laura Del Prete, Erminia Francesca Romeo, Simona Faraci, Valerio Balassone, Anna Chiara Iolanda Contini, and Giovanni Federici di Abriola

15.1 Study Technique and Interpretation

15.1.1 Gastric Emptying Scintigraphy

Gastric emptying is a radionuclide technique with a low effective radiation dose (maximum 0.3 mSv for 37 MBq) that is frequently used for measuring gastric emptying. In addition, other important clinical information achievable by this simple test are identifying repetitive reflux episodes, quantifying reflux level, duration and frequency, and evaluating possible lung aspiration.

The unique preparation required for this test is a fasting of 4 h.

Gastric emptying study is performed for 60 min duration (180 frames × 20 s) after meal administration: liquid, semi-liquid, or semisolid meal with an adequate caloric intake can be radiolabeled according to child habits (as milk with or without biscuits, yogurt, homogenized) to achieve a functional evaluation in physiological conditions. For more details about meal administration, see in capital 1. The administered activity of radiotracer is adjusted to the patient's weight (0.55 MBq/kg of technetium-99 m-diethylene-triamine-pentaacetate – 99mTc-DTPA), with a minimum suggested activity of 7.4 MBq and a maximum dose of 37 MBq).

Posterior view registration (with gamma camera centered on the chest and upper abdomen region) allows to achieve a better quality imaging in pediatric patients. With this arrangement of the gamma camera, the child can see and feel near to parents, and the team staff can more easily block (when necessary) the patient or assist the patient in case of vomiting or aspiration. Dedicated software for movement correction is useful, using careful evaluation to exclude possible artifacts.

The qualitative (displayed 600 s per frame) and time/activity curves analyses of dynamic study allow evaluating measurement of gastric emptying velocity (for this end point, gastric emptying scan is considered the gold-standard technique). Excessive gastric emptying delay is a major mechanism in facilitating gastroesophageal reflux, because it causes prolonged gastric wall distension, ending with lower esophageal sphincter dysfunction.

After motion correction, the gastric region of interest (ROI) is drawn to achieve time/activity curves, and all data are corrected for time decay. Gastric emptying is expressed by quantitative parameters (calculated by A/T curve analysis) as lag time, gastric emptying half-time (GE T1/2), and percent of gastric retention at 1 h. Normal values are not established for pediatric population, but in our experience a normal gastric emptying pattern is characterized by gastric emptying >30 % at 1 h and/or GE T1/2<90 min with lag time <10 min.

Accurate qualitative and quantitative evaluation of scintigraphic study also allow detecting and quantifying

T. Caldaro • P. De Angelis (✉) • F. Torroni • F. Rea • G. Angelino
L. Del Prete • E.F. Romeo • S. Faraci • V. Balassone
A.C.L. Contini • G. Federici di Abriola
Unit of Endoscopic Surgery, "Bambino Gesù" Children Hospital, Rome, Italy
e-mail: paola.deangelis@opbg.net

G. Federici di Abriola
Digestive Surgery and Endoscopy Unit, Bambino Gesù Children's Hospital, Rome, Italy

© Springer International Publishing Switzerland 2017

M.C. Garganese, G.F.L. D'Errico (eds.), *Conventional Nuclear Medicine in Pediatrics*, DOI 10.1007/978-3-319-43181-9_15

gastroesophageal reflux; all of these information give important contribution to the diagnostic assessment and therapeutic management of gastroesophageal reflux disease.

Lung fields evaluation is useful to detect ab ingestis inhalation of labeled meal (if orally assumed) or pulmonary aspiration secondary to reflux episodes. Gastroesophageal studies in relationship to respiratory problems are reported in clinical teaching cases of capitol 20.

15.1.2 Scintigraphy of the Esophageal Transit

The transit of a radiolabeled solid or liquid bolus is recorded by fast dynamic scintigraphy (0.1–0.5 s/frame); results can be described as reframed dynamic series or by means of activity/time curves obtained in multiple regions. Assessment of swallowing by oropharyngoesophageal scintigraphy is feasible in cooperative children and helpful in patients with history of dysphagia, for the evaluation of esophageal motility, in primary or acquired structural esophageal abnormalities. Scintigraphy of the esophageal transit can be performed after gastric emptying study, and it is considered as normal if total transit time is 4–6 s for liquid bolus or 6–10 s for solid bolus. Normal clearance time of esophageal activity is less than 15 s with a percentage of clearance equal to 90 %.

15.2 Teaching Cases

15.2.1 Gastric Emtying Scintigraphy in Management of Children with Gastrointestinal Motility Disorders and Clinical Suspect of Gastroesophageal Reflux Disease

15.2.1.1 Case 15.1 Normal Scintigraphic Pattern of Gastric Emptying and Esophageal Transit

A 6-year-old girl, born at term, onset of recurrent respiratory infections with wheezing since the first year of life. The patient experienced several episodes of pneumonia (mainly clinical diagnoses) treated with antibiotics. Diagnostic workup, including immunological and allergological evaluation sweat test, Mantoux test, thoracic CT, and lung scintigraphy, was negative. Therapy with inhaled steroids and oral leukotriene receptor antagonists was partially beneficial. At the age of 4 years, esophageal pH-monitoring was suggestive for moderate-severe gastroesophageal reflux. Treatment with proton pump inhibitor (PPI) was started with marked clinical improvement. Disruption of the therapy after 10 months was followed by one episode of pneumonia. PPI was restarted, and the patient only presented sporadic episodes of cough and dysphagia. At the age of 6 years, definitive treatment discontinuation was well tolerated. Gastric emptying scintigraphy showed normal clearance of the radiolabeled meal without any gastroesophageal reflux and normal esophageal transit. Subsequent follow-up was uneventful (Fig. 15.1).

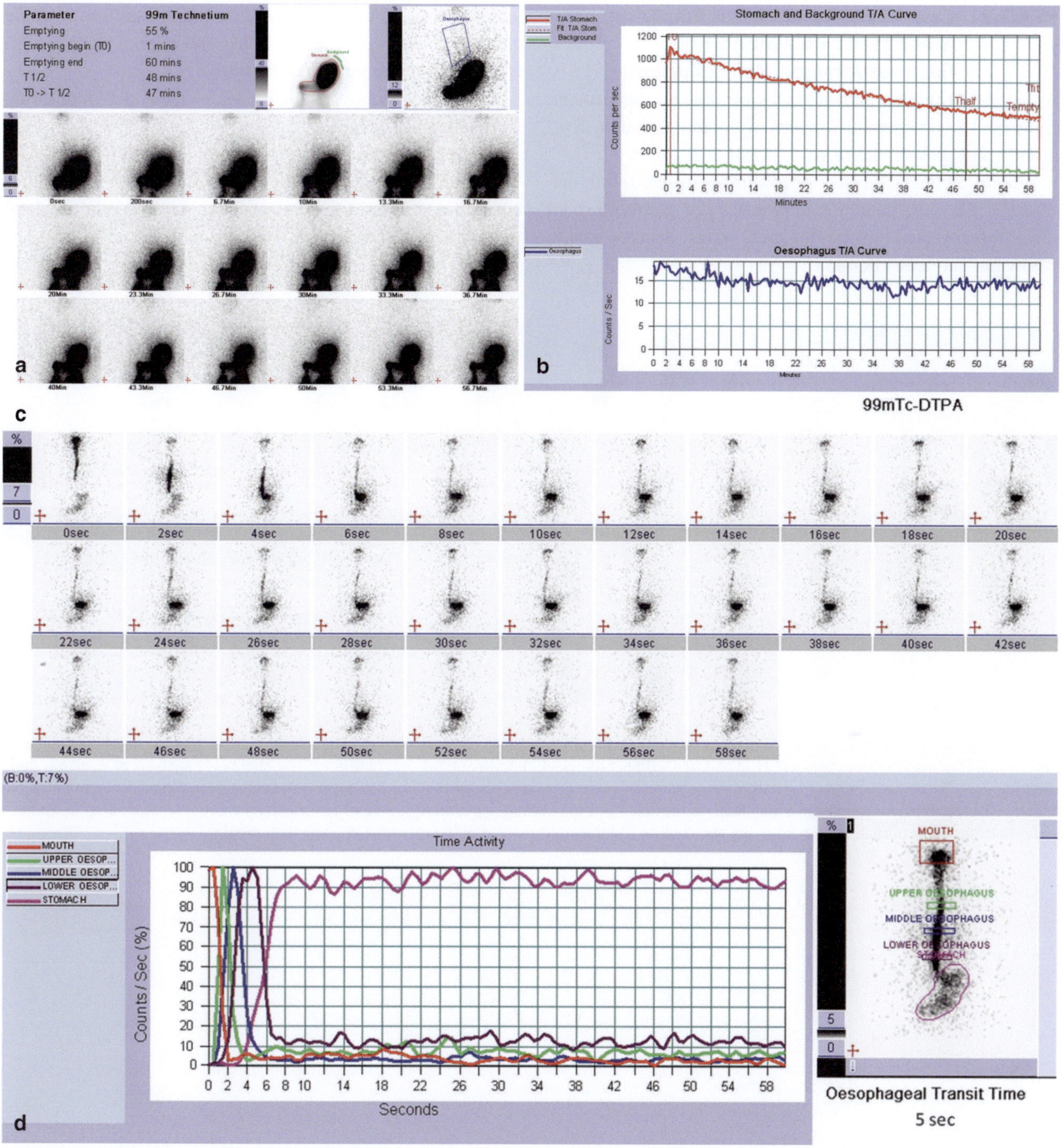

Fig. 15.1 (**a**, **b**) Scintigraphic study is performed after oral liquid meal administration revealing a progressive gastric emptying without gastroesophageal reflux. Time/activity curves corresponding to stomach and esophagus allow to calculate quantitative parameters (showing normal gastric emptying) and to confirm absence of gastroesophageal reflux, respectively. (**c**) The qualitative evaluation of dynamic study shows a normal oropharyngoesophageal transit after a single and complete swallowing. This finding is confirmed by time/activity curves analysis showing normal pattern of each curve and the sequential coordinated peaks of the T/A curves derived from upper, middle, and lower esophagus. Complete clearance of activity from the esophagus at the end of dynamic sequence is evident with a normal transit time (inferior than 5–6 s from upper esophagus tract to stomach)

15.2.1.2 Case 15.2 Normal Gastric Emptying Associated with a Mild Single Gastroesophageal Reflux Episode

A 3-year-old female patient with neurological impairment, congenital hydrocephalus, recurrent nocturnal cough, food refusal, and growth failure.

Due to a clinical suspect of gastroesophageal reflux disease (GERD), the patient underwent *upper* gastrointestinal series that revealed gastroesophageal reflux, delayed gastric emptying, and hiatal hernia.

Conversely, Tc99m gastric scintigraphy showed a single episode of gastroesophageal reflux and normal gastric emptying (46% in 60 min, T/2 = 66 min).

Upper endoscopy and 24-h esophageal pH monitoring were negative for GERD.

Therefore, the patient stopped proton pump inhibitors.

In this case, the complete assessment for GERD has ensured a correct diagnosis and has modified the medical treatment (Fig. 15.2).

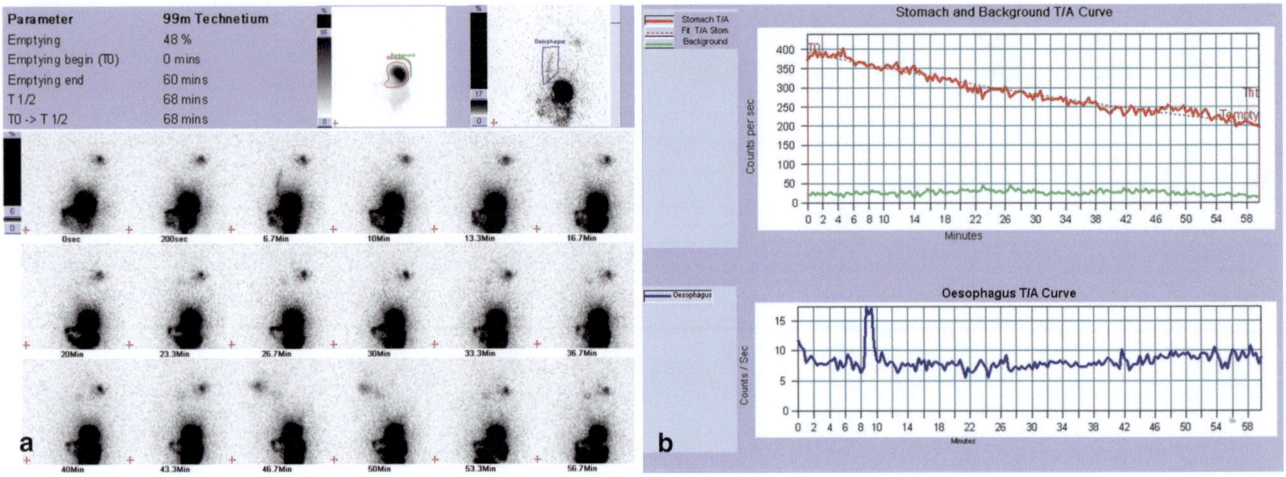

Fig. 15.2 (**a**, **b**) Gastric emptying study is performed after oral milk administration, and first dynamic study image allows to assess possible evidence of ab-ingestis inhalation (especially in children with neurological impairment and oral nutrition). The qualitative analysis of dynamic study reveals a progressive gastric emptying with a single gastroesophageal reflux episode that reaches upper esophageal tract. No evidence of abnormal activity is detectable corresponding to lung fields in the first frame and during dynamic registration. Time/activity curves corresponding to stomach and esophagus show normal gastric emptying and confirm a single mild gastroesophageal reflux episode with rapid washout

15.2.1.3 Case 15.3 Mild Delayed Gastric Emptying Associated with Severe Gastroesophageal Reflux Disease

A 4-year-old boy, born at term, cesarean section for polyhydramnios, postnatal diagnosis of esophageal atresia type C. The patient underwent surgical repair on the second day of life. The postoperative course was uneventful, and progressive oral alimentation was well tolerated. Treatment with H2 blocker was started and continued after discharge. After 2 months, anastomotic esophageal stenosis occurred, requiring endoscopic dilation. At the age of 4 months, H2 blocker was substituted by proton pump inhibitor (PPI). At the age of 14 months, the patient was evaluated for recurrent vomiting and cough. Upper GI endoscopy was unremarkable (patent esophageal anastomosis and normal gastric and esophageal mucosa), and esophageal pH monitoring was suggestive for moderate gastroesophageal reflux. PPI treatment cycles were beneficial. One year later, upper GI endoscopy revealed hiatal hernia, with positive histology for mild esophagitis, and still abnormal esophageal pH monitoring. Subsequent clinical course was good on PPI continuous treatment. However, at the age of 4 years, upper GI endoscopy showed macroscopic distal esophagitis and confirmed hiatal hernia. Gastric emptying scintigraphy showed slightly delayed clearance of the labeled food, in association to frequent episodes of gastroesophageal reflux. Therefore, the patient underwent laparoscopic antireflux surgery (Nissen fundoplication) associated to pyloromyotomy, with uneventful postoperative course and follow-up (Fig. 15.3).

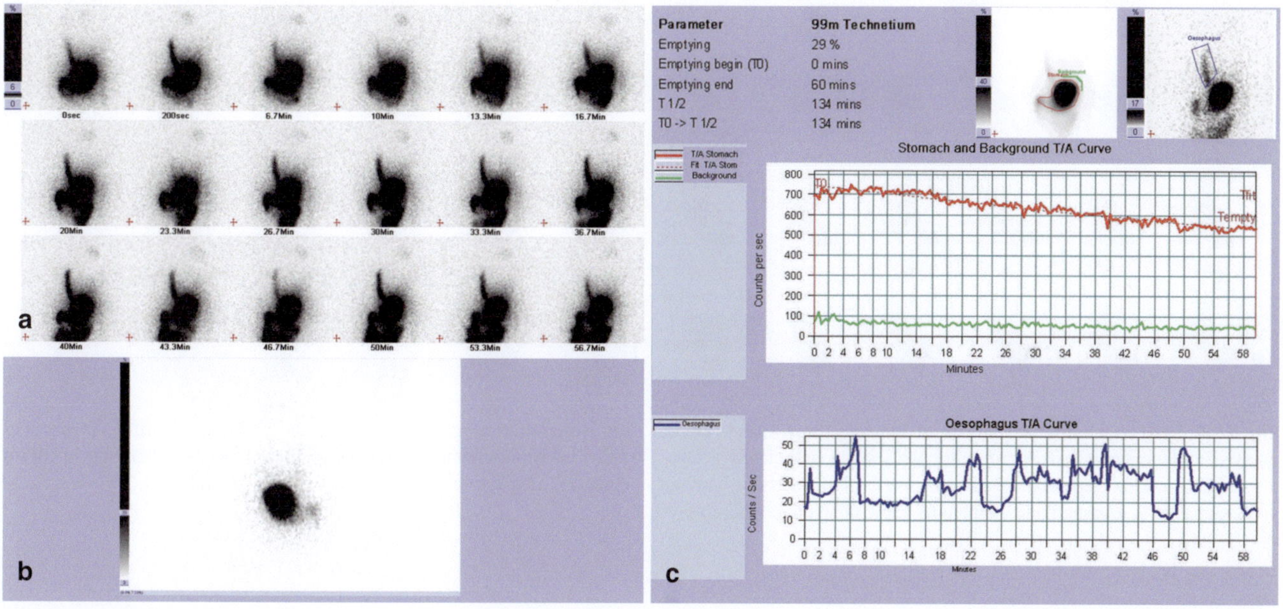

Fig. 15.3 (**a–c**) Qualitative analysis of dynamic study reveals a progressive gastric emptying with severe and frequent gastroesophageal reflux. Time/activity curves corresponding to stomach and esophagus show mild delayed gastric emptying (quantitative parameters: 29 % in 60 min, T/2 = 134 min) confirming evidence of numerous gastroesophageal reflux episodes. When gastric/esophagus activity ratio is higher than 3 %, gastroesophageal reflux is considered of large quantity. Number and volume of reflux help to define the grade of gastroesophageal reflux disease: in this clinical case, gastroesophageal reflux is considered as severe. Frame-by-frame assessment of dynamic study is necessary to evaluate reflux clearance (numerous gastroesophageal reflux episodes can be incorrectly detected by A/T curves and qualitative imaging as prolonged and slow reflux washout). (**b**) First study frame evaluation is important to highlight residual esophageal stasis after oral meal administration (in particular, in case of esophageal atresia history or surgical gastroesophageal treatment) differentiating from early reflux episode. It is always necessary for a careful assessment of possible evidence of activity corresponding to lung fields to exclude (or detect) ab-ingestis inhalation episodes

15.2.1.4 Case 15.4 Delayed Gastric Emptying Associated with Mild Gastroesophageal Reflux Disease (Scintigraphic Pretreatment Assessment)

A 3-year-old female, preterm (GE 24° sett, weight: 725 g; spontaneous delivery), polyhydramnios. Periventricular leukomalacia, bronchial dysplasia, retinopathy (laser therapy). Mild malnutrition, food refusal, dysphagia, chronic vomiting, and regurgitation.

Upper gastrointestinal (UGI) series: no UGI alterations, no gastroesophageal reflux (GER), delayed gastric emptying.

US pylorus: no alterations.

Tc99m gastric scintigraphy (*prepyloric dilation*): 17 % in 60 min, T/2 = 3.9 h, mild GER

Pyloric dilation: 12 mm hydrostatic pyloric dilation throughout endoscopy.

Clinical improvement and scintigraphic control after dilation were indicative of complete therapeutic efficacy, confirming diagnostic role of scintigraphy in pretreatment evaluation and monitoring therapeutic effect of pyloric dilation (Fig. 15.4).

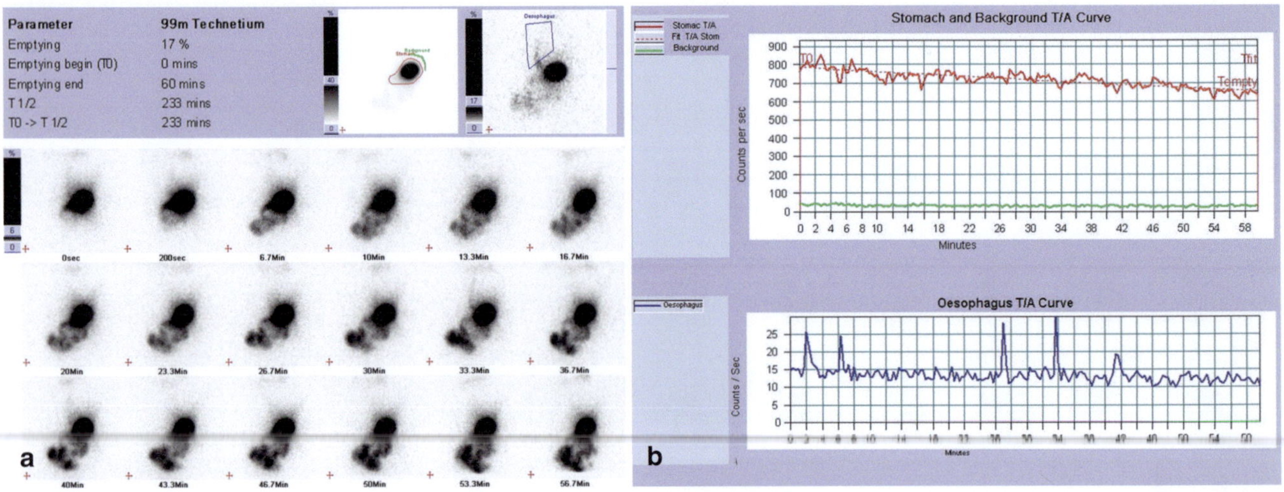

Fig. 15.4 (**a**) The qualitative analysis of dynamic study reveals a progressive but delayed gastric emptying with some associated gastroesophageal reflux episodes (almost five). Time/activity curves corresponding to stomach and esophagus show delayed gastric emptying (quantitative gastric parameters: 17 % in 60 min, theoretical T/2 = 3.9 h), confirming evidence of five mild gastroesophageal reflux episodes, respectively

15.2.1.5 Case 15.5 Delayed Gastric Emptying Associated with Severe Gastroesophageal Reflux Disease (Presurgical Assessment in Child Who Underwent Nissen Fundoplication and Pyloromyotomy)

An 8-year-old male patient with history of chronic iron-deficiency anemia (Hb 7.5 g/dl) and heartburn.

Upper endoscopy documented severe erosive esophagitis and hiatal hernia, and pH-multichannel intraluminal impedance (pH-MII) confirmed the diagnosis of severe gastroesophageal reflux disease (GERD). Treatment with proton pump inhibitors (PPI) was administered for 6 months with good clinical response and improvement of anemia.

An endoscopic re-evaluation without PPI documented esophagitis in the lower third of the esophagus.

Because of the dependence on medical therapy, surgical treatment was carried out.

In the preoperative period, patient underwent scintigraphy to evaluate gastric emptying and define the surgical procedure (Nissen fundoplication ± pyloromyotomy, (Fig. 15.5a, b).

Tc99m gastric scintigraphy detected delayed gastric emptying (14 % in 60 min; T/= 2.4 h) associated to GER.

Laparoscopic Nissen fundoplication and pyloromyotomy were performed to treat GERD and improve gastric emptying. Currently, the patient is in good clinical condition with normal value of hemoglobin (Hb 12.5 g/dl).

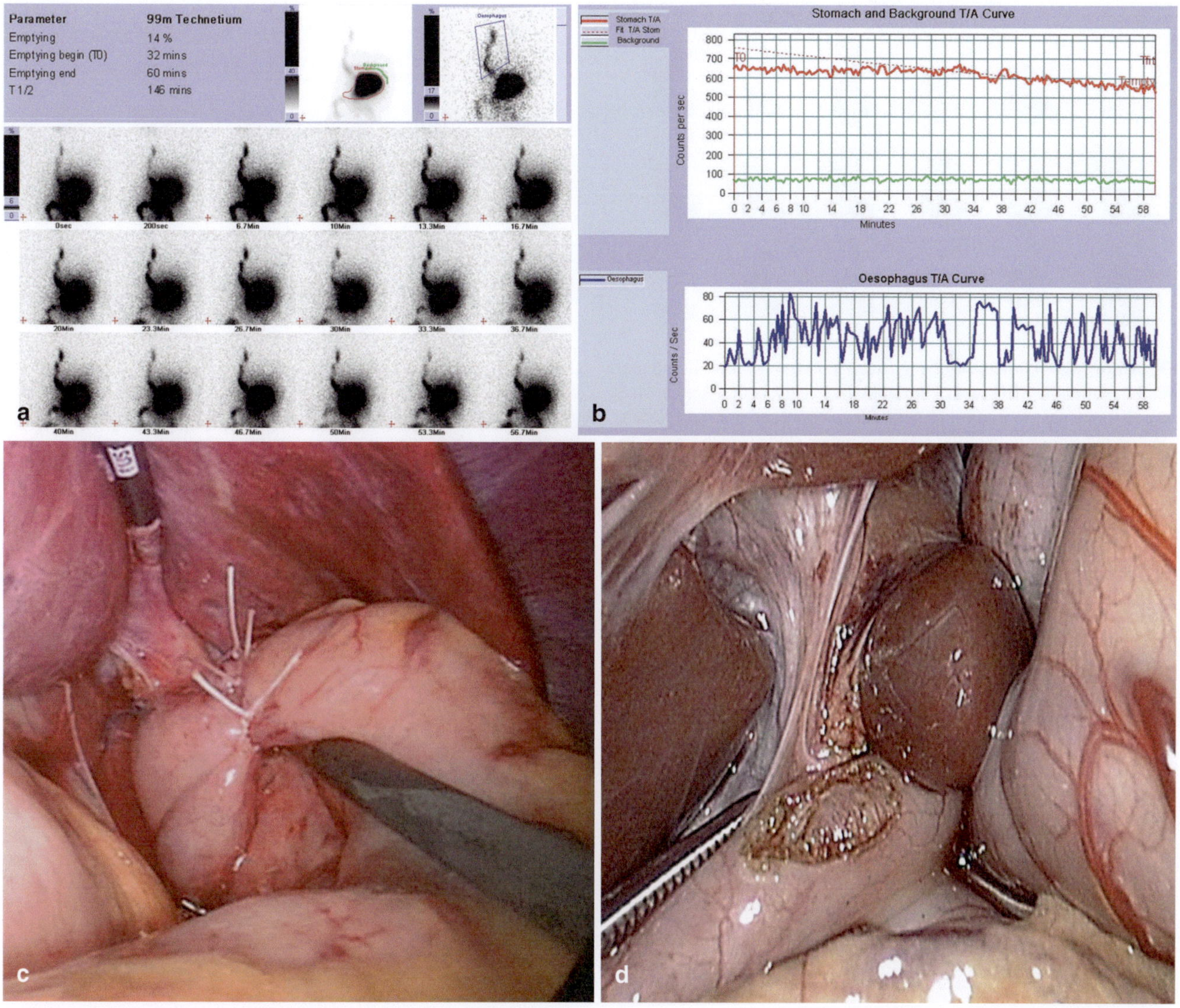

Fig. 15.5 (**a**, **b**) Qualitative analysis of dynamic study reveals a progressive but delayed gastric emptying with labeled meal stasis corresponding to stomach, up to the end of dynamic study. Numerous and severe gastroesophageal reflux episodes are also detectable without evidence of activity corresponding to lung fields. Time/activity curve corresponding to stomach shows delayed and irregular gastric emptying: after 32 min of latency time, gastric parameters are slower than normal (14 % in 60 min and theoretical T/2 = 2.4 h). Frame-by-frame and T/A esophagus curve analyses reveal numerous gastroesophageal reflux episodes: some of these show prolonged clearance, other ones rapid washout. (**c**, **d**) Laparoscopic Nissen fundoplication and pyloromyotomy

15.2.1.6 Case 15.6 Delayed Gastric Emptying Associated with Severe Gastroesophageal Reflux Disease (In Child Who Underwent Nissen Fundoplication Without Scintigraphic Gastric Motility Assessment in the Preoperative Planning)

A 5-year-old male patient with history of severe gastroesophageal reflux disease (GERD) underwent Nissen fundoplication with placing of percutaneous endoscopic gastrostomy (PEG). A previous scintigraphic gastric emptying assessment was not performed. Persisting GERD symptoms, the child was referred to our center, and a gastric emptying scintigraphy was performed in the preoperative planning to choose adequate medical or surgical treatment. Delayed gastric emptying detected by gastric scintigraphy was considered the principal cause of failed previous Nissen fundoplication; a subsequent antireflux surgery associated with pyloromyotomy was necessary (Fig. 15.6).

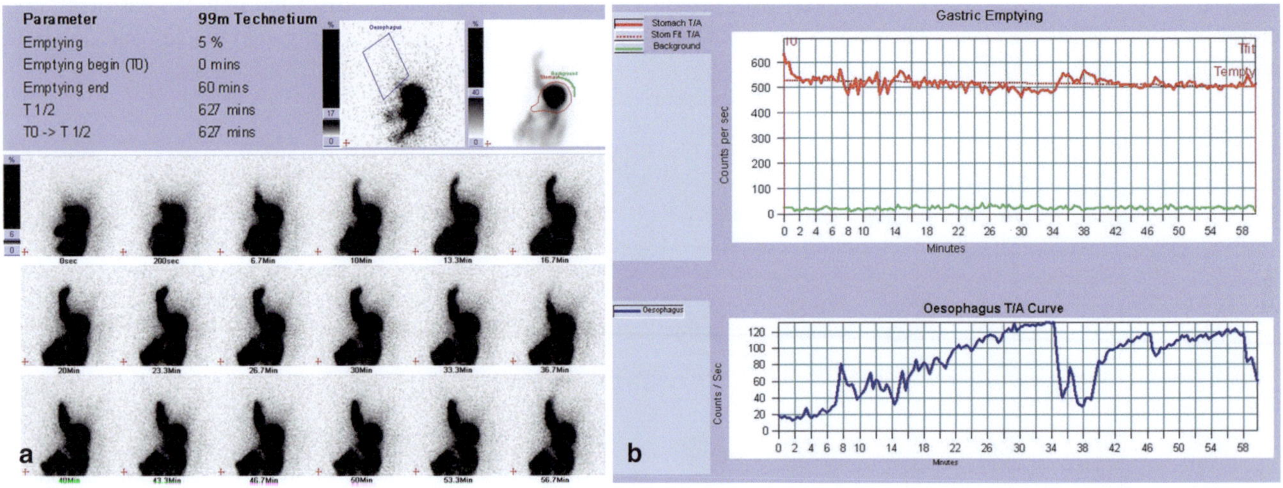

Fig. 15.6 (**a**, **b**) Gastric emptying study is performed after liquid meal administration by PEG tube. The qualitative analysis of dynamic study reveals poor gastric emptying with considerable retention of labeled meal in the stomach up to the end of dynamic study. Three severe gastroesophageal reflux episodes are also detectable without evidence of complete washout up to the end of dynamic registration. Time/activity curve corresponding to stomach shows severely delayed and irregular gastric emptying (5 % in 60 min with nonassessable T/2). Frame-by-frame and T/A esophagus curve analyses confirm evidence of three severe gastroesophageal reflux episodes with slow and partial washout

15.2.1.7 Case 15.7 Delayed Gastric Emptying and Intestinal Transit Without Gastroesophageal Reflux Disease Associated

A 4-year-old female, diagnosis of chronic idiopathic intestinal pseudo-obstruction (POIC) and megacystis. ACTG2 gene "de novo" mutation, no inbreeding. In order to confirm the clinical diagnosis of POIC, to assess bowel anatomy and motility, and to rule out secondary causes of POIC, the child underwent several diagnostic examinations. Abdominal US showed marked fecal impaction with significant bladder distention, marked gastric distention, mesenteric nodes, and accessory spleen. Upper gastrointestinal (UGI) series showed marked bowel distention with no mechanical obstruction; contrast enema noticed moderately dilated colon with no haustrations. Spinal magnetic resonance imaging was normal. The anorectal manometry showed RAIR, with no evidence of Hirschsprung's or spinal neuropathy. The antro-duodenal manometry showed no migrating motor complex (MMC) during fasting, and after challenge with erythromycin and octreotide, her antrum also did not respond to erythromycin; the colonic manometry showed no colonic activity during fasting, no response to a meal, and no response to bisacodyl instillated via the catheter. The upper and lower gastrointestinal endoscopy showed mild esophagitis and a normal colon. Full thickness small bowel, colonic, and rectal biopsies showed marked depletion of interstitial cells of Cajal, but normal neural markers (beta-S100 and alpha-SMA) and normal ganglion cells. In this patient, feeding intolerance, vomiting, failure to thrive, and intestinal obstruction leading to intestinal failure needed a cecostomy tube, percutaneous endoscopic gastrostomy (PEG), and central venous catheter (CVC). In spite of these therapeutic tools, persistence of abdominal obstruction occurred. A gastric and colonic scintigraphy was done to better study total intestinal and colonic transit, before a more aggressive therapeutic option. Tc99m gastric scintigraphy showed delayed gastric emptying (22 % in 60 min, T/2 = 3 h) and no gastroesophageal reflux. 67Ga-citrate intestinal and colonic scintigraphy showed delayed intestinal transit, stasis at ileal terminal loop (terminal ileum, ileocecal region), without images referred to altered intestinal permeability. Then, our patient underwent ileostomy-colostomy and stopped parenteral nutrition. She had gastrojejunal nutrition for 6 months; now, she is continuing gastric enteral nutrition (nocturnal enteral nutrition for 11 h, 40 ml/h) via PEG, gluten-free diet *per os*. She has daily colonic irrigations, she gets bladder catheterization every 3 h, she has a good growth, with a BMI of 13.8. Every mild recurrent episodes of intestinal distention are managed at home by parents with tube opening and intestinal decontaminations. The role of scintigraphy in our case was confirmed by therapeutic choices: scintigraphy findings helped to guide the correct stoma placement and to decide a better nutritional planning, promoting enteral feeding (Fig. 15.7).

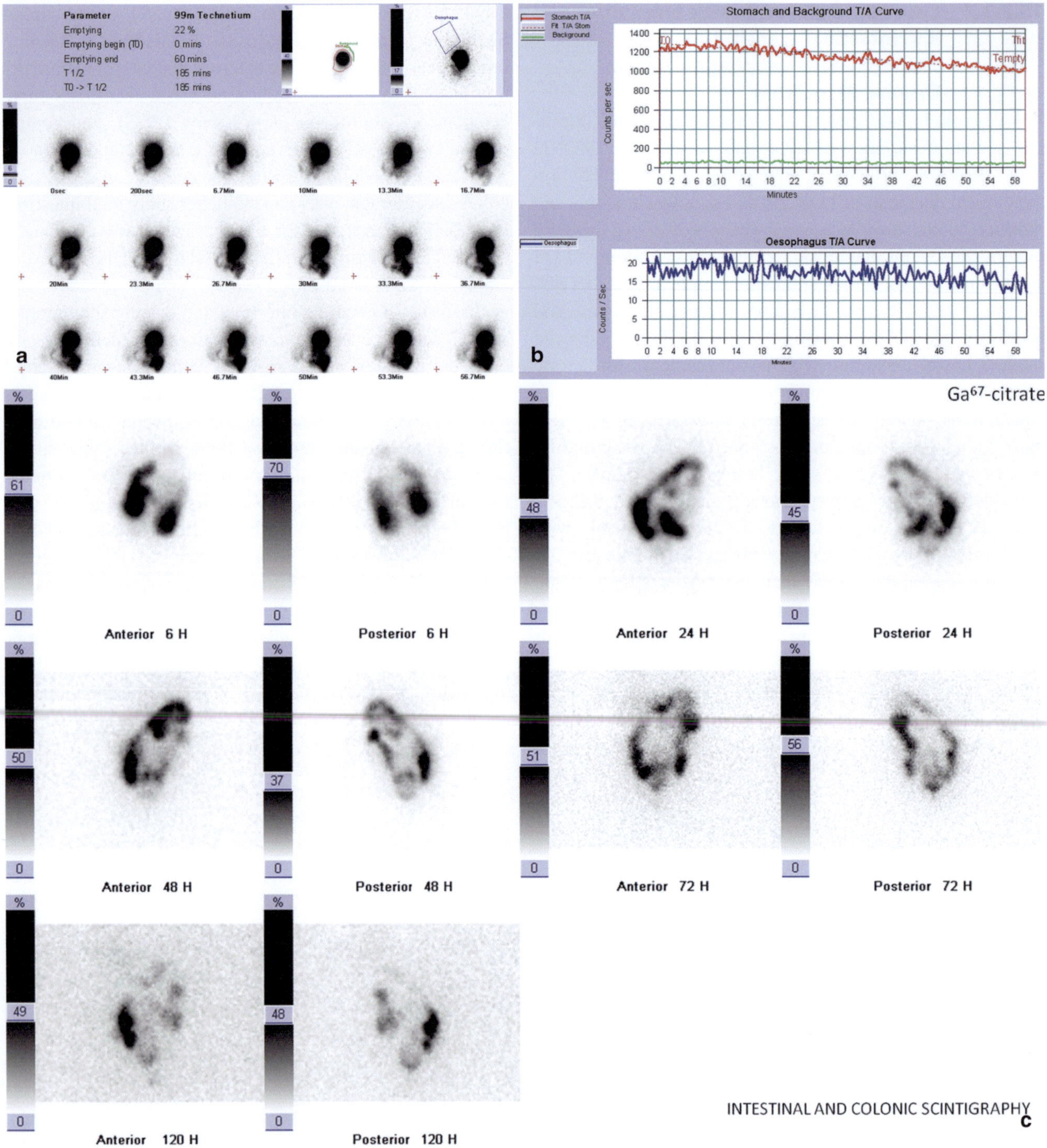

Fig. 15.7 (**a**, **b**) Gastric emptying study is performed after labeled milk administration by PEG tube. Qualitative analysis of dynamic study reveals a progressive gastric emptying with no evidence of gastroesophageal reflux. Time/activity curves corresponding to stomach and esophagus show delayed gastric emptying parameters (22 % in 60 min, theoretical T/2 = 3 h), confirming absence of significative gastroesophageal reflux. (**c**) Intestinal and colonic scintigraphy is performed administering ^{67}Ga-citrate by PEJ tube. Static image performed at 6 h shows tracer stasis corresponding to ileal terminal loop (terminal ileum-ileocecal region) and distal descending/sigmoid colon. In the following images, progressive tracer transit throughout the colon is detectable up to static acquisition performed at 72 h. Delayed intestinal transit is evident up to the last image (at 120 h), with persistent stasis corresponding to proximal ascending colon and poor residual activity in the other intestinal segments. No evidence of altered intestinal permeability is detectable

15.2.1.8 Case 15.8 Rapid Gastric Emptying Associated with Gastroesophageal Reflux Disease

A 9-year-old girl patient with history of diaphragmatic rhabdomyosarcoma (off-therapy). She underwent multiple operations for diaphragmatic herniation of stomach and part of intestine. Symptoms as vomiting, diarrhea, and cramping that occurred after the last surgical treatment (especially right after eating), and gastric emptying scintigraphy was performed to assess gastric motility in relation to clinical suspicion of Dumping syndrome (Fig. 15.8).

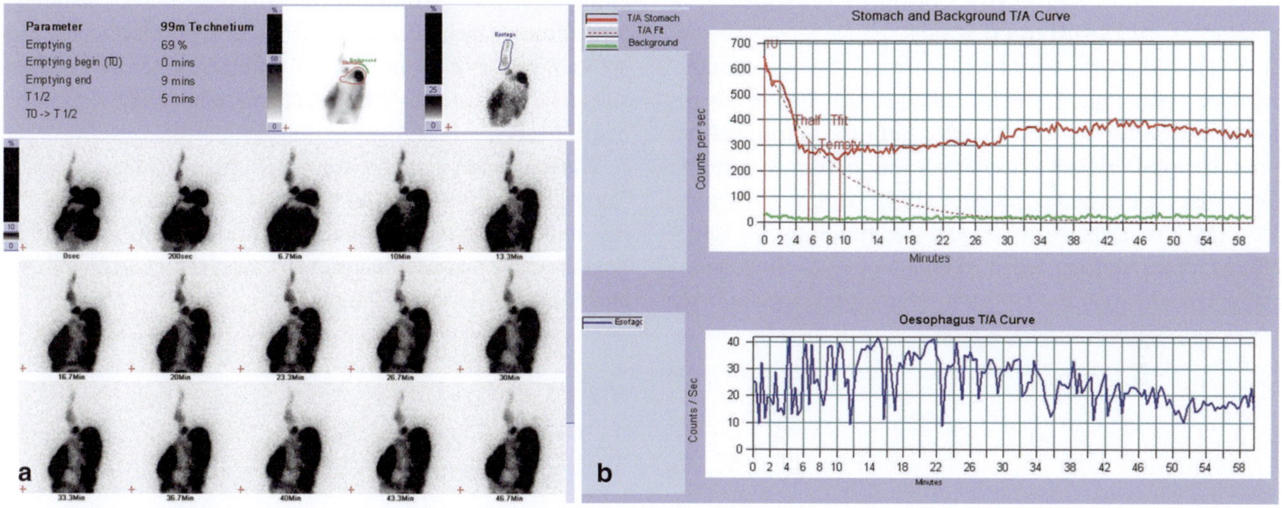

Fig. 15.8 (**a**, **b**) Qualitative and time/activity curve analyses of dynamic study reveal an irregular gastric emptying. Calculating intestinal versus total activity ratio in the first frame of dynamic registration, a share of 47 % of administered meal is already present in the intestine. In the following minutes, gastric parameters are more rapid than normal (69 % in 60 min and T/2 = 5 min), with associated numerous and severe gastroesophageal reflux episodes (especially in the first 30 min of the study). A persistent esophageal stasis is evident up to the end of registration, depicting moderate dilatation of distal esophagus and a hiatal hernia, endoscopically detected

15.2.2 Gastric Emptying Scintigraphy in the Follow-Up of Children Affected by Esophageal Atresia

15.2.2.1 Case 15.9 Normal Gastric Emptying Associated with a Mild Gastroesophageal Reflux Episodes and Progressive Complete Washout of Esophageal Stasis

A 5-year-old male patient was born at 38-week gestation with long-gap, type A esophageal atresia. A Stamm gastrostomy was performed shortly after birth for nutritional purpose. Delayed primary anastomosis was performed 3 months later, and proton pump inhibitor (PPI) therapy was started. He had recurrent esophageal anastomotic strictures (Fig. 15.9a) requiring repeated endoscopic dilations and, at the age of 14 months, a custom esophageal dynamic stent was placed. Gastroesophageal reflux disease was suspected based on the history of recurrent vomiting and feeding difficulties with inadequate weight gain. A 24-h pH monitoring showed prolonged esophageal acid exposure time and increased number of reflux episodes. Antireflux surgery was needed, and Tc99m gastroesophageal scintigraphy, showing mild gastroesophageal reflux episodes and normal gastric emptying, was performed as a preoperative planning. Sometimes, a lack of correlation between pH monitoring and scintigraphy is evident, due to different kinds of refluxes selectively detected by two tests (acid reflux and food reflux, respectively).

Nissen fundoplication was performed at the age of 2. Significant improvement in symptoms was observed, and the last upper endoscopy (4-year-old) was normal (no esophageal stricture and esophagitis). To date, the child is off PPI and clinically asymptomatic.

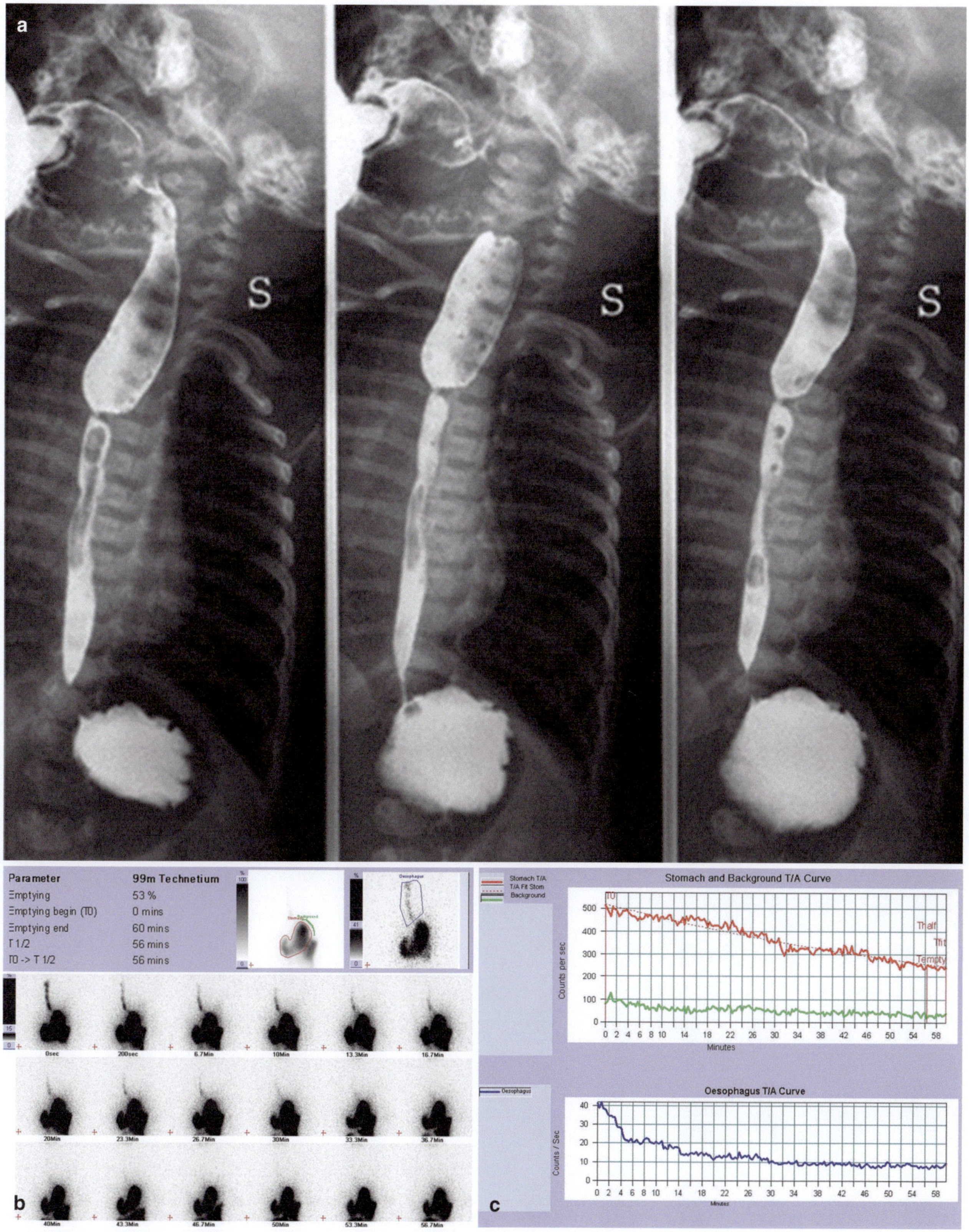

Fig. 15.9 (**a**) Esophageal anastomotic stricture. (**b, c**) Gastric emptying study is performed after oral milk intake (suitable in case of previous esophageal atresia – when clinically possible – to assess residual esophageal stasis after meal administration). The qualitative analysis of dynamic study reveals a progressive gastric emptying with several mild gastroesophageal reflux episodes (some of which reach the mouth). By first frame qualitative evaluation, esophageal stasis is detected, with evidence of subsequent slow but progressive washout (within first 30 min). No evidence of abnormal activity is detectable corresponding to lung fields in the first frame and during dynamic registration. Time/activity curve corresponding to stomach shows slightly irregular gastric emptying with normal gastric clearance parameters (53 % in 60 min and T/2 = 56 min). Esophageal T/A curve analysis confirms evidence of progressive esophageal stasis resolution, while mild gastroesophageal reflux episodes are better assessed by qualitative and frame-by-frame evaluation

15.2.2.2 Case 15.10 Mild Delayed Gastric Emptying not Associated with Gastroesophageal Reflux Episodes and Evidence of Progressive but Partial Washout of Esophageal Stasis (Esophagus-Esophageal Anastomosis)

A 3-year-old boy born with esophageal atresia and tracheoesophageal fistula (type C) underwent surgical repair within the first week of life. Shortly after the procedure, the clinical course was complicated by the occurrence of pneumothorax and hydrothorax, and a barium swallow showed an anastomotic leak. Therefore, a gastrostomy was performed, while esophageal leak was treated conservatively. Afterward, repeated endoscopic dilations were needed in order to manage recurrent esophageal anastomotic strictures (Fig. 15.10a), leading to severe dysphagia. During diagnostic assessment, Tc99m gastroesophageal scintigraphy showed a mild delayed gastric emptying (28 % at 1 h) without associated reflux episodes. Based on these results, the child underwent pyloromyotomy (2 years of age). Significant improvement of clinical symptoms was observed.

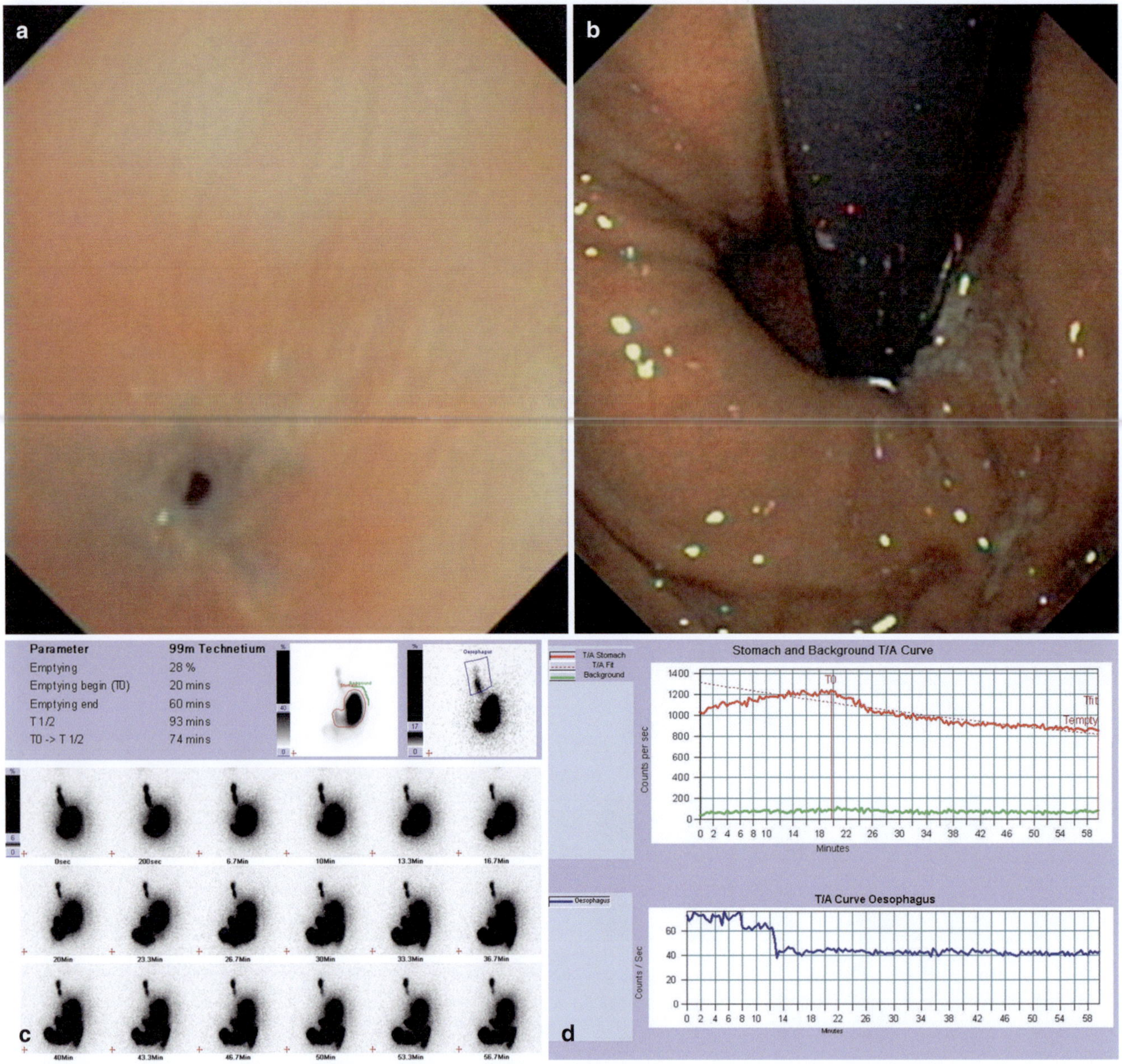

Fig. 15.10 (**a**, **b**) Upper endoscopy: esophageal anastomotic stricture (**a**) and hiatal hernia (**b**). (**c**, **d**) Gastric emptying study is performed after oral semiliquid meal intake. Qualitative analysis of dynamic study reveals esophageal stasis with evidence of partial washout in early registration phase; persisting residual activity corresponding to upper and middle esophagus is evident up to the end of dynamic registration with no associated abnormal activity in lung fields. The qualitative and time/activity curves (corresponding to stomach and esophagus) analyses reveal an irregular gastric emptying (partially due to labeled meal refill from esophagus into stomach): after 20 min of latency time, gastric emptying shows slightly delayed gastric clearance parameters (28 % in 60 min). Frame-by-frame and esophageal T/A curve analyses show absence of significant gastroesophageal reflux episodes

15.2.2.3 Case 15.11 Markedly Delayed Gastric Emptying Associated with Vomiting Episode (In a Child with Gastric Pull-up Reconstruction for Esophageal Atresia)

A 6-year-old female child born with congenital cardiac disease, esophageal atresia type C, tracheomalacia, and congenital subglottic stenosis. The patient was first operated in another hospital, where a gastric pull-up reconstruction and a tracheoplasty were performed.

At the age of 4, the child was referred to our center for recurrent pneumonia (three episodes in 6 months), cough during meal, food refusal, and poor weight gain.

An upper endoscopy and a laryngotracheal endoscopy excluded an esophageal anastomotic stricture and a subglottic stenosis, respectively. However, a difficult passage of the endoscope through the pylorus was documented. On this basis, in order to evaluate the gastric emptying, a Tc99m gastric scintigraphy was mandatory; scintigraphic examination detected severe delayed gastric emptying and an episode of vomiting during the investigation.

After three endoscopic pneumatic dilations of the pylorus, a progressive increase in appetite and weight gain was found.

During follow-up, a further scintigraphic evaluation will be repeated to quantify the improvement of gastric emptying (Fig. 15.11).

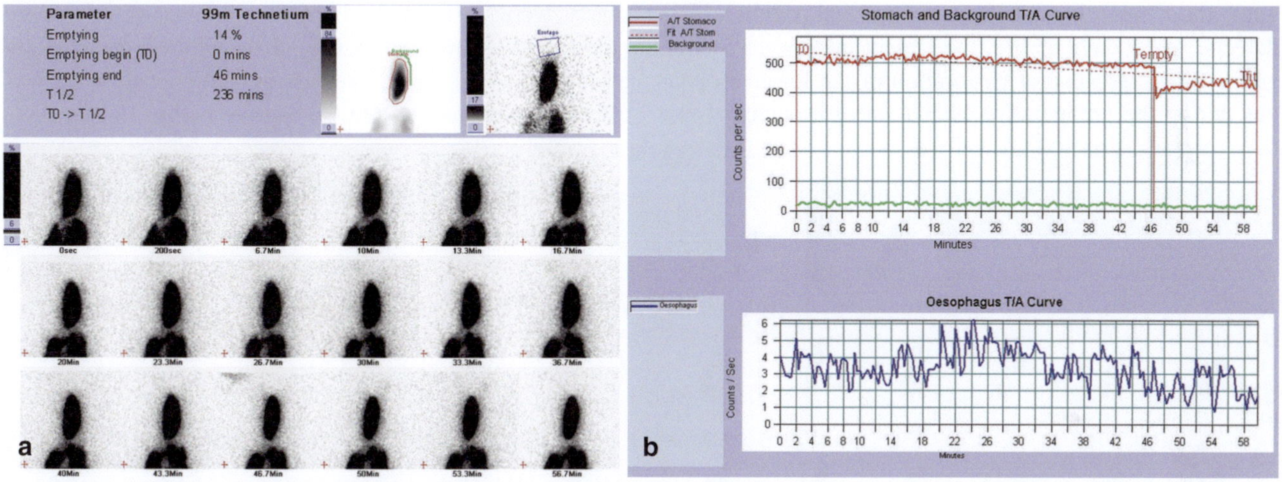

Fig. 15.11 (**a**, **b**) Gastric emptying study is performed after oral liquid meal intake. By the qualitative imaging evaluation, stomach is dislocated in thorax in relation to surgical outcomes of gastric pull-up reconstruction. Gastric emptying is markedly irregular: a share of about 45 % of administered meal is already present in the intestine in the first frame of dynamic registration. During dynamic registration, qualitative images and time/activity curve analysis show severely poor gastric emptying with considerable retention of labeled meal in the stomach (stomach T/A curve appeared flattened) up to the end of the study. At 46th min of registration, a vomiting episode is evident with excretion of about 14 % and without further gastric clearance in the rest part of the study. No evidence of significant gastroesophageal reflux episodes (previous or post vomiting) or pulmonary aspiration are detected, even if intense gastric activity does not allow an optimal imaging evaluation

15.2.2.4 Case 15.12 Markedly Irregular and Delayed Gastric Emptying Associated with Severe Gastroesophageal Reflux and Stasis of Labeled Material into the Dilated Colonic Graft (In a Child with Esophageal Atresia Who Underwent Esophageal Colonic Anastomosis)

A 4-year-old male child. Preterm birth at 34 weeks due to pregnancy complicated by polyhydramnios. Prenatal ultrasound diagnosis of esophageal atresia confirmed postnatally (esophageal atresia without tracheoesophageal fistula, Type A) and subsequent diagnosis of DiGeorge syndrome with mild neurological impairment and cardiological defects. At 10 days of life, the patient underwent Stamm gastrostomy. Because of perforation of the lower esophagus during the preoperative evaluation of esophageal gap length using Hegar dilator, an esophagostomy was performed; tracheostomy was added for glottic stenosis. In 2014, after three ineffective Kimura's procedures to lengthen the esophagus, the proposal for an esophageal substitution by colonic graft was submitted. One month after colonic interposition, the patient presented recurrent vomiting and weight loss. An upper gastrointestinal series documented persistence of contrast medium into the colonic graft without stenosis of the upper and lower anastomoses. Tc99m gastric scintigraphy (radiolabeled meal via gastrostomy) showed markedly irregular and delayed gastric emptying with severe gastroesophageal reflux and stasis of labeled material into the dilated colonic graft. Consequently, tailoring of the colonic graft and pyloroplasty were performed to improve transit of interposed colon and gastric emptying, that resulted beneficially affected. In this case, the scintigraphic evaluation was effective to define the surgical approach (Fig. 15.12).

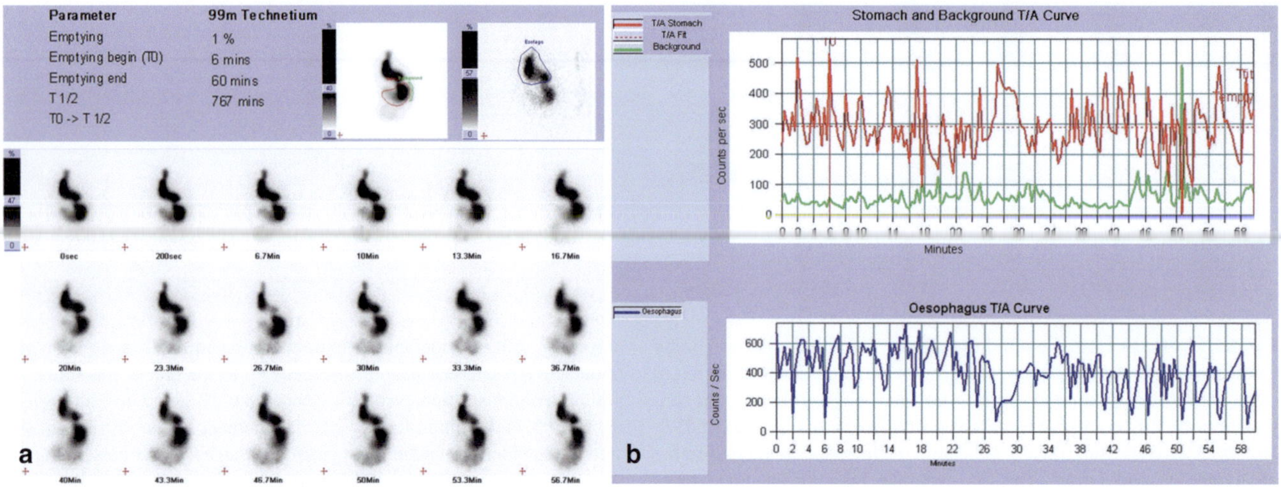

Fig. 15.12 (**a**, **b**) Gastric emptying study is performed after labeled milk administration by PEG tube. During meal administration (performed under persistence monitor control) is evident a reflux and stasis of labeled material into the dilated colonic graft. During dynamic registration, qualitative and time/activity curve analyses show severely irregular and poor gastric emptying with considerable retention of labeled meal in the stomach (stomach T/A curve shows that T/2 is not evaluable). Labeled meal stasis persists into the dilated colonic graft with evidence of activity decrease and increase, secondary to washout and reflux, respectively (as for junctional steno-insufficient pattern). No evidence of pulmonary aspiration is detected, even if labeled milk stasis corresponding to neo-esophagus reconstructed does not allow an optimal imaging evaluation

15.2.2.5 Case 15.13 Markedly Irregular and Delayed Gastric Emptying Associated with Stasis of Labeled Material into the Dilated Colonic Graft (In a Child with Long-Gap Esophageal Atresia Associated with Diaphragmatic Hernia Who Underwent Esophageal Colonic Anastomosis)

A 10-year-old male patient, with prenatal ultrasound diagnosis of left congenital diaphragmatic hernia, long-gap esophageal atresia with tracheoesophageal fistula (type C), left hemifacial hypoplasia and scleral show left eye. Repair of diaphragmatic defect, closure of tracheoesophageal fistula by clips, and placement of gastrostomy tube were performed at birth in another hospital. In the postoperative period, due to a mediastinitis following perforation of the lower esophagus, a cervicotomy and a tracheostomy were necessary. At the age of 1 year, the baby underwent esophagocoloplasty with closure of gastrostomy and tracheostomy. Since 2012, the clinical history was characterized by recurrent ab ingestis pneumonia with frequent nocturnal episodes of acute respiratory failure. In 2015, the patient was admitted in our hospital for severe malnutrition, dysphagia, and decline in pulmonary function. During the hospitalization, a complete anatomical and functional evaluation of the colonic graft was planned, as is better described below:

Upper gastrointestinal series (Fig. 15.13a): dilated colonic graft with passage of the contrast medium into the stomach only in orthostatic position. Delayed gastric emptying.

Tc99m esophagogastric scintigraphy (Fig. 15.13c, d): delayed transit with retention of labeled material in the colonic graft; delayed gastric emptying (4 % in 1 h; T/2 = not evaluable), no evidence of gastroesophageal reflux.

Upper endoscopy: dilated colon with residual food; no mucosal inflammation. Normal diameter of the esophagocolic and cologastric anastomoses. Wide pylorus. No evidence of gastroduodenal mucosal lesions.

According to the radiological, scintigraphic, and endoscopic findings that documented delayed esophagocolonic transit and delayed gastric emptying in the absence of stomach obstruction, a gastrojejunostomy with gastrostomy for enteral nutrition was performed. The child is now asymptomatic with progressive improvement of nutritional conditions.

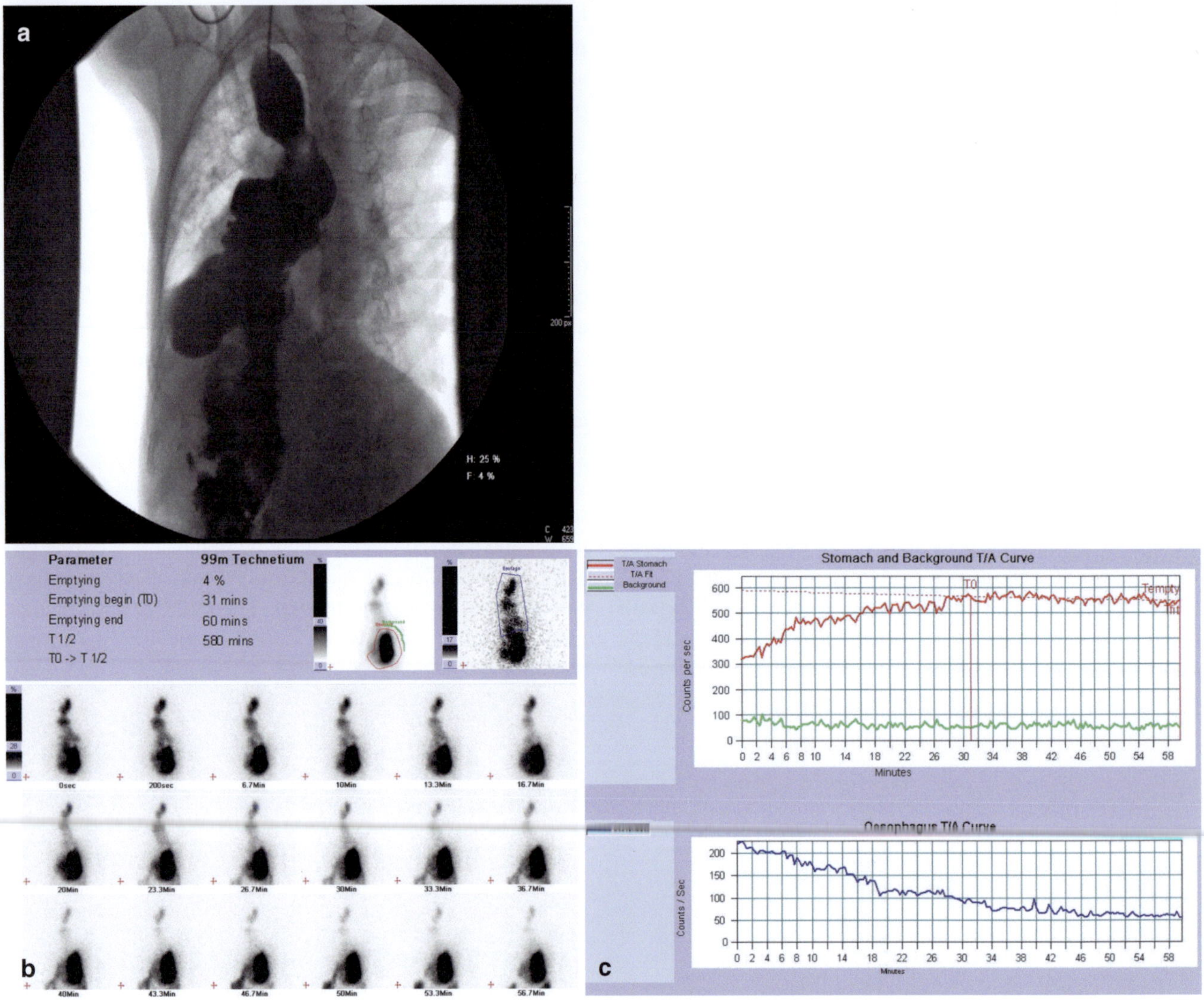

Fig. 15.13 (**a, b**) Dilatated colonic graft. (**c**) Gastric emptying study is performed after oral liquid meal intake. The qualitative analysis of dynamic study reveals meal stasis with evidence of progressive washout in 30 min of registration confirmed by time/activity curves (corresponding to stomach and esophagus) analysis revealing a labeled meal refill from esophagus into stomach. Colonic graft appears dilated and tortuous with evidence of a hypoactive deficient ring corresponding to esophageal colonic anastomosis (as for a relative stenosis). After 30 min, gastric emptying shows markedly delayed gastric clearance parameters, with considerable retention of labeled meal in the stomach (with not evaluable T/2). No evidence of significant gastroesophageal reflux episodes or pulmonary aspiration are detected up to the end of the study

15.2.3 Scintigraphic Contribution in the Management of Children Affected by Cystic Fibrosis

15.2.3.1 Case 15.14 Delayed Gastric Emptying with Associated Mild Gastroesophageal Reflux Disease and Transient Stasis Detected by Esophagus Transit (In Child Affected by Cystic Fibrosis)

A 10-year-old boy affected by cystic fibrosis with a CFTR gene mutation, pancreatic insufficiency, chronic pulmonary colonization, with recurrent acute pulmonary infections.

Onset of heart burn, regurgitation, epigastric pain, and feeling of early satiety at the age of 5.

Upper endoscopy documented mild esophagitis and gastritis, histologically confirmed.

pH-multichannel intraluminal impedance detected a moderate gastroesophageal reflux disease with acid and weak acid reflux episodes.

99mTc gastric scintigraphy showed mild gastroesophageal reflux events, absence of inhalations, and delayed gastric emptying (17 % in 1 h; T/2 = 4.3 h), with transient stasis into the distal esophagus.

According to these procedures that were positive for a moderate gastroesophageal reflux disease, therapy with proton pump inhibitors (two cycles per year) and prokinetic drugs was administered with good clinical response (Fig. 15.14).

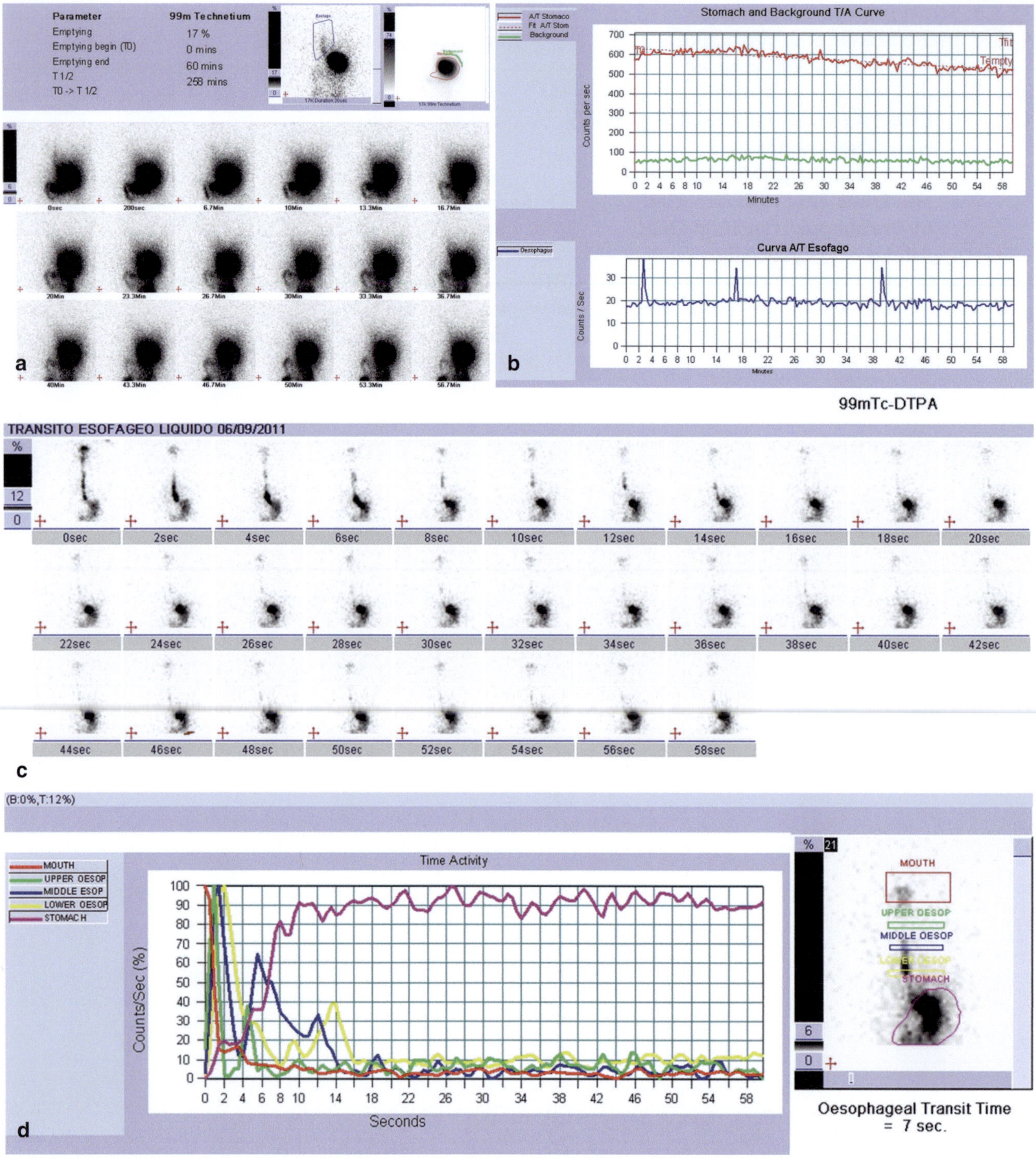

Fig. 15.14 (**a**, **b**) Gastric emptying study is performed after oral liquid meal administration. The qualitative analysis of dynamic study reveals poor gastric emptying with considerable retention of labeled meal in the stomach up to the end of dynamic study. Three mild gastroesophageal reflux episodes are also detectable with evidence of rapid and complete washout. Time/activity curves corresponding to stomach show delayed and irregular gastric emptying (17 % in 60 min, T/2 = 4.3 h). Frame-by-frame and esophageal T/A curve analyses confirm evidence of three mild gastroesophageal reflux episodes with complete and rapid washout. (**c**) Assessment of swallowing by oropharyngoesophageal scintigraphy is helpful in patient with history of cystic fibrosis. Qualitative evaluation of dynamic study shows a slightly delayed oropharyngoesophageal transit after swallowing due to mild and transient stasis corresponding to distal esophagus (total transit time is slightly higher than normal: 7 s from upper esophagus tract to stomach). This finding is confirmed by time/activity curves analysis showing sequential coordinated peaks of the T/A curves derived from upper, middle, and lower esophagus, even if distal esophagus curve shows mildly large width

Bibliography

1. Garganese MC, Knafelz D. Chapter 24. "Manuale SIGENP di gastroenterologia ed epatologia pediatrica" (Il pensiero scientifico editore Ed 2014). p. 103–4.

Gastroenterology: Intestinal Bleeding

16

Milena Pizzoferro, Maria Felicia Villani, Tamara Caldaro, Valerio Balassone, Anna Chiara Iolanda Contini, Erminia Francesca Romeo, Simona Faraci, and Maria Carmen Garganese

16.1 Study Technique and Interpretation

16.1.1 Meckel's Diverticulum Scintigraphy

Gastrointestinal (GI) bleeding in infants and children is a fairly common problem, and it could be related to several clinical pathology according to patient age; however, it is usually limited in volume allowing time for diagnosis and treatment. One of the most frequent causes of lower gastrointestinal bleeding in pediatrics is Meckel's diverticulum.

In patients with clinical suspicion of Meckel's diverticulum, technetium-99m (99m Tc) pertechnetate scanning is a simple investigative study that can identify ectopic gastric mucosa, responsible for intestinal bleeding in acute or subacute phase. Previous administration of H2 blockers (30 min before tracer administration) improves the sensibility and the accuracy of this test. The administered activity of radiotracer is adjusted to the patient's weight (3.7 MBq/kg of 99mTc pertechnetate), with a minimum suggested activity of 7.4 MBq. Main preparation required for this test is a fasting of 4 h; a frequent bladder voiding is preferable when child is toilet trained. Scintigraphy must be performed few days after radiological examination to ensure the absence of barium in the abdomen; thus, residual contrast in bowel from previous barium studies may hinder scintigraphic detection of ectopic gastric mucosa with false-negative results. Scintigraphy is acquired using seriated images of the abdomen and pelvis (at 5′, 15′, 30′, 45′, and 60′ after the intravenous administration of Tc99m-pertechnetate) in anterior view, with the child in supine position. In case of uncooperative children, it is also helpful turning the child in prone position, setting the head of gamma camera rotated below the patient. Lateral image should be performed as soon as a suspicious focal uptake is detected avoiding subsequent overlap with physiological tracer progression. Delayed imaging (more than 1 h after administration of radiotracer) could be helpful to confirm doubtful abdominal uptake suggestive of Meckel's diverticulum.

Characteristic scintigraphic pattern of Meckel's diverticulum is a focal tracer uptake (generally within 30 min in the lower right quadrant) visualized at the same time and with the same intensity of gastric tracer concentration. In addition to normal pattern, the focal uptake may modify its position in relation to bowel loop movements, or tracer activity in the lesion may fluctuate in relation to wash out (secondary to intestinal secretions or hemorrhage). Some cases could be challenging, and suspicious finding could be false-positive result.

16.1.2 Radiolabeled Red Blood Cell Scintigraphy

Nuclear imaging with technetium-labeled red blood cells can be used to detect bleeding at a rate as low as 0.1 mL per minute (in anatomical region with low background activity) or 0.4 mL per minute (in case of higher background activity).

In vivo or in vitro RBC labeling has a good binding stability, allowing to perform delayed imaging up to 24 h. For this reason, nuclear medicine imaging can detect obscure or intermittent intestinal bleeding; however, the patient must be actively bleeding at the time of investigation to provide useful information.

In children under 18 years old, the recommended administered activity is based on the EANM Pediatric Dosage Card

M. Pizzoferro • M.F. Villani
Nuclear Medicine Unit, Imaging Departement – "Bambino Gesù" Children's Hospital, Rome, Italy

T. Caldaro (✉) • V. Balassone • A.C.I. Contini • E.F. Romeo
S. Faraci
Digestive Surgery and Endoscopy Unit,
"Bambino Gesù" Children's Hospital, Rome, Italy
e-mail: tamara.caldaro@opbg.net

M.C. Garganese
Department of Diagnostic Imaging of Nuclear Medicine,
IRCCS Bambino Gesù Children's Hospital, Rome, Italy

© Springer International Publishing Switzerland 2017

M.C. Garganese, G.F.L. D'Errico (eds.), *Conventional Nuclear Medicine in Pediatrics*, DOI 10.1007/978-3-319-43181-9_16

(with a minimum administered activity of 80 MBq for a 3-kg patient and a maximum administered activity of 784 MBq for a 68-kg patient). Registration of radiolabeled red blood cell scintigraphy is performed by a dynamic acquisition, followed by time-sequential static images up to 24 h; in case of uncooperative infants, time-sequential static images can replace dynamic study. In case of sleeping or cooperative child, SPECT acquisition should be performed as soon as an abnormal finding is detected to localize bleeding position. Delayed SPECT imaging is useful to detect other bleeding sites discriminating from labeled red blood cell progression in the gut lumen.

99mTc-labeled RBC scintigraphy is useful to assist in the localization of the site of bleeding (revealing abnormal accumulation of labeled RBC) and to select the best time to perform angiography that is determinant to diagnosis confirmation and bleeding treatment by embolization.

16.2 Teaching Cases

Case 16.1 Meckel's Diverticulum Scintigraphy in Child with Rectal Bleeding: Negative Pattern

A 4-year-old boy, with constipation and rectal bleeding, came to visit, and no anal polyps or blood traces at the digital rectal exploration were found. Blood tests were negative for anemia. An abdominal scintigraphy for the research of ectopic gastric mucosa was required, and no abnormal tracer uptake was detected by scintigraphy. Therefore, a colonoscopy was required. Due to the resolution of the constipation, obtained with changes in the dietary habit, no new episodes of rectal bleeding were referred, and the patient is actually in health. The role of the abdominal scintigraphy in this case was to exclude Meckel's diverticulum, which is one of the most common reasons for rectal bleeding in children (Fig.16.1).

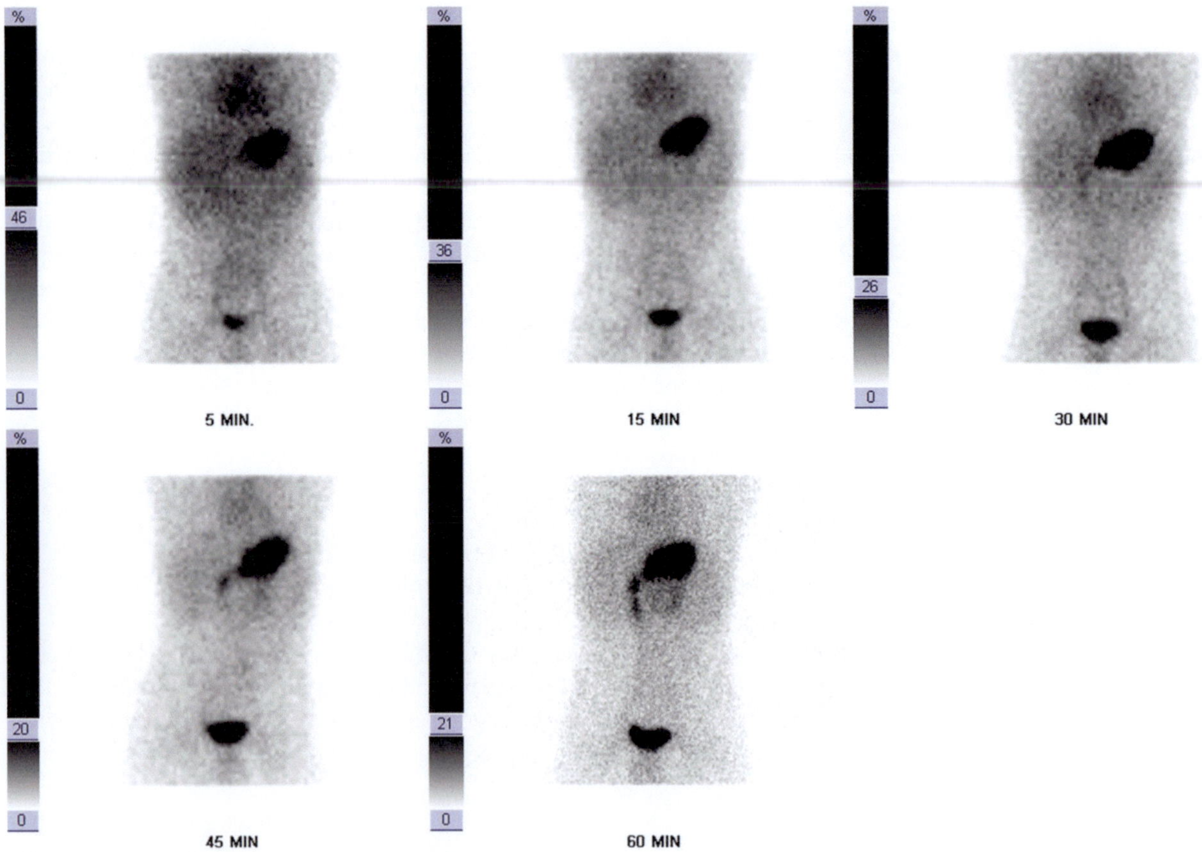

Fig. 16.1 Scintigraphy is performed using seriated images (at 5′, 15′, 30′, 45′, and 60′ after the intravenous administration of Tc99m pertechnetate) in anterior view, with the child in supine position. In case of uncooperative children, it is also helpful turning the child in prone position, setting the head of gamma camera rotated below the patient. In the first image is evident a physiological tracer distribution in the stomach, cardiac blood pool, liver, spleen, and bladder; urinary tracer excretion could also be seen in the renal pelvis and ureters. There is no ectopic site of focal tracer accumulation suspicious for Meckel's diverticulum. A normal rapid gastric uptake followed by a progressive increased and a physiological intestinal tracer progression appreciable during images acquisition is evident. In early phase, a slight and diffuse tracer uptake is detectable in lower abdomen, as for nonspecific intestinal inflammation

Case 16.2 A Scintigraphic Pattern Indicative of Meckel's Diverticulum in Child with Rectal Bleeding

A 15-month-old male child was admitted to our emergency department after several episodes of rectal bleeding and a moderate anemia. An abdominal scintigraphy with 99m Tc-pertechnetate was performed showing an oval area of pathological pooling of the marker at the level of the middle-right abdomen, and a Meckel's diverticulum was suspected. The patient underwent a laparoscopic-assisted resection of Meckel's diverticulum, and the histology confirmed the presence of ectopic gastric mucosa at the level of the bowel resection. The ^{99m}Tc pertechnetate abdominal scintigraphy confirmed also in this case its role in the diagnosis of Meckel's diverticulum (Fig. 16.2).

Case 16.3 A Scintigraphic Pattern Indicative of Meckel's Diverticulum After Intravenous Ranitidine Administration

An 8-year-old male child was referred to our unit after three episodes of melena. The esophagogastroduodenoscopy was negative, and the colonoscopy demonstrated a slight, nonspecific inflammation of the right colon. A previous standard ^{99m} Tc abdominal scintigraphy performed in another institution was negative for radiomarker pooling. Due to the persistence of episodes of melena, despite the administration of mesalamine, we decided to repeat the Tc-99m abdominal scintigraphy. To improve the sensitivity, intravenous ranitidine was previously administrated, and an abnormal oval pooling of the radiotracer in the right abdomen was demonstrated suspicious for Meckel's diverticulum. The patient underwent a minimally invasive laparotomic resection of the diverticulum, confirmed by the histopathology of the specimen. In this case, the previous administration of H2 inhibitors improved the sensitivity of the Tc99m scintigraphy and helped to confirm the clinical suspect of a Meckel's diverticulum (Fig. 16.3).

Case 16.4 Characteristic Scintigraphic Pattern of Meckel's Diverticulum with Progressive Increasing Focal Uptake

A 14-year-old boy was admitted to our emergency department for syncopal episode and 2 days long history of abdominal pain and black stool, suspected for melena. The patient was sick and pale; no history of prematurity and previous NSAIDs consumption. Blood tests showed worsening anemia that was treated with blood transfusion; abdominal ultrasound was normal. An upper gastrointestinal endoscopy excluded esophagitis, gastritis and duodenitis, and active bleeding. A 99mTc-pertechnetate scintigraphy detected a focal accumulation of radionuclide near the iliac bifurcation. In order to confirm the scintigraphic suspect of Meckel's diverticulum, a minimally invasive laparotomic approach was performed with resection of the diverticulum. The postoperative period and follow-up were without complications (Fig. 16.4).

Case 16.5 Scintigraphic Findings of Meckel's Diverticulum with Variable Positions of Focal Tracer Uptake

A 6-year-old male child was admitted in our hospital for a Kawasaki syndrome, without cardiac complications. During hospitalization, the patient presented blood and mucus into the stool, progressive anemia, absence of abdominal pain. The routine laboratory tests and the levels of fecal calprotectin and anti-*Saccharomyces cerevisiae* antibody (ASCA) were normal. A colonoscopy excluded active bleedings. A 99mTc pertechnetate scintigraphy documented a focal accumulation of the radionuclide near the terminal ileum. On the basis of the scintigraphic findings, a surgical exploration was performed showing a Meckel's diverticulum 30 cm above the ileocecal valve. Presence of ectopic gastric mucosa into the specimen was histologically confirmed. No complications occurred in the postoperative period and during the follow-up (Fig. 16.5).

Case 16.6 Diagnostic Imaging of Meckel's Diverticulum: Scintigraphic and Radiological Findings

An 11-year-old boy admitted in our pediatric emergency department after an onset of abdominal pain associated to diarrhea with blood and mucus into the stool. His past clinical history was characterized by recurrent abdominal pain and one episode of subacute proximal small bowel obstruction at the age of 5. During hospitalization, laboratory tests were normal, but the level of fecal calprotectin was increased. An upper gastrointestinal series showed a suspect of Meckel's diverticulum. To confirm the diagnosis and identify ectopic gastric mucosa, a 99mTc pertechnetate scintigraphy was performed. The scintigraphic pattern was characterized by a round focal accumulation of pertechnetate below iliac bifurcation. During a laparoscopic-assisted exploration, a Meckel's diverticulum with a thick inflammatory band linked to the appendix was found. Resection of the diverticulum and appendectomy were performed without complications (Fig. 16.6).

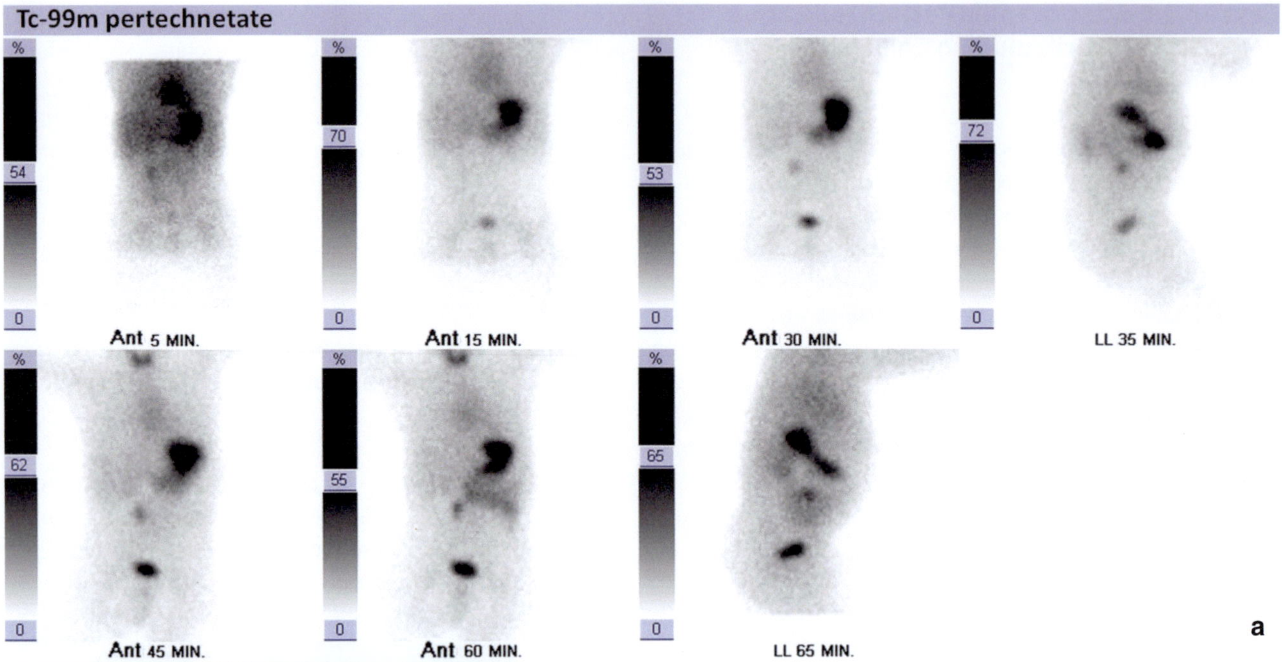

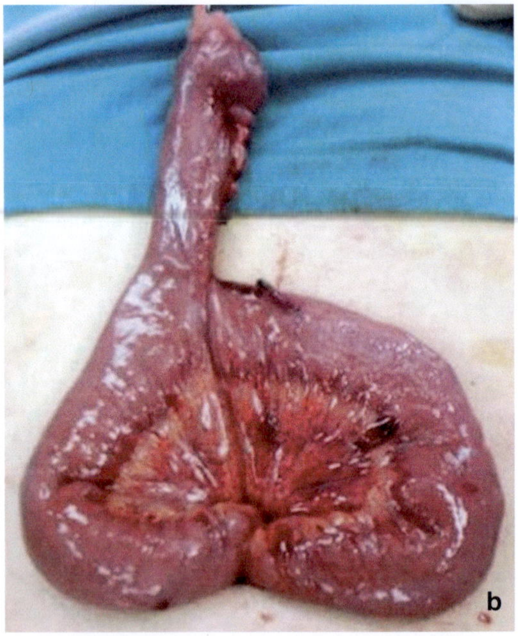

Fig. 16.2 (**a**) Scintigraphy is performed using seriated images (at 5′, 15′, 30′, 45′, and 60′ after the intravenous administration of Tc99m-pertechnetate). In the first image, an abnormal area of focal uptake can be seen in the middle-right abdomen that fades at 15 min but reveals a following tracer increasing concentration up to the last image. An early and transient uptake in right abdomen could be a false-positive result caused by urinary retention activity in the right kidney (sometimes in lower position than usual), but following increasing concentration and anterior localization in lateral view are indicative of scintigraphic pattern of Meckel's diverticulum. Lateral image should be performed as soon as a suspicious focal uptake is detected to avoid subsequent overlap with physiological tracer progression. (**b**) Intraoperative image of Meckel's diverticulum during laparoscopic-assisted resection. Histology confirmed the presence of ectopic gastric mucosa at the level of the surgical specimen

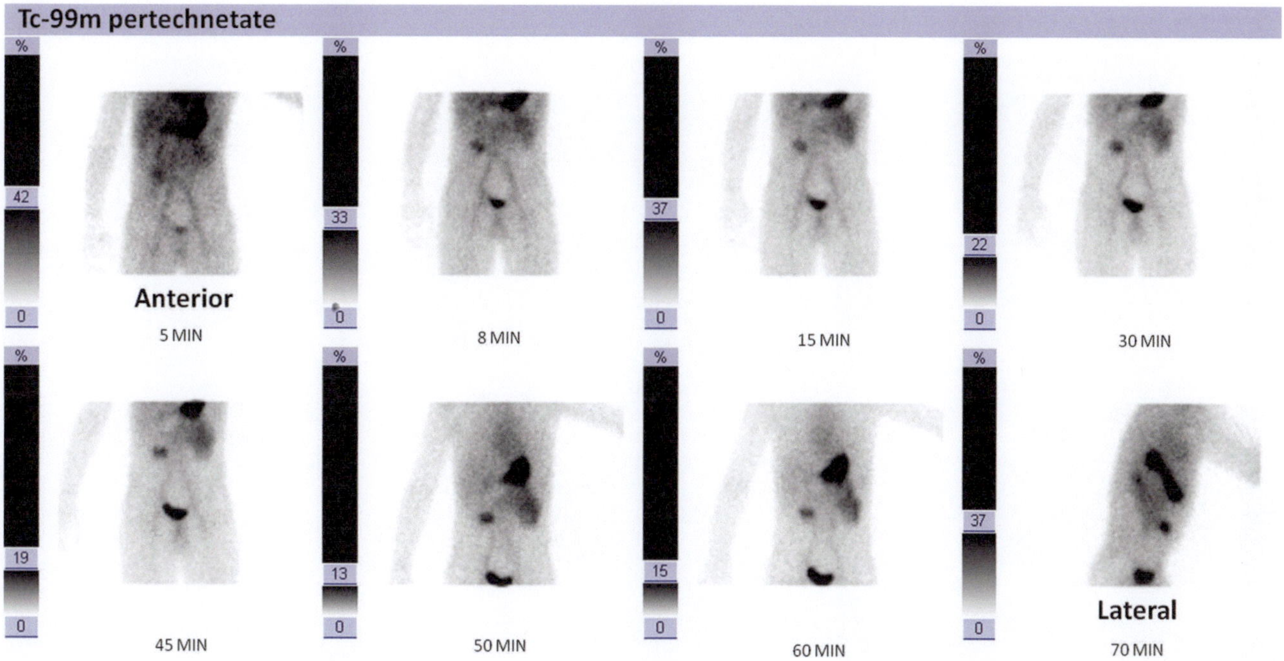

Fig. 16.3 Tc^{99m} pertechnetate abdominal scintigraphy is performed after previous intravenous ranitidine administration. Ranitidine premedication allows to inhibit acid secretion by parietal cells, thus limiting release of Tc^{99m} pertechnetate by the mucosal cells and improving the sensitivity of the Meckel scan. The study shows an intense focus of increased tracer uptake in the right upper abdominal quadrant, seen simultaneously to stomach visualization and persisting up to the last static acquisition. In the first image, physiological tracer uptake in the right renal pelvis is evident in the region above focal area of intense pertechnetate concentration. A lateral image confirms anterior localization of focal abnormal uptake within intestine. This finding is strongly suspicious for Meckel's diverticulum even if nonspecific inflammation of the right colon (especially when ulcerations are evident as detected by colonoscopy) could be the cause of false positive

Case 16.7 False-Positive Scintigraphic Findings due to Severe Ulcerative Bowel Inflammation

A 2-year-old male patient was admitted in our hospital after an episode of intestinal bleeding. Laboratory tests documented: Hb 13.2 g/dL, WBC 11330/mmc; negative stool cultures. An abdominal ultrasonography showed bowel distension with liquid into the intestinal loops; no lesions in liver, pancreas, and spleen. Due to persistence of hematochezia, a 99mTc pertechnetate scintigraphy was performed with a suspect of ectopic gastric mucosa. Whereupon, a surgical exploration excluded a Meckel's diverticulum. In order to complete the intestinal assessment, a colonoscopy showing severe ulcerative pancolitis was performed. At first, the child was treated with steroids and immunosuppressant drugs, but then a total colectomy was necessary because of the aggressive course of the disease (Fig.16.7).

Case 16.8 Normal Pattern of Tc99m Red Blood Cell Scintigraphy in Child with Sideropenic Anemia

A 3-year-old female patient was admitted in our hospital with diagnosis of sideropenic anemia (Hb 8 g/dl) during investigations performed for fatigue. Investigations performed to exclude malabsorption were negative, while blood traces in stools were positive for more than one sample. No evidence of intestinal lesions with bleeding was detected by upper endoscopy, colonoscopy, and wireless capsule endoscopy. 99mTc pertechnetate scintigraphy was performed without evidence of images attributable to Meckel's diverticulum. Tc99m red blood cell (RBC) study was performed to detect intestinal dripping or intermittent bleeding. Scintigraphic study showed a negative pattern. After martial therapy, she improved general conditions; no further blood tests were indicative of sideropenic anemia, and the patient is actually in health (Fig.16.8).

Case 16.9 ^{99m}Tc-Labeled RBC Scintigraphy in the Diagnostic Workup of Intestinal Bleeding

A 11-year-old girl who underwent surgery for duodenal duplication in the first year of life. The patient was admitted in our hospital for recurrent, obscure gastrointestinal bleeding with acute epigastric pain and anemia. In order to define the causes of bleeding, the following procedures were performed:

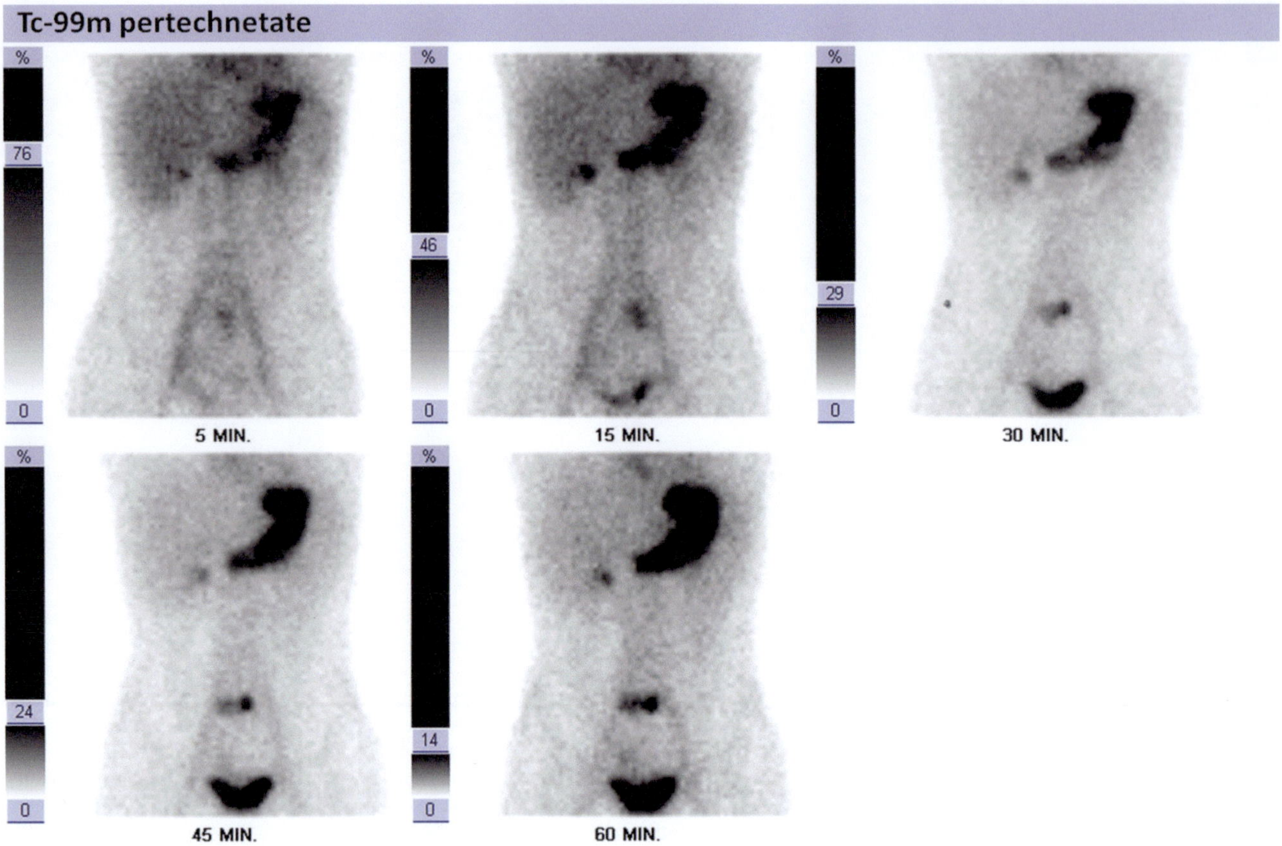

Fig. 16.4 ^{99m}Tc-pertechnetate abdominal scintigraphy reveals a minimal focus of mild abnormal tracer uptake corresponding to inferior lower quadrants (at 5 min) with progressive tracer increasing concentration, up to the last image. This scintigraphic pattern is characteristic of Meckel's diverticulum, confirmed by surgical and histological findings

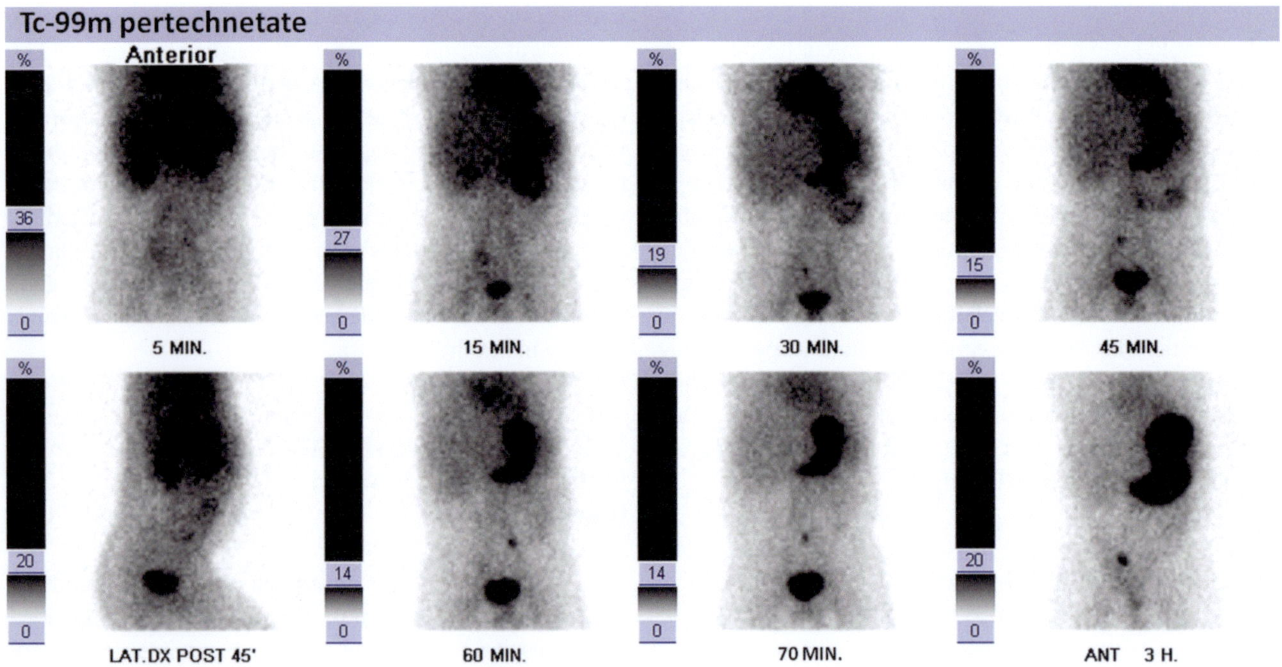

Fig. 16.5 ^{99m}Tc-pertechnetate abdominal scintigraphy reveals an abnormal focus of tracer uptake corresponding to lower quadrants. This finding changes position in relation to bowel loop movements showing partial wash out at 30 and 70 min, and increasing concentration on the following images. A prolonged imaging (delayed image at 3 h) with empty bladder is helpful to confirm focal abdominal uptake strongly suggestive of Meckel's diverticulum. Surgical resection of Meckel's diverticulum is performed confirming the presence of ectopic gastric mucosa in the resected intestinal segment. However, a similar scintigraphic pattern could be due to gastrointestinal bleeding nonrelated to Meckel's diverticulum or presence of severe bowel inflammation

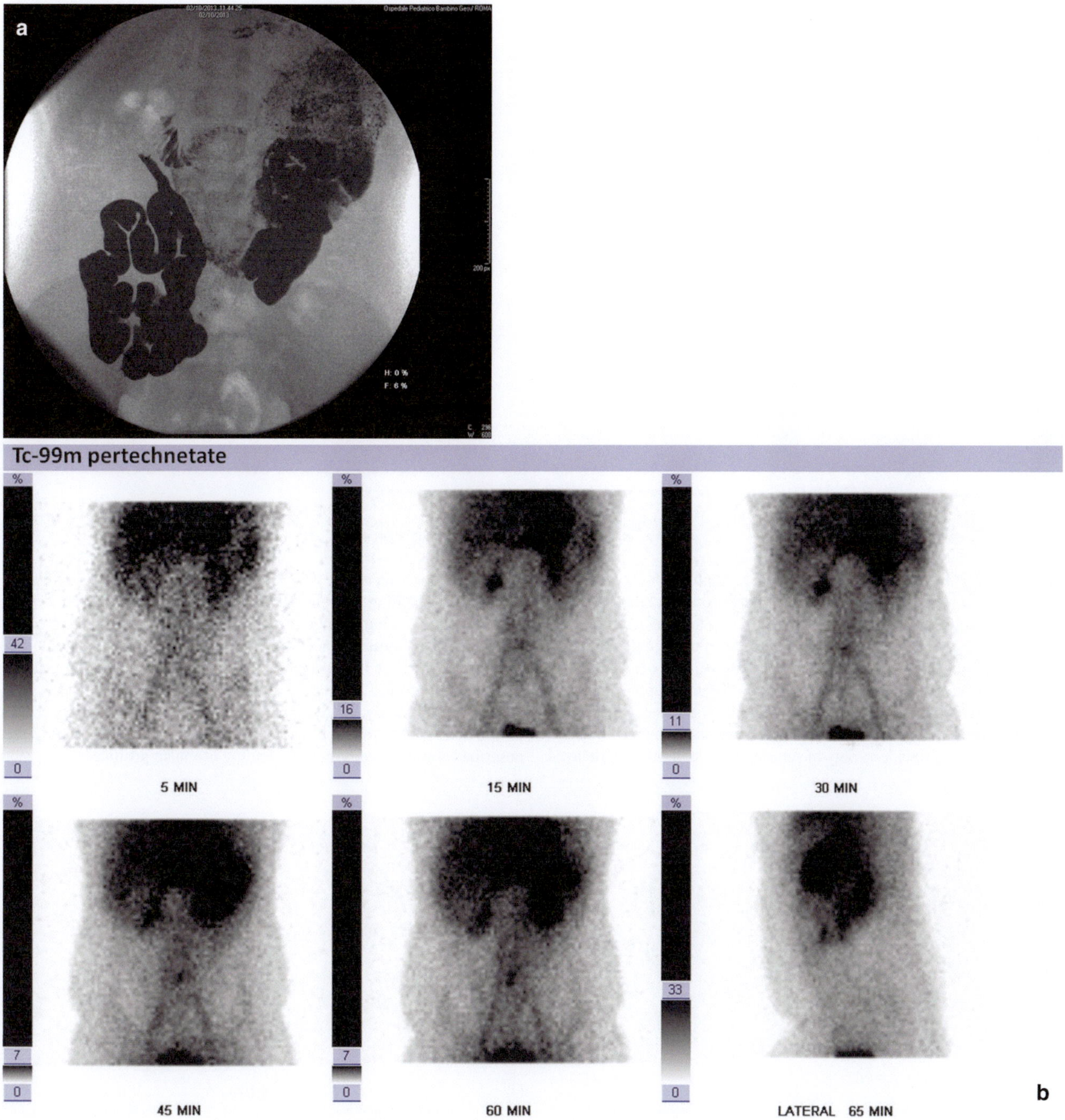

Fig. 16.6 (**a**) Upper GI series documented an image at the level of distal ileum that strongly suggested a Meckel's diverticulum. (**b**) Tc^{99m}pertechnetate abdominal scintigraphy is performed few days after radiological examination to ensure the absence of barium in the abdomen. Residual contrast in bowel from previous barium studies may hinder scintigraphic detection of ectopic gastric mucosa with false-negative results. In early phase, a slight and diffuse tracer uptake is evident in the abdomen corresponding to the lower side, as for nonspecific intestinal inflammation. Since image performed at 15 min, a focal area of tracer uptake is evident corresponding to lower quadrants, in median side, with following increasing concentration up to the last image. Approximately, 57 % of Meckel's diverticula contain ectopic gastric mucosa which actively secretes hydrochloric acid responsible for mucosal ulcerations within the diverticulum and unprotected wall of adjacent ileum (causing gastrointestinal bleeding). This scintigraphic result reveals uptake of radiopertechnetate by functioning ectopic gastric mucosa in the diverticulum, detected by radiological imaging; for such reason, it is important to perform scintigraphic evaluation in acute or subacute bleeding phase

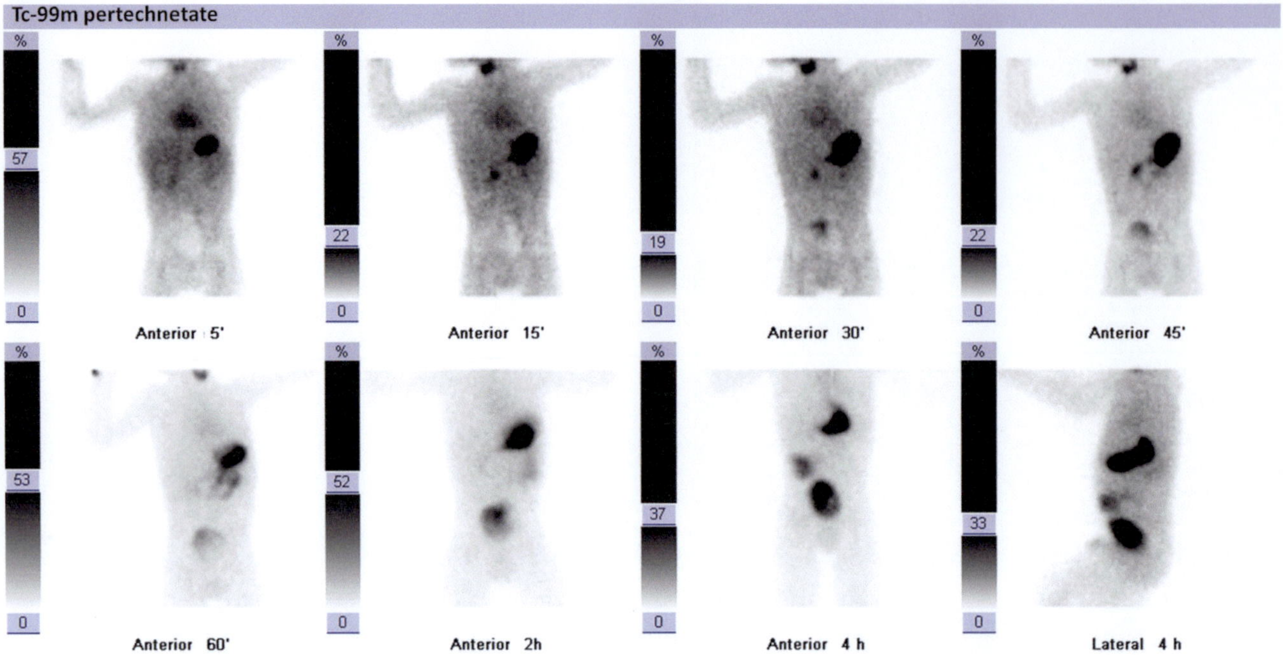

Fig. 16.7 ^{99m}Tc-pertechnetate abdominal scintigraphy reveals an abnormal focus of tracer uptake corresponding to lower right quadrant (nearby the bladder). This finding appears on static acquisition performed at 30 min, showing progressive wash out up to 2 h and subsequent increasing concentration on the following images at 4 h (in anterior and lateral views). This is not a typical scintigraphic pattern of Meckel's diverticulum, because focal uptake is not visualized simultaneously with the stomach, and progressive wash out is evident. However, there is a wide variety of scintigraphic patterns, and delayed focal uptake or evidence of tracer wash out (due to large focus of hyperfunctioning bleeding ectopic gastric mucosa) could be associated to Meckel's diverticulum. Otherwise, a similar scintigraphic pattern could be due to gastrointestinal bleeding nonrelated to Meckel's diverticulum or presence of severe inflammation that may cause nonspecific activity accumulation owing to hypervascularity, increased blood pool, and elevated permeability. Delayed images are usually helpful in discriminating equivocal findings, but some cases are challenging because the described abnormal scintigraphic finding is a false-positive result

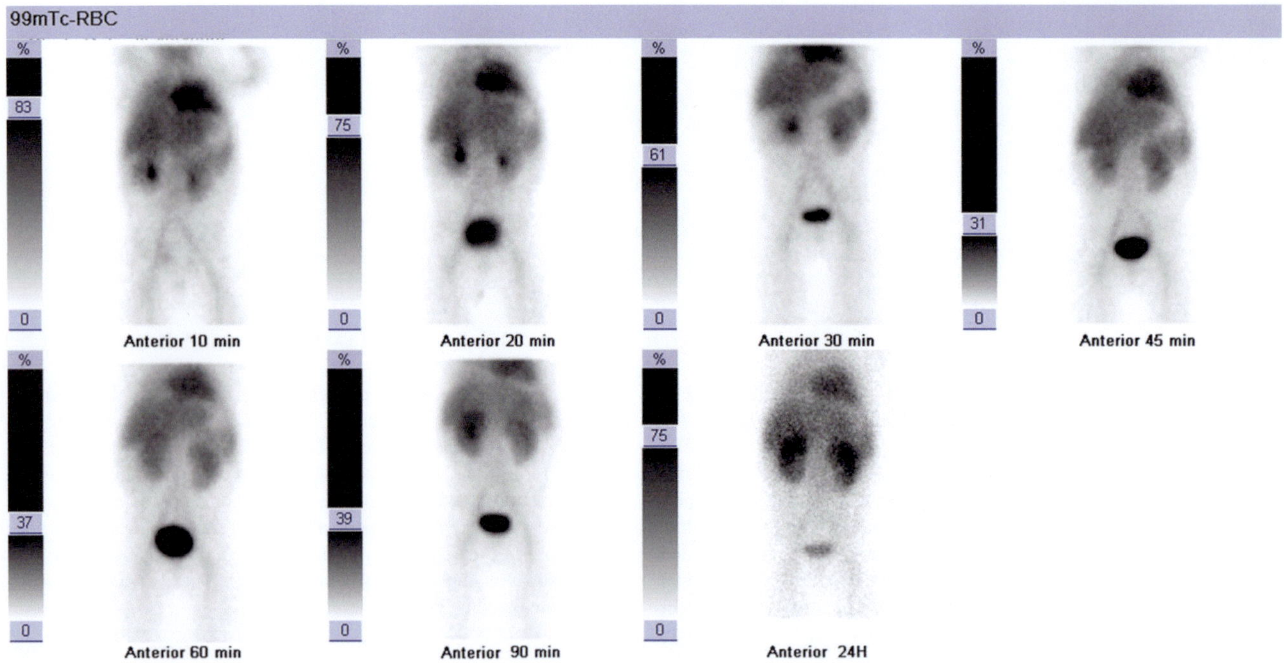

Fig. 16.8 Time-sequential static images are usually performed (as an alternative to dynamic study) in infants; delayed image up to 24 h is suggested. Red blood cells are labeled with Tc^{99m} using an in vivo method by a previous treatment with stannous ion via intravenous administration (cold pyrophosphate kit). This is a normal study with no evidence of any active gastrointestinal bleeding. Images reveal physiological visualization of blood pool compartment (heart, aorta, and iliac arteries), abdominal parenchymal organs (liver, spleen, and kidneys), and urinary excretion activity. No abnormal uptake of radiolabeled RBC is evident in abdomen, outside vascular compartment

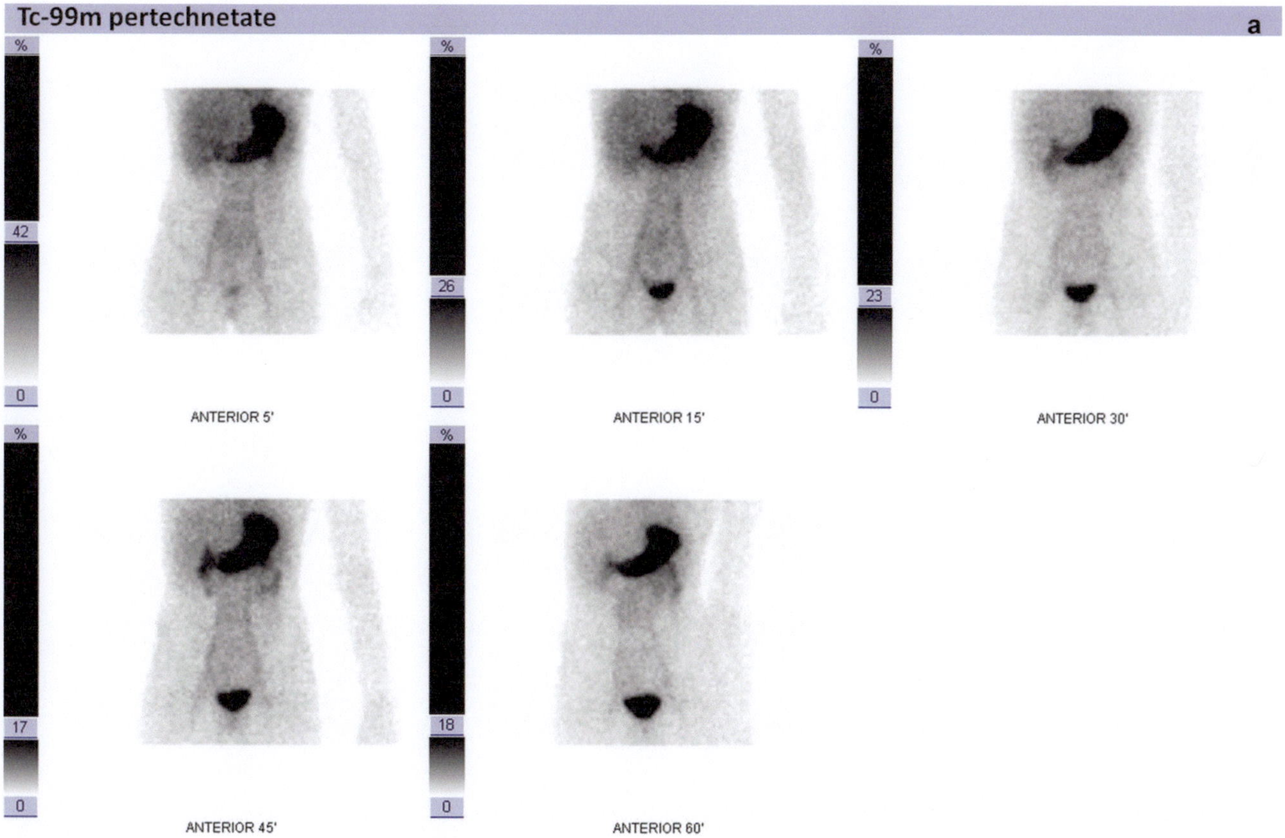

Fig. 16.9 (**a**) Tc^{99m} pertechnetate abdominal scintigraphy reveals no abnormality (**b–c**) ^{99m}Tc-labeled RBC scintigraphy is performed using an in vivo labeling method (by a previous treatment with stannous ion administration). In the figures are reported dynamic acquisition (duration of 5 min) and following time-sequential static images up to 24 h. A diffuse and inconstant area of mildly increased activity is evident in the lower abdominal region (above bladder), since 60 min of registration. This finding appears more intense at 2 and 6 h, as for intestinal bleeding; delayed image performed at 24 h confirms labeled RBC uptake associated with activity progression. ^{99m}Tc-labeled RBC scintigraphy is positive for intestinal bleeding and is helpful in the management of a patient who is actively bleeding to detect the right time for furthermore invasive investigations

- Upper endoscopy, colonoscopy, and wireless capsule endoscopy: no signs of intestinal lesions with bleeding;
- 99mTc-pertechnetate scintigraphy: no evidence of images attributable to Meckel's diverticulum;
- 99mTc-labeled RBC scintigraphy (during episode of bleeding): radiolabeled RBC accumulation in distal ileum;
- *Percutaneous* selective arteriography of superior mesenteric artery: negative for vascular anomalies; abdominal angina similar to the one of the acute bleeding during procedure;
- Endoscopic retrograde cholangiopancreatography: detection of a pancreatic pseudocyst.

On the basis of the scintigraphic and endoscopic results, a surgical exploration was necessary to identify the source of bleeding. A bloody branch of the pancreatic-duodenal artery, which was directly in contact with the pancreatic pseudocyst, was detected during the operation. The repair of the blood vessel resolved the gastrointestinal bleeding. In conclusion, in cases of obscure intestinal bleeding, scanning radionuclide and angiography may help localize and/or identify the source of bleeding. Unfortunately, the patient must be actively bleeding at the time of investigation to provide useful information (Fig.16.9).

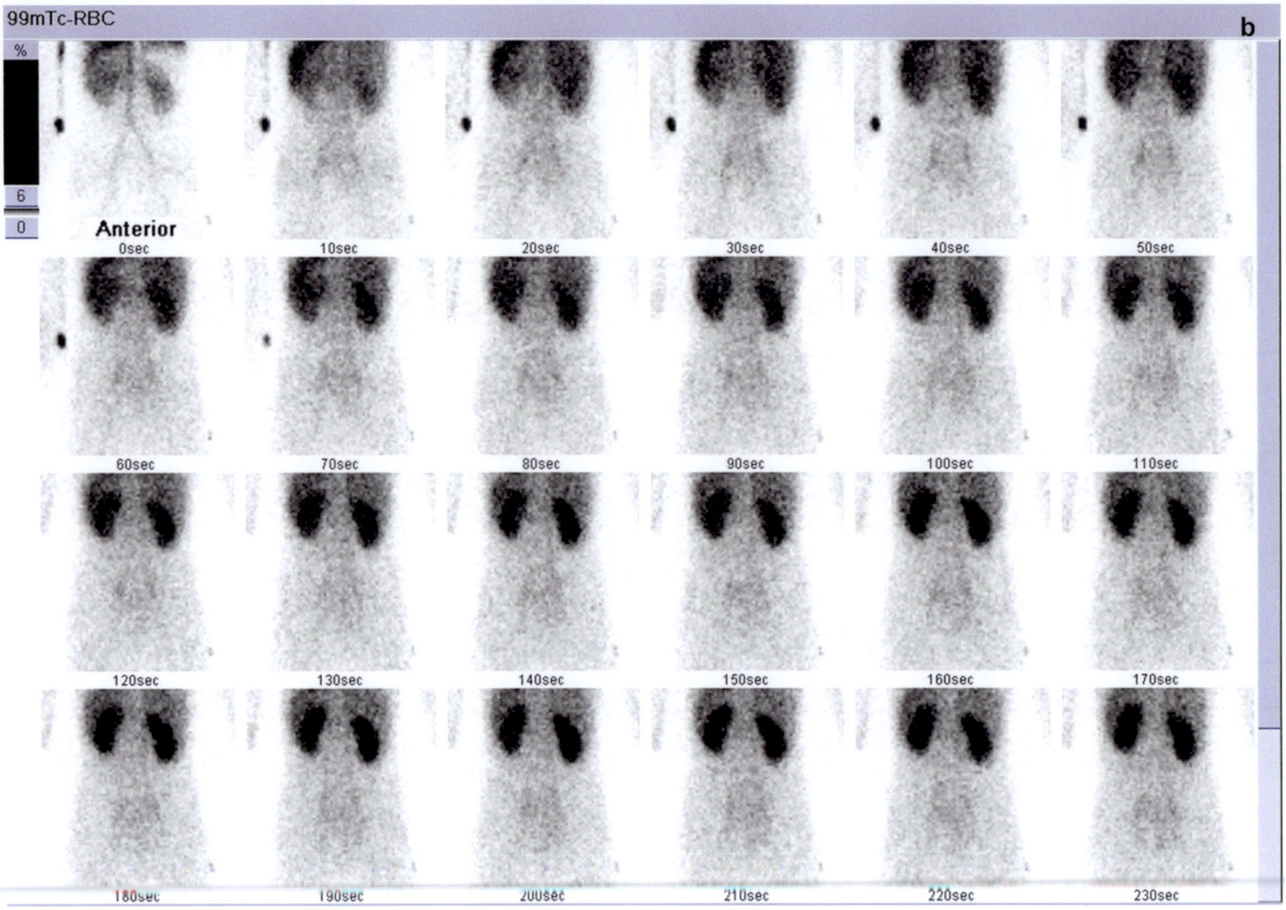

Fig. 16.9 (continued)

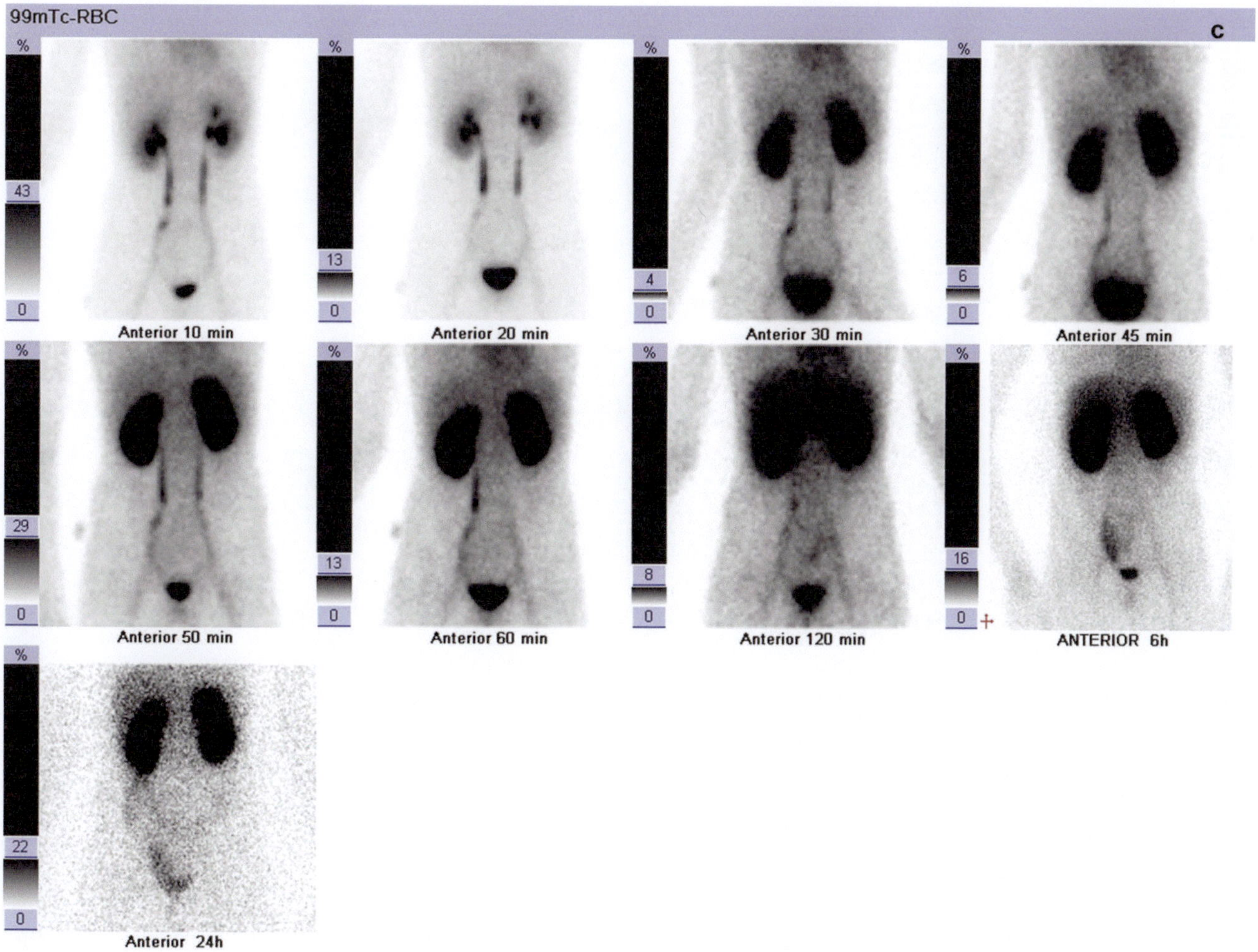

Fig. 16.9 (continued)

Case 16.10 ^{99m}Tc-Labeled RBC Scintigraphy in a Case of Chronic Idiopathic Intestinal Pseudo-Obstruction (POIC) with Intestinal Muscle Involvement

A 3-year-old female patient, preterm delivery at 35 weeks of gestational age, diagnosis of chronic idiopathic intestinal pseudo-obstruction (POIC) with involvement of gastrointestinal and bladder muscle component. In this complex clinical phenotype, there is a substitution of normal smooth tissue with connective tissue. The child was affected by megacystis and adhesions of intestinal wall due to the impossibility of intestinal motor activity. The patient underwent gastrostomy and two ileostomies due to occlusive/subocclusive abdominal episodes. Clinical course was further characterized by recurrent sepsis, neurological damage, progressive renal failure, and hepatic cirrhosis, with secondary portal hypertension and diffuse intestinal varices. At the age of 2 years, the patient was admitted for hematochezia with severe anemia, requiring transfusion. Trans-stomal ileoscopy, upper and lower gastrointestinal endoscopy did not show any active bleeding lesion. The patient underwent 99mTc-RBC scintigraphy revealing abnormal accumulation of labeled RBC in the lower right quadrant of the abdomen, compatible with active bleeding from terminal ileum, and subsequent progressive peritoneal labeled RBC diffusion. Percutaneous selective arteriography of inferior mesenteric artery was performed confirming vascular lesion and had a curative efficacy by embolization. ^{99m}Tc-labeled RBC scintigraphy was useful to assist in the localization of the site of bleeding, helping to select the best time to perform angiography that was determinant to diagnosis confirmation and bleeding treatment (Fig.16.10).

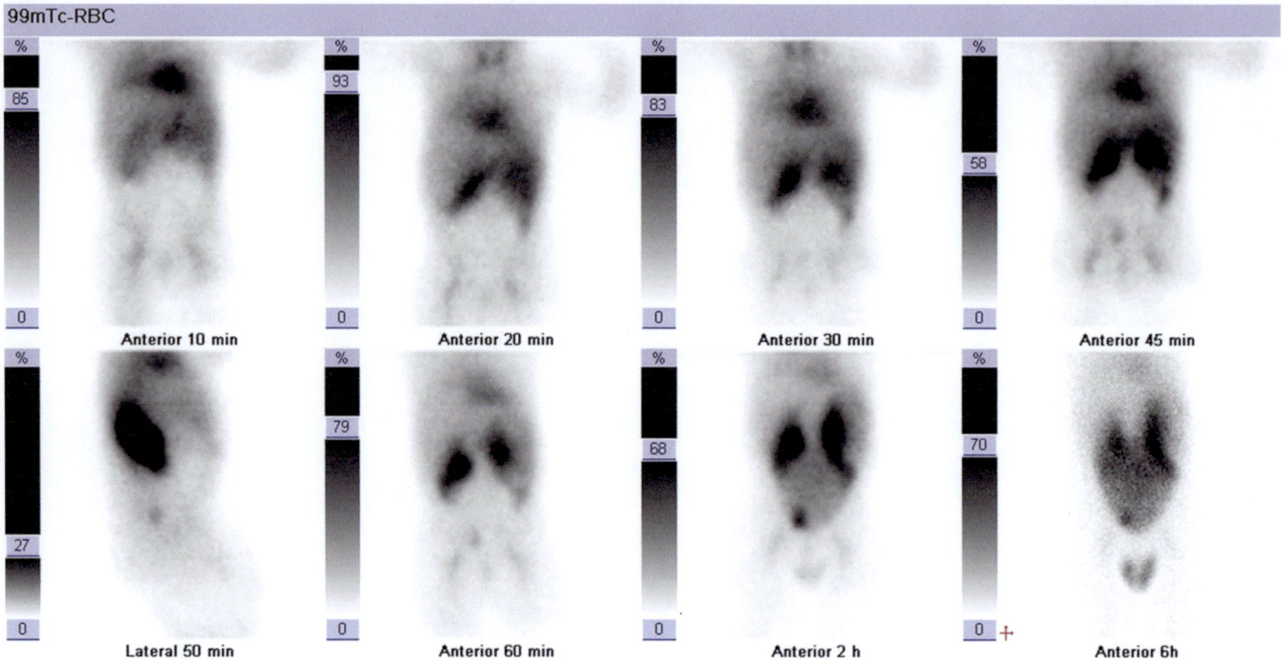

Fig. 16.10 ^{99m}Tc-labeled RBC scintigraphy is performed using an in vivo labeling method (by a previous treatment with stannous ion administration). In figure are displayed time-sequential static images up to 6 h. Since early images, a wide area devoid of tracer corresponding to abdomen region is evident (without visualization of aorta and iliac arteries), as for indirect sign of severe ascites. By evaluation of static images performed at 45, 50, and 60 min, a mild area of labeled RBC is evident in the lower right quadrant. This finding appears more intense at 2 and 6 h, as for active bleeding from terminal ileum, associated with diffuse uptake in the abdominal region. Up to the last image, urinary activity is observed bilaterally, corresponding to dilated pelvis and ureters

Case 16.11 ^{99m}Tc-Labeled RBC Scintigraphy in the Detection of Large Bowel Inflammation Associated with Flowing Ulcers

A 13-year-old boy with an iron-related chronic anemia resistant to therapy and a slight elevation of the C-reactive protein came to visit. Fecal occult blood test was positive, but no symptoms were referred except for a single episode of syncope. His familiar history was positive for celiac disease, but his tests were always negative.

An abdominal scintigraphy with TC-99m labeled blood cells showed an abnormal collection of labeled RBC at the right, transverse, and left colon, as a possible consequence of a large bowel inflammation associated with intestinal dripping episode. The patient underwent an esophagogastroduodenoscopy and a colonoscopy. Colonic mucosa was markedly inflamed, and flowing ulcers were present, especially at the level of right colon, ileocecal valve, and distal ileus. The histopathology was strongly suggestive for a Crohn's disease, and the administration of mesalamine, elementary diet, budesonide, and iron supply was started.

Due to the persistence of anemia and inflammation, in July 2013, an immunosuppressive therapy was undertaken. The therapy was promptly reduced as a consequence of a lymphopenia.

The patient is actually in good condition, and a satisfactory control of the inflammatory bowel disease was demonstrated during the last clinical and endoscopic follow up.

In this clinical case, the scintigraphy was helpful to suppose the inflammatory bowel disease diagnosis, which was subsequently confirmed by endoscopy (Fig.16.11).

Case 16.12 ^{99m}Tc-Labeled RBC Scintigraphy in a Case of Intestinal GVHD

A 23-year-old female patient affected by a chronic T-lymphoproliferative disease (CD4+CD3+) diagnosed when she was 19, and she underwent an allogenic bone marrow transplantation with hematopoietic stem cells from a compatible unfamiliar HLA donor. The treatment was complicated by an early intestinal GVHD, treated with a number of immunosuppressive therapy lines according to the endoscopic biopsies. She was admitted in our hospital due to a worsening of bowel symptoms; a daily blood transfusion regimen and pain control therapy were necessary.

Abdominal US showed fluid-particulate collection surrounding moderately thickened-wall bowel loops, especially in the left and sigmoid colon.

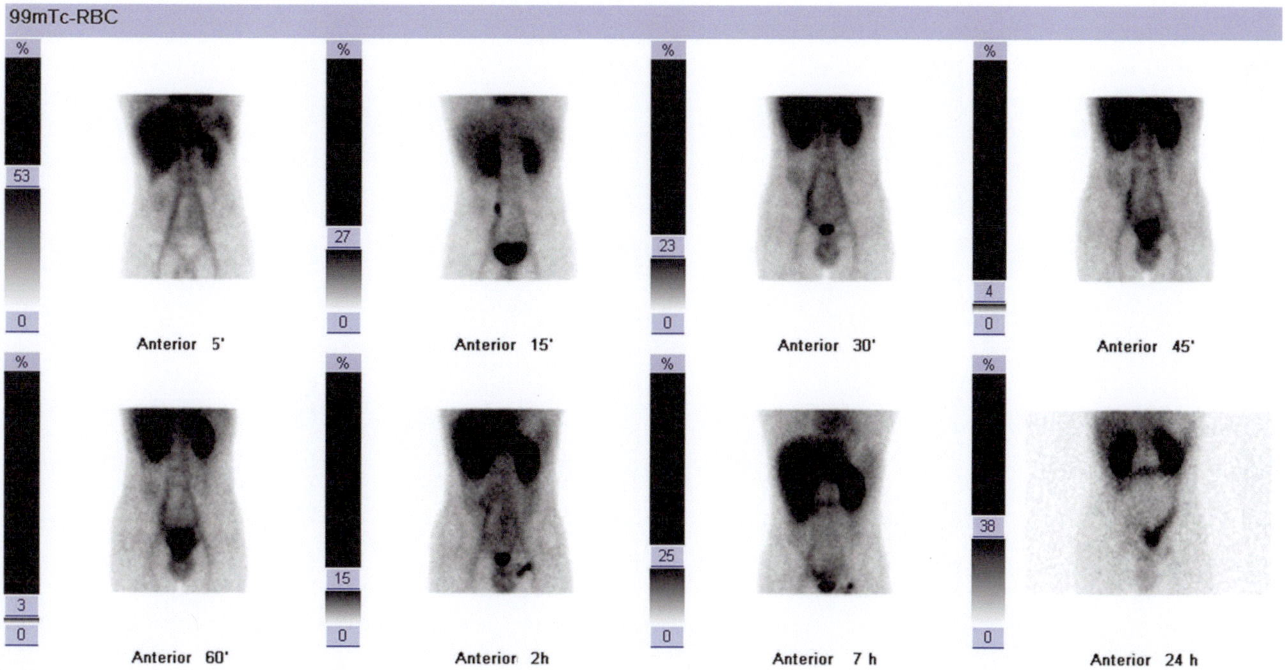

Fig. 16.11 ^{99m}Tc-labeled RBC scintigraphy is performed using an in vivo labeling method (by a previous treatment with stannous ion administration) by time-sequential static images up to 24 h. An abnormal area of labeled RBC uptake is evident in the right abdominal region persisting up to the static image performed at 2 h. In the delayed images performed at 7 and 24 h, abnormal activity corresponding to transverse and descending colon is also evident. These findings are considered suggestive of extended bowel inflammation with dripping or intermittent bleeding

An abdominal scintigraphy with TC-99m labeled blood cells was compatible with an impaired widespread intestinal permeability with an intestinal bleeding at the level of the distal jejunum.

An endoscopic evaluation was repeated and multiple biopsies were taken (stomach, ileum, duodenum, colon, rectum). An intestinal GVHD, especially at the level of the ileus, once again was confirmed (Fig.16.12).

Case 16.13 ^{99m}Tc-Labeled RBC Scintigraphy in the Detection of Intermittent Bleeding

An 11-year-old male child with a diagnosis of hyperphenylalaninemia by newborn screening and confirmed by molecular analysis was visited. A normal diet for his age with a controlled protein intake and a previous history of renal calculi was referred. Due to necrotizing enterocolitis, a bowel resection was performed, resulting in a 27 cm remaining bowel. As a consequence of a positive fecal occult blood test, an intestinal decontamination was prescribed. Subsequently, a symptomatic severe anemia was diagnosed, and a transfusion of red blood cells was necessary. An emergency upper endoscopy and colonoscopy in a poor bowel prep conditions were performed, and no digestive bleeding was demonstrated. Due to the persistence of anemia, a scintigraphy was performed showing an abnormal uptake of labeled red blood cells in the lower left abdominal quadrant. Thanks to the postprocessing and the fusion with CT scan images, it was possible to suppose a left colon intermittent bleeding.

A colonoscopy after adequate bowel prep showed a large ulceration with a spontaneous bleeding at the level of the previous surgical anastomosis. An anti-inflammatory, decontaminating, and iron-supply therapy was established.

Despite the stabilization of hemoglobin at the subsequent blood tests, the iron-deficit and positive fecal obscure blood test was persistent. Abdominal ultrasounds were normal.

A colonoscopy was repeated, and a platelet gel was applied on the ulcerated anastomosis.

The patient is still under medical treatment for occasional episodes of iron deficit.

In this case, the scintigraphy confirmed a higher level of sensitivity compared to an emergency colonoscopy that is often performed under poor bowel preparation (Fig.16.13).

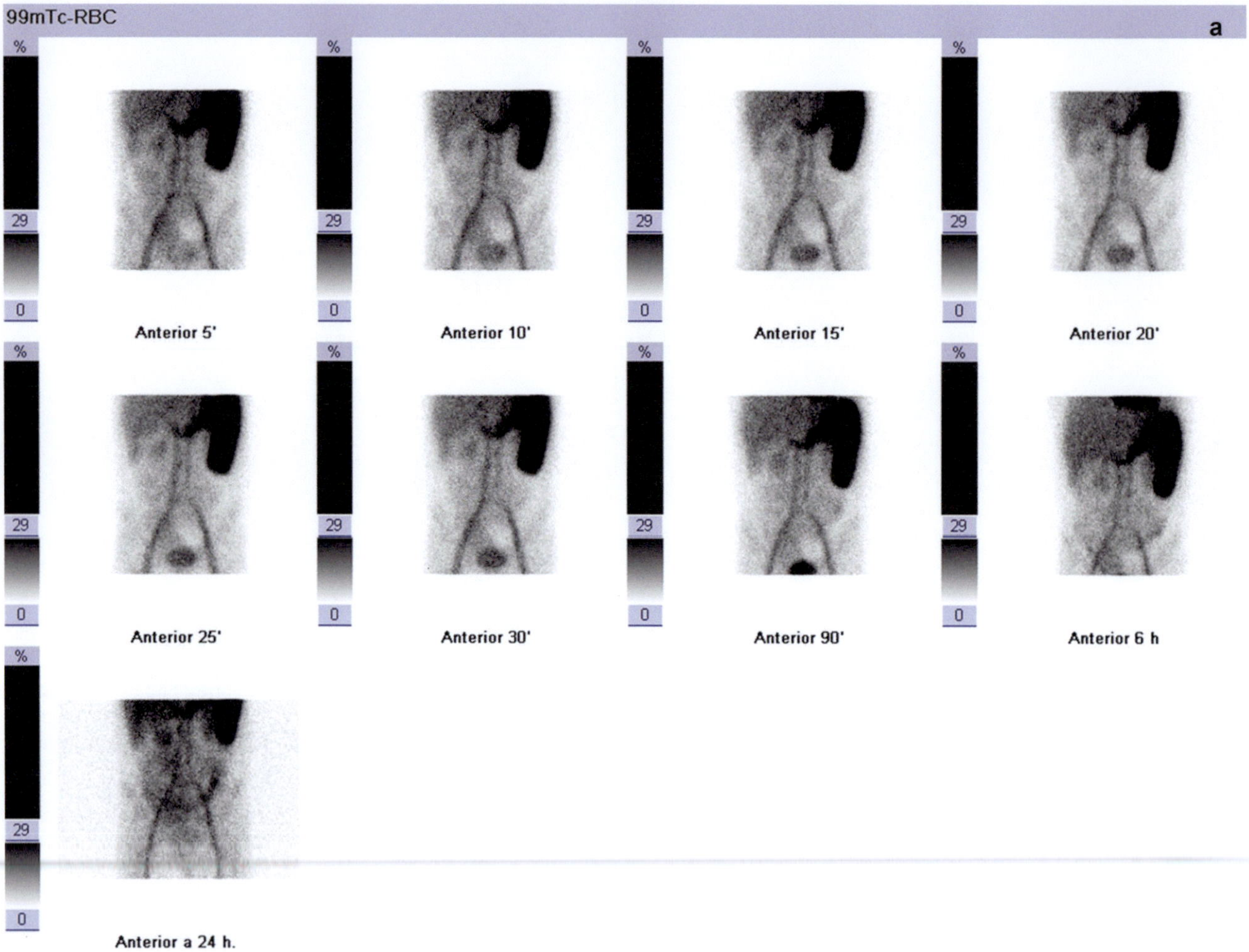

Fig. 16.12 (**a–c**) ^{99m}Tc-labeled RBC scintigraphy is performed (using an in vivo labeling method) by time-sequential abdominal static images up to 24 h (**a**); the study was completed with SPECT acquisition of abdominal region (**b**), and a postprocessing fusion of SPECT/CT images (**c**) was performed. Already in the early images and for the whole duration of the study, a diffuse signal activity of the intestine was observed, as a possible consequence of an altered permeability. In the static image performed at 90 min is evident an abnormal area of labeled RBC uptake in the left lower abdominal quadrant. This finding is more intense and extended on static image at 6 h when a SPECT acquisition is performed with postprocessing fusion of SPECT/CT images. Considering loop intestinal movements between two examinations, fusion processing is a critical point, but it could be helpful to assist in the localization of intestinal bleeding site. The labeled RBC area of uptake is localized at the level of the distal jejunum; in the delayed images performed at 24 h, intestinal activity is evident, as for labeled RBC progression. In all images, an intense and diffuse spleen uptake is visualized (probably due to labeled hemoglobin fragments)

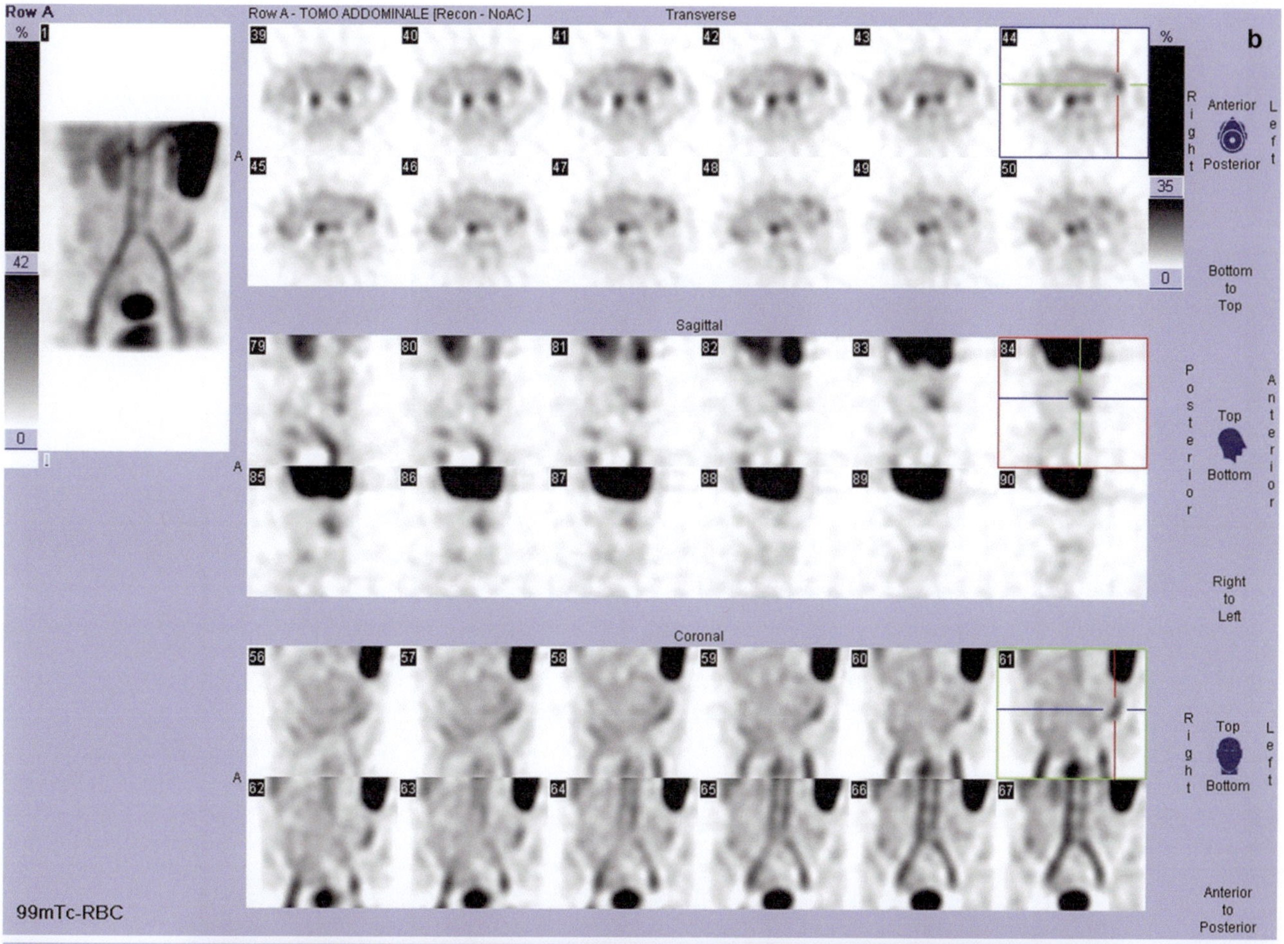

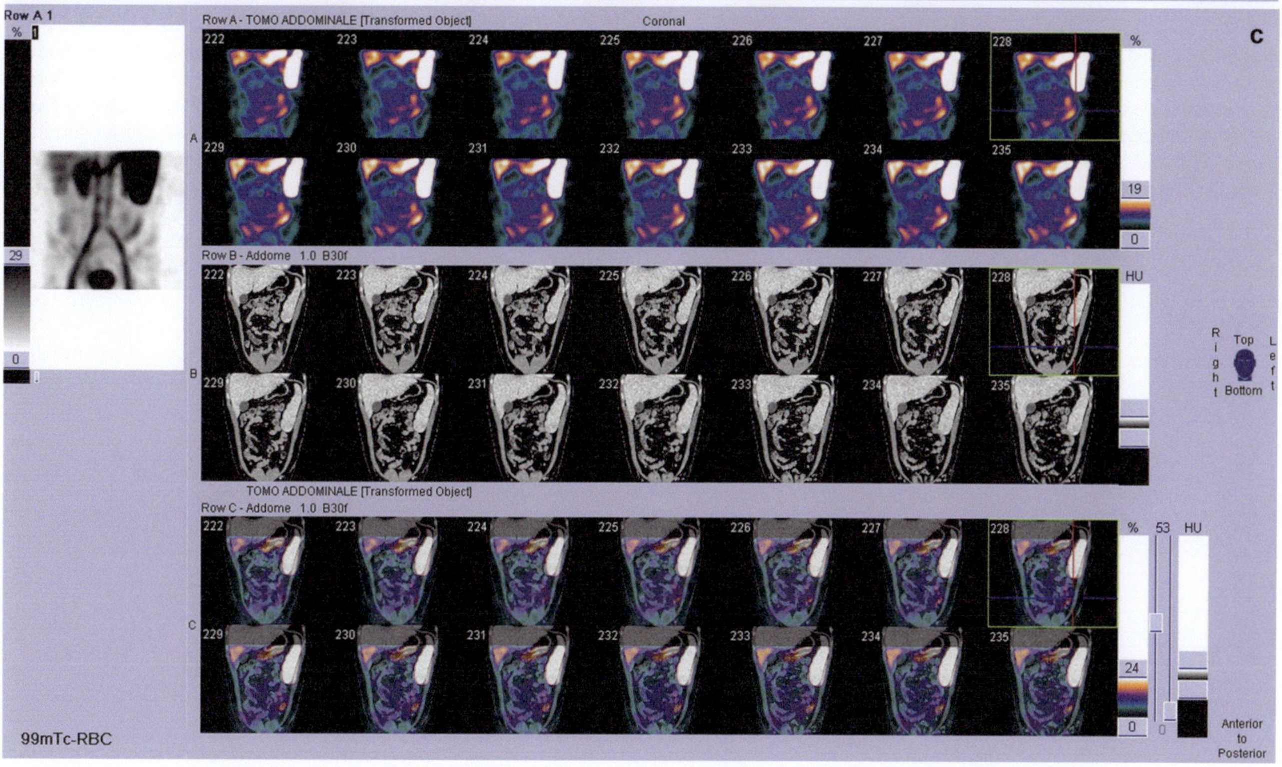

Fig. 16.12 (continued)

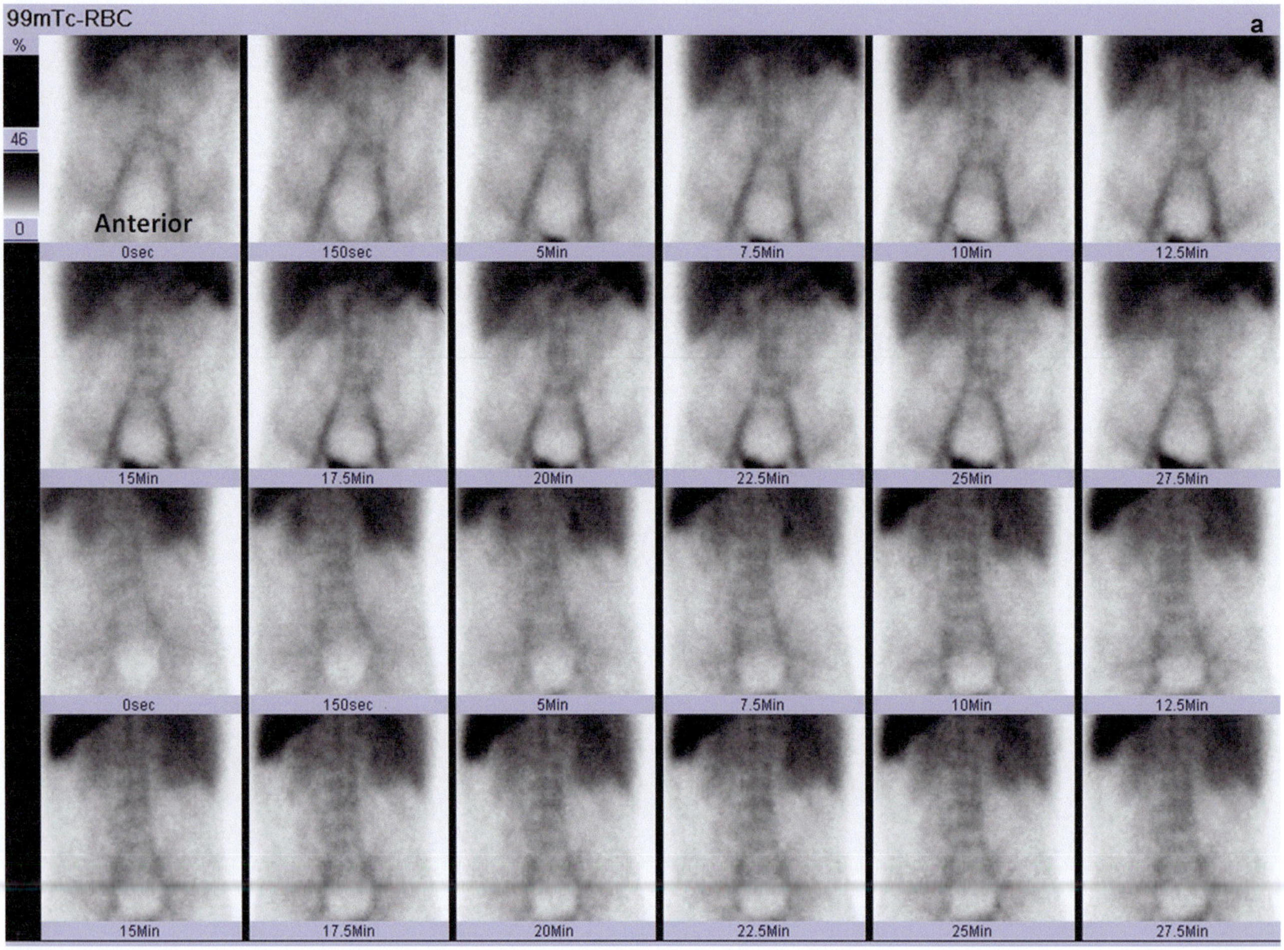

Fig. 16.13 (**a–d**) ^{99m}Tc-labeled RBC scintigraphy is performed (using an in vivo labeling method) by dynamic acquisition (**a**) and following time-sequential static images up to 24 h (**b**). A SPECT imaging (**c**) of the abdominal region at 4, 6, and 24 h after the "in vivo" labeling of red blood cells and a postprocessing fusion of SPECT/CT images (**d**). Since the first projections in the dynamic phase, an abnormal pooling of labeled red blood cells in the lower left abdominal quadrant is evident. In the following static images, a linear area of RBC uptake is observed (at 100 min, 4 h, and 6 h); by fusion imaging analysis, this finding is localized at the level of sigmoid bowel corresponding to the intestinal wall (without activity inside gut lumen). No evidence of increased RBC is detected at 24 h

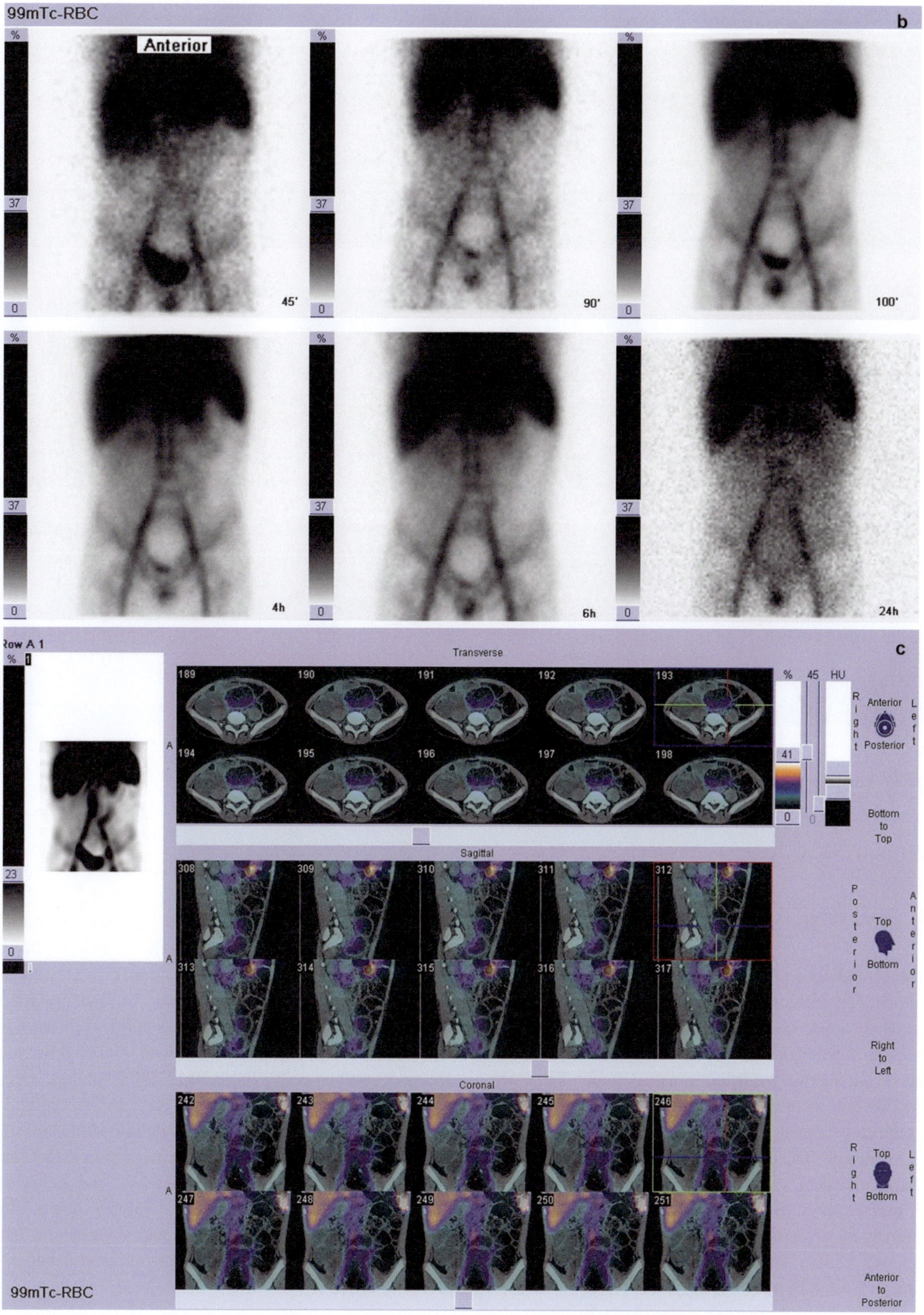

Fig. 16.13 (continued)

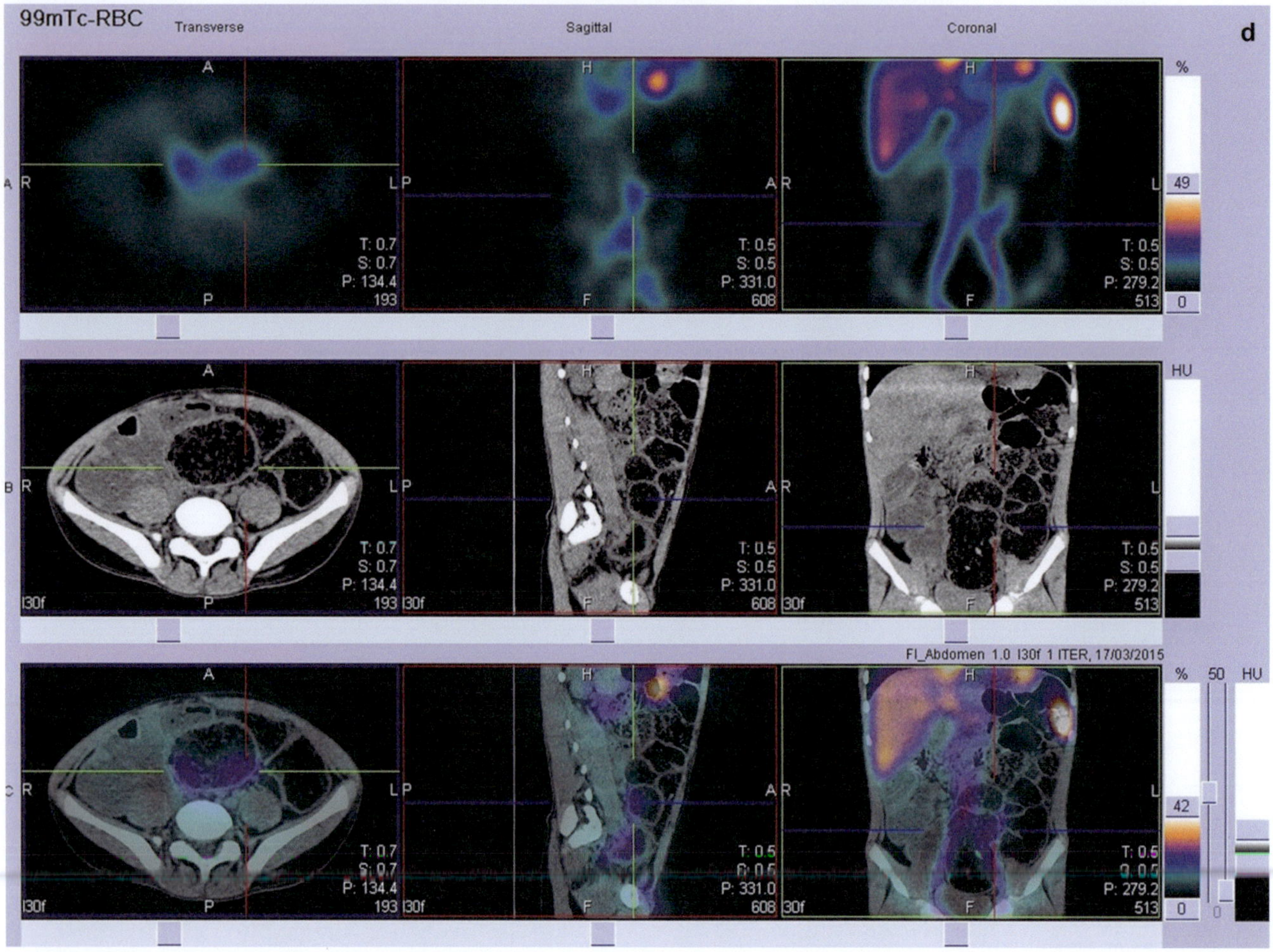

Fig. 16.13 (continued)

Case 16.14 ^{99m}Tc-Labeled RBC Scintigraphy

A 7-month-old male patient, preterm delivery at 32 weeks of gestational age, clinical features suggestive for plurimalformative syndrome/congenital infection (cardiac and cerebral anomalies, hepatosplenomegaly). At birth, the child presented severe anemia requiring transfusion and developed a necrotizing enterocolitis (NEC) stage III by the 15th day of life, requiring extended bowel resection, leading to short bowel syndrome. The residual intestinal segments (first jejunal loop, ileocecal valve, and colon) were anastomosed. Total parenteral nutrition was administered, and enteral nutrition by a gastrostomy tube was later introduced. Clinical course was further complicated by sepsis, cardiac arrest requiring resuscitation and anaphylaxis to cow's milk protein. After discharge, at the age of 7 months, the baby presented melena with severe anemia (Hb 7.1 g/dL). Abdominal ultrasound was unremarkable. First upper and lower gastrointestinal endoscopy was negative for actively bleeding lesions, but showed a suspected postsurgical kinking of the ileocecal valve. The patient underwent 99mTc-RBC scintigraphy accompanied by fused SPECT/CT images, revealing abnormal accumulation of labeled RBC in the middle/lower right quadrant of the abdomen, compatible with active bleeding from an intestinal loop. Laparoscopic-assisted enteroscopy confirmed ileocecal valve stenosis and ileitis of the prestenotic intestinal tract (mucosal damage due to chronic stasis). The stenosis was treated with hydrostatic balloon dilatation, and medical treatment was started with budesonide and antibiotics (Fig. 16.14).

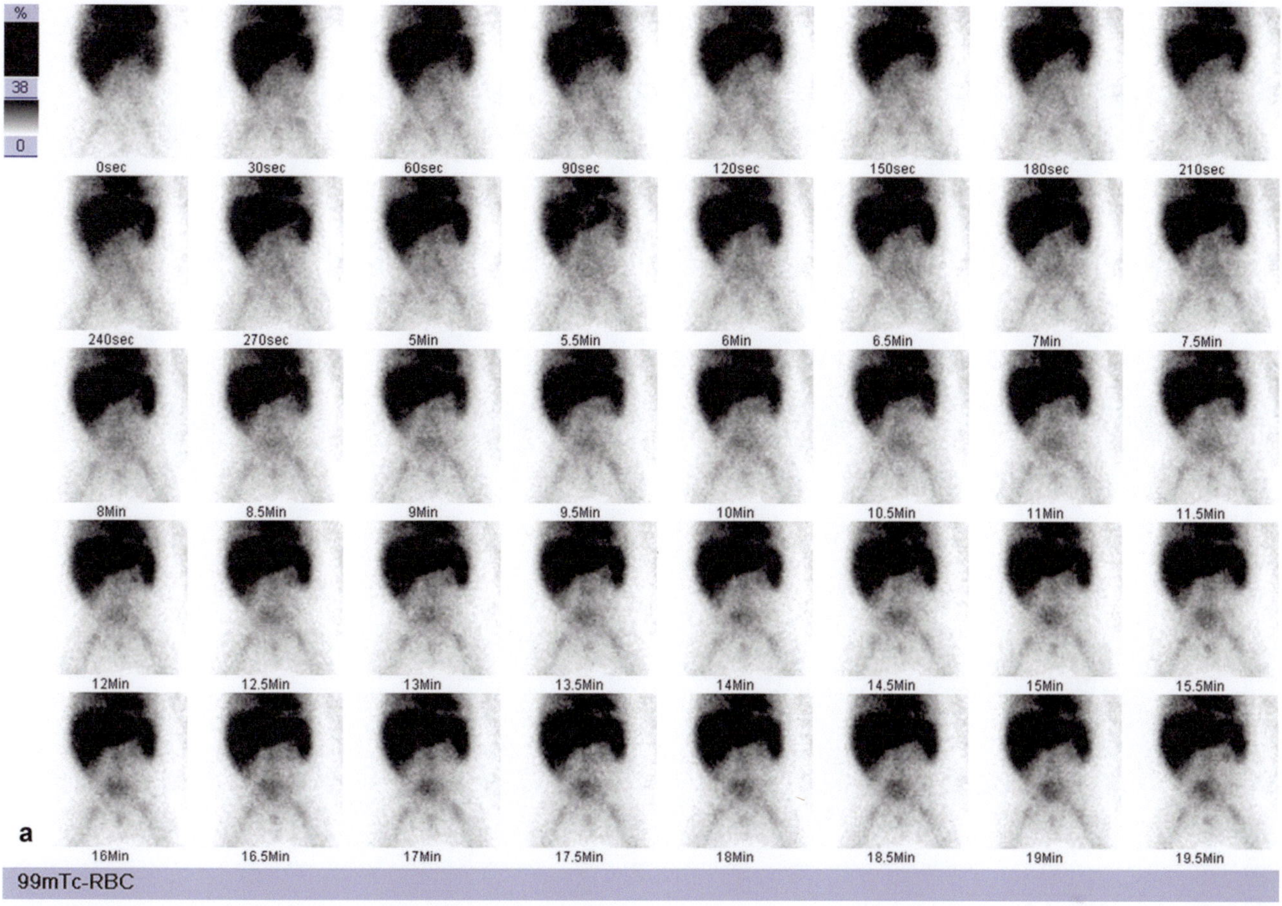

Fig. 16.14 (**a**–**e**) ^{99m}Tc-labeled RBC scintigraphy is performed (using an in vivo labeling method) by dynamic acquisition (**a**) and following time-sequential static images up to 24 h (**b**). A SPECT imaging (**c**) of the abdominal region at 4, 6, and 24 h after the "in vivo" labeling of red blood cells and a postprocessing fusion of SPECT/CT images (**d**). A doubtful abnormal accumulation of labeled RBC in the middle/lower right quadrant of the abdomen is evident on static image at 2 and 7 h, confirmed by SPECT images. By fusion imaging analysis, this finding is localized at the level of an intestinal loop and is considered indicative of active bleeding. As known, SPECT images improve diagnostic accuracy

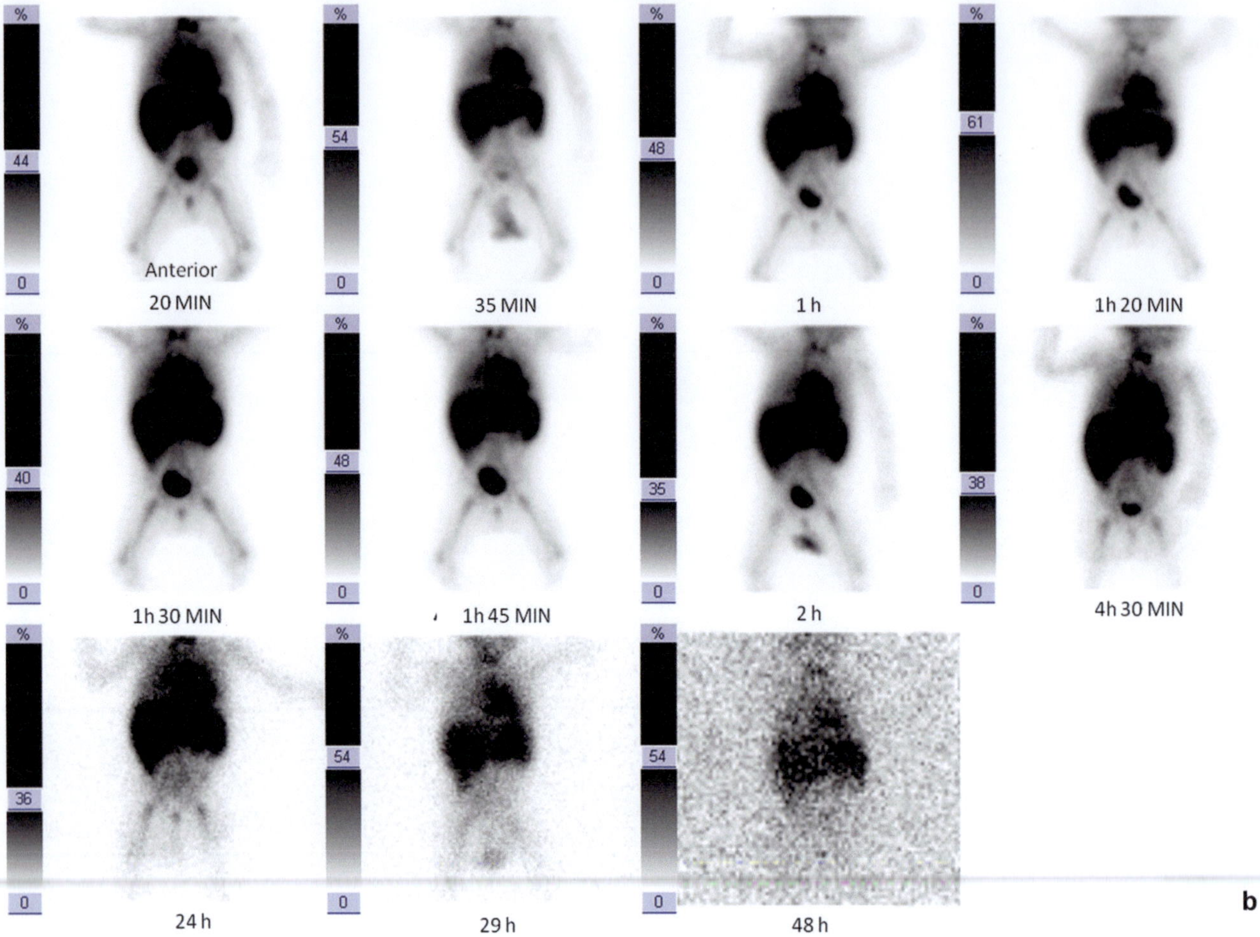

Fig. 16.14 (continued)

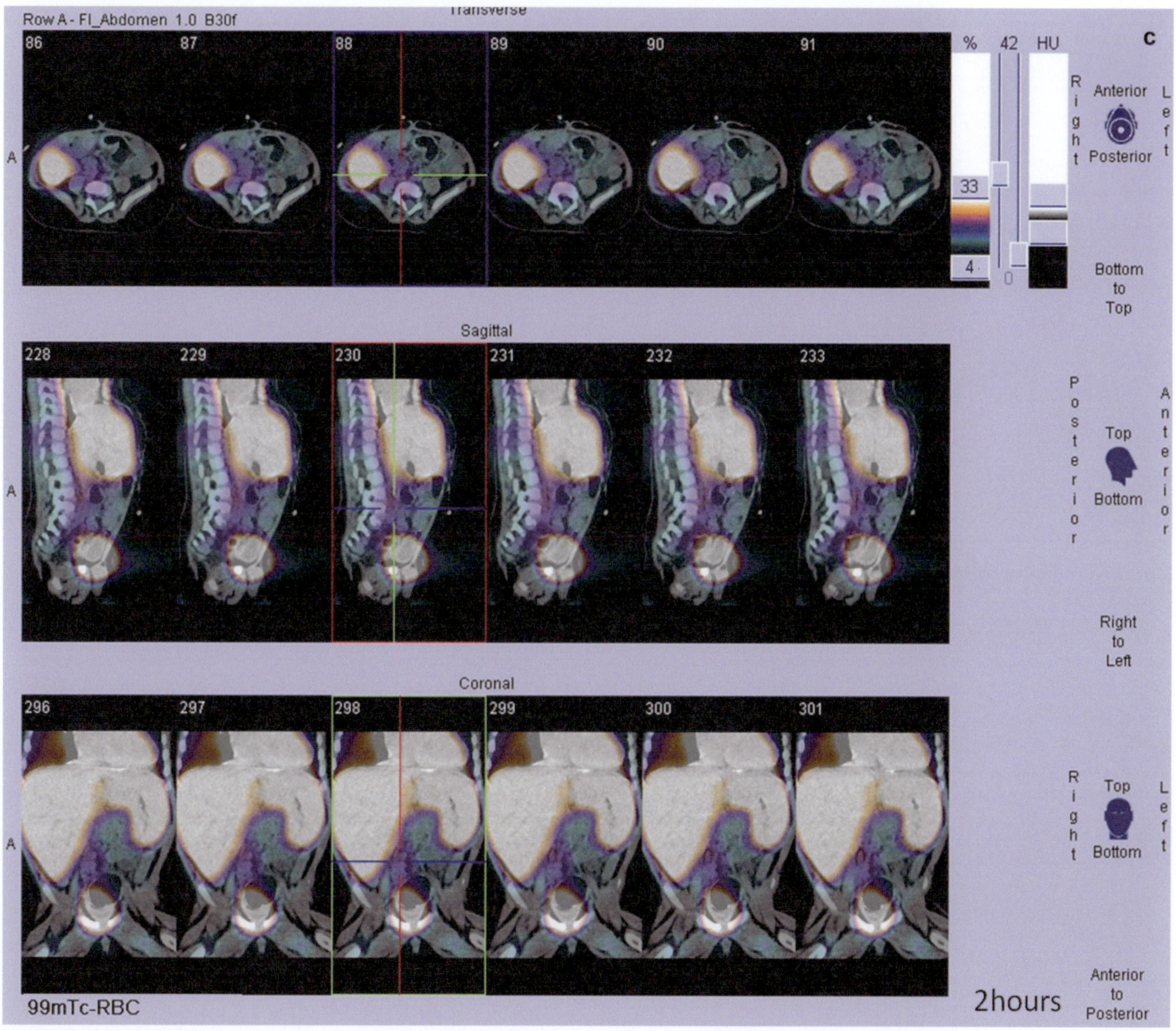

Fig. 16.14 (continued)

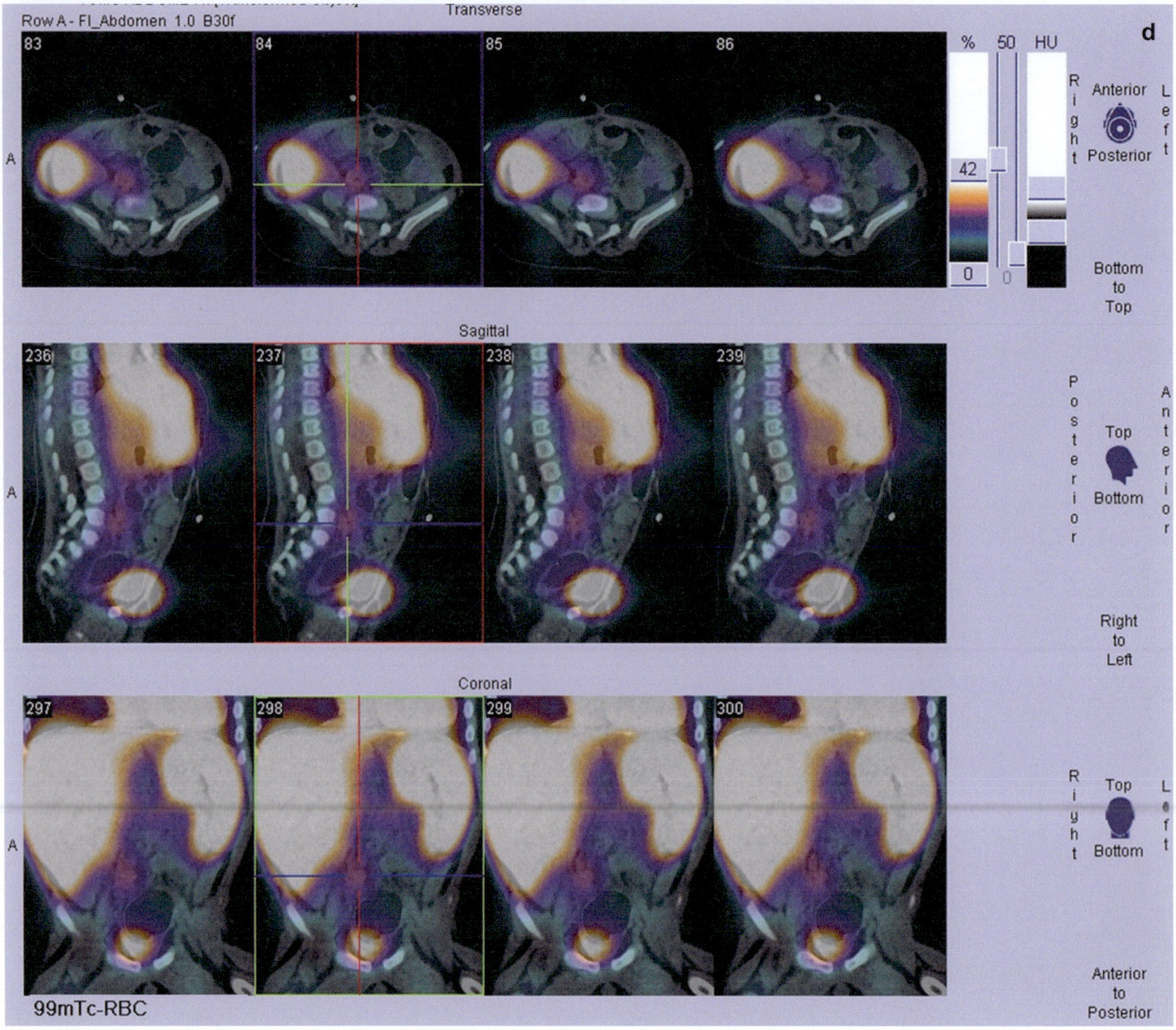

Fig. 16.14 (continued)

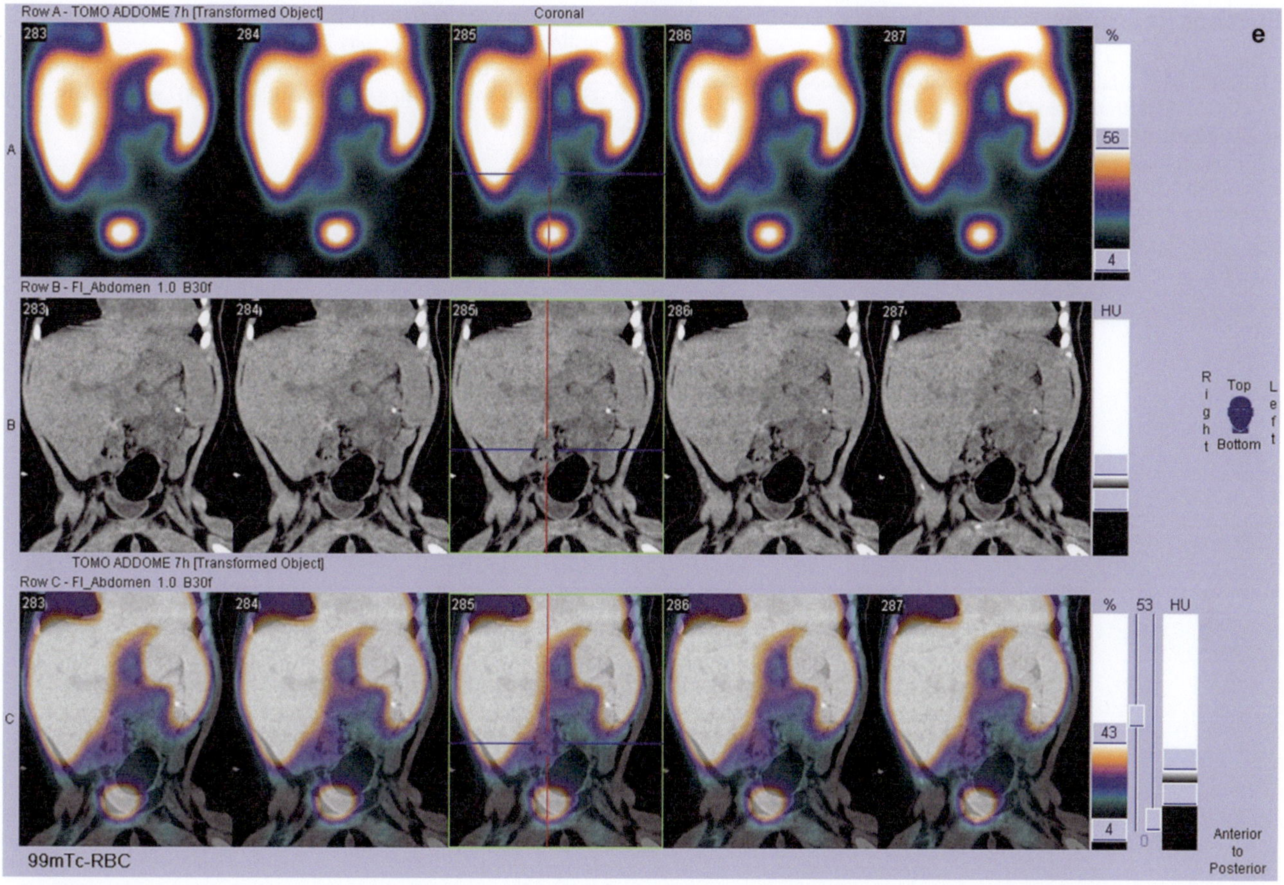

Fig. 16.14 (continued)

Further Readings

1. Fogelman I, Maisey MN, Clarke SEM. Chapter 9. "An Atlas of clinical nuclear medicine". 2nd ed. p. 685–92.
2. Garganese MC, Knafelz D. Chapter 24. "Manuale SIGENP di gastroenterologia ed epatologia pediatrica" (Il pensiero scientifico editore Ed 2014). p. 103–4.
3. SNMMI procedure standard/EANM practice guideline for gastrointestinal bleeding scintigraphy 2.0.
4. Treves ST, Grand RJ. Pediatric nuclear medicine. In Chapter 8. Gastrointestinal bleeding. 3rd ed. Springer; 2007. p. 192–208.

17 Gastroenterology: Bronchoaspiration: Neurological Child

Milena Pizzoferro, Maria Felicia Villani, Francesco De Peppo, and Maria Carmen Garganese

Recurrent pneumonia secondary to bronchial aspiration is typical of neurologically impaired children; both radionuclide salivagram and gastroesophageal reflux scintigraphy are commonly used in the detection of pulmonary aspiration. Radionuclide salivagram visualizes activity in trachea and bronchi secondary to salivary aspiration, while gastroesophageal scintigraphy detects labeled meal in respiratory airway. Furthermore, aspiration can occur by two routes (anterograde and retrograde), and each nuclear medicine imaging targeting different types of pulmonary aspiration should be required according to specific clinical suspicion. Sometimes, it could be helpful to perform both examinations, beginning by gastric emptying and performing salivagram in case of no evidence of aspiration during gastric emptying test. It is crucial to perform gastroesophageal scintigraphy administering an appropriate amount of labeled meal to reduce the risk of false-negative tests due to poor filling of the stomach.

In the following clinical cases, different nuclear medicine patterns of examinations performed in neurologically impaired children with recurrent chest infections are reported. In patients with clinical suspicion of pulmonary aspiration, an oximeter should be placed, and all that necessary for aspiration should be feasible in the diagnostic room. Nuclear medicine staff should annotate eventual episodes of cough or desaturation.

M. Pizzoferro • M.F. Villani
Nuclear Medicine Unit, Imaging Departement – "Bambino Gesù" Children Hospital, Rome, Italy

F. De Peppo (✉)
Unit of Pediatric Surgery, "Bambino Gesù" Children Hospital, Rome, Italy
e-mail: francesco.depeppo@opbg.net

M.C. Garganese
Diagnostic Imaging Department of Nuclear Medicine, IRCCS Bambino Gesù Paediatric Hospital, Rome, Italy

17.1 Study Technique and Interpretation

17.1.1 Detection of Aspiration During Gastric Emptying Scintigraphy

Study technique has been reported in Chap. 15. The study phase and aspiration magnitude should be considered in interpretation of gastroesophageal studies when related to evaluation of respiratory problems. In order to characterize pulmonary aspiration type, it is important to evaluate if respiratory airway visualization is evident early after oral meal intake or secondly after a reflux episode. Other useful information on the severity of pulmonary aspiration are achievable by nuclear medicine imaging evaluating the level of tracer (visualization of main bronchi (mono or bilateral) rather than entire bronchial tree (mono or bilateral)), amount of refluxate inhalation, and aspirated clearance capability.

17.1.2 Detection of Aspiration During Radionuclide Salivagram

Radionuclide salivagram is a simple investigative study that can be used to detect aspiration of radiolabeled saliva into the airways. A small amount (ranging from 0.1 to 0.2 mL) of radiotracer (99mTc DTPA) is administered under the patient's tongue, with the patient placed in supine position and the camera in posterior view, centered on patient's chest, including oral cavity and upper stomach. The radionuclide salivagram is recorded by fast dynamic scintigraphy (15 s/frame), and the registration should start some seconds before tracer administration, avoiding to miss the swallowing phase. No specific preparations are required for the test. In patients with neurological dysphagia, risk of salivary aspiration is related to swallowing incoordination, and scintigraphic study interpretation must include a careful frame-by-frame evaluation. Regions-of-interest (ROI)s, corresponding to esophagus and lung fields, are drawn on a summed image of dynamic frames using a dedicated software; thus, time/activity curves are obtained and analyzed. Registration

© Springer International Publishing Switzerland 2017

M.C. Garganese, G.F.L. D'Errico (eds.), *Conventional Nuclear Medicine in Pediatrics*, DOI 10.1007/978-3-319-43181-9_17

of 30 min is useful for several reasons: to have enough time in case of delayed swallowing, to detect delayed episodes of aspiration (in case of multiple swallowing), to detect persistence or clearance of aspirated tracer. If persistent tracer activity is present, delayed scanning after repositioning the children in upright position may detect aspiration, extending the period of scanning until after the esophagus is cleared of all material. Moreover, prolonged registration can detect delayed aspiration of labeled saliva refluxate from the stomach.

Severity of aspiration interpretation: criteria of pulmonary aspiration evaluation are the same as those reported for gastric emptying study.

17.1.3 Detection of Lung Impairment Secondary to Aspiration by Lung Perfusion Scan

Study technique will be reported in Chap. 23. In this group of patients, perfusion lung scan is useful for a quantitative and qualitative evaluation of pulmonary impairment due to chronic pulmonary aspiration.

17.2 Teaching Cases

17.2.1 Case 17.1 "Radionuclide Salivagram: Normal Pattern"

A 10-year-old boy in gastrostomy tube feeding affected by genetic syndrome, neuromotor deficits, and severe gastroesophageal reflux disease, with frequent hospitalizations for respiratory infections. A radionuclide salivagram was required for the salivary swallowing evaluation to schedule a laparoscopic Nissen fundoplication integrated with salivary duct ligation.

17.2.2 Case 17.2 "Radionuclide Salivagram: Massive Pulmonary Aspiration with Partial Clearance"

A 2-year-old infant affected by severe postasphyxia cerebropathy and tetraparesis. Clinical course was further characterized by pathological fractures (secondary to osteoporosis), surgical gastroesophageal reflux correction with gastrostomy tube feeding placement, salivary duct ligation, and tracheotomy. In this complex clinical case, despite these therapies, persistent episodes of pneumonitis occurred and a radionuclide salivagram was required to confirm clinical suspicion of salivary aspiration.

17.2.3 Case 17.3 "Radionuclide Salivagram: Massive Pulmonary Aspiration with Progressive Increased Concentration"

A 4-year-old child affected by epileptogenic encephalopathy, dysphagia, and inability to manage salivary secretions with the need of frequent pharyngeal aspirations. After radionuclide salivagram showing severe chronic aspiration, salivary duct ligation procedure and tracheotomy were performed.

17.2.4 Case 17.4 "Radionuclide Salivagram: Salivary Micro-aspiration Pattern"

A 5-year-old child with neurological postasphyxia impairment and previous history of chronic pulmonary aspiration, He underwent surgical gastroesophageal reflux correction with gastrostomy tube feeding placement and a retraining swallowing function program. Before restarting oral feeding, radionuclide salivagram was required showing salivary micro-aspiration in right lung.

17.2.5 Case 17.5 "Radionuclide Salivagram: Pulmonary Aspiration by Anterograde and Retrograde Routes"

A 10-year-old boy with a complex clinical status due to multiple pathologies (neurological, orthopedic, and respiratory pathology) secondary to epileptogenic encephalopathy. After a multispecialty consultation, a radionuclide salivagram was included in a complex preoperative diagnostic workup. Salivagram allowed to detect aspiration of saliva (anterograde route) associated with refluxate inhalation (retrograde route) during exam registration. A combined surgical treatment of gastroesophageal reflux disease and salivary aspiration was carried out with Nissen fundoplication and salivary ducts ligation.

17.2.6 Case 17.6 "Radionuclide Salivagram: Absence of Swallowing as a Severe Dysfunction Pattern"

Eleven-month-old infant affected by cerebral palsy. A radionuclide salivagram was required to assess salivary secretions management ability.

17.2.7 Case 17.7 "Gastric Emptying: Pulmonary Aspiration of Discrete Labeled Meal"

A 10-year-old child affected by postasphyxia cerebropathy underwent laparoscopic antireflux surgery (Nissen fundoplication) associated with pyloromyotomy. Two years later, several respiratory infections occurred, and postoperative scintigraphic control was required to achieve a functional gastric evaluation allowing investigating pulmonary respiratory problems. Gastric emptying scintigraphy ruled out gastroesophageal reflux or delayed clearance of the radiolabeled meal, but detected severe pulmonary aspiration of discrete labeled meal (early after meal administration).

17.2.8 Case 17.8 "Delayed Gastric Emptying Associated with Gastroesophageal Reflux Disease and Pulmonary Aspiration"

A 1-year-infant, affected by postasphyxia cerebropathy with poor weight gain and respiratory infections despite gastrostomy tube feeding. Gastric emptying scintigraphy revealed delayed gastric emptying associated with gastroesophageal reflux disease and pulmonary aspiration. Laparoscopic antireflux surgery (Nissen fundoplication) associated to pyloromyotomy was performed with significant clinical improvement. In this case, gastric emptying scintigraphy gave an important contribution to the diagnostic assessment and therapeutical management of a child with gastroesophageal reflux (GER) disease complicated by GER-related respiratory disease.

17.2.9 Case 17.9 "Scintigraphic Assessment of Pulmonary Impairment in a Child Treated at Birth for Esophageal Atresia Associated with Tracheoesophageal Fistula"

A 5-year-old child, treated at birth for esophageal atresia associated with tracheoesophageal fistula, with neonatal respiratory distress and neurological impairment. A gastric emptying scintigraphy revealed mildly delayed gastric emptying associated with gastroesophageal reflux disease and pulmonary aspiration of discrete labeled meal (early after oral meal administration). An endoscopic control ruled out tracheoesophageal fistula relapse. Considering previous history of recurrent episodes of bronchopneumonia and radiological worsening of right lung parenchyma, a functional assessment of lung perfusion was required to achieve a quantitative data of pulmonary impairment (Figs. 17.1, 17.2, 17.3, 17.4, 17.5, 17.6, 17.7, 17.8, and 17.9).

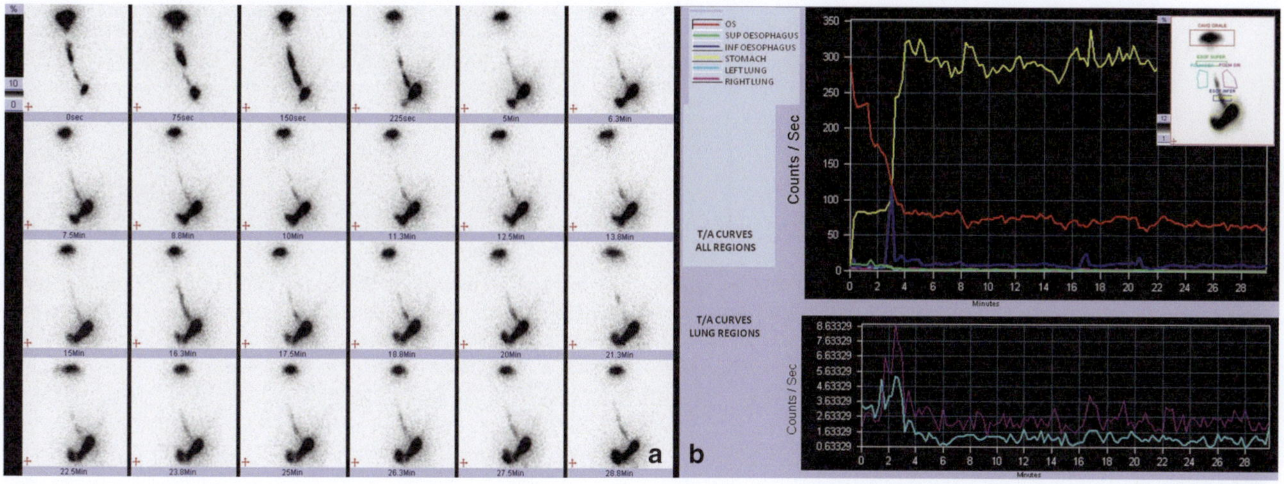

Fig. 17.1 (**a**, **b**) By qualitative imaging and time/activity curves evaluation, a normal swallowing is observed with a regular passage of the radioactive bolus through the esophagus. No evidence of pulmonary aspiration episodes is detected during the registration. Some episodes of gastroesophageal reflux are evident, also with a small amount of labeled tracer

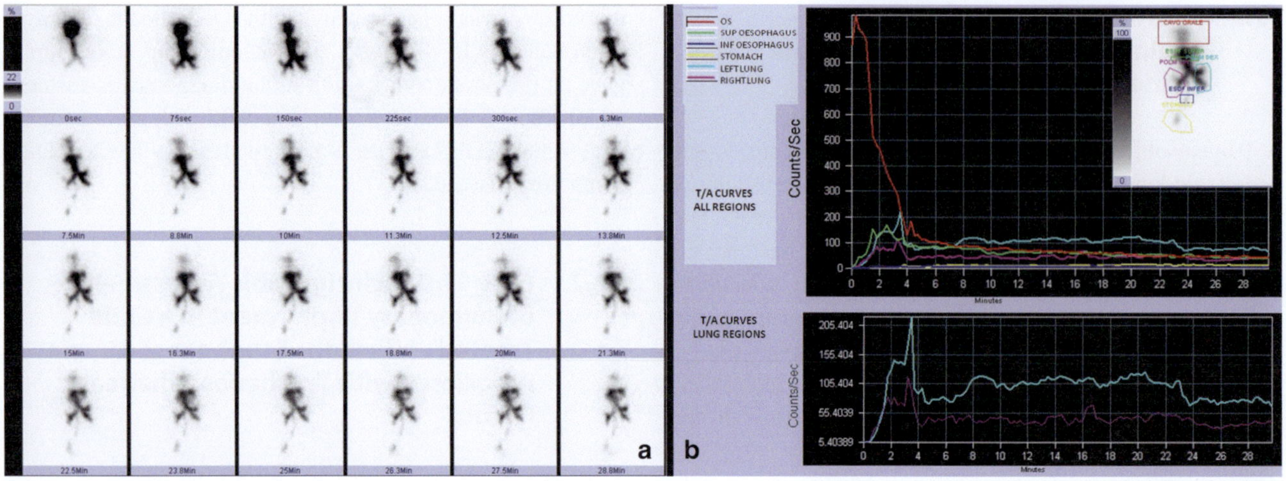

Fig. 17.2 (**a**, **b**) Radionuclide salivagram shows massive and bilateral salivary aspiration in tracheal cannula and both lungs. A large amount of administered labeled bolus is visualized in the respiratory airways (proximal and distal), with evidence of mild tracer activity in the lower tract of esophagus and in the stomach. Partial clearance of aspirated tracer is evident at 4th and 23rd minute of registration in relation to tracheobronchial aspiration (necessary for breathing difficulties associated with desaturation). Eventually caught episodes or tracheobronchial aspiration procedure must be annotated and considered for a correct evaluation of aspirated clearance mechanism. This finding is considered as massive pulmonary aspiration

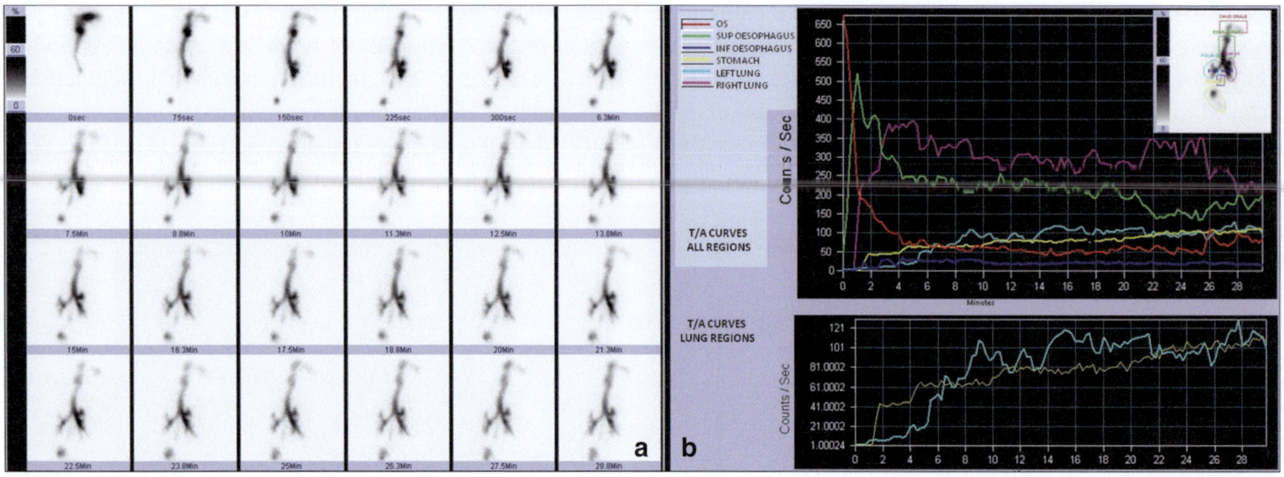

Fig. 17.3 (**a**, **b**) After swallowing, fast progression of salivary secretion is evident in upper esophageal tract, and most of the salivary secretion passes directly into the trachea and in the right bronchus. Tracer penetration is subsequently evident into the left bronchus and in the distal airways of both lungs. Qualitative and T/A curves analyses show a progressive increased concentration of aspirated tracer (*especially on the right*). Low amount of labeled saliva is evident in the lower esophagus and in the stomach

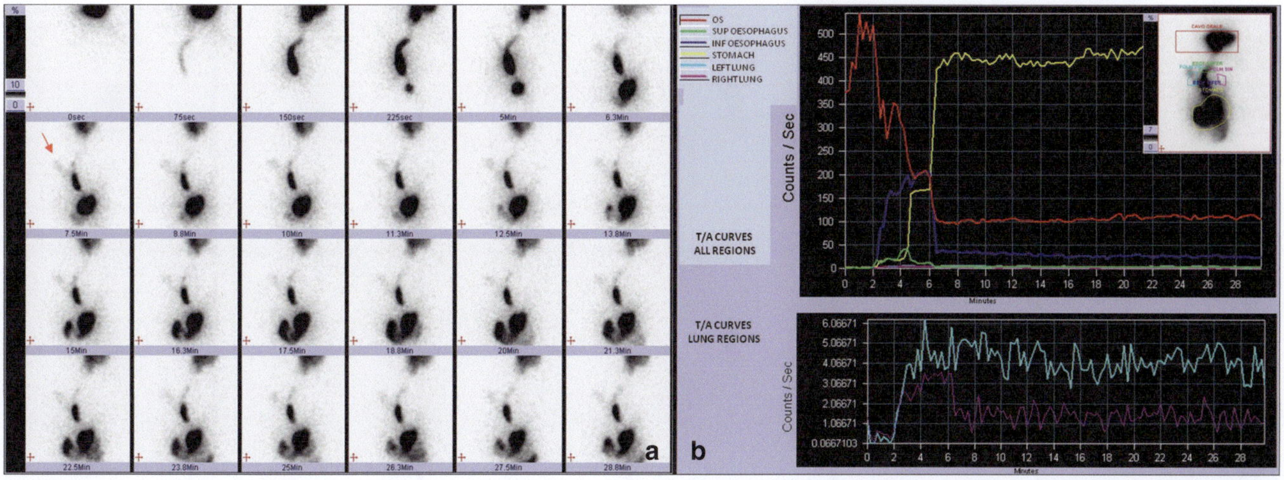

Fig. 17.4 (**a**, **b**) After swallowing, progression of salivary secretion is evident in the esophagus showing a significant deviation of its course (secondary to a severe scoliosis) and a persistent tracer stasis in the distal tract due to a tight gastric fundoplication. A weak signal activity is documented in the right lung field, as for micro-aspiration scintigraphic sign

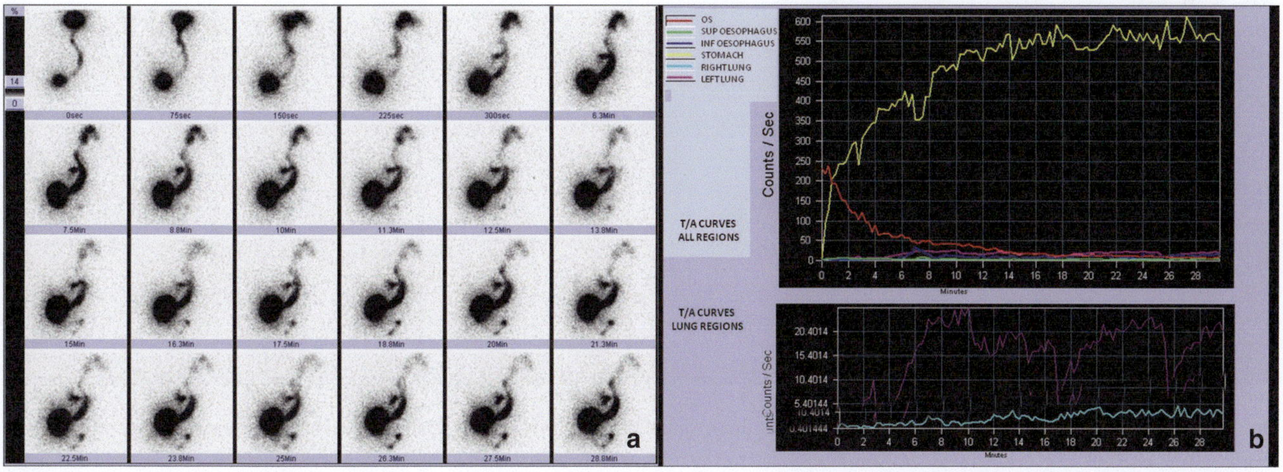

Fig. 17.5 (**a**, **b**) After swallowing, progression of salivary secretion is evident in the esophagus associated with pulmonary aspiration in the left bronchial airway system that increases early after a gastroesophageal reflux episode (appreciable at 6th minute of registration). In the following part of registration, cyclic decreased and increased tracer activities are detectable in relation to other reflux episodes. These findings are indicative of salivary aspiration associated with bronchial refluxate aspiration

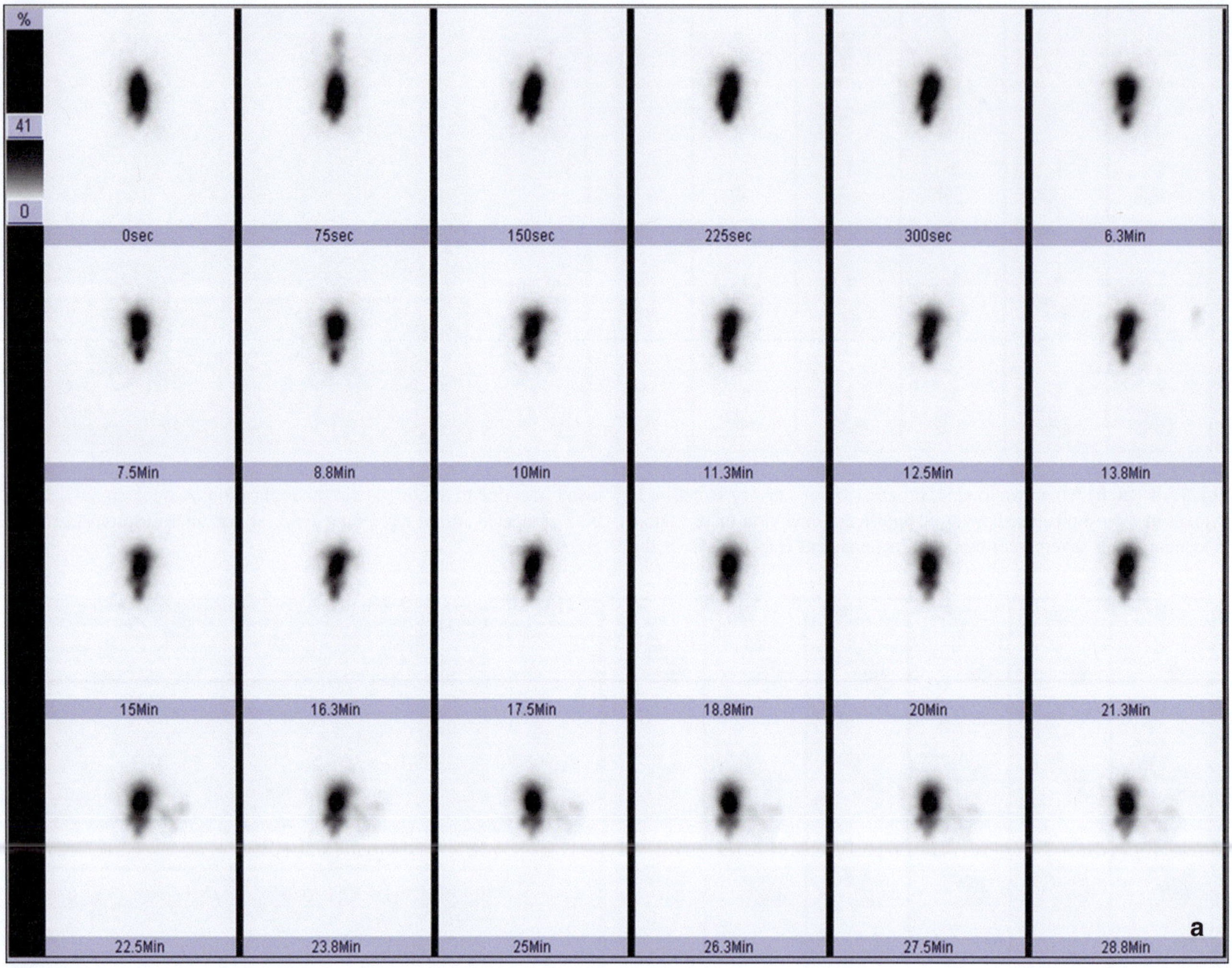

Fig. 17.6 Even after prolonged mechanical and sensitive stimulation, there is no evidence of labeled saliva (and oropharyngeal secretions) progression through esophagus. This finding represents a severe swallowing dysfunction, giving a useful clinical information

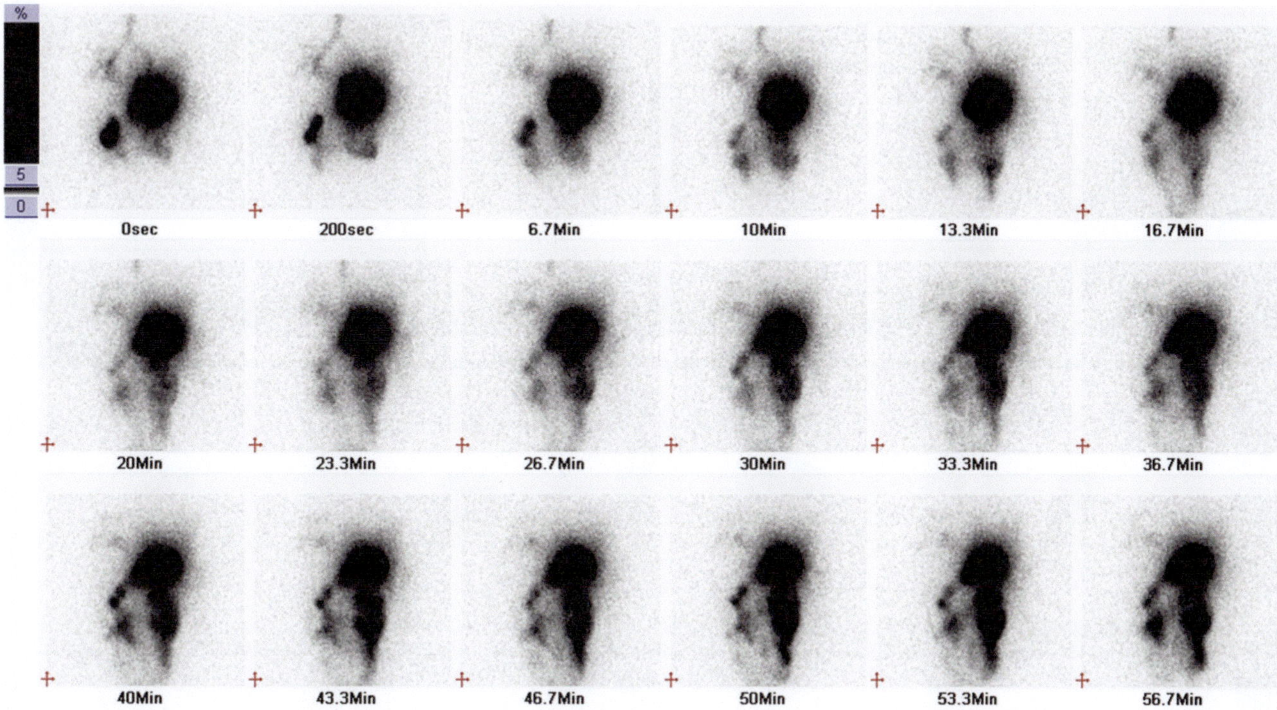

Fig. 17.7 Gastric emptying study is performed after oral milk administration; since the first frame of registration, pulmonary aspiration of discrete labeled meal is bilaterally evident in the proximal and distal airways (*especially on the right*). A progressive but partial clearance of aspirated meal is noted without evidence of following significant gastroesophageal reflux associated with normal gastric emptying

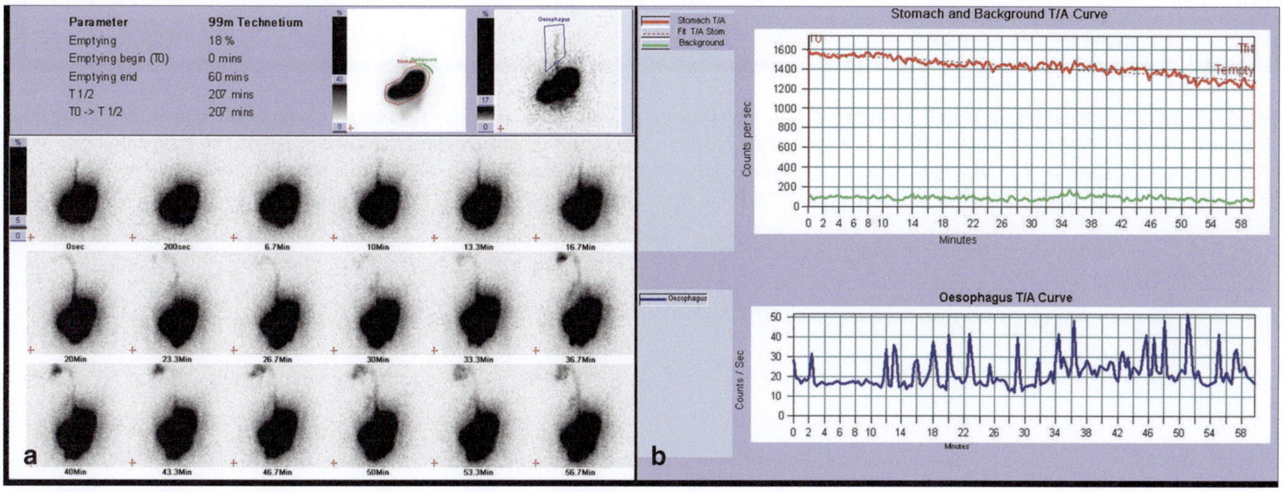

Fig. 17.8 (**a**, **b**) Gastric emptying study is performed after labeled milk administration by PEG tube. After meal administration (performed under persistence monitor control), several gastroesophageal reflux episodes are evident, associated with delayed gastric emptying. Some reflux episodes reach the oral cavity with subsequent visualization of the respiratory airways (*especially on the right*), as for multiple pulmonary aspiration

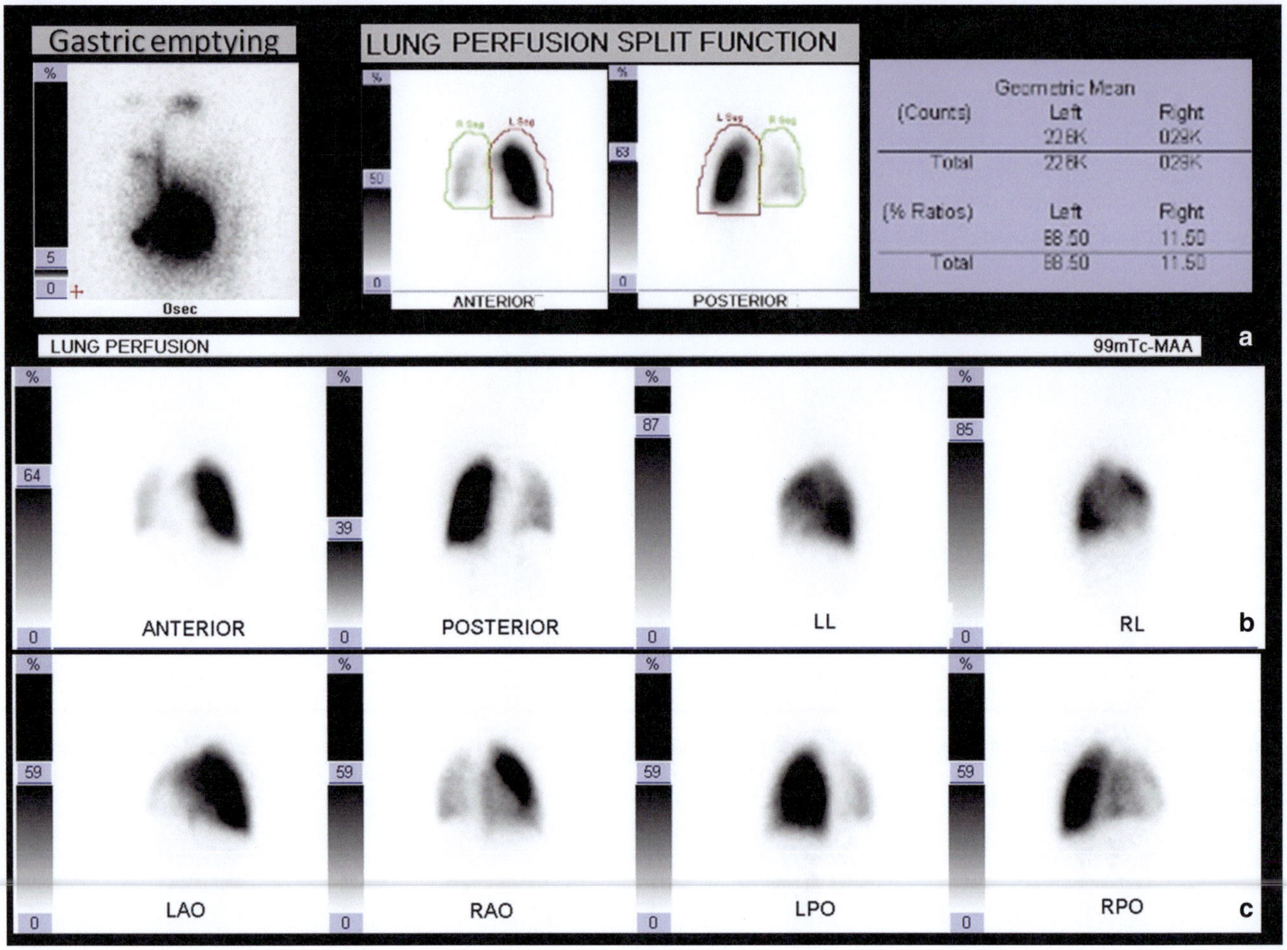

Fig. 17.9 (**a**) Gastric emptying study is performed after oral milk administration; the first frame of registration shows pulmonary aspiration of discrete labeled meal in the right lung. (**b**, **c**) Scintigraphy of lung perfusion shows left lung normal dimension, tracer uptake, and distribution; right lung is small with poor tracer uptake and diffuse nonhomogeneous distribution (without evidence of segmental defects of lung perfusion). By quantitative analysis, functional contribution of right lung is markedly low (11.5 %)

Bibliography

1. Ciofetta G. Gastro-esophageal studies in relationship to respiratory problems. Q J Nucl Med Mol Imaging. 2010;54(4):372–8. Review. Nucl Med Mol.
2. Garganese MC, Knafelz D. "Manuale SIGENP di gastroenterologia ed epatologia pediatrica" Il pensiero scientifico editore (Ed 2014) Chapter 24. 101–3.
3. Yang J, Codreanu I, Servaes S, Zhuang H. Radionuclide salivagram and gastroesophageal reflux scintigraphy in pediatric patients: targeting different types of pulmonary aspiration. Clin Nucl Med. 2015;40(7):559–63.

Gastroenterology: Focus on Children with Liver Problems

18

Giuliano Torre

18.1 Introduction

Hepatobiliary scintigraphy is a radionuclide diagnostic imaging study that evaluates hepatocellular function and the biliary system by tracing the production and flow of bile from the formative phase in the liver and its passage through the biliary system into the small intestine.

Sequential (or dynamic) images of the liver, biliary tree, and gut are obtained. Computed acquisition and analysis, including pharmacological interventions, are used according to varying indications and an individual patient's needs.

Scintigraphy today works in combination with other methods of hepatobiliary imaging, mainly sonography and echocolor Doppler, magnetic resonance, and Colangio-RM, bringing the advantage of a dynamic display of the tracer extraction phases, concentration, and excretion in the bile duct.

In adult hepatobiliary disease, main indications of hepatobiliary scintigraphy are acute and chronic cholecystitis, evaluation of patency and integrity of biliary tree, dysfunction of the sphincter of Oddi, functional biliary pain syndromes, or chronic pain localized at the right hypochondrium. In case of ongoing surgical liver resection, hepatobiliary scintigraphy is employed for the functional preoperative evaluation. After liver transplant, it is used for the study of the biliary tree and of the functional hepatic reserve.

In childhood, the above indications are less frequent, while more often hepatobiliary scintigraphy is used in the differential diagnosis of neonatal cholestasis, in particular, to distinguish between obstructive jaundice depending on anatomical malformations (biliary atresia, choledochal cysts) and medical cholestatic jaundice resulting from a defective hepatocellular function (due to infectious, metabolic, hormonal causes). It also allows to evaluate the patency and the function of hepatic–jejunal anastomosis (Kasai surgery) after surgery for atresia and the possible presence of leak of the bile duct. Similar to adulthood, it has a role in anatomical and functional aspects of the transplanted liver.

Main hepatobiliary clinical problems and indications in pediatrics:

1. Neonatal cholestasis and suspicion of biliary atresia:
   Neonatal cholestasis has an incidence of 1:2500 newborns and is more common in premature babies. It can be recognized by various causes: infectious/septic, genetic/metabolic, endocrine, hematological. Liver and biliary congenital malformations must always be considered and excluded: among them, the most typical is biliary atresia. It is a progressive fibro-obliterative condition of extrahepatic and intrahepatic bile ducts, resulting in the obstruction of bile flow to the intestine, intrahepatic retention of bile and bile salts, leading to structural liver damage. From the clinical point of view, biliary atresia usually affects a full-term infant (of few weeks of age) generally in good clinical conditions and regular growth, who is referred for jaundice, hyperchromic urine, and hypo-acholic stools. In suspicion of biliary atresia (incidence 1:8000–15,000 births, depending on the ethnic groups), the differential diagnosis versus other causes of neonatal cholestasis is absolutely urgent, for the possibility in case of biliary atresia of an early surgical correction, before the development of biliary cirrhosis and portal hypertension. The sooner the surgery (Kasai portoenterostomy) is performed, better is the outcome and chances of an effective and lasting biliary drainage.

   Hepatobiliary scintigraphy is the investigation of choice to confirm a suspected sonographic diagnosis of biliary atresia (Sonography can show gallbladder agenesis or dysmorphic features, hyperechoic and irregular profiles of liver, presence of triangular cord, failure visualization of the biliary tract, altered distribution of intrahepatic blood flow.).

G. Torre
Pediatric Hepatology Gastroenterology Nuriition Unit, "Bambino Gesù" Children Hospital, Rome, Italy
e-mail: giuliano.torre@opbg.net

© Springer International Publishing Switzerland 2017

M.C. Garganese, G.F.L. D'Errico (eds.), *Conventional Nuclear Medicine in Pediatrics*, DOI 10.1007/978-3-319-43181-9_18

The sensitivity of scintigraphy for biliary atresia is virtually 100 % (the suspicion of atresia is ruled out if there is passage of the tracer in the gut); the specificity is much lower (on average 70 %), that is, if it is proved passage of the tracer, it is possible that this is due to the causes different from biliary atresia. In addition, specificity is higher for the full-term baby compared to preterm. It is possible to increase the scintigraphic performances with a pretreatment of the newborn with phenobarbital (5 mg/kg/day) administered for 3–5 days before the test; alternative to barbiturate, similar results have been reported with ursodeoxycholic acid (20 mg/kg/day for 2–3 days). In case of no bowel elimination of the radiopharmaceutical tracer in the physiological time, it is appropriate to prolong the examination even up to 24 h after injection to highlight a condition of late biliary transit (it can depend on a reduced liver function, especially in the premature infant). In the case hepatobiliary scintigraphy was not diriment for a differential diagnosis, it is necessary to perform liver biopsy or intraoperative cholangiography during exploratory laparotomy. Even after surgery for biliary atresia (Kasai procedure), if doubts exist coming from the persistence of jaundice or its slow clearance, hepatobiliary scintigraphy can verify the patency and function of the anastomosis, with the demonstration and quantification of bile flow from its origin (intrahepatic bile) until bowel, and any remaining barriers.

2. Malformations of the extrahepatic bile ducts:
   The choledochal cyst is the most common malformation and can manifest with cholestatic jaundice (similar to biliary atresia), vomiting, and pain after meals, depending on bowel compression or bacterial infection (cholangitis secondary to intrahepatic bile retention). It can occur in the neonatal period as well as in subsequent ages. Clinical suspicion is usually sonographic, and hepatobiliary scintigraphy is useful for confirmation: it is possible to highlight the collection of the radiopharmaceutical in a cystic mass corresponding to the malformation of extrahepatic bile duct, define the morphological and dimensional characteristics, its relationship with the bile duct system, and the way and timing of the intestinal transit. Treatment is surgical.

   A possible complication of cystic malformations is the spontaneous perforation of the bile duct leading to bile peritoneum (localized or widespread). More rarely, perforation affects a normal bile duct, either spontaneously or as a result of abdominal trauma.

   In the case of biliary leak, hepatobiliary scintigraphy traces the biliary transit of the radiopharmaceutical and indicates the site and extent of the possible extravasation in the abdominal cavity. This clinical information provides the surgeon the better choice between attitudes – conservative or interventional.

3. Familial progressive cholestasis (PFIC 1-2-3):
   It is a group of congenital cholestatic diseases depending on molecular defects of enzymes involved in excretion of bile salts and phosphatidylcholine in the bile canaliculus (PFIC-1, BSEP deficiency, MDR3 deficiency). They are rare diseases (1:50,000–100,000 births), currently well recognized in the differential diagnosis of neonatal and infantile cholestasis, owing to the availability of genetic diagnosis. The phenotype and the clinical picture are variable in severity of progressive chronic cholestatic liver disease (up to biliary cirrhosis, leading to liver transplantation even in early childhood). A common clinical element of progressive familial cholestasis, together with jaundice and nutritional effects of chronic cholestasis on growth, is itching, often extremely severe and difficult to treat: it depends on the blocked secretion of bile salts into the bile, their overflow into the blood stream, and stimulation of specific nerve receptors for itching stimulus.

   Recently, for situations of itching not or poorly responsive to medical treatment, surgical biliocutaneous shunt (ostomy skin) as well as internal bypass surgery (anastomosis between the biliary tract and colon with interposition of jejunal loop) have been proposed: the final goal is to divert outside the bile salts, or prevent their intestinal reabsorption, and consequently to decrease the blood level and the itching trigger.

   Hepatobiliary scintigraphy is used to evaluate the efficacy of these surgical procedures through the study of excretion of the radiopharmaceutical tracer: it allows a quantitative assessment of flow and serial monitoring of biliary elimination over time, especially if there are suspects of complications at the anastomotic level. The information obtained allows, also in this case, to program the medical or the surgical option.

4. Liver transplantation:
   Liver transplantation is the therapeutic choice for irreversible liver failure, both acute fulminant and chronic progressive. It is now available for children with a greater than 90 % survival for elective transplant. Given the age of the children who are in need of a transplant (more than 50 % are less than 2 years old), the surgical technique used in most cases is the split liver technique from adult donor (dead or alive). This surgery implies the use of a portion of the donor's liver (usually the left lobe).

   After pediatric liver transplant, a possible complication of surgery is anastomotic biliary stricture between the very thin bile duct of the graft and intestinal loop of the receiver.

   Hepatobiliary scintigraphy is employed to confirm the sonographic suspicion of biliary anastomotic stenosis, showing the level of the obstruction and dilation of the biliary tree.

As another possible application in liver transplant, a recent pediatric experience shows an early diagnosis of hepatic infarction as a result of hepatic artery thrombosis.

Scintigraphy was able to demonstrate the infarction areas through localized reduced tracer extraction. In this case, previous sonography was not enough to diagnose; subsequent PET TC confirmed the diagnosis.

Bibliography

1. Arnell H, Fischler B, et al. Hepatobiliary scintigraphy during cholestatic and non cholestatic periods in patients with progressive familial intrahepatic cholestasis after partial external biliary diversion. J Pediatr Surg. 2011;46:467–72.
2. Fukuda A, Sakamoto S, et al. Hepatobiliary scintigraphy for the assessment of biliary stricture after pediatric living donor liver transplantation for hepaticojejunostomy reconstruction: the value of the excretion rate at 60 min. Pediatr Transplant. 2011;15:594–600.
3. Kianifar HR, Tehranian S, et al. Accuracy of hepatobiliary scintigraphy for differentiation of neonatal hepatitis from biliary atresia: systematic review and meta-analysis of the literature. Pediatr Radiol. 2013;43:905–19.
4. Kwatra N, Shalaby-Rana E, et al. Phenobarbital-enhanced hepatobiliary scintigraphy in the diagnosis of biliary atresia: two decades of experience at a tertiary center. Pediatr Radiol. 2013;43:1365–75.
5. Poddar U, Bhattacharya A, et al. Ursodeoxycholic acid–augmented hepatobiliary scintigraphy in the evaluation of neonatal jaundice. J Nucl Med. 2004;45:1488–92.
6. Tulchinsky M, Ciak BW, et al. SNM practice guideline for hepatobiliary scintigraphy 4.0. J Nucl Med Technol. 2010;38:210–8.

19 Gastroenterology: Biliary Atresia, Choledochal Cyst, Cystic Fibrosis

Milena Pizzoferro, Maria Felicia Villani, Lidia Monti, Amato Infante, Manila Candusso, Maria Sole Basso, Andrea Pietrobattista, and Maria Carmen Garganese

19.1 Study Technique and Interpretation

19.1.1 Hepatobiliary Scintigraphy

Hepatobiliary imaging evaluates the function of the liver showing whether there are any blockages in the gallbladder or biliary duct system.

Hepatobiliary scintigraphy is performed using a radiotracer (99mTc HIDA or derivatives) after a fasting of 4 h. The administered activity of radiotracer is very low (1.85 MBq/kg) with a minimum suggested activity of 9 MBq and a maximum dose of 111 MBq. Immediately after tracer injection, hepatobiliary scan is recorded by dynamic study of 45 min or by time-sequential static images (in uncooperative child). In suspicion of biliary leak, severe hepatic dysfunction, obstruction of the common bile duct or biliary atresia, or in presence of severe hepatic dysfunction, it is appropriate to have a more prolonged observation (2–4 h, up to 24 h).

A specific element of the hepatobiliary scintigraphy in pediatrics is its prevalent application in children under the first year of life.

Radiotracer is taken up and excreted by hepatocytes allowing to image intrahepatic and extrahepatic biliary drainage. The normal findings of hepatobiliary scintigraphy are characterized by an immediate visualization of the liver parenchyma (with rapid clearance of blood and heart), followed by visualization of the biliary system in sequence (intrahepatic and extrahepatic, gallbladder, and intestine). All these structures are to be displayed within 45 min. A correct filling of the gallbladder requires the patency of the cystic duct: in adults, this excludes acute cholecystitis, in the newborn agenesis or dysmorphic gallbladder, which are usually present in biliary atresia.

Physiological urinary excretion is observed, especially when a biliary duct's obstruction is evident.

All hepatobiliary scans presented in this chapter are performed with ^{99m}Tc-BRIDA, and we report in Table 19.1 normal values of the main hepatogram parameters for a correct scintigraphy interpretation. Normal values are mildly different, using other tracers (Table 19.1).

Table 19.1 BRIDA, pharmacokinetic characteristics

	^{99m}Tc-BRIDA (mins)
Hepatic Tmax	12
Hepatic T ½	15–20
Principal bile duct visualization	5–20
Gallbladder visualization	10–40
Tracer appearing in the bowel	15–45

M. Pizzoferro • M.F. Villani
Nuclear Medicine Unit, Imaging Departement – "Bambino Gesù" Children Hospital, Rome, Italy

L. Monti • A. Infante
Imaging Department, "Bambino Gesù" Children Hospital, Rome, Italy

M. Candusso • M.S. Basso • A. Pietrobattista (✉)
Unit of Epathology, "Bambino Gesù" Children Hospital, Rome, Italy
e-mail: andrea.pietrobattista@opbg.net

M.C. Garganese
Diagnostic Imaging Department of Nuclear Medicine, IRCCS Bambino Gesù Paediatric Hospital, Rome, Italy

© Springer International Publishing Switzerland 2017

M.C. Garganese, G.F.L. D'Errico (eds.), *Conventional Nuclear Medicine in Pediatrics*, DOI 10.1007/978-3-319-43181-9_19

19.2 Teaching Cases

Case 19.1 Hepatobiliary Scintigraphy in Diagnostic Workup of Recurrent Pancreatitis

A 9-year-old girl with Crohn's disease diagnosed at the age of 5 years. Subsequently, she had recurrent episodes of acute pancreatitis secondary to papillary stenosis and underwent surgical treatment. Three years after treatment, she had relapsed episodes of pancreatitis. Ultrasonography and magnetic resonance imaging showed severe chronic pancreatitis with pancreatic ducts dilatation, splenomegaly, and increased gallbladder wall thickening without biliary ducts dilatation. A hepatobiliary scintigraphy was performed to evaluate liver function and biliary system excretion before further surgical treatment. A normal hepatic function was detected with regular parenchymal transit and transient tracer stasis in the gallbladder (as for gallbladder atonia).

Radiological imaging plays a major role in the diagnostic workup of children with hepatobiliary or pancreatic diseases, while hepatobiliary scintigraphy is performed in selected cases to achieve functional and biliary drainage data (Fig. 19.1).

Case 19.2 Biliary Atresia in a Newborn with Prolonged Neonatal Cholestasis

A 4-week-old boy with tetralogy of Fallot, cholestatic jaundice, and pale stool. Laboratory examination showed elevated total bilirubin with an increased conjugated portion, slightly elevated gGT. Hepatobiliary scintigraphy reported, "no drainage" of the radiolabeled tracer in the small bowel within 24 h as in extrahepatic biliary atresia (BA) patients. A percutaneous liver biopsy showed obstructive cholestasis. Diagnosis of BA was confirmed at 2 months of age by intraoperative cholangiography during Kasai portoenterostomy. Diagnosis of BA and performance of a hepatoportoenterostomy (Kasai Procedure) by 8–10 weeks of age are optimal for transplant-free survival beyond early childhood (Fig. 19.2).

Case 19.3 Late Diagnosis of Biliary Atresia with Secondary Liver Impairment

A 6-month-old boy referred to our hospital presenting with chronic cholestatic jaundice, high bilirubin level, splenomegaly, and acholic stool. Abdominal ultrasound and hepatobiliary scintigraphy were promptly performed, establishing the diagnosis of biliary atresia. Biliary atresia (BA) is universally fatal if untreated and is the single most common cause of liver disease leading to liver transplantation in children. In BA, bile flow from the liver to the gallbladder is blocked, and bile trapped inside the liver progressively causes damage and scarring of the liver cells (cirrhosis) and liver failure. Hepatobiliary scintigraphy revealed liver impairment in this patient due to late diagnosis of BA, and liver transplantation was necessary after few months (Fig. 19.3).

Case 19.4 Progressive Liver Failure After Performance of Hepatoportoenterostomy (Kasai Procedure) with Scintigraphic Finding of Bile Ascites

A 5-month-old boy diagnosed with biliary atresia at 4 weeks of age. At 2 months of age, a Kasai portoenterostomy was performed. He did not afford the restoration of the bile flow after the procedure and developed cirrhosis and ascites. In addition to radiological imaging, a hepatobiliary scintigraphy was performed showing liver disease progression with low hepatic function and biliary ascites (confirmed by ascitic fluid analysis). He underwent a liver transplant after 4 months.

Infants with biliary atresia who undergo a successful Kasai procedure regain good health and no longer have jaundice or major liver problems. When Kasai procedure is not successful, infants usually need a liver transplant within 1–2 years. Even after a successful surgery, most infants with biliary atresia could slowly develop cirrhosis over the years requiring a liver transplant by adulthood (Fig. 19.4).

Case 19.5 Diagnostic Imaging for Differential Diagnosis Between Cystic Biliary Atresia and a Congenital Choledochal Malformation

A 5-week-old female presented with jaundice and acholic stools to our center. She underwent a complete hepatology assessment that ruled out metabolic or infectious causes of her cholestasis. Ultrasound scan of the abdomen showed evidence of a choledochal cyst and sonographic signs suspicious of biliary atresia. Therefore, hepatobiliary scintigraphy was performed, and "no draining" of the radiolabed tracer in the small bowel within 24 h was seen, as in keeping with extrahepatic biliary atresia. Soon after the nuclear imaging, an intraoperative cholangiography confirmed the diagnosis of biliary atresia, and a portoenterostomy was done. In a small number of cases, biliary atresia may be associated with choledochal cyst, and preoperative diagnostic workup is crucial to select the right surgical approach (Fig. 19.5).

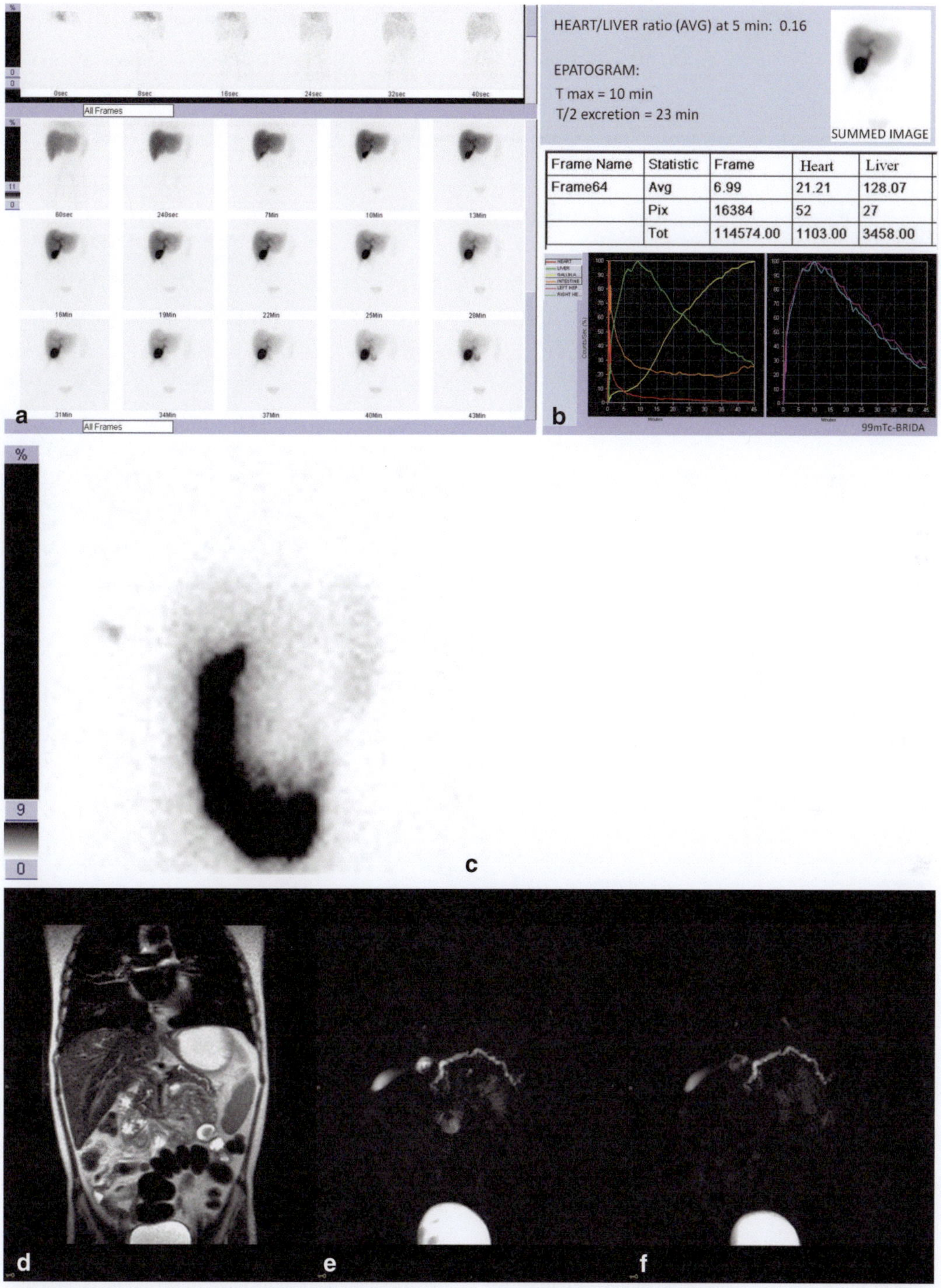

Fig. 19.1 (**a**, **b**) Dynamic study and time/activity curves reveal adequate hepatic uptake of the tracer and normal parenchymal transit time. Tracer is visualized in the gallbladder at approximately 7 min of the dynamic acquisition, with ever-increased concentration. No evidence of bowel activity up to 45 min of dynamic study. (**c**) Static image at 90 min demonstrates complete tracer transit in the bowel. (**d**) (Coronal) A 3-month-old girl with hereditary pancreatitis (*SPINK1* mutation) presented with chronic pancreatitis. MRI scans show the main features in chronic pancreatitis in children. (**e**, **f**). Maximum intensity projection three-dimensional magnetic resonance cholangiopancreatography (MRCP) image showing diffuse dilatation of the pancreatic duct. Note the irregular stricture of the pancreatic duct. Single-shot radial acquisition with relaxation enhancement magnetic resonance cholangiopancreatography (MRCP) image showing three pancreatoliths in the downstream minor pancreatic duct. The irregularity of the upstream duct can also be seen (*curved arrow*). Images obtained with fast T2-weighted sequences, usually constituting a coronal slab along the pancreatic duct, are acquired every 30 s for 10 min. MR cholangiopancreatography is limited by small-caliber ducts, poor signal, and patient motion, which create artifacts. The smaller duct caliber in children makes it difficult to visualize nondilated ducts at MR cholangiopancreatography, especially when evaluating intrahepatic duct caliber. MRI accurately depicts the pathology, leading to a better understanding of the disease process with optimal patient management and follow-up, without the use of ionizing radiation

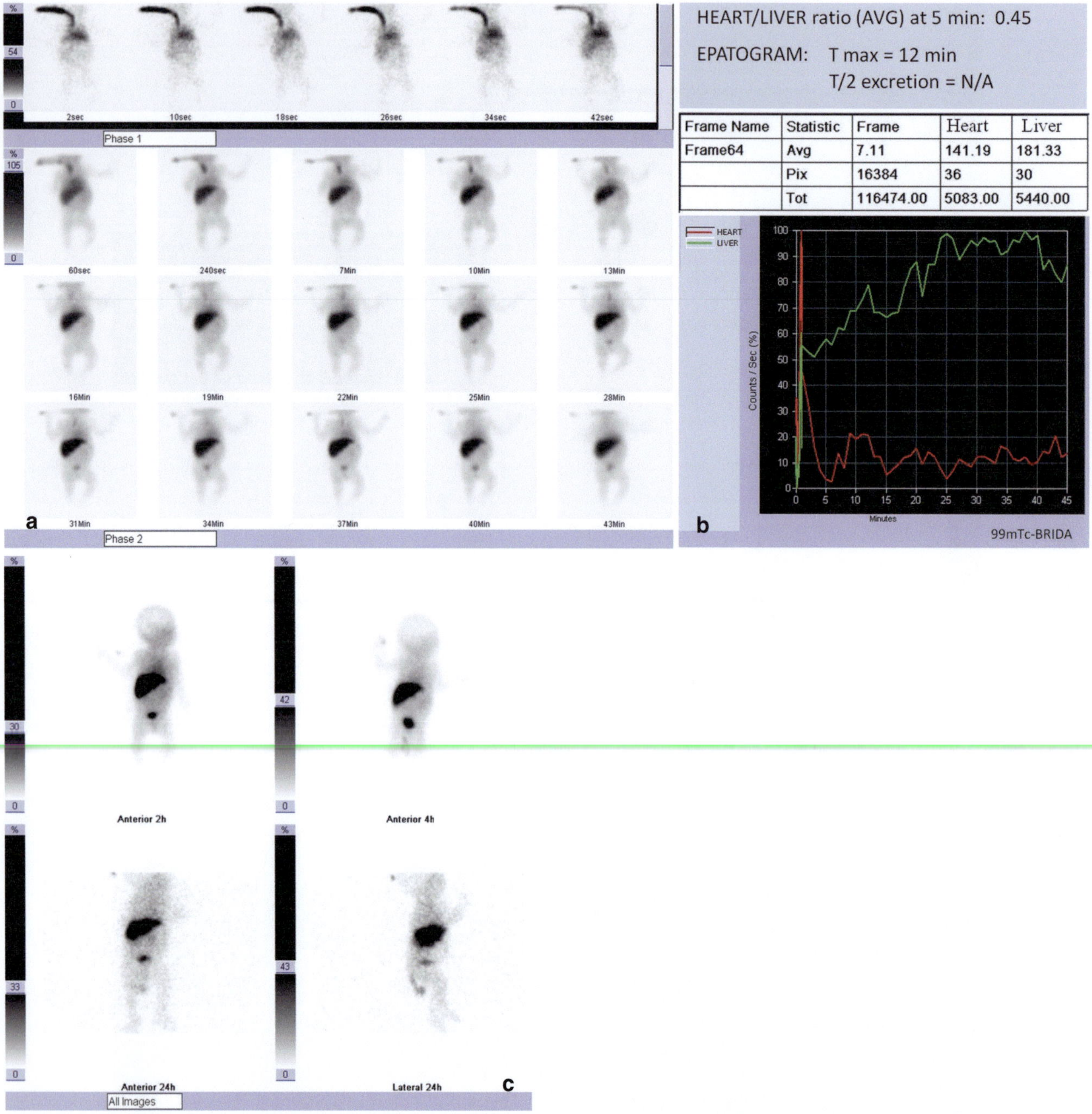

Fig. 19.2 (**a, b**) Dynamic study shows rapid and intense hepatic uptake of tracer with normal heart/liver ratio (maximum normal value is 0.5). No evidence of tracer in the intestine during the initial 45 min of the dynamic study is detectable. Physiological urinary excretion is observed. (**c**) Delayed static images performed at 2, 4, and 24 h confirm absence of tracer passage in the bowel. Lateral projection is useful when a faint abdominal activity is evident. Persistent neonatal cholestasis: sonographic scans show features in BA diagnosis. (**d**) High-frequency ultrasound with linear probe is used to evaluate the hepatic parenchyma. Transverse scan shows the inhomogeneous hepatic parenchyma, with a marked increase in periportal echoes due to fibrosis. (**e**) The thickness of the anterior wall of the right portal vein just proximal to the bifurcation site is greater than 4 mm. (**f**) Longitudinal ultrasound scan shows a normal gallbladder length >2 cm. (**g**) Transverse ultrasound scan depicts an irregular lining and wall of the gallbladder

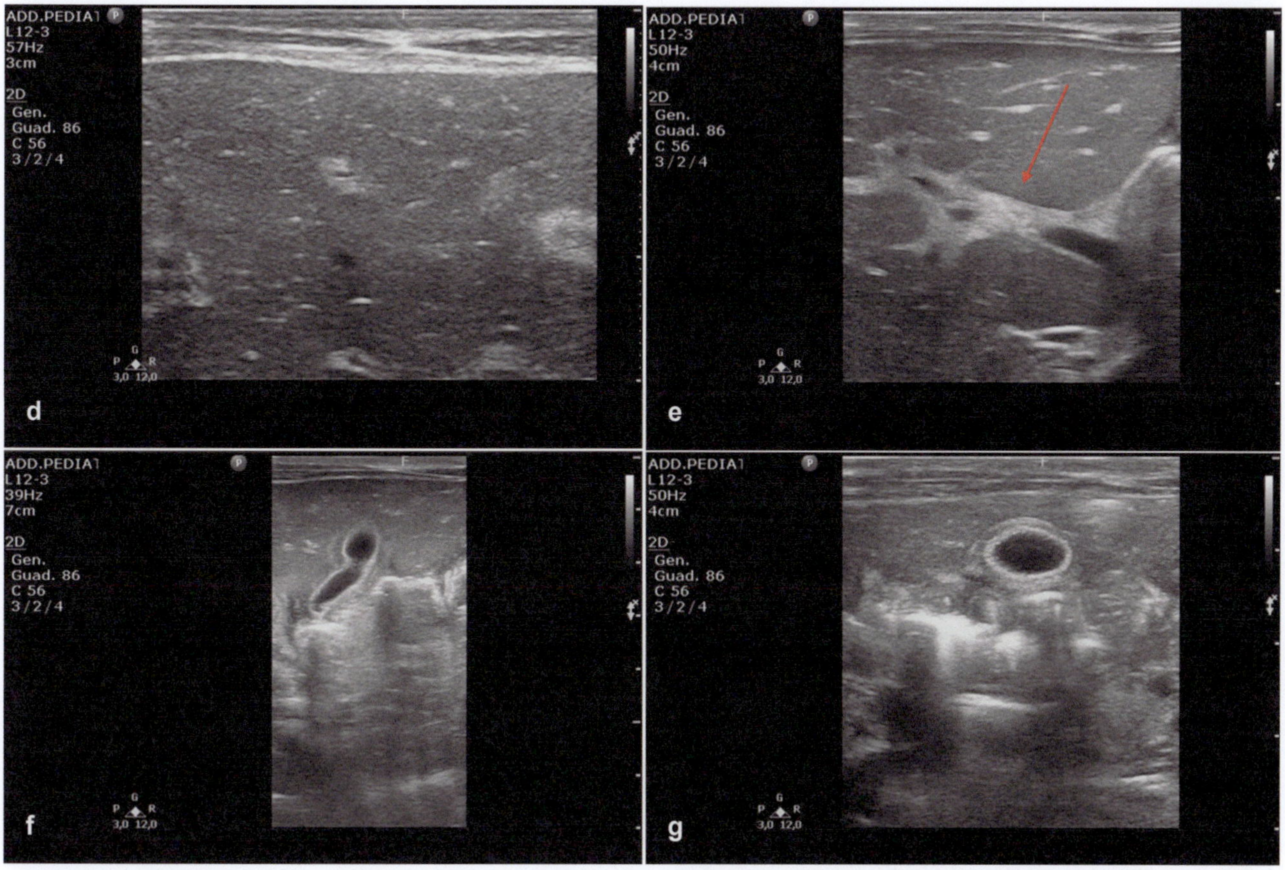

Fig. 19.2 (continued)

Case 19.6 Diagnostic Workup in a Case of a Choledochal Cyst

A 1-month-old boy, with no picture of cholestasis, underwent an abdominal ultrasound scan during the workup for intestinal motility disorders. Ultrasound abdominal scan revealed the presence of biliary dilatation, and hepatobiliary scintigraphy was performed to rule out the less likelihood hypothesis of a biliary atresia associated with choledochal cyst. Nuclear medicine imaging revealed a normal liver function and further clarified the biliary excretion, showing an early photon-deficient area in the porta hepatis with biliary tracer filling on late images (as for choledochal cysts); physiological gut activity was detected excluding biliary atresia association. A diagnosis of choledochal cyst was made and surgery planned (Fig. 19.6).

Case 19.7 Hepatobiliary Scintigraphy in Diagnostic Workup of Choledochal Cyst Complicated by Perforation of Bile Duct

A 2-month-old boy came to Emergency with clinical presentation of ascites and acholic stools. Previous history was uneventful with physiological neonatal jaundice and a prenatal ultrasonography referred as normal. Radiological imaging showed evidence of a large choledochal cyst, and a drainage tube was placed to evacuate and characterize the nature of abdominal fluid. By macroscopic analysis, the abdominal fluid had biliary color; chemical analysis confirmed high bilirubin level (12.9 mg/dL), whereas blood bilirubin level was quite normal (1.4 mg/dL), and all cultures performed were negative. These findings were indicative of perforation of bile duct that is an uncommon but possible event, consequent to different causes (trauma, ischemia, necrotizing enterocolitis, congenital malformation of bile ducts, or spontaneous breakage). Hepatobiliary scintigraphy was performed to achieve a complete evaluation of biliary drainage in relation to malformation of biliary tree complicated by abdominal leak (Fig. 19.7).

Case 19.8 Hepatobiliary Scintigraphy for Differential Diagnosis Between Hepatic Cyst and Biliary Origin Lesion

A 3-month-old boy with prenatal diagnosis of hepatic cyst (maximum axial diameter of 13 mm) in the VIII segment. Ultrasound postnatal abdominal scan confirmed the

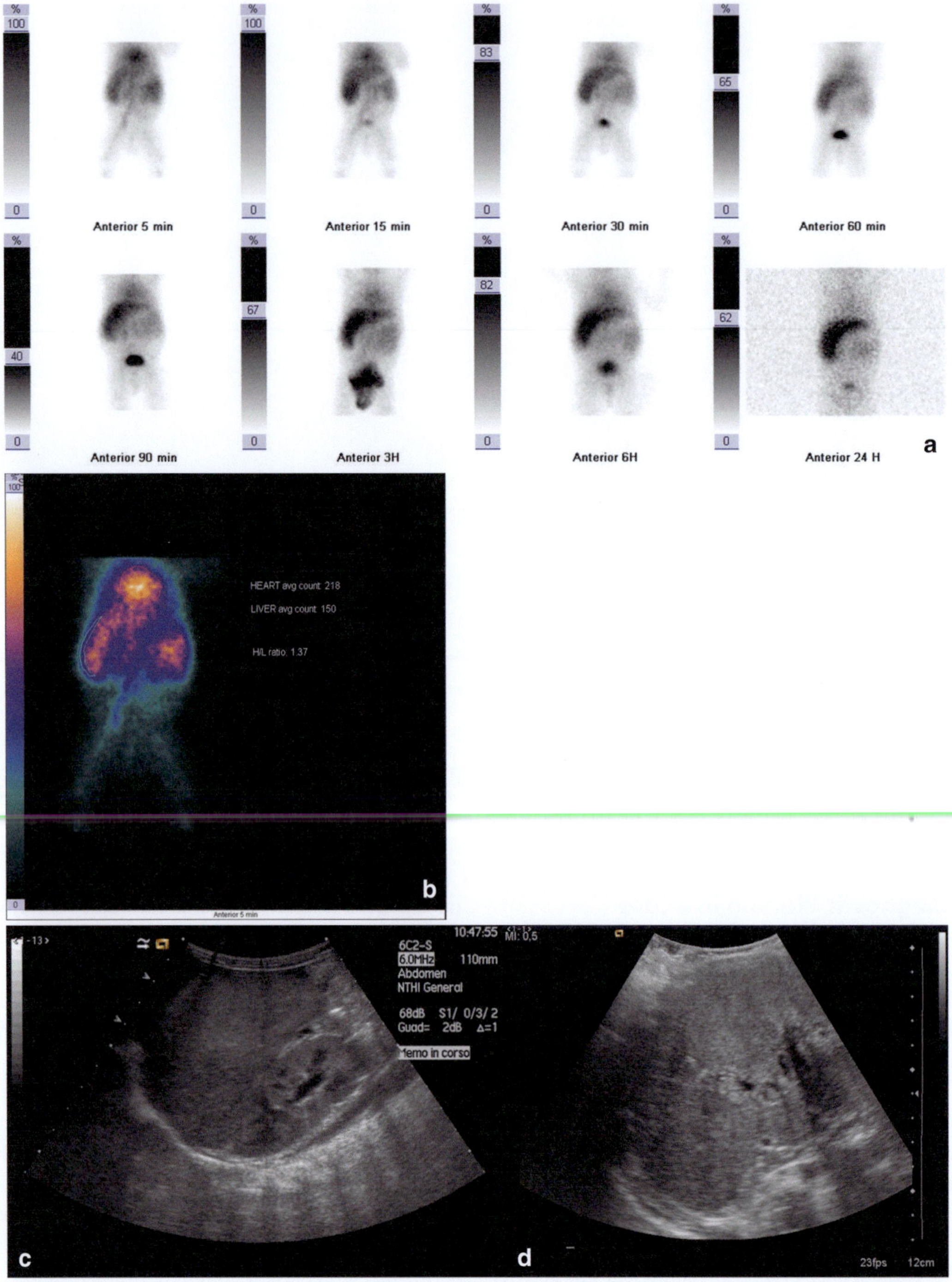

Fig. 19.3 (**a**) As an alternative to dynamic study in uncooperative child, time-sequential static images are performed. Images reveal poor extraction by the liver and high blood level (abnormal residual activity is evident in heart, enlarged spleen and aorta, and iliac arteries). Intraparenchymal liver distribution is nonhomogeneous with an area devoid of tracer corresponding to hepatic hilum region, as for indirect sign of ascites. No evidence of tracer in the intestine is detectable up to the last delayed image at 24 h. Physiological urinary excretion is observed. (**b**) Heart/liver ratio at 5 min (normal maximum value = 0.5) is calculated to obtain a semiquantitative parameter showing tracer extraction capability by the liver. Hepatic activity sample is determined by drawing a thin region of interest in peripheral marginal region, avoiding inclusion of biliary ducts; heart/liver ratio at 5 min is higher than normal (1.37), confirming low hepatic function observed by qualitative imaging evaluation. (**c**) An enlarged liver and splenomegaly are statistically significant features in infants with BA. (**d**) The liver has a nodular and cirrhotic surface. The triangular cord (TC) sign is observed as a focal area of increased echogenicity anterior to the bifurcation of the portal vein representing the fibrotic remnant of the extrahepatic biliary tree in BA. Images reveal poor extraction by the liver and high blood level (abnormal residual activity is evident in heart, enlarged spleen and aorta, and iliac arteries). Intraparenchymal liver distribution is nonhomogeneous, with an area devoid of tracer corresponding to hepatic hilum region, as for indirect sign of ascites. No evidence of tracer in the intestine is detectable up to the last delayed image at 24 h. Physiological urinary excretion is observed

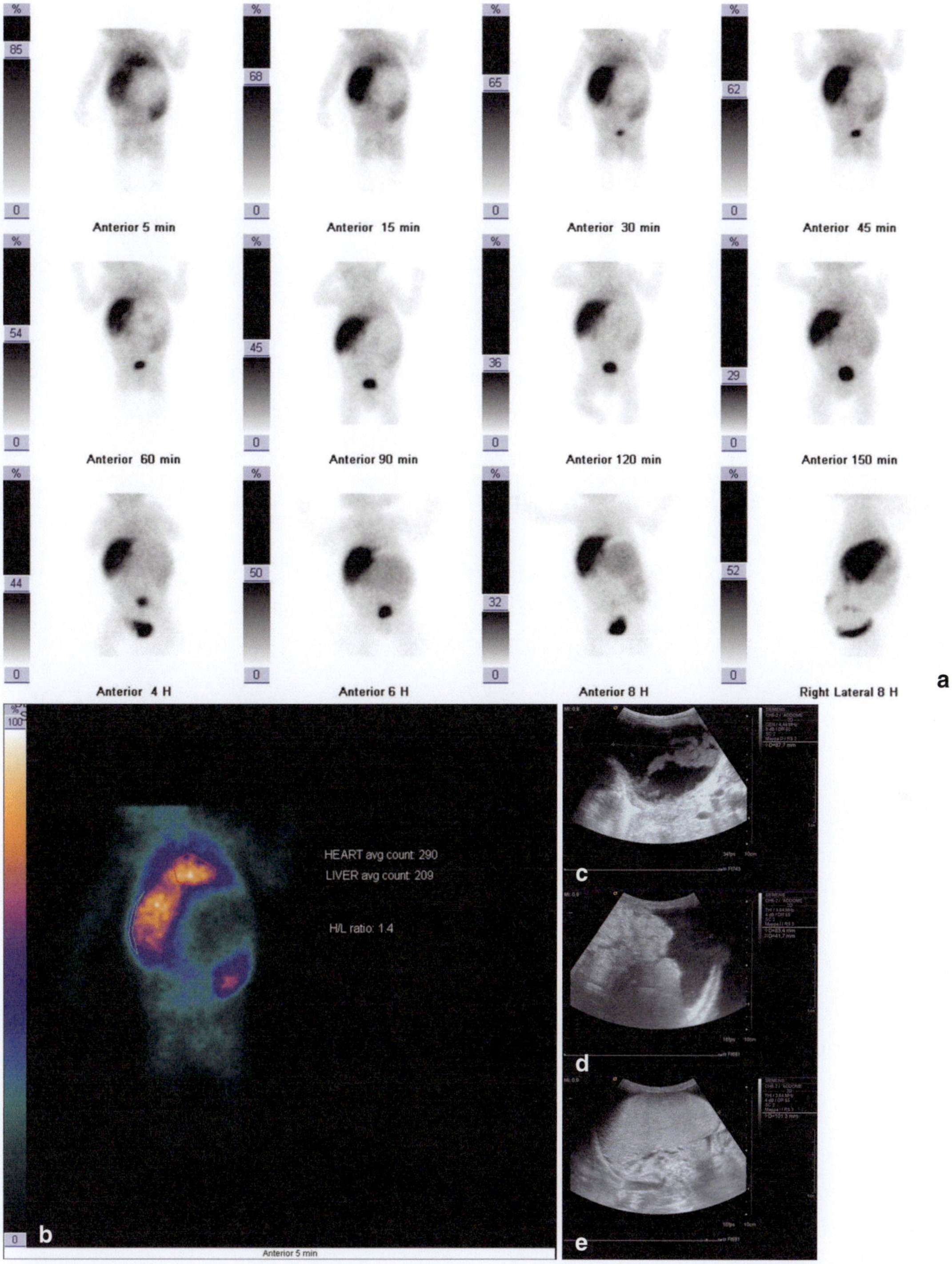

Fig. 19.4 (**a**, **b**) Time-sequential static images are performed up to 8 h after tracer administration. Images reveal poor extraction by the liver and high blood level (abnormal residual activity is evident in heart and enlarged spleen). Heart/liver ratio at 5 min is higher than normal (1.4). Since early images, a wide area devoid of tracer corresponding to left abdomen region is evident as for indirect sign of severe ascites. By evaluation of images performed at 30, 45, and 60 min, poor biliary tracer uptake is detectable in the middle of photopenic area, decreasing in the following images. In the latest images (at 150 min, 4 h, and 6 h), progressive and diffuse uptake is observed in left abdomen, as for bile ascites. Physiological urinary excretion is evident. Diagnosis of BA and performance of a hepatoportoenterostomy (Kasai procedure) by 8–10 weeks of age are optimal for transplant-free survival beyond early childhood. Prompt diagnosis ensures early treatment and results in improved prognosis. (**c**, **d**) Nevertheless, in some cases, progression to cirrhosis with portal hypertension, ascites, splenic varices, and splenomegaly. Features of portal hypertension. (**e**) Ultrasound: images of the liver with ascites is an early occurrence, following hepatoportoenterostomy

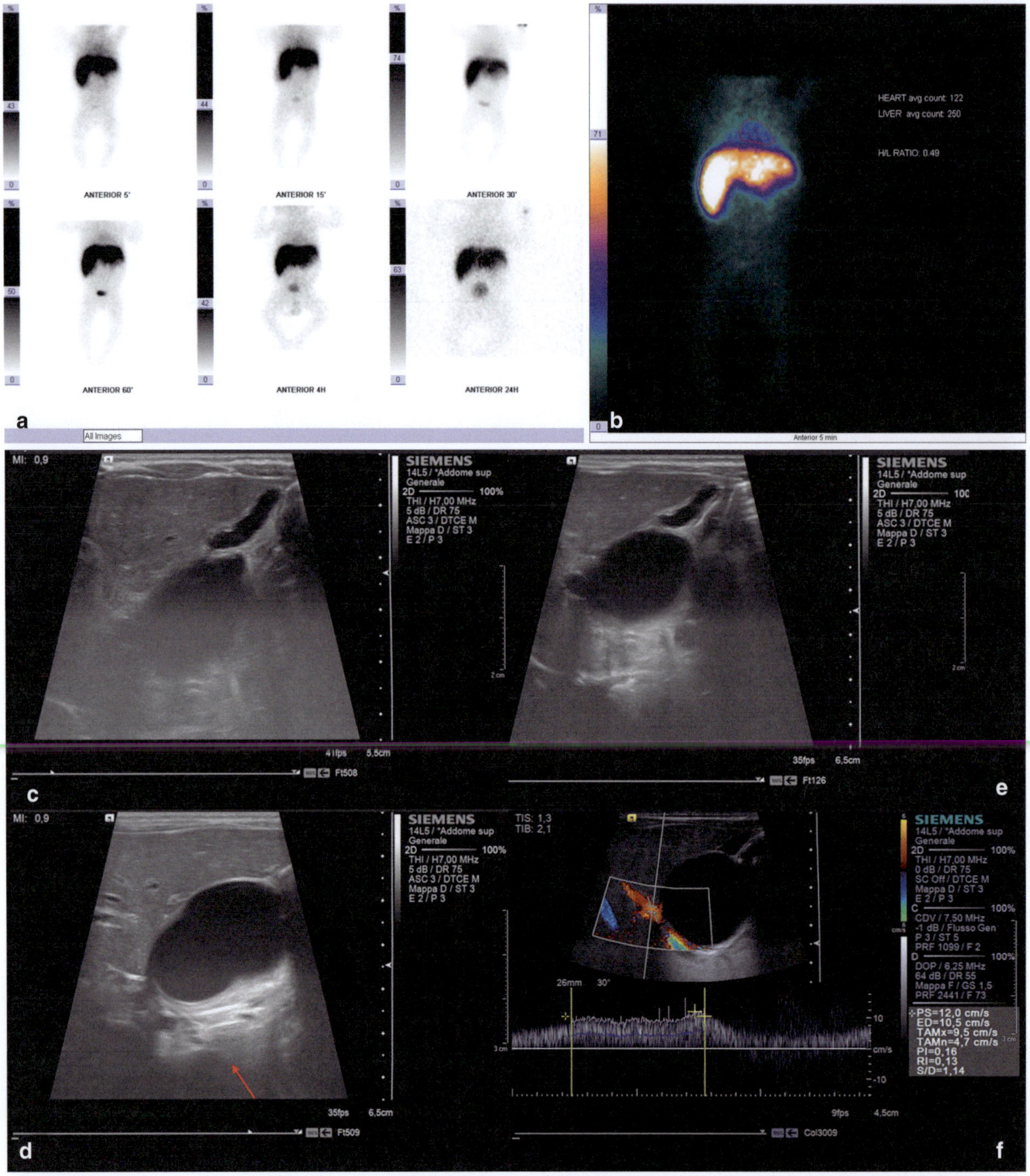

Fig. 19.5 (**a**, **b**) Time-sequential static images are performed up to 24 h after tracer administration showing intense and homogeneous hepatic uptake of tracer with normal heart/liver ratio at 5 min. By visual imaging evaluation, an area devoid of tracer corresponding to choledochal cyst (detected by ultrasound scan) is appreciable without biliary activity up to the study end. No evidence of tracer in the intestine up to 24 h is also detectable. Physiological urinary excretion is observed. Cystic biliary atresia (CBA). (**c**–**e**) US shows a cystic structure is in the right upper quadrant at the site of CBD apart from the gallbladder, irregularly elongated. The cystic dilation of the common bile duct does not involve the intrahepatic bile ducts. The cystic duct and gallbladder arise from the dilated common bile duct. (**d**–**f**) US shows the presence of a triangular cord sign in the porta hepatis and the enlargement of the hepatic artery diameter. The portal flow is reduced. Choledochal cyst in the newborn may be associated with atresia of the distal common bile duct; CBA is an uncommon variant of BA in which prognosis may be relatively favorable but liable to misdiagnosis as CDC. It is classified into three types according to the Japanese classification system based on the atretic segment of bile duct into type 1 (distal atresia), type 2 (proximal atresia), and type 3 (complete atresia). The cyst can occur anywhere along the atretic segment and is proximal to atresia in types 1 and 2 and distal to it in type 3

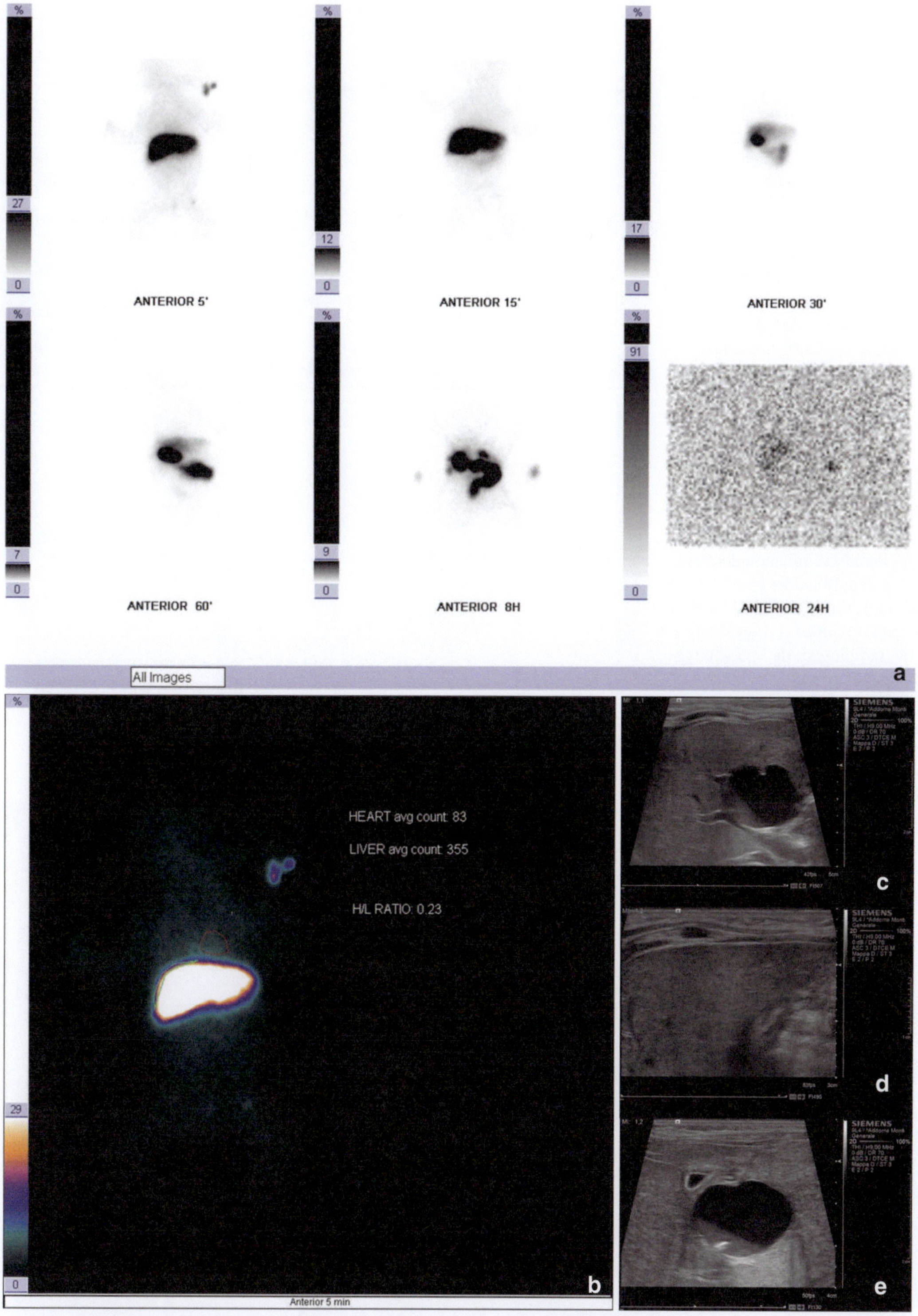

Fig. 19.6 (**a**, **b**) Time-sequential static images are performed up to 4 h after tracer administration showing intense and homogeneous hepatic uptake of tracer with normal heart/liver ratio at 5 min. By visual imaging evaluation, a photon-deficient area in the porta hepatis is detected with progressive biliary tracer filling up to the late image (performed at 8 h) and subsequent decreased activity at 24 h. Tracer transit in the bowel is observed at 30 min after tracer administration, whereas gallbladder was not clearly seen, probably due to the compression of the large choledochal cysts. Physiological urinary excretion is observed. According to the ultrasound scan, the nuclear medicine finding is compatible with choledochal cysts. (**c**, **d**) US scans: dilated intrahepatic ducts and normal gallbladder above the cyst demonstrate the continuity with the bile duct. Type I choledochal cyst: cyst is associated with sludge deposits. (**e**) US: treatment of choice is complete excision of the involved portion of the extrahepatic bile duct; a Roux-en-Y hepaticojejunostomy is performed to restore biliary–enteric continuity. Postoperative follow-up was uneventful, and US showed normal appearance of liver after hepaticojejunostomy

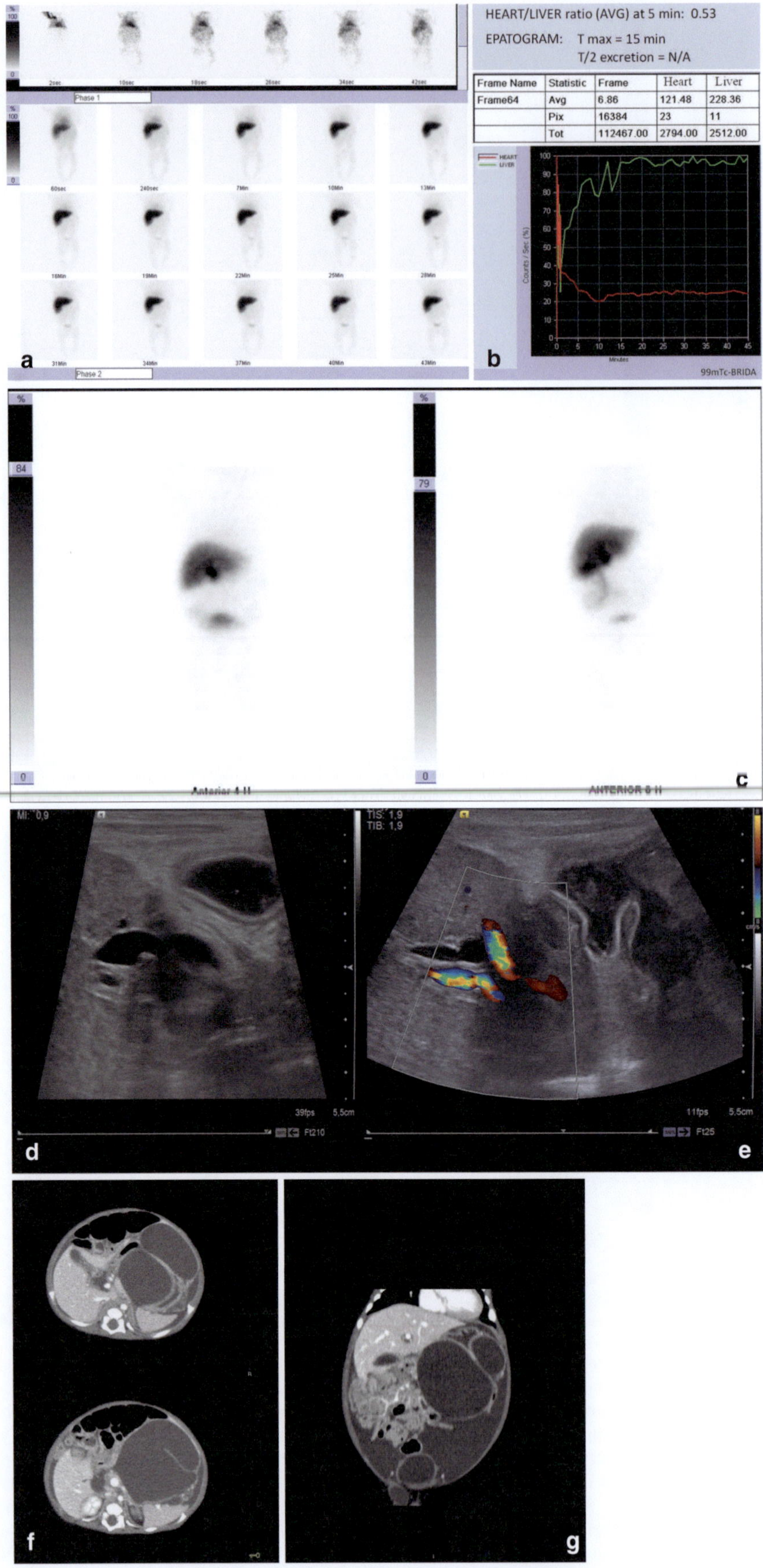

Fig. 19.7 (**a**, **b**) Dynamic study showed intense and homogeneous hepatic uptake of tracer with normal heart/liver ratio at 5 min. Qualitative images and time/activity curves analysis revealed abnormal parenchymal transit time with no evidence of biliary activity corresponding to extrahepatic bile ducts or intestinal region up to 45 min of dynamic study. (**c**) Static images at 4 and 6 h demonstrate biliary tracer stasis corresponding to fusiform dilatation of extrahepatic bile ducts without evidence of transit in the bowel. Biliary activity is also observed in the lower right quadrant (likely in peritoneal cavity) that increases in the last static image with evidence of tracer biliary stasis corresponding to drainage tube. (**d**, **e**): US scanning is the initial screening examination of choice in patients with choledochal cysts. Type-IC cysts are smooth fusiform dilations of the entire extrahepatic bile duct, usually extending from the pancreatic–biliary junction to the intrahepatic biliary tree. Ultrasound examination detects periportal edema and gallbladder and coledochal wall thickening. The intrahepatic biliary ducts are slightly dilated. Depending on the skill of the radiologist, the specific type or class of choledochal cyst may be identified. (**f**, **g**) Axial and coronal CT scans shows compartmentalized accumulation of fluid in the peritoneal cavity. CT is useful in detecting a large amount of ascitic fluid. Ultrasound examination is an invaluable guide for localizing a safe and useful site for paracentesis

presence of hepatic lesion with significant increased dimension (maximum axial diameter of 2.8 cm). The newborn presented good clinical condition even if jaundice with high indirect bilirubin component was present (6.7 vs. 0.28 mg/dL total vs direct respectively). Two further abdominal ultrasounds were performed showing a dimensional increase of hepatic lesion (up to 4.3 × 3 × 3 cm) corresponding to the hepatic segments VIII, V, and IV. No evidence of pale stools was reported. Alpha-1 fetoprotein level was normal for age. Hepatobiliary scintigraphy was performed to rule out the biliary origin of the lesion by biliary drainage evaluation, but no evidence of biliary tracer uptake was observed corresponding to the hepatic lesion detected by ultrasound scan.

In the following years, the child remained asymptomatic, and a strict sonographic follow-up revealed stable morphological features of the lesion, excluding (up to the last clinical control) surgical treatment indications (Fig. 19.8).

Case 19.9 Hepatobiliary Scintigraphy in Liver Disease Assessment of Children with Cystic Fibrosis and Signs of Cirrhotic Evolution

A 9-year-old boy with cystic fibrosis had a full hepatological review for assessment of his liver disease. The child was in poor clinical conditions presenting severe cirrhosis associated with chronic liver failure with signs of portal hypertension, protein synthesis defects, and mixed hyperbilirubinemia. Hepatobiliary scintigraphy was part of the assessment, and the result was in keeping with the previous laboratory, clinical, and radiological evaluations of severe chronic liver disease with signs of cirrhotic evolution. The patient was scheduled for liver transplantation (Fig. 19.9).

Case 19.10 Hepatobiliary Scintigraphy in Biliary Drainage Assessment of Children with Hepatic Angiomatosis and Intractable Pruritus

A 13-year-old girl with cutaneous and hepatic angiomatosis at birth. By interferon treatment, she had regression of dermal component but persistence of hepatic impairment. The child was clinically followed up with periodical blood analysis and ultrasonography scans until the age of 11 when itching appeared without any response to medical treatment. Hepatobiliary scintigraphy was performed showing moderately reduced liver function and biliary stasis secondary to intrahepatic bile ducts compression and distortion by vascular malformation. The girl underwent liver transplantation with an uneventful follow-up. Biopsy performed at 5 years after transplantation did not show any significant abnormalities Fig. 19.10.

Case 19.11 Hepatobiliary Scintigraphy in Biliary Drainage Assessment of Children with Congenital Bile Duct Paucity and Relapse of Intractable Pruritus After Internal Biliary Diversion Treatment

A 12-year-old girl with progressive intrahepatic cholestasis type II (PFIC II, secondary to congenital bile duct paucity detected by biopsy) underwent internal biliary diversion (direct biliary–enteric bypass) because of intractable pruritus after all medications failed to control the symptom. Soon after surgery, she clinically improved; however, after 12 months, pruritus was intense as much as before. A hepatobiliary scintigraphy was performed to investigate biliary drainage and in particular gallbladder biliary excretion into the diversion (bowel loop) to rule out obstruction as surgical complications (Fig. 19.11).

Case 19.12 Hepatobiliary Scintigraphy in Biliary Drainage Assessment of Children Underwent Liver Transplantation with Suspect of Biliary Stasis

A 2-year-old boy with liver transplantation for cryptogenic cirrhosis. After liver transplantation, he had constant increase of cholestasis indices with suspect of biliary stasis. Hepatobiliary scintigraphy was performed to rule out obstruction as surgical complications by biliary drainage assessment (Fig. 19.12).

Case 19.13

A 10-year-old boy with LLA and hepatic GVHD. Laboratory examination showed elevated total bilirubin (54.4 mg/dL), with an increased conjugated portion, with elevated Ggt, and liver enzyme. Hepatobiliary scintigraphy was performed in relation to clinical and radiological suspicion of bilioportal fistula (Fig. 19.13).

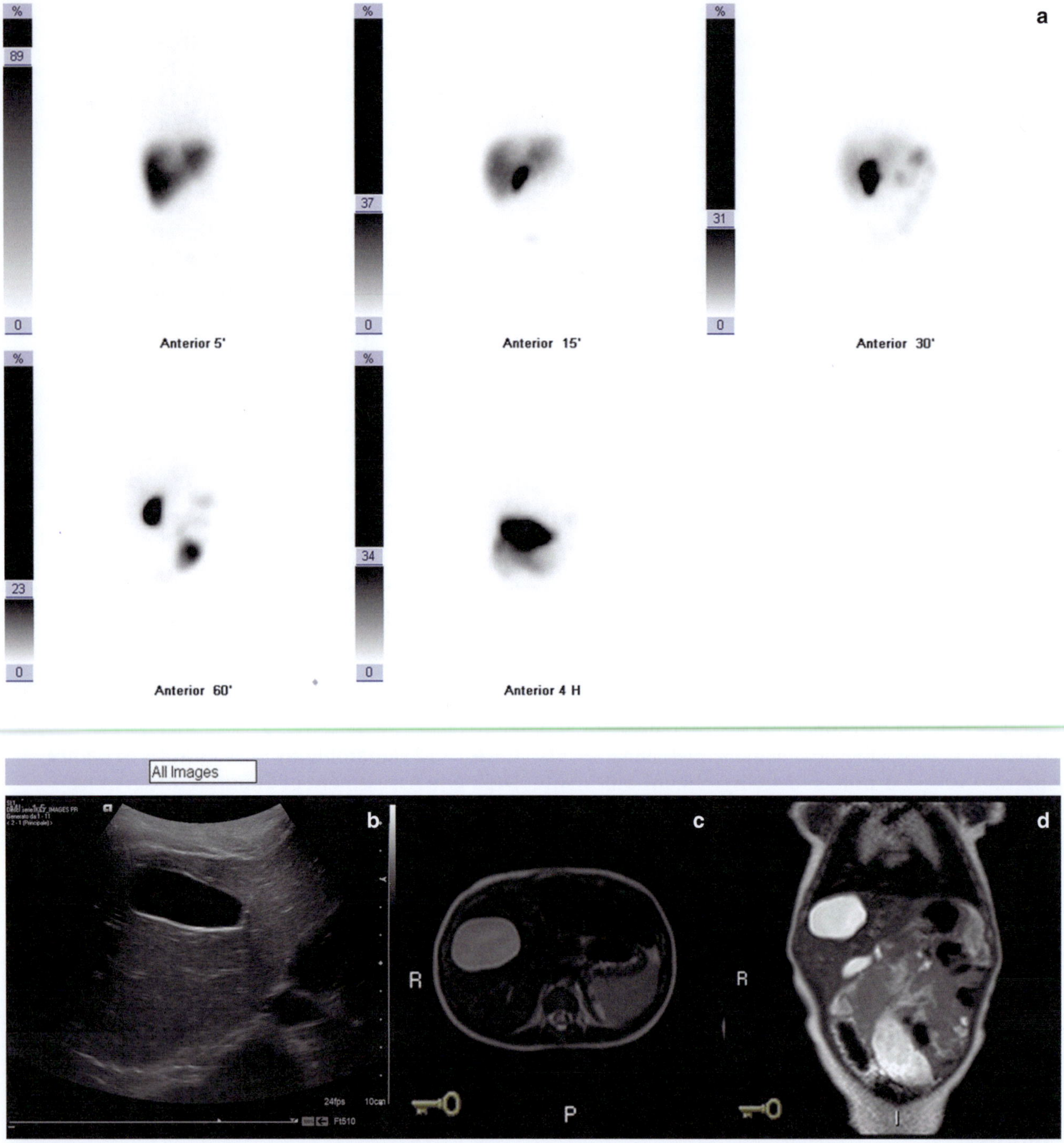

Fig. 19.8 (**a**) Time-sequential static images are performed up to 4 h after tracer administration showing intense hepatic uptake of tracer. Intraparenchymal liver distribution is not homogeneous with evidence of photon-deficient area in VIII, V, and IV segments, without subsequent biliary tracer filling up to the last image (performed at 4 h due to complete hepatocytes tracer clearance). Tracer is visualized in the gallbladder at 15 min, and transit in the bowel is observed at 30 min after tracer administration. A mild biliary tracer activity is evident in the upper left abdominal quadrant, as for biliary reflux from the duodenum into the stomach. (**b**) US examination shows rounded anechoic cyst in VIII segment of the liver with subtle wall. (**c**, **d**) Axial and coronal plane T2-weighted MRI high-intensity cyst lying along without communicating with biliary tree

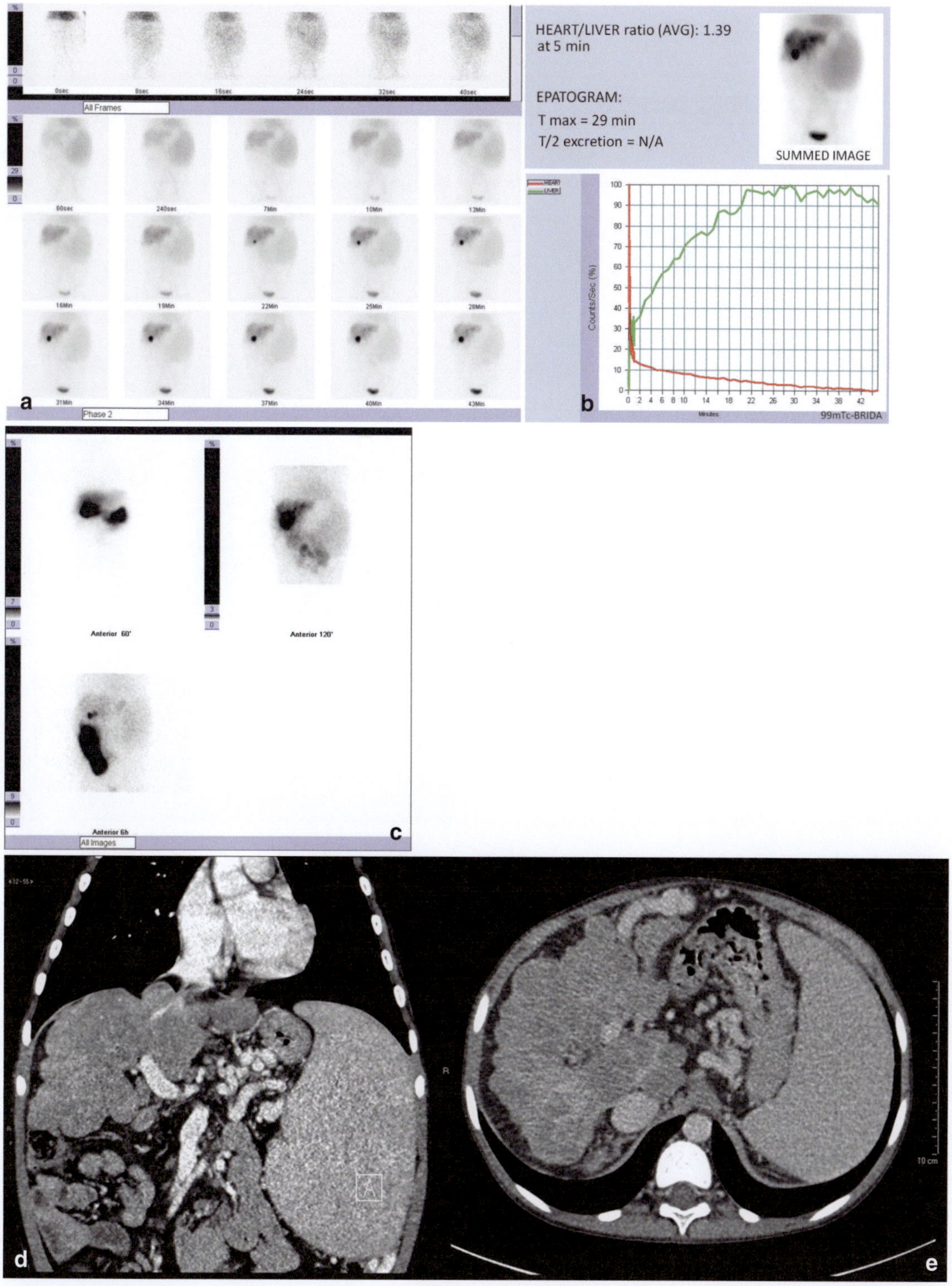

Fig. 19.9 (**a**, **b**) Dynamic study shows small liver with irregular margins and poor hepatocytes uptake of tracer (confirmed by heart/liver ratio at 5 min higher than normal). Intraparenchymal liver distribution is not homogeneous with evidence of multiple areas devoid of tracer due to cirrhotic nodules. Time/activity curves analysis reveals slow hepatocytes extraction, abnormal parenchymal transit time (T/2 > 20), and poor biliary tracer excretion. Tracer is visualized in the gallbladder at 22 min without evidence of transit in the bowel up to 45 min of dynamic study registration. (**c**) Static images performed at 1, 2, and 6 h demonstrate delayed but quite complete biliary tracer excretion from the gallbladder to the bowel. *Cirrhosis in FC.* (**d**, **e**) CT: coronal and axial scans show macronodular cirrhosis and the changes secondary to portal hypertension. The gastrointestinal manifestations of cystic fibrosis are primarily caused by the resultant abnormally viscous luminal secretions. Liver disease is the third leading cause of death in patients with cystic fibrosis (CF). Obstruction of the small intrahepatic biliary ducts induces ductal proliferation and hyperplasia, and that together with periductal inflammation results in fibrosis. Focal biliary cirrhosis, characterized by focal portal fibrosis and cholestasis, is pathognomonic of CF-related liver disease

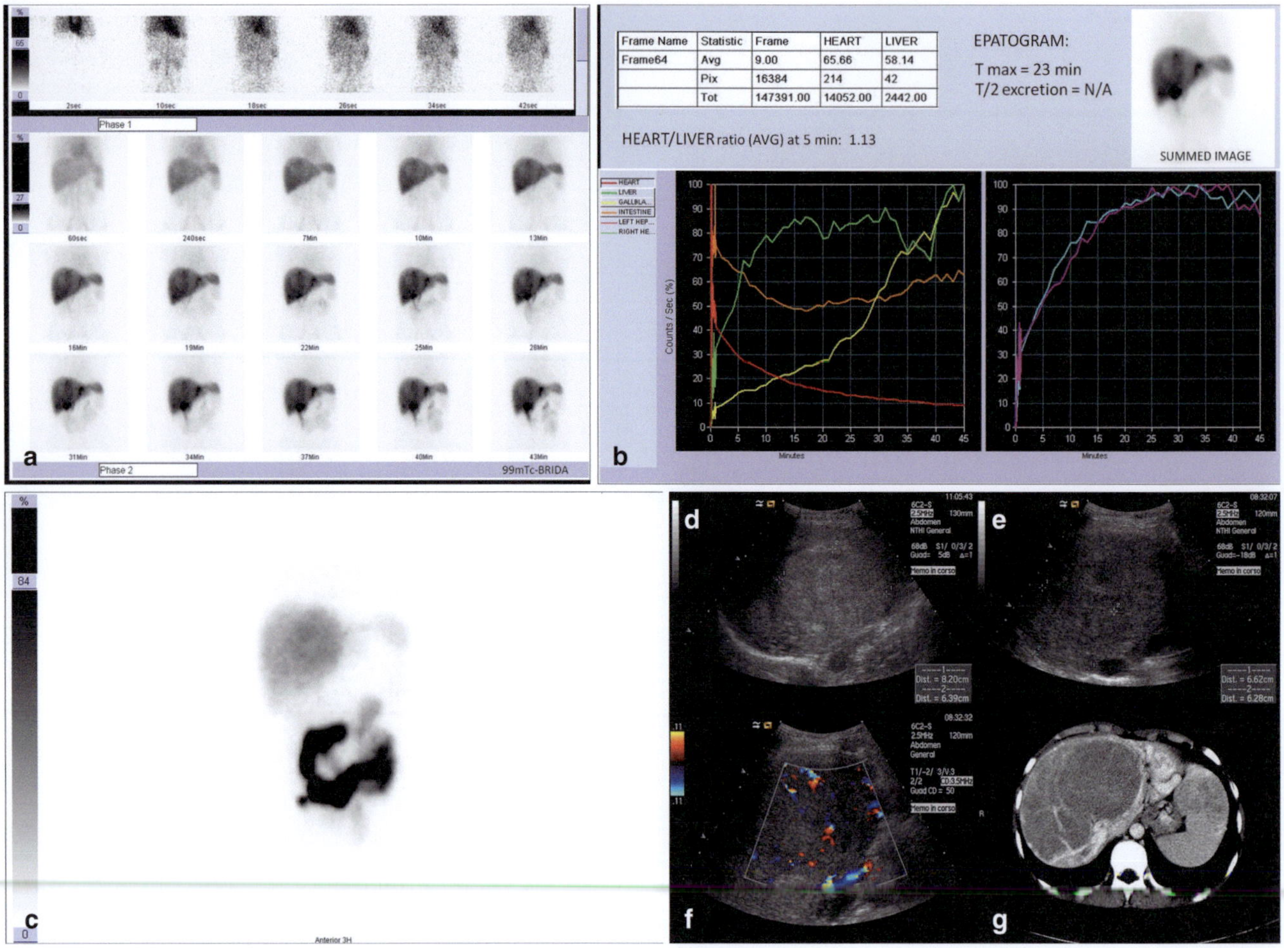

Fig. 19.10 (**a**, **b**) Dynamic study shows moderately reduced liver uptake of tracer with heart/liver ratio at 5 min higher than normal. Intraparenchymal liver tracer distribution is not homogeneous with evidence of two wide areas devoid of tracer due to vascular malformation detected by radiological imaging. Time/activity curves analysis reveals moderately slow hepatocytes extraction (T_{max} = 23 min), abnormal parenchymal transit time (T/2 > 20), and poor biliary tracer excretion. Multiple areas of biliary stasis are detectable in the dome of the liver (between the two areas devoid of tracer), in the left hepatic lobe (corresponding to the left biliary duct that appears irregularly distorted), in the inferior and lateral parts of right hepatic lobe (corresponding to V–VI liver segments). Tracer is belatedly visualized in the gallbladder at 25 min with evidence of transit in the bowel during the dynamic study registration. A mild biliary tracer activity is evident in the upper left abdominal quadrant, as for biliary reflux from the duodenum into the stomach. (**c**) Static image performed at 3 h demonstrates good biliary tracer excretion in the bowel. (**d**, **e**) US examination shows changes of the parenchymal structure with multiple intrahepatic nodules becoming identifiable, widespread throughout the whole liver (two large masses in the right liver associated with multiple small lesions). (**f**) Color Doppler: the hepatic nodules were heterogeneous and hypervascularized, and the diagnostic of multiple hemangiomas was evoked. (**g**) Angio-CT (*left*) showing a progression of the lesions in size with most lesions having merged together in the central area of the liver, replacing most of the normal liver parenchyma with the latter remaining areas being spread in periphery

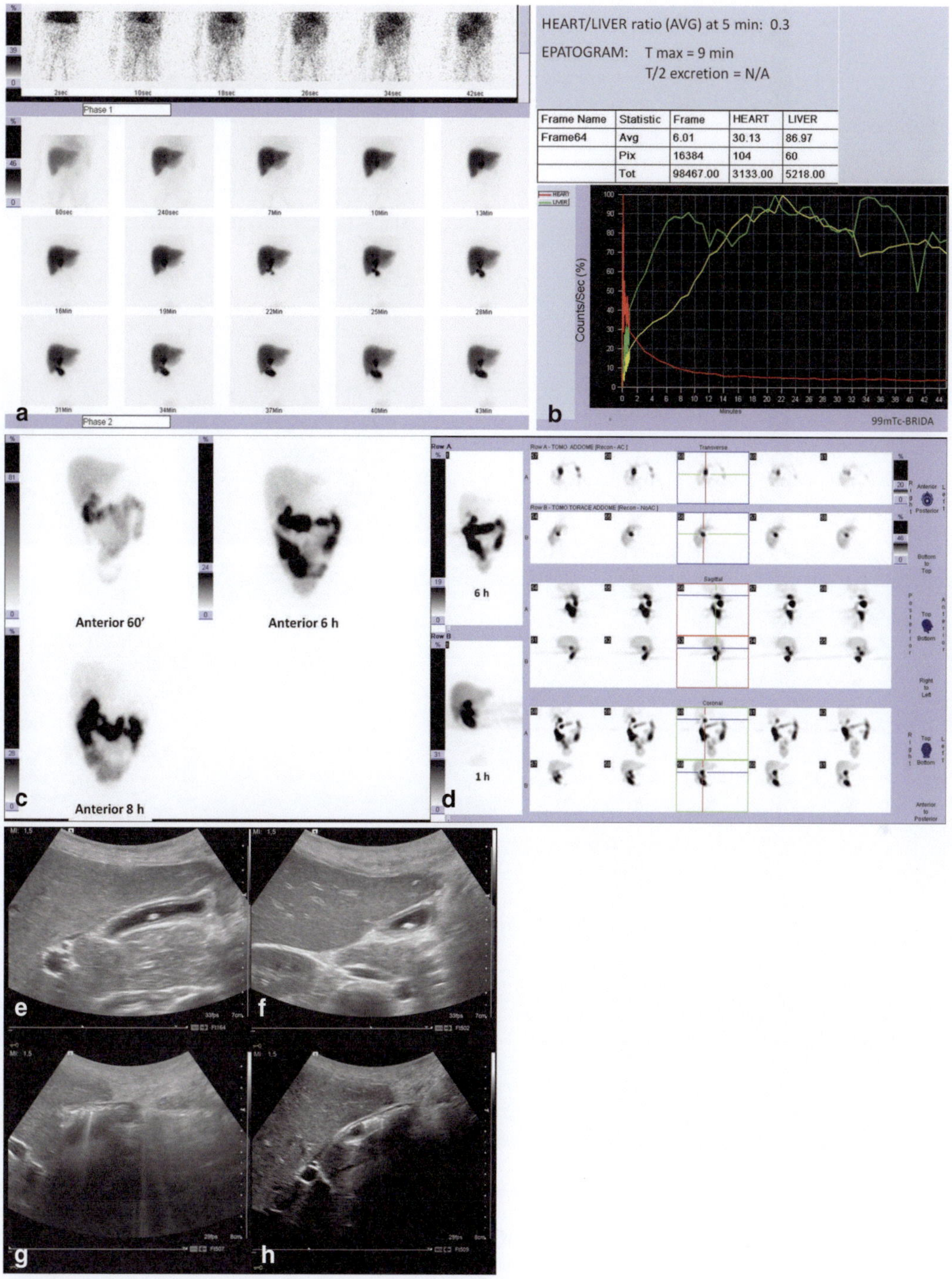

Fig. 19.11 (**a**, **b**) Dynamic study shows intense and homogeneous hepatic uptake of tracer with normal heart/liver ratio at 5 min. Qualitative images and time/activity curves analysis reveal good hepatocytes extraction (Tmax = 9 min), abnormal parenchymal transit time with slow biliary tracer excretion. Tracer is visualized in the gallbladder in physiological time with ever-increased concentration (up to 25th min of dynamic study) and partial intestinal transit. (**c**) Static images at 6 and 8 h demonstrate evidence of biliary tracer transit in the bowel and persistence of moderate activity stasis corresponding to gallbladder. (**d**) SPECT acquisition improves biliary excretion evaluation, achieving a better visualization of gallbladder, intrahepatic and extrahepatic bile ducts, and bowel activity. SPECT images (performed at 1 and 6 h) comparison helps to perform a better biliary excretion time-analysis when persisting stasis is evident. (**e**, **f**) Ultrasonography is the "modality of choice" for differentiating between obstructive and nonobstructive causes of cholestasis. High-resolution ultrasound examination (using 9–14 MHz high frequency linear transducer) shows coarsened texture of the liver without nodular contour and bile ducts dilatation. (**g**, **h**) The current first-line therapy is bile diversion in patients with severe pruritus. This therapy appears to work by creating a relatively hydrophilic bile acid composition, thus improving bile formation. Ultrasound scans after the palliative biliary diversion procedures are useful to assess for patency and depict the cholejejunostomy with air in the lumen and no stricture or obstruction

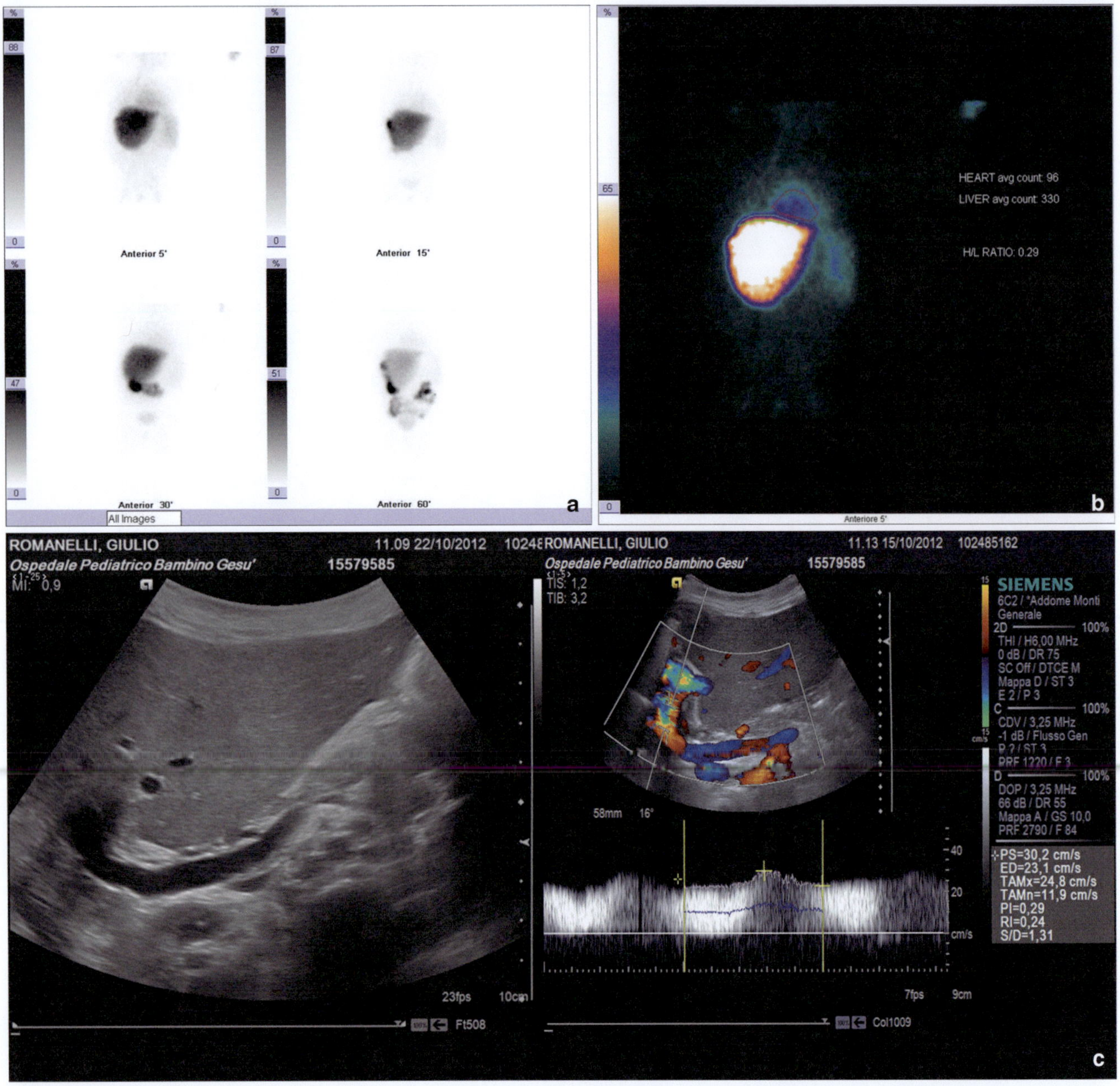

Fig. 19.12 (**a**, **b**) Time-sequential static images are performed up to 1 h after tracer administration showing intense hepatocytes uptake of tracer (confirmed by normal heart/liver ratio at 5 min) and good biliary drainage with biliary tracer excretion in the bowel. Transient tracer stasis is evident corresponding to cystic dilatation of bile duct detected by radiological imaging, without scintigraphic signs of postsurgical obstruction. *Split liver transplantation ultrasound scans.* (**c**) In children, liver transplantation often makes use of a reduced-sized or segmental transplant, which may consist of a lateral segment, left lobe, right lobe, or extended right lobe, so that the graft is size appropriate for the child. When a segmental graft is used, some mild heterogeneity may be visible on sonographic gray-scale imaging along the cut edge in the immediate postoperative period, and mild periportal edema may be evident. The vascular anastomoses typically consist of a hepatic artery end-to-end anastomosis, a portal vein end-to-end anastomosis, and a "piggy-back" side-to-side or end-to-side cavocaval anastomosis. The biliary anastomosis typically consists of a choledochojejunostomy, particularly in the setting of biliary atresia

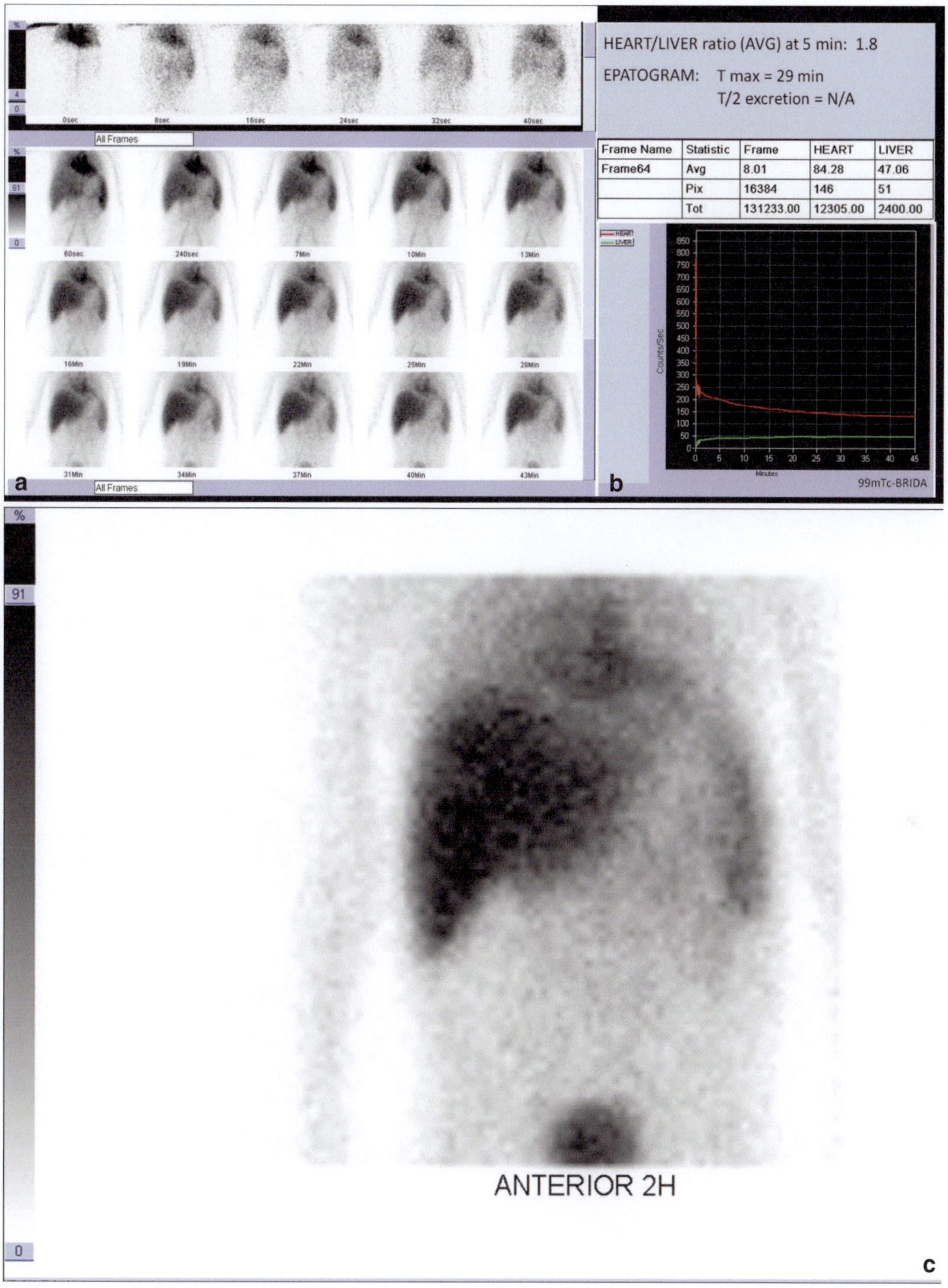

Fig. 19.13 (**a**, **b**) Dynamic study shows homogeneous hepatic uptake of tracer and high blood level up to the end of dynamic study (abnormal residual activity is evident in the heart and enlarged spleen). Heart/liver ratio at 5 min is severely higher than normal (1.8), excluding biliary atresia hypothesis. No evidence of tracer in the intestine during the initial 45 min of the dynamic study is detectable. Physiological urinary excretion is observed. (**c**) Delayed static images performed at 2 h confirm absence of tracer passage in the bowel. This scintigraphic pattern could be due to a possible bilioportal fistula if clinically suspected. (**d**, **e**) Arterioportal fistula secondary to liver biopsy performed utilizing ultrasound guidance and percutaneous procedures in Graft-versus-host disease (GVH). The arterioportal fistula was diagnosed using ultrasonography.(**f**) Color Doppler US of the liver parenchyma was performed to directly identify the APF, defined as an echo-free focal hepatic lesion, which contained fast and turbulent flow at Doppler examinations. The flow directions in the main trunk and in the two main branches of the portal vein were evaluated to verify the reversal of portal blood flow. Color Doppler US of the liver parenchyma was also performed to directly identify the APF, defined as an echo-free focal hepatic lesion, which contained fast and turbulent flow at Doppler and color Doppler US examinations. The arterioportal fistula was treated with endovascular percutaneous procedures. Color Doppler examination in GVH shows bowel wall thickening with increase of neovascularization in the early stages of gastrointestinal (GI) acute GVHD

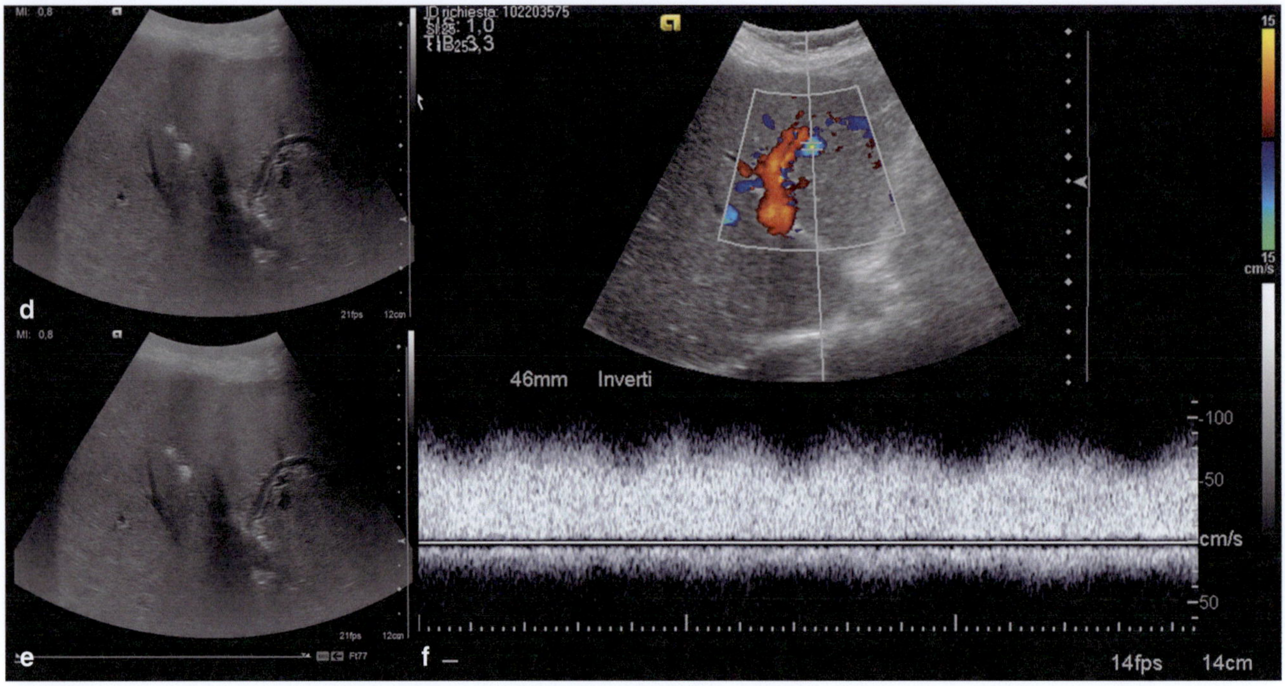

Fig. 19.13 (continued)

Bibliography

1. ^{99m}Tc-mebrofenin (^{99m}Tc-BRIDA): summary of product characteristics
2. Fogelman I, Maisey MN, Clarke SEM. "An Atlas of clinical nuclear medicine" (Second Edition). Liver and Spleen. Chapter 8. 577–85.
3. Garganese MC, Knafelz D. "Manuale SIGENP di gastroenterologia ed epatologia pediatrica" (Il pensiero scientifico editore Ed 2014) Chapter 24. 104.
4. Treves ST, Grand RJ. Pediatric Nuclear Medicine (Springer Third Edition 2007). Liver and Spleen. Chapter 9. 192–208.

20 Rheumatology

Fabrizio De Benedetti and Antonella Insalaco

20.1 Introduction

Skeletal disorders can be grouped by their etiology and pathophysiology into a variety of entities, including metabolic diseases, tumors, matrix disorders, and inflammatory conditions. The pathophysiological spectrum of chronic inflammatory disorders of bone tissue ranges from autoimmune diseases to diseases which present with autoinflammatory characteristics [31]. In general, autoinflammatory diseases are characterized by chronic inflammation without evidence of autoimmunity (e.g., autoantibodies or autoreactive T cells) and may affect various tissues, including the skeletal system [28]. Autoinflammatory bone disorders result from a dysregulation of the innate immune system with subsequent inflammatory cellular infiltration of the bone, increased osteoclast activity, osteolysis, and bone remodeling [9, 15]. Chronic/recurrent noninfectious osteomyelitis is the common denominator of all autoinflammatory bone diseases. The recurrent disease course in the absence of microorganisms at the site of inflammation and the lack of high-titer autoantibodies and/or autoreactive T lymphocytes have led to the inclusion of this disease in the group of autoinflammatory conditions.

Sporadic chronic nonbacterial osteomyelitis is the most common disease subtype. It is an inflammatory, noninfectious disorder of the musculoskeletal system that primarily affects children. Its hallmark is recurring episodes of sterile osteomyelitis [12, 14, 15, 22, 38, 44]. Multiple names are used in the literature to describe this disorder; these include chronic nonbacterial osteomyelitis (CNO), chronic recurrent multifocal osteomyelitis (CRMO) in cases with extended multifocal involvement (often symmetric) and synovitis, acne, pustulosis, hyperostosis, and osteitis syndrome (SAPHO) which usually manifests in adolescent and adult patients. In the pediatric literature, the terms CRMO and CNO are often used interchangeably. It is still unclear if SAPHO and CRMO/CNO are the same different diseases presenting in different age groups, or if they represent the spectrum of the same disease [7, 14, 22].

20.2 Pathogenesis

The etiology of sporadic CNO is still unknown [12, 14, 15, 22, 38, 44]. For chronic CNO, infectious versus noninfectious etiology has been the subject of an intense debate; however, extensive microbiological analyses have not demonstrated a microbial pathogenesis of CNO [13]. There is an accumulating evidence for a genetic contribution to CNO disease susceptibility. The strongest evidence comes from the so-called *syndromic forms of CNO*: Majeed syndrome [8, 27], cherubism [34], hypophosphatasia [43], primary hypertrophic osteoarthropathy (PHO) [5]. In addition, chronic osteomyelitis is a typical feature of two diseases caused by mutations affecting the inflammasome and Il-1b activity [pyogenic arthritis, pyoderma gangrenosum, and acne (PAPA) syndrome [40], and the deficiency of IL-1 receptor antagonist (DIRA)] [1]. There is also evidence that nonsyndromic or sporadic CRMO has a genetic basis. Golla et al. [17] reported a susceptibility locus on human chromosome 18q21.3-18q22 in a small German CNO cohort. Several reports have described families with multiple affected members or have reported a high incidence of psoriasis, inflammatory bowel disease, and other chronic inflammatory conditions in first-degree family members of individuals with CNO, which suggests that there is a significant genetic component to disease susceptibility [9, 17, 22]. Additional evidence of a possible genetic contribution to disease comes from studying the role of interleukin (IL)-10 in disease pathogenesis. One small study reported the association of CNO with polymorphism of the IL-10 promoter, and functional data suggest that IL-10 deregulation may play a role in the disease [18, 19]. Other candidate genes, including

F. De Benedetti • A. Insalaco (✉)
Unit of Rheumatology, "Bambino Gesù" Children Hospital, Rome, Italy
e-mail: antonella.insalaco@opbg.net

© Springer International Publishing Switzerland 2017

M.C. Garganese, G.F.L. D'Errico (eds.), *Conventional Nuclear Medicine in Pediatrics*, DOI 10.1007/978-3-319-43181-9_20

PSTPIP1, PSTPIP2, CARD15/NOD2, and *IL1RN*, have been analyzed in small CRMO/CNO cohorts [3, 22, 30], but no definitive disease-causing mutations have been identified.

20.3 Clinical Presentation

The clinical manifestations of CNO are highly variable. CNO typically presents with bone pain that is worse at night and occurs in the presence or absence of fever [7, 21, 22]. The onset is typically insidious, and most children appear well. Swelling and warmth can occur in the affected areas, but there may be no objective findings on physical examination. One to twenty sites can be affected at one time. The disease may follow a chronic or recurrent disease course. In childhood and adolescence, CNO predominantly affects the metaphyses of long bones, the pelvis, clavicles, and vertebral bodies [7, 24, 38]. However, lesions can occur at almost any site of the skeleton, including the mandible and the small bones of the hands and feet, except for the neurocranium. Extraosseous organs including skin, eyes, gastrointestinal tract, and lungs can be affected. Current estimates suggest that approximately 25 % of individuals with CNO have manifestations involving organ/systems other than bone. Most frequently palmoplantar pustulosis (PPP) [33], psoriasis vulgaris [26], pyoderma gangrenosum, sweet syndrome, or inflammatory bowel disease (Crohn disease more so than ulcerative colitis, but also celiac disease) [15, 21, 22, 30]. Other less-frequent associations include acne, generalized pustulosis, sclerosing cholangitis, arthritis, and sacroiliac joint involvement. Anecdotal reports of associations with Takayasu arteritis [25], antineutrophil cytoplasmic antibody-positive vasculitis [1, 3, 5, 7, 8, 12–14, 17–19, 21, 22, 27, 30, 34, 38, 40, 43, 44], parenchymal lung disease [35], or dermatomyositis [10].

20.4 Diagnosis

CNO is a diagnosis of exclusion [14, 17, 22]. Differential diagnoses include infections (septic osteomyelitis, typical and atypical mycobacterial infections, etc.), malignancies (primary bone tumors and leukemia/lymphoma), benign bone tumors (osteoid osteoma), trauma, metabolic disorders (including hypophosphatasia), other autoinflammatory disorders (DIRA, PAPA, cherubism, etc.), osteonecrosis, and osteopetrosis. Laboratory investigations may reveal mild elevations in white blood cell count and in inflammatory parameters (C-reactive protein, ESR), but often these abnormalities are absent in CNO patients [7, 22, 38]. Cultures of blood and bone are invariably negative, and sophisticated assays to identify evidence of a microbial etiology have been unsuccessful. Autoantibodies (antinuclear antibodies, rheumatoid factor), as well as carriage of the HLAB27 allele, have the same prevalence in CNO patients when compared to healthy individuals. At present, no specific biomarkers are available for the diagnosis or prediction of flares in CNO patients. A crucial role, in the diagnosis of this condition, is provided by imaging. Radiology findings can be quite variable. Inflammatory lesions in CNO may be detected by conventional radiographs as radiolucent, osteolytic lesions with a sclerotic edge. Clavicular lesions and mandibular lesions often have a more prominent sclerotic appearance [24] (Fig. 20.1). Vertebral involvement can lead to collapse with subsequent vertebra plana or other deformity [21, 24, 38] (Figs. 20.2 and 20.3). It should be pointed out that plain X-rays can be negative in the early stages of the disease [24]. Since CNO is a systemic disorder that can affect multiple skeletal sites, whole-body imaging techniques (Tc-99 bone scintigraphy or MRI) provide major contribution to the initial diagnostic approach, as well as during follow-up (Fig. 20.4). MRI is particularly sensitive in (a) detecting bone edema during the early stages of inflammation, before osteolysis and/or sclerosis can be detected (b) showing adjacent inflammatory reactions, e.g., periostitis or synovitis, and (c) determining the extent of soft tissue involvement (Figs 20.5 and 20.6), [11, 32]. Although no formal studies are available, in order to confirm diagnosis, a biopsy of the bone lesion is, at present, required. Bone biopsies show signs of inflammation in the absence of infection. The composition of cellular infiltrates at the sites of inflammation depends on the "age" of biopsied lesions. Neutrophils are predominant in early lesions, whereas lymphocytes, macrophages, and plasma cells can be detected during the later course of the inflammatory process. Osteolysis with concomitant sclerosis and fibrosis is regarded as a later stage of the inflammatory lesion [13].

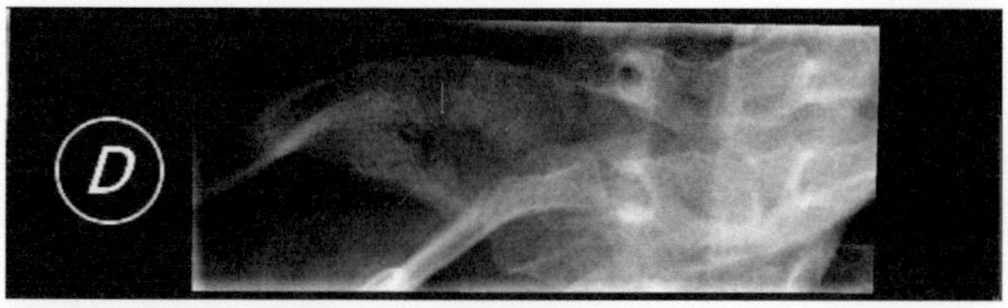

Fig. 20.1 Thickening of the clavicle (proximal part) with marked apposition and central osteolytic lesion with irregular edges

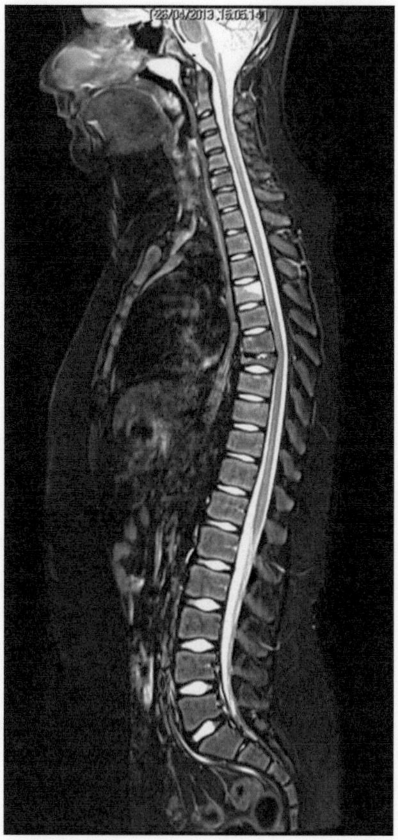

Fig. 20.2 MRI shows initial inflammatory edema of the D4 vertebral body, and prominent collapse of D7 vertebral body (late lesion), as well as initial reduction of height and anterior wedging of D8, D9 e D10

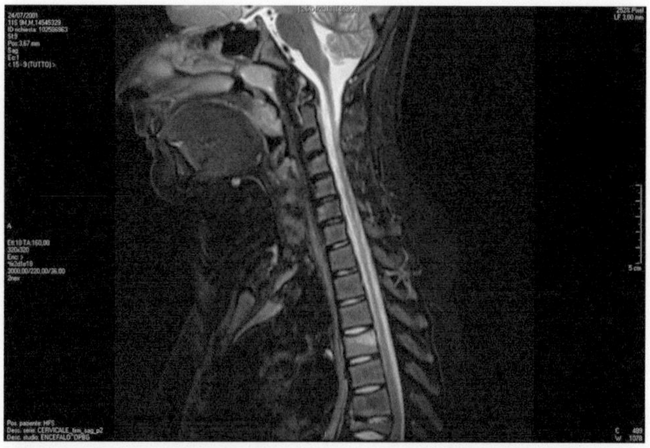

Fig. 20.3 MRI shows initial inflammatory edema of the D4 vertebral body, and prominent collapse of D7 vertebral body (late lesion), as well as initial reduction of height and anterior wedging of D8, D9 e D10

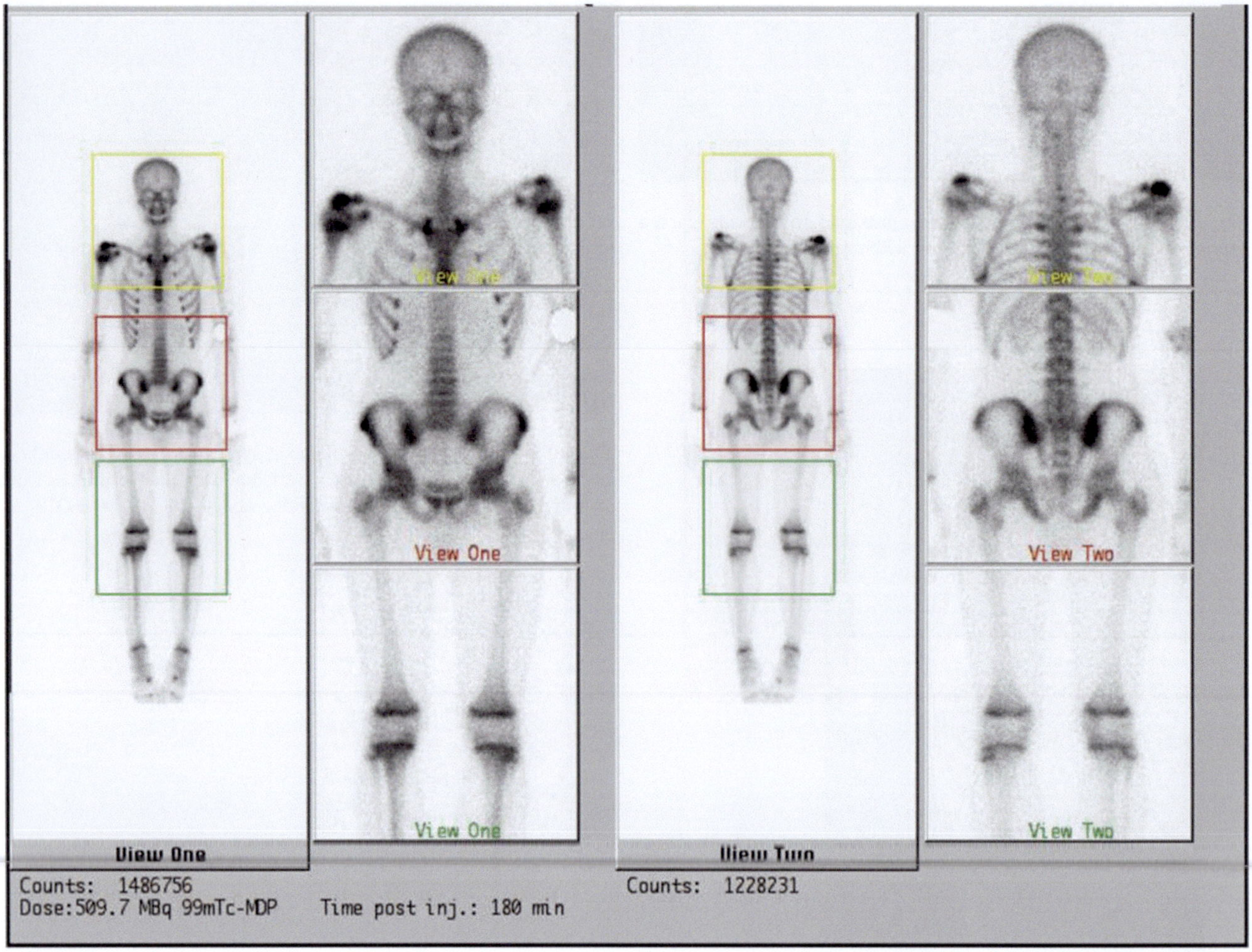

Fig. 20.4 Tc-99 bone scintigraphy shows increased uptake of the right shoulder, the right ileus, of the sternum and of the sternoclavicular joints

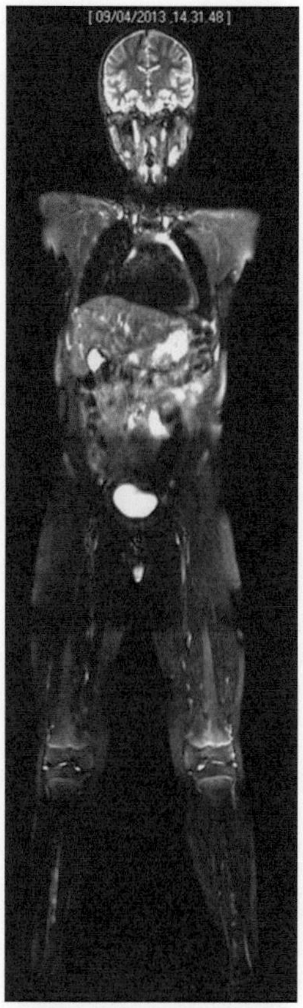

Fig. 20.5 Whole-body MRI shows symmetrical bilateral involvement of tibial diaphysis

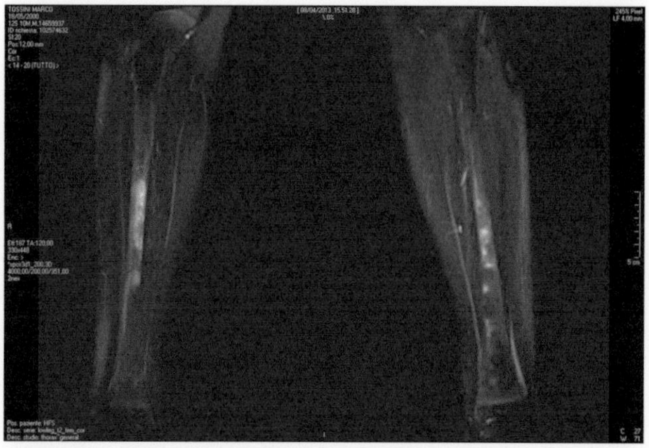

Fig. 20.6 Whole-body MRI shows symmetrical bilateral involvement of tibial diaphysis

20.5 Treatment

Generally accepted treatment protocols for CNO do not exist, and the treatment of CNO has been largely empiric. A number of retrospective assessments of response to treatment in case reports or small series is available in the literature. There are a few prospective studies of response to treatment in CRMO/CNO, with no randomized trials having been performed, primarily because of the rarity of the disease. NSAIDs are commonly used as first-line treatment and provide pain reduction in most patients (reported response rates up to 80 %) [4]. Even when used chronically throughout the first year of disease, NSAIDs have been proven to be safe and considerably effective in CNO patients. However, a significant proportion of patients (varying from 20 to 60 % in the different series) requires additional treatment. Additional treatment should be considered in the presence of (a) lack of response to NSAIDs, (b) persistence of active bone lesions on imaging, and (c) lesions on structural sites (e.g., active lesion in vertebral bodies, active lesions in proximity or invading the growth plate). Second-line treatment includes short courses of oral glucocorticoids, chronic oral glucocorticoids, or classical DMARDs such as methotrexate and sulfasalazine [42]. More recently, TNF-blocking agents and bisphosphonates have been increasingly utilized. TNF-α blocking agents are the most frequently used cytokine-targeting drugs. Although TNF-α blockade has been reported in case reports and in a small series of CNO patients to improve the disease course [4, 6, 42], a significant fraction of treated patients do not benefit from this treatment. Intravenous bisphosphonates (e.g., pamidronate) have been demonstrated to reduce pain and bone inflammation in CNO patients [16, 20, 29] in a large proportion of patients. However, there might be safety concerns for long-term treatment with bisphosphonates and for their deposition in the bone matrix. Many patients who failed TNF inhibitors had a response to pamidronate, and vice versa. There is considerably less evidence pointing to a role of IL-1 blockade in CNO [2]. The optimal treatment strategy remains to be determined.

Conclusion

CNO pathogenesis is still unclear. Accumulating evidence points to a potential role of inflammasome and cytokine production deregulation [18, 19, 39]. The prominent role of interleukin-1 in the development of skin and bone manifestations in DIRA suggests a potential role for interleukin-1 in the pathophysiology of autoinflammatory bone disorders.

Bibliography

1. Aksentijevich I, Masters SL, Ferguson PJ, Dancey P, Frenkel J, van Royen-Kerkhoff A, Laxer R, Tedgård U, Cowen EW, Pham TH, Booty M, Estes JD, Sandler NG, Plass N, Stone DL, Turner ML, Hill S, Butman JA, Schneider R, Babyn P, El-Shanti HI, Pope E, Barron K, Bing X, Laurence A, Lee C-CR, Chapelle D, Clarke GI, Ohson K, Nicholson M, Gadina M, Yang B, Korman BD, Gregersen PK, van Hagen PM, Hak AE, Huizing M, Rahman P, Douek DC, Remmers EF, Kastner DL, Goldbach-Mansky R. An autoinflammatory disease with deficiency of the interleukin-1-receptor antagonist. N Engl J Med. 2009;360(23):2426–37.
2. Almeida de Jesus A, Goldbach-Mansky R. Monogenic autoinflammatory diseases:concept and clinical manifestations. Clin Immunol. 2013;147(3):155–74.
3. Beck C, Girschick HJ, Morbach H, Schwarz T, Yimam T, Frenkel J, van Gijn ME. Mutation screening of the IL-1 receptor antagonist gene in chronic non-bacterial osteomyelitis of childhood and adolescence. Clin Exp Rheumatol. 2011;29(6):1040–3.
4. Beck C, Morbach H, Beer M, Stenzel M, Tappe D, Gattenlohner S, Hofmann U, Raab P, Girschick HJ. Chronic nonbacterial osteomyelitis in childhood: prospective follow-up during the first year of anti-inflammatory treatment. Arthritis Res Ther. 2010;12:R74.
5. Castori M, Sinibaldi L, Mingarelli R, Lachman RS, Rimoin DL, Dallapiccola B. Pachydermoperiostosis: an update. Clin Genet. 2005;68:6477–86.
6. Eleftheriou D, Gerschman T, Sebire N, Woo P, Pilkington CA, Brogan PA. Biologic therapy in refractory chronic non-bacterial osteomyelitis of childhood. Rheumatology. 2010;49(8):1505–12.
7. El-Shanti HI, Ferguson PJ. Chronic recurrent multifocal osteomyelitis: a concise review and genetic update. Clin Orthop Relat Res. 2007;462:11–9.
8. Ferguson PJ. Homozygous mutations in LPIN2 are responsible for the syndrome of chronic recurrent multifocal osteomyelitis and congenital dyserythropoietic anaemia (Majeed syndrome). J Med Genet. 2005;42(7):551–7.
9. Ferguson PJ, El-Shanti HI. Autoinflammatory bone disorders. Curr Opin Rheumatol. 2007;19(5):492–8.
10. Ferguson PJ, Sandu M. Current understanding of the pathogenesis and management of chronic recurrent multifocal osteomyelitis. Curr Rheumatol Rep. 2012;14(2):130–41.
11. Fritz J, Tzaribatchev N, Claussen CD, Carrino JA, Horger MS. Chronic recurrent multifocal osteomyelitis: comparison of whole-body MR imaging with radiography and correlation with clinical and laboratory data. Radiology. 2009;252(3):842–8.
12. Gikas PD, Islam L, Aston W, Tirabosco R, Saifuddin A, Briggs TWR, Cannon SR, O'Donnell P, Jacobs B, Flanagan AM. Nonbacterial osteitis: a clinical, histopathological, and imaging study with a proposal for protocol-based management of patients with this diagnosis. J Orthop Sci. 2009;14(5):505–16.
13. Girschick HJ, Huppertz HI, Harmsen D, Krauspe R, Müller-Hermelink HK, Papadopoulos T. Chronic recurrent multifocal osteomyelitis in children: diagnostic value of histopathology and microbial testing. Hum Pathol. 1999;30(1):59–65.
14. Girschick HJ, Raab P, Surbaum S, Trusen A, Kirschner S, Schneider P, Papadopoulos T, Müller-Hermelink HK, Lipsky PE. Chronic non-bacterial osteomyelitis in children. Ann Rheum Dis. 2005;64(2):279–85.
15. Girschick HJ, Zimmer C, Klaus G, Darge K, Dick A, Morbach H. Chronic recurrent multifocal osteomyelitis: what is it and how should it be treated? Nat Clin Pract Rheumatol. 2007;3(12):733–8.
16. Gleeson H, Wiltshire E, Briody J, Hall J, Chaitow J, Sillence D, Cowell C, Munns C. Childhood chronic recurrent multifocal osteomyelitis: pamidronate therapy decreases pain and improves vertebral shape. J Rheumatol. 2008;35:707–12.
17. Golla A, Jansson A, Ramser J, Hellebrand H, Zahn R, Meitinger T, Belohradsky BH, Meindl A. Chronic recurrent multifocal osteomyelitis (CRMO): evidence for a susceptibility gene located on chromosome 18q21.3-18q22. Eur J Hum Genet. 2002;10:217–21.
18. Hamel J, Paul D, Gahr M, Hedrich CM. Pilot study: possible association of IL10 promoter polymorphisms with CRMO. Rheumatol Int. 2011. doi:10.1007/s00296-010-1768-8.

19. Hofmann SR, Schwarz T, Moller JC, Morbach H, Schnabel A, Rosen-Wolff A, Girschick HJ, Hedrich CM. Chronic non-bacterial osteomyelitis is associated with impaired Sp1 signaling, reduced IL10 promoter phosphorylation, and reduced myeloid IL-10 expression. Clin Immunol. 2011;141:317–27.
20. Hospach T, Langendoerfer M, von Kalle T, Maier J, Dannecker GE. Spinal involvement in chronic recurrent multifocal osteomyelitis (CRMO) in childhood and effect of pamidronate. Eur J Pediatr. 2010;169:1105–11.
21. Huber AM, Lam PY, Duffy CM, Yeung RS, Ditchfield M, Laxer D, Cole WG, Kerr Graham H, Allen RC, Laxer RM. Chronic recurrent multifocal osteomyelitis: clinical outcomes after more than five years of follow-up. J Pediatr. 2002;141:198–203.
22. Jansson A, Renner ED, Ramser J, Mayer A, Haban M, Meindl A, Grote V, Diebold J, Jansson V, Schneider K, Belohradsky BH. Classification of non-bacterial osteitis: retrospective study of clinical, immunological and genetic aspects in 89 patients. Rheumatology (Oxford). 2007;46(1):154–60.
23. Jesus AA, Osman M, Silva CA, Kim PW, Pham TH, Gadina M, et al. A novel mutation of IL1RN in the deficiency of interleukin-1 receptor antagonist syndrome: description of two unrelated cases from Brazil. Arthritis Rheum. 2011;63(12):4007–17.
24. Khanna G, Sato TS, Ferguson P. Imaging of chronic recurrent multifocal osteomyelitis. Radiographics. 2009;29:1159–77.
25. Kim JE, Kolh EM, Kim DK. Takayasu's arteritis presenting with focal periostitis affecting two limbs. Int J Cardiol. 1998;67:267–70.
26. Laxer RM, Shore AD, Manson D, King S, Silverman ED, Wilmot DM. Chronic recurrent multifocal osteomyelitis and psoriasis—a report of a new association and review of related disorders. Semin Arthritis Rheum. 1988;17:260–70.
27. Majeed HA, Kalaawi M, Mohanty D, Teebi AS, Tunjekar MF, al-Gharbawy F, Majeed SA, al-Gazzar AH. Congenital dyserythropoietic anemia and chronic recurrent multifocal osteomyelitis in three related children and the association with Sweet syndrome in two siblings. J Pediatr. 1989;115(5):730–4.
28. Master SL, Simon A, Aksentijevich I, Kastner DL. Horror autoinflammaticus: the molecular pathophysiology of autoinflammatory disease. Annu Rev Immunol. 2009;27(1):621–68.
29. Miettunen PM, Wei X, Kaura D, Reslan WA, Aguirre AN, Kellner JD. Dramatic pain relief and resolution of bone inflammation following pamidronate in 9 pediatric patients with persistent chronic recurrent multifocal osteomyelitis (CRMO). Pediatr Rheumatol Online J. 2009;7:2. This is a prospective analysis of response to bisophosphonates in nine children with CRMO.
30. Morbach H, Dick A, Beck C, Stenzel M, Muller-Hermelink HK, Raab P, Girschick HJ. Association of chronic non-bacterial osteomyelitis with Crohn's disease but not with CARD15 gene variants. Rheumatol Int. 2010;30:617–21.
31. Morbach H, Hedrich CM, Beer M, Girschick HJ. Autoinflammatory bone disorders. Clin Immunol. 2013;147(3):185–96.
32. Morbach H, Schneider P, Schwarz T, Hofmann C, Raab P, Neubauer H, Düren C, Beer M, Girschick HJ. Comparison of magnetic resonance imaging and 99mTechnetium-labelled methylene diphosphonate bone scintigraphy in the initial assessment of chronic non-bacterial osteomyelitis of childhood and adolescents. Clin Exp Rheumatol. 2012;30(4):578–82.
33. Paller AS, Pachman L, Rich K, Esterly NB, Gonzalez-Crussi F. Pustulosis palmaris et plantaris: its association with chronic recurrent multifocal osteomyelitis. J Am Acad Dermatol. 1985;12:927–30.
34. Papadaki ME, Lietman SA, Levine MA, Olsen BR, Kaban LB, Reichenberge EJ. Cherubism: best clinical practice. Orphanet J Rare Dis. 2012;7(1):S6.
35. Ravelli A, Marseglia GL, Viola S, Ruperto N, Martini A. Chronic recurrent multifocal osteomyelitis with unusual features. Acta Paediatr. 1995;84:222–5.
36. Reddy S, Jia S, Geoffrey R, Lorier R, Suchi M, Broeckel U, et al. An autoinflammatory disease due to homozygous deletion of the IL1RN locus. N Engl J Med. 2009;360(23):2438–44.
37. Schnellbacher C, Ciocca G, Menendez R, Aksentijevich I, Goldbach-Mansky R, Duarte AM, et al. Deficiency of interleukin-1 receptor antagonist responsive to anakinra. Pediatr Dermatol. 2012:1–2.
38. Schultz C, Holterhus PM, Seidel A, Jonas S, Barthel M, Kruse K, Bucsky P. Chronic recurrent multifocal osteomyelitis in children. Pediatr Infect Dis J. 1999;18(11):1008–13.
39. Scianaro R, Insalaco A, Bracci-Laudiero L, Teti A, De Benedetti F, Prencipe G. Deregulation of the IL-1β axis in the monocyte-macrophage lineage in chronic recurrent multifocal osteomyelitis. Pediatr Rheumatol Online J. 2014;12:30.
40. Smith EJ, Allantaz F, Bennett L, Zhang D, Gao X, Wood G, Kastner DL, Punaro M, Aksentijevich I, Pascual V, Wise CA. Clinical, molecular, and genetic characteristics of PAPA syndrome: a review. Curr Genomics. 2010;11(7):519–27.
41. Stenerson M, Dufendach K, Aksentijevich I, Brady J, Austin J, Reed AM. The first reported case of compound heterozygous IL1RN mutations causing deficiency of the interleukin-1 receptor antagonist. Arthritis Rheum. 2011;63(12):4018–22.
42. Twilt M, Laxer RM. Clinical care of children with sterile bone inflammation. Curr Opin Rheumatol. 2011;23:424–31.
43. Whyte MP. Physiological role of alkaline phosphatase explored in hypophosphatasia. Ann N Y Acad Sci. 2010;1192:190–200.
44. Wipff J, Adamsbaum C, Kahan A, Job-Deslandre C. Chronic recurrent multifocal osteomyelitis. Joint Bone Spine. 2011;78(6):555–60.

Benign Skeletal Disease: Bone Infection and Inflammation

21

Maria Felicia Villani, Milena Pizzoferro, Antonella Insalaco, Andrzej Krzysztofiak, and Maria Carmen Garganese

21.1 Study Technique and Interpretation

21.1.1 Three-Phase Bone Scintigraphy

Phase I (angiographic phase): a dynamic scan is obtained after an intravenous bolus injection of 99mTc-methylene diphosphonate (MDP)

Phase II ("blood pool" or early phase): a static scan is acquired over 5 min after injection.

Phase III ("bone metabolism" or delayed phase): a static scan of the affected site is taken 2–3 h after injecting the radiotracer, followed by a whole-body acquisition in all patients.

A single photon emission tomography (SPECT) was also performed, when required.

The administered activity of the radiotracer was adjusted to the patient's weight, according to the EANM dosage card and Italian regulations (Fig. 21.1).

21.1.2 Dual Phase Bone Scintigraphy

Early whole-body scan ("blood pool" whole-body scan): whole-body acquisition is performed about 5 min after intravenous injection of 99mTc-MDP.

Delayed whole-body scan ("bone metabolism" whole-body scan): whole-body acquisition is performed about 2–3 h later and completed with spot views and/or SPECT images of interested segments, when required.

SPECT images are also manually fused with CT and/or MRI when available.

21.2 Teaching Cases

Case 21.1: Three-Phase Bone Scintigraphy in Arthritis

A 10-year-old boy referred to our institution for fever and pain in right shoulder. C-reactive protein was 16.02 mg/dl (normal value <0.5), but plain radiography of right shoulder did not show any lesion in bone and/or joint.

Suspecting an arthritis, a bone scan was performed, and scintigraphy detected a subacute arthritis (Fig. 21.2).

Case 21.2: Bone Scintigraphy in Sacroiliitis

Normal distribution in hips and pelvis and scintigraphic patterns of sacroilitis.

Case 21.3: Scintigraphic Pattern of Osteomyelitis of Left Tibia in an 11-Year-Old Boy

Fever and pain in the left ankle region developed in an 11-year-old boy who did not have prior trauma. For several days, he presented limping. Plain radiography showed structural alterations of left tibia and swelling of the soft tissue around malleolus.

Laboratory investigations showed white blood cell count of 11.720/mm^3 and a C-reactive protein of 2.23 mg/dl (normal value <0.5). Blood culture was negative.

M.F. Villani • M. Pizzoferro
Nuclear Medicine Unit, Imaging Department, "Bambino Gesù" Children Hospital, Rome, Italy

A. Insalaco (✉)
Unit of Rheumatology, "Bambino Gesù" Children Hospital, Rome, Italy
e-mail: antonella.insalaco@opbg.net

A. Krzysztofiak
Unit of Infettivology, "Bambino Gesù" Children Hospital, Rome, Italy

M.C. Garganese
Department of Diagnostic Imaging-Nuclear Medicine, IRCCS Bambino Gesù Paediatric Hospital, Rome, Italy

© Springer International Publishing Switzerland 2017

M.C. Garganese, G.F.L. D'Errico (eds.), *Conventional Nuclear Medicine in Pediatrics*, DOI 10.1007/978-3-319-43181-9_21

A three-phase bone scintigraphy was performed in order to exclude osteomyelitis in interested region and in other skeletal segments; the examination showed left tibial osteomyelitis and tibiotarsal arthritis; therefore, the boy carried specific antibiotic therapy and discharged after 3 weeks in improved clinical conditions (Fig. 21.3).

Case 21.4: Arthritis of Left Knee Complicated by Ipsilateral Distal Femoral Osteomyelitis in Child with *Staphylococcus aureus* Sepsis

A 3-year-old child presented fever and pain in left knee. Laboratory investigations showed white blood cell count of 9.390/mm^3, a C-reactive protein of 4.53 mg/dl (normal value <0.5), and an erythrocyte sedimentation rate of 60 mm/h (normal value <20 mm/h).

A bone scintigraphy was then asked in order to verify the presence of osteomyelitis in interested region and/or in other skeletal segments and showed arthritis of left knee complicated by ipsilateral distal femoral osteomyelitis.

MRI findings were indicative in the first hypothesis to Brodie abscess. Blood cultures were positive for *Staphylococcus aureus*.

She started therapy with intravenous antibiotic, with gradual improvement up to resolution of pain.

The clinical course was complicated by a Rotavirus enteritis. She was discharged in good general condition with follow-up program (Fig. 21.4).

Case 21.5: Bone Scintigraphy in *Staphylococcus aureus* Sepsis Complicated by Myositis and Osteomyelitis of Left Femur

Fever and pain in the left femur region developed in a 4-year-old boy who had no prior trauma. Plain radiography was normal. Laboratory investigations showed a marked leukocytosis (white blood cell count of 14.390/mm^3), a C-reactive protein of 10 mg/dl (normal value <0.5), an erythrocyte sedimentation rate of 67 mm/h (normal value <20 mm/h). Therefore, the child was hospitalized. MRI showed massive edema around the head of proximal femur with modest joint effusion. Blood culture was positive for *Staphylococcus aureus* (MSSA). Suspecting an osteomyelitis, a three-phase bone scintigraphy was performed and showed osteomyelitis in the suspected site.

The patient was discharged after a month of antibiotic therapy in good clinical condition (Fig. 21.5).

Case 21.6: Three-Phase Bone Scan in Posttraumatic Spondyloscitis in a 2-Year-Old Child

A 2-year-old child presented pain after trauma due to an accidental fall. For the persistence of pain in the lumbar region and difficulty in walking, he has made a plain radiography of the spine and pelvis showing a reduction of the L2–L3 intervertebral space. Laboratory investigations did not

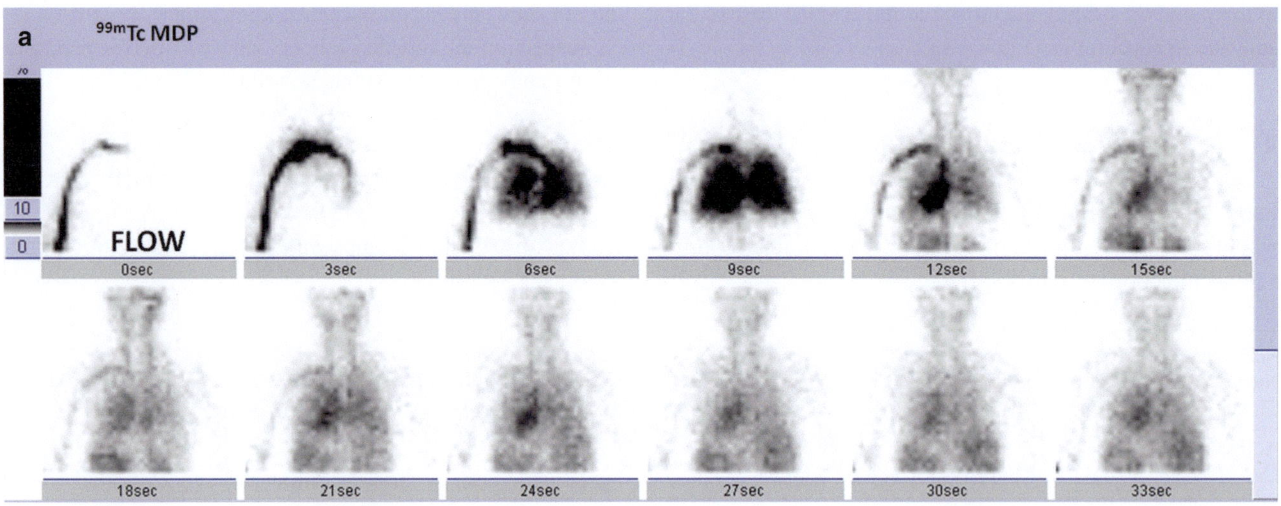

Fig. 21.1 (**a–c**) Three-phase bone scintigraphy: Phase I (**a**) showed symmetric flow in the shoulders; in phase II (early phase, **b**, *left image*), a mild radiotracer uptake was evident in right shoulder, expression of cellulites; phase III (delayed phase, **b**, *right image*) showed moderate radiotracer uptake in right scapulohumeral joint. Whole-body bone scan (**c**) showed no foci of pathological uptake in other skeletal segments

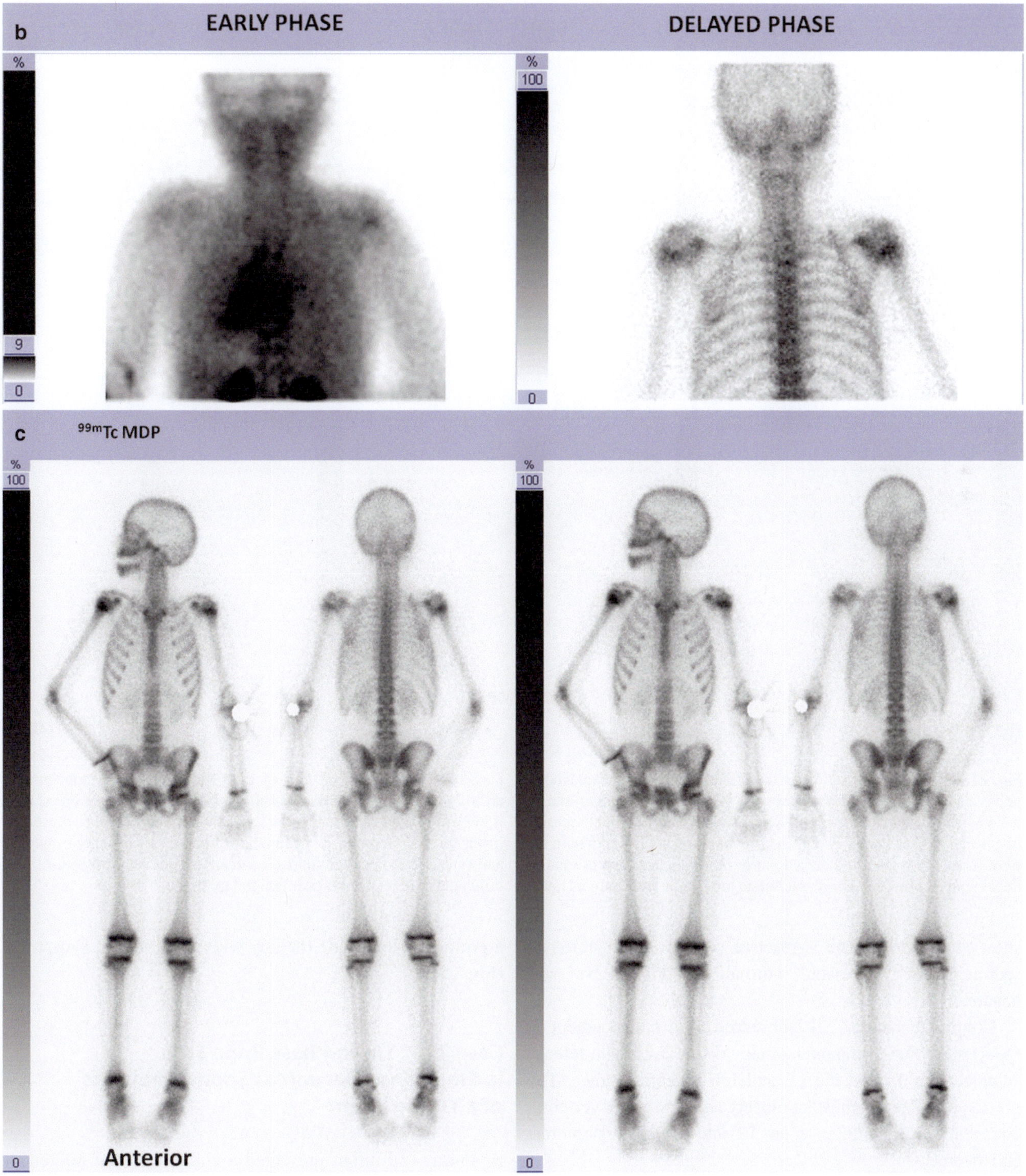

Fig. 21.1 (continued)

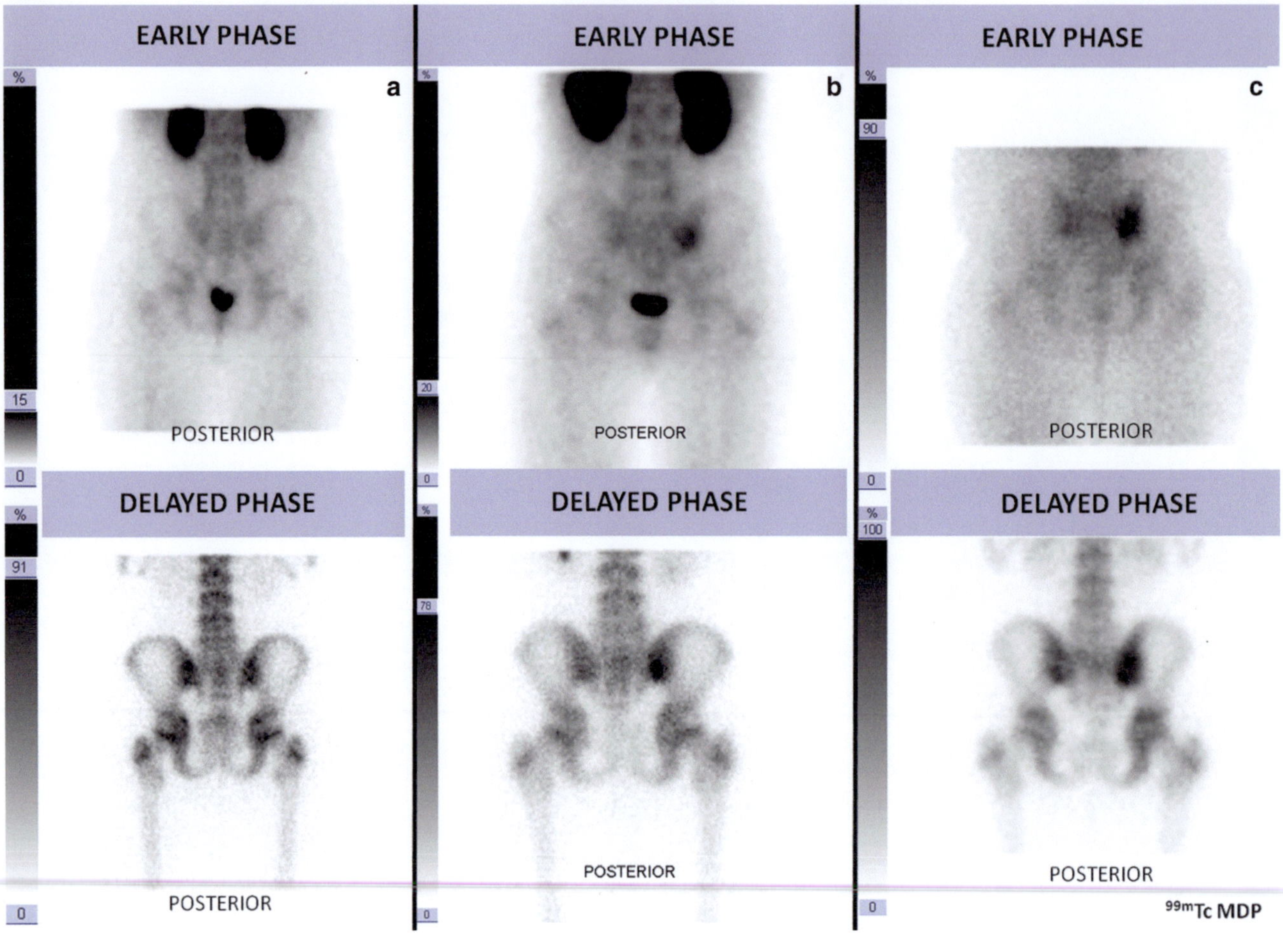

Fig. 21.2 (**a**) A normal pattern of radiotracer distribution displayed in pelvis and sacroiliac joint both in early phase (*upper image*) and in delayed phase (*lower image*). (**b**) Scintigraphic pattern of right sacroiliitis: in early phase (*upper image*), increased blood pool is evident in the right sacroiliac region; in delayed phase (*lower image*), intense radiotracer uptake is present in right sacroiliac joint, in particular, in its lower part. (**c**) Scintigraphic pattern of right sacroiliitis, with concomitant arthritis of the hip: in early phase (*upper image*), increased blood pool is evident in right sacroiliac region; mild radiotracer uptake is present in ipsilateral coxofemoral joint; in delayed phase (*lower image*), intense and extended radiotracer uptake is evident in right sacroiliac joint, with mild uptake in ipsilateral coxofemoral joint, too

show leukocytosis, and C-reactive protein and erythrocyte sedimentation rate were normal. Blood culture was negative.

Contrast-enhanced MRI observed mild enhancement in the front portion of the intersomatic disk L2–L3 with intense enhancement around the L2 and L3 vertebral bodies. The portion of the psoas muscles closely adjacent to the vertebral changes was hyperintense on T2 and shows postcontrast enhancement.

A three-phase bone scintigraphy was then performed in order to confirm the clinical suspicion of spondyloscitis and showed intense radiotracer uptake in L2 soma, upper border of L3, and spinous process of L2 and L3; for this reason, a biopsy was suggested.

Histopathological examination of tissue obtained after surgical curettage was consistent with a diagnosis of osteomyelitis without bacterial growth. The patient has carried out a prolonged antibiotic therapy with resolution of symptoms (Fig. 21.6).

Case 21.7: Three-Phase Bone Scan in *Staphylococcus aureus* Spondylodiscitis of a Young Infant

A 45-day-old infant presented a circumferential nontender swelling of 3 cm in the paradorsal region. Laboratory investigations showed a marked leukocytosis (white blood cell count: 31.390/mm^3), a C-reactive protein of 27.83 mg/dl (normal value <0.5), and an erythrocyte sedimentation rate of 127 mm/h (normal value <20 mm/h). Blood culture was positive for *Staphylococcus aureus*. Dorsal swelling increased in its dimension, with normal rose skin. Radiograph of spine showed a pulmonary infiltrate and a disk narrowing of the D8–D9 space, compatible with intervertebral disk space infection.

Bone scintigraphy, performed for detecting multiple foci of infection, revealed increased signal intensity at the body and at the end plate of D9. Contrast-enhanced MRI was performed in order to provide a specific diagnosis and to define the anatomic extent of vertebral and soft tissue involvement. It was highly suggestive of both disk and vertebral infection of two dorsal vertebrae, with involvement of adjacent paraspinal soft tissue and spinal cord compression. Because of the improvement in clinical condition and radiological findings, therapy was stopped, and during follow-up (3 years later), stepwise bony consolidation of the vertebral defect and partial remodeling was observed (Fig. 21.7).

Case 21.8 Chronic Recurrent Multifocal Osteomyelitis: Good Response to Therapy

A 7-year-old girl referred to our institution for fever and migrating arthralgia; C-reactive protein value was 17 mg/dl and erythrocyte sedimentation rate was 84 mm/h (normal value <20 mm/h). Suspecting an inflammatory disease, a bone scintigraphy was performed and showed areas of radiotracer uptake in multiple skeletal segments, so that clinical suspicion is supported; a bone biopsy was scheduled to confirm the diagnosis, and distal left femur was identified as a site eligible for biopsy. Histological examination detected a chronic nonbacterial osteomyelitis.

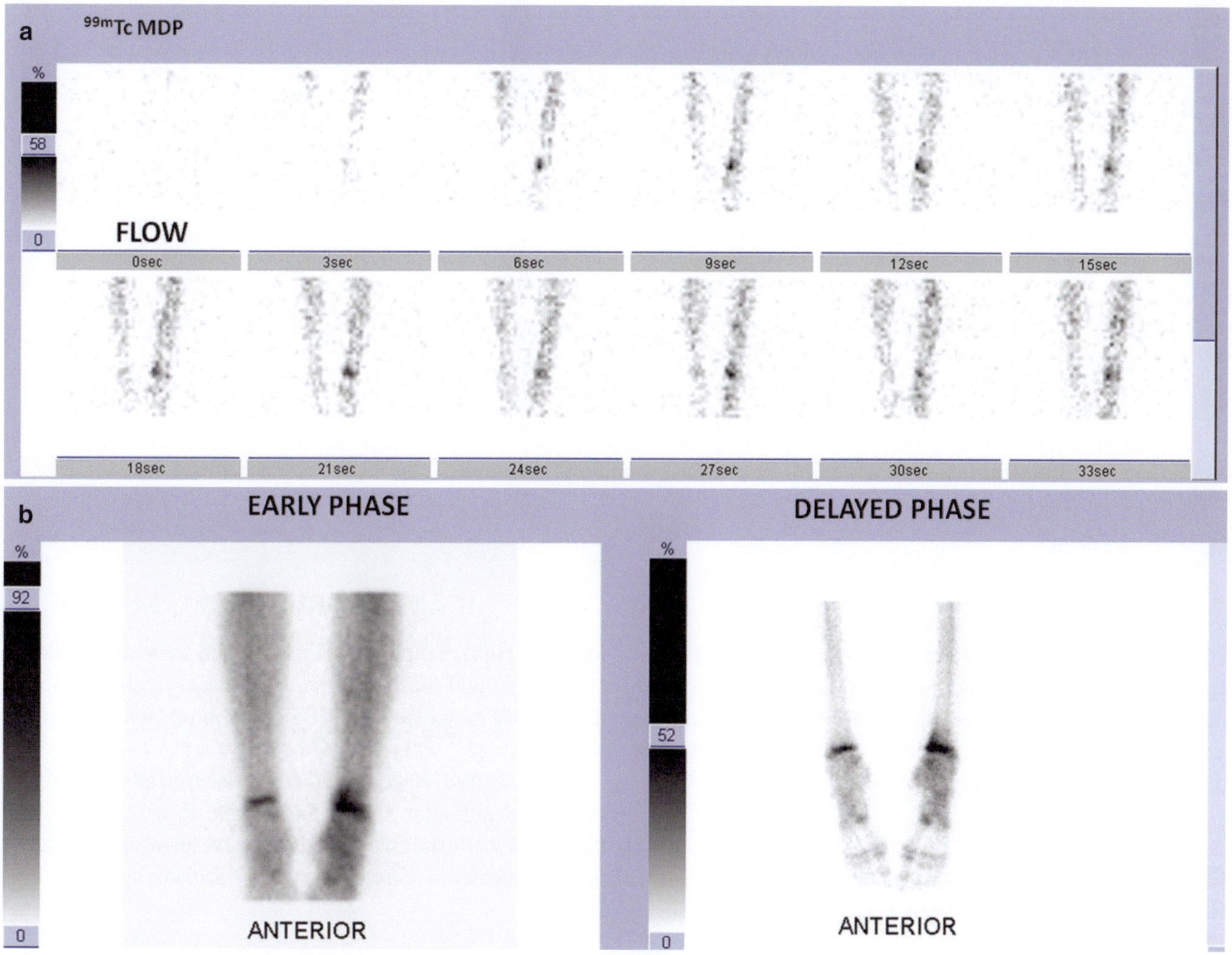

Fig. 21.3 (**a**–**e**) Three-phase bone scintigraphy: Phase I (**a**) showed increased flow in left distal tibia; in phase II (early phase, **b**, *left image*), radiotracer uptake in the same site was evident, expression of cellulites; phase III (delayed phase, **b**, *right image*) showed intense radiotracer uptake in left tibiotarsal joint, extending to medial malleolus of left tibia; this finding was better defined in lateral (**d**) and anterior static views of the feet (**e**). Whole-body bone scan showed no foci of pathological uptake in other skeletal segments (**c**)

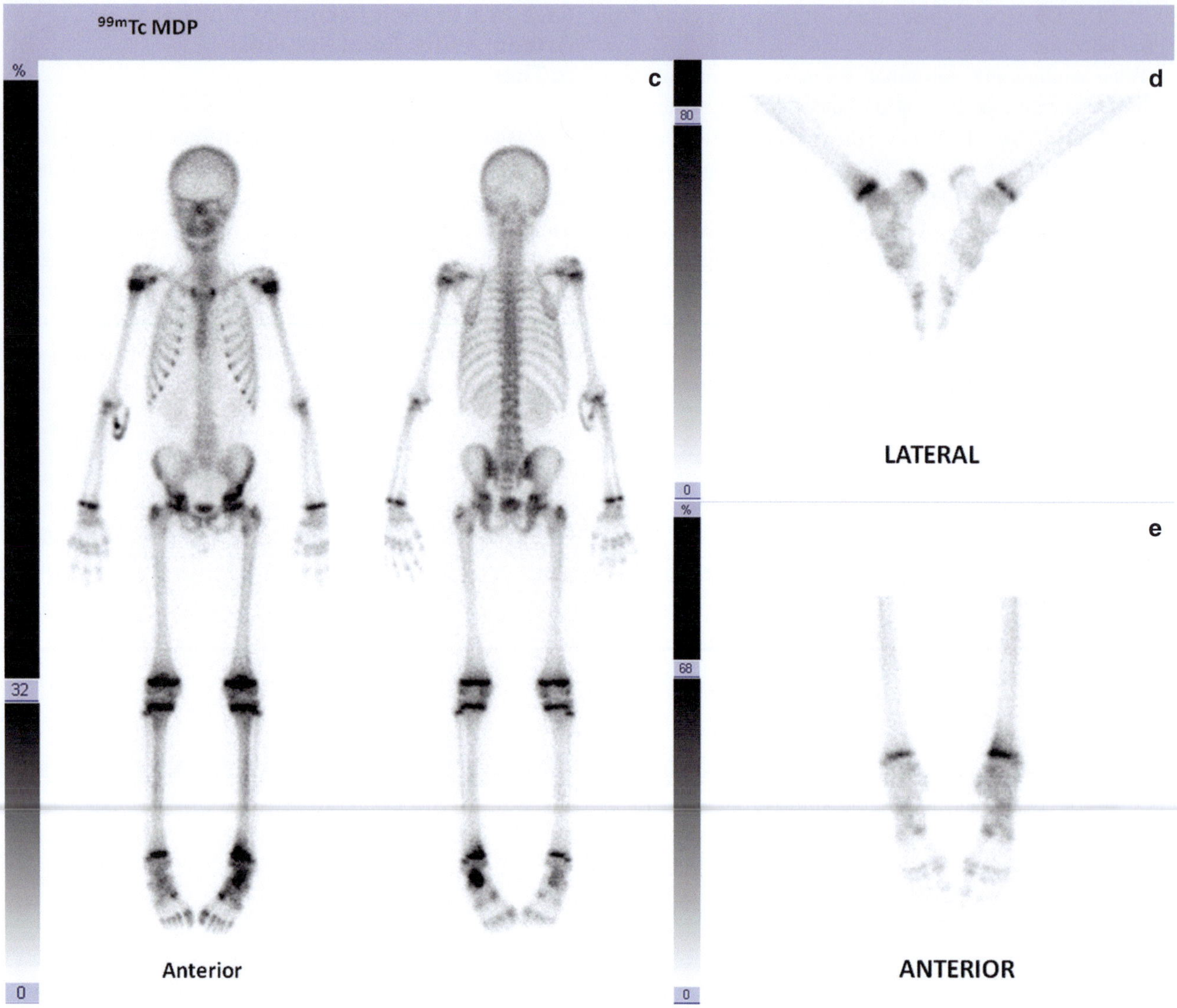

Fig. 21.3 (continued)

The girl began appropriate therapy, and a further bone scan was performed in order to assess the response to treatment. Scintigraphy showed disappearance of most of the areas of increased osteometabolism previously evident, such that indicating a good response to therapy (Fig. 21.8).

Case 21.9 Rare Presentation of Chronic Recurrent Multifocal Osteomyelitis: A Case of Unifocal Disease

A 5-year-old boy was treated in another center with antibiotics and steroids for a suspected dental abscess. For the persistence of pain and swelling in right emimandibula, nonresponsive to treatment, the child referred to our institution. A CT was performed and showed a large lytic lesion in right mandibular ramus; on the basis of radiological and clinical findings, a bacterial osteomyelitis of mandibula was suspected, and a bone scintigraphy was then scheduled.

Bone scan revealed an increased osteometabolic activity in right mandibular ramus, attributable to osteomyelitis; a biopsy of the lesion was suggested, and histological examination detected a chronic nonbacterial osteomyelitis (Fig. 21.9).

Case 21.10 Chronic Recurrent Multifocal Osteomyelitis: Partial Response to Therapy

A 12-year-old girl referred to our institution for swelling in right clavicle, with no history of pain or fever; plain radiogra-

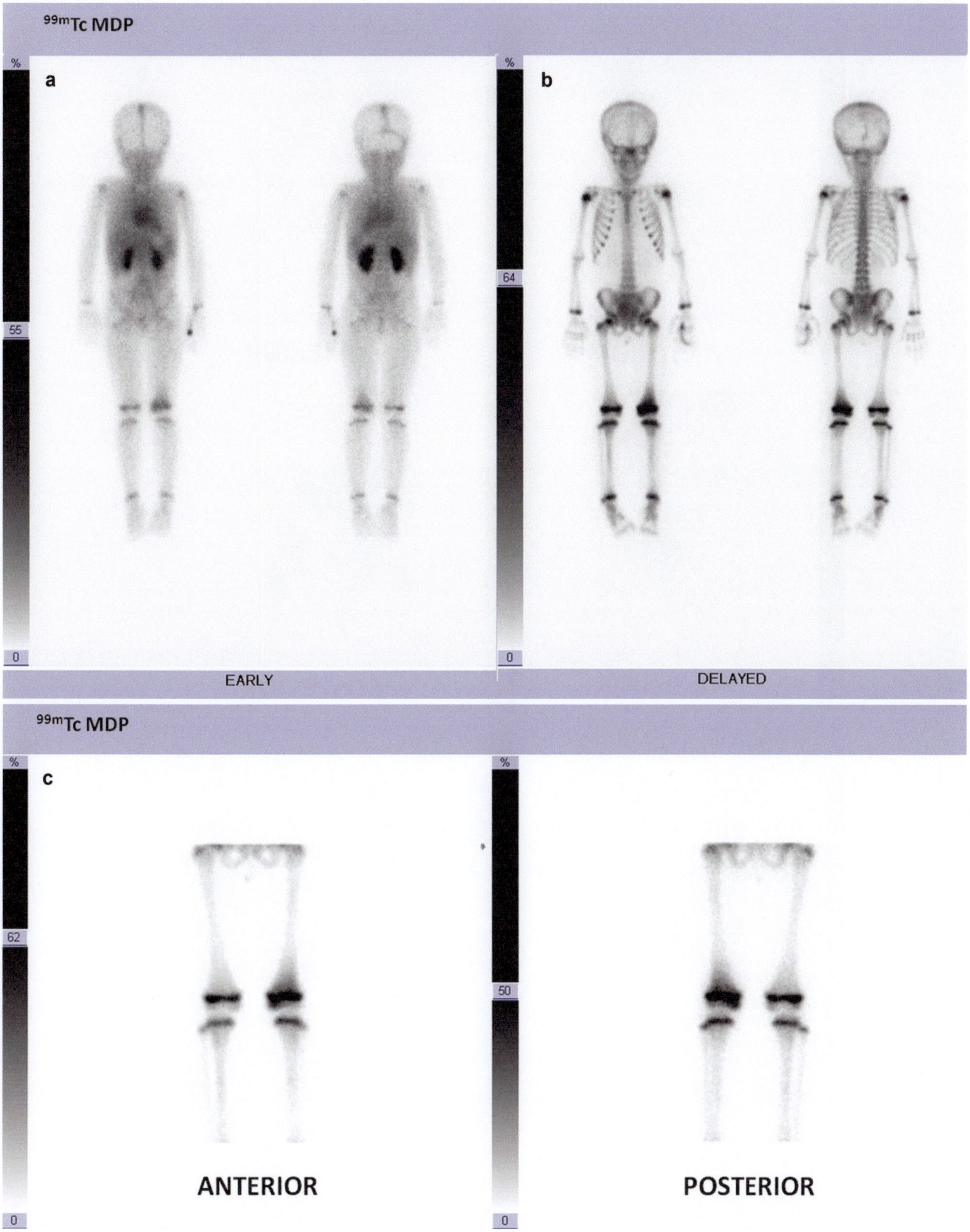

Fig. 21.4 (**a–c**) Early phase whole-body scan. (**a**) Increased radiotracer uptake in left knee was evident, indicating cellulitis; delayed phase whole-body scan (**b**) showed radiotracer uptake in the same site, extending to the region above the metaphysis in ipsilateral distal femur, indicating arthritis complicated by osteomyelitis. This finding was better defined in static views of the knees (**c**). Delayed whole-body scan (**b**) showed no foci of pathological uptake in other skeletal segments

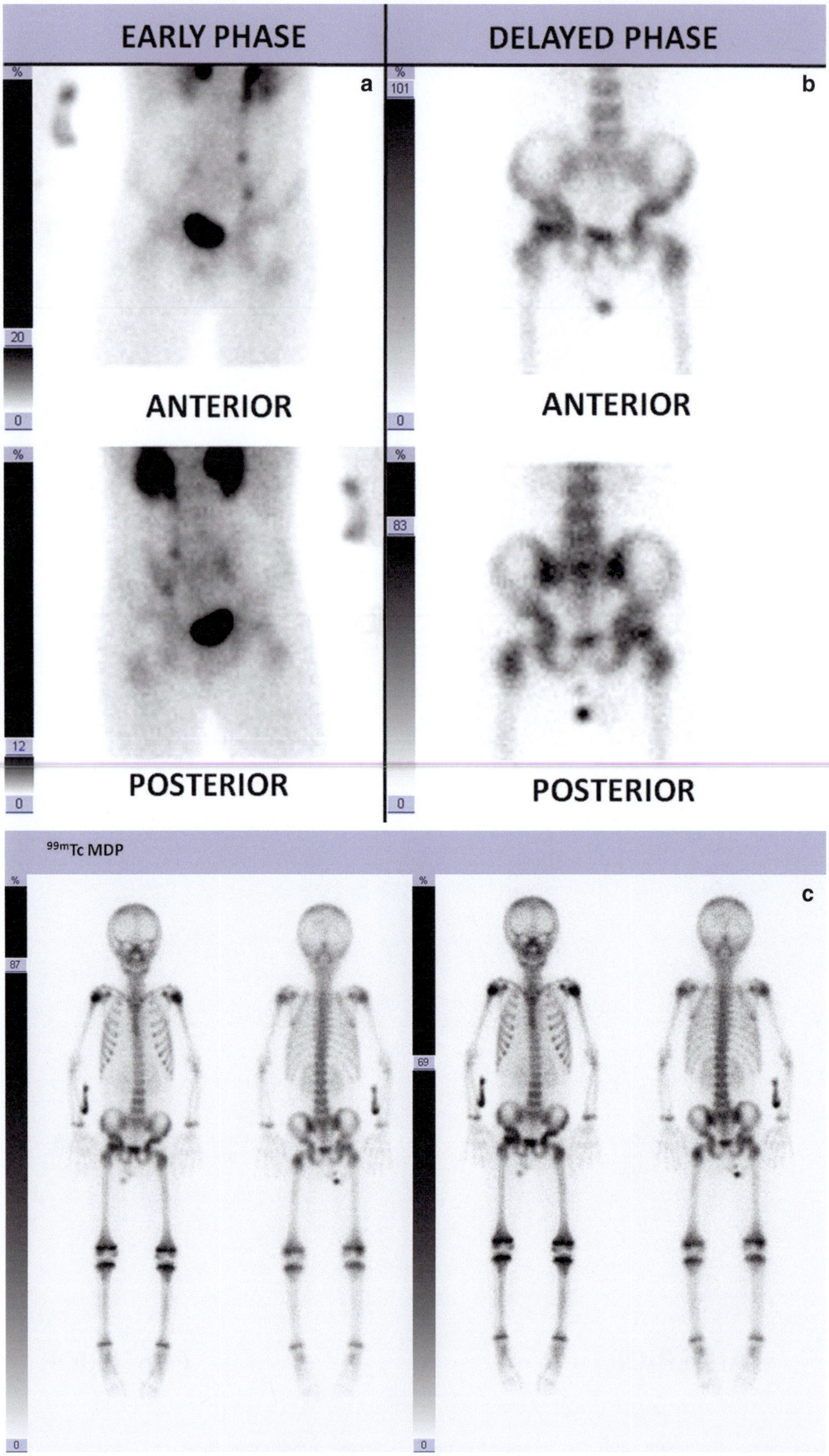

Fig. 21.5 (**a–c**) Three-phase bone scintigraphy: in phase II (early phase, **a**, images on the *left*), severe and extended reduction of radiotracer uptake was evident in left hip joint, as in extended edema; phase III (delayed phase, **b**, images on the *right*) showed severe reduction of radiotracer uptake in head and neck of left femur, because of severe compressive surrounding edema. Whole-body bone scan (**c**) showed mild increased radiotracer uptake in the region above the metaphysis in ipsilateral distal femur, indicating another focus of osteomyelitis

phy showed structural alterations of right proximal clavicle, and markers of inflammation were elevated. MRI detected swelling of proximal clavicle near the sternoclavicular joint involving bone and soft tissue; similar alterations were also evident in the sternum and were possibly attributable to inflammatory disease. For this reason, a bone scintigraphy was performed to confirm the diagnostic suspicion and, moreover, to evaluate the whole skeleton; the scan showed increased osteometabolic activity in right proximal clavicle, ipsilateral sternoclavicular joint, sternum, and in several segments of feet, confirming clinical suspicion. A CT-guided biopsy of clavicular lesion was done, and histological examination detected a chronic nonbacterial osteomyelitis.

Considering this finding and the multifocality of disease, diagnosis of CRMO was made, and the girl began treatment (Fig. 21.10).

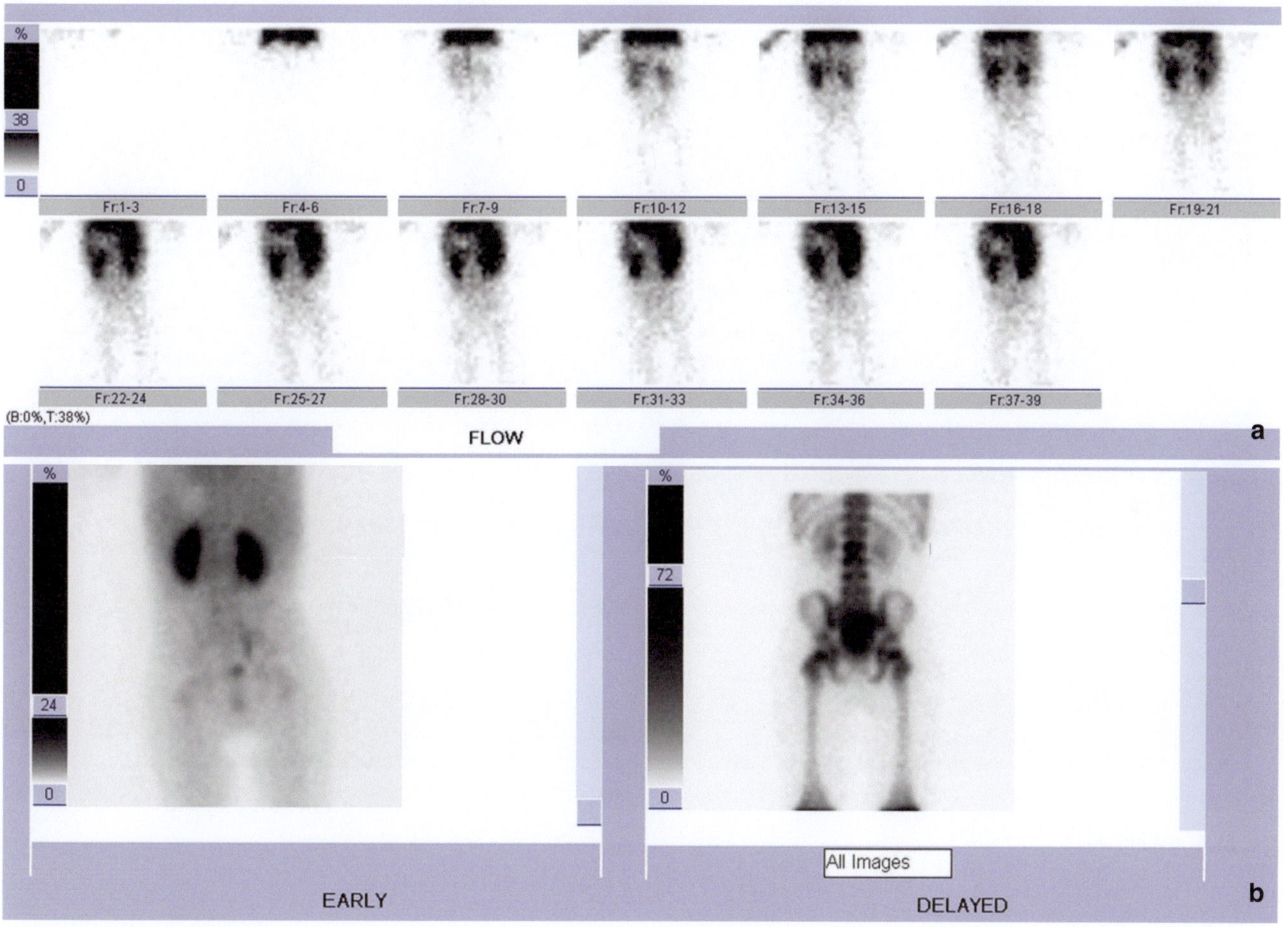

Fig. 21.6 (**a**–**c**) Three-phase bone scintigraphy: Phase I (**a**) and phase II (early phase, **b**, *left image*) showed normal flow and normal blood pool in lumbar–sacral region, respectively; phase III (delayed phase, **b**, *right image*) showed intense radiotracer uptake in L2 soma, upper border of L3, and spinous process of L2 and L3. A SPECT acquisition was also obtained, and SPECT images were manually fused with MRI; SPECT–MRI fused image allowed to better define vertebral uptake (**c**). Considering this finding, a vertebral biopsy was suggested

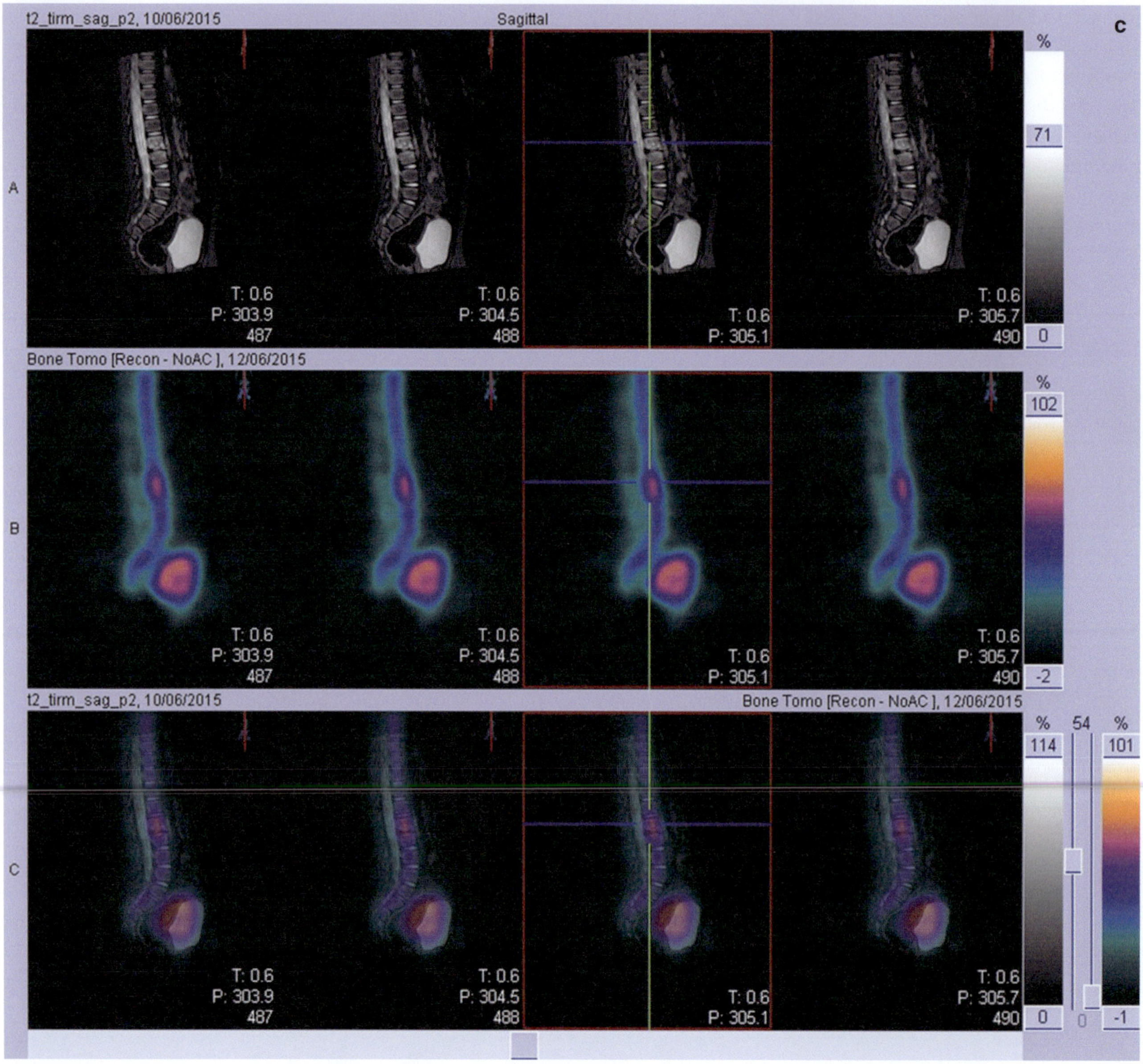

Fig. 21.6 (continued)

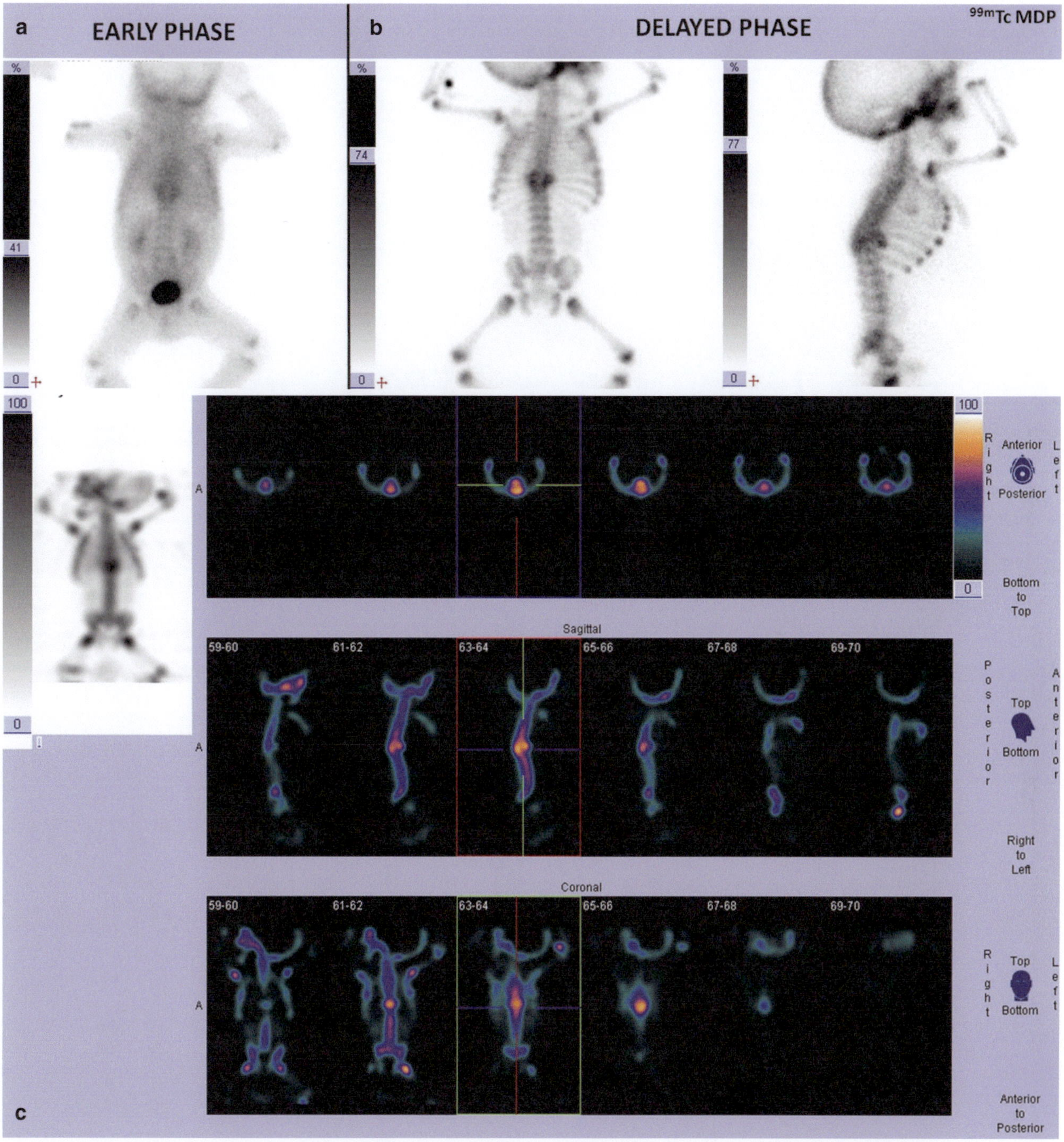

Fig. 21.7 (**a**–**d**) Whole-body bone scan in early phase (**a**) showed increased blood pool in correspondence of middle dorsal region. Whole-body bone scan in delayed phase (**b**) shows increased radiotracer uptake in a dorsal vertebra (possibly D9) and no foci of pathological uptake in other skeletal segments. A SPECT acquisition was also obtained, and SPECT images were manually fused with CT; SPECT (**c**) and SPECT–CT fused image (**d**) allowed to locate radiotracer uptake in body (mainly in its *right* part) and posterior vertebral arch (in particular pedicles) of D9, respectively

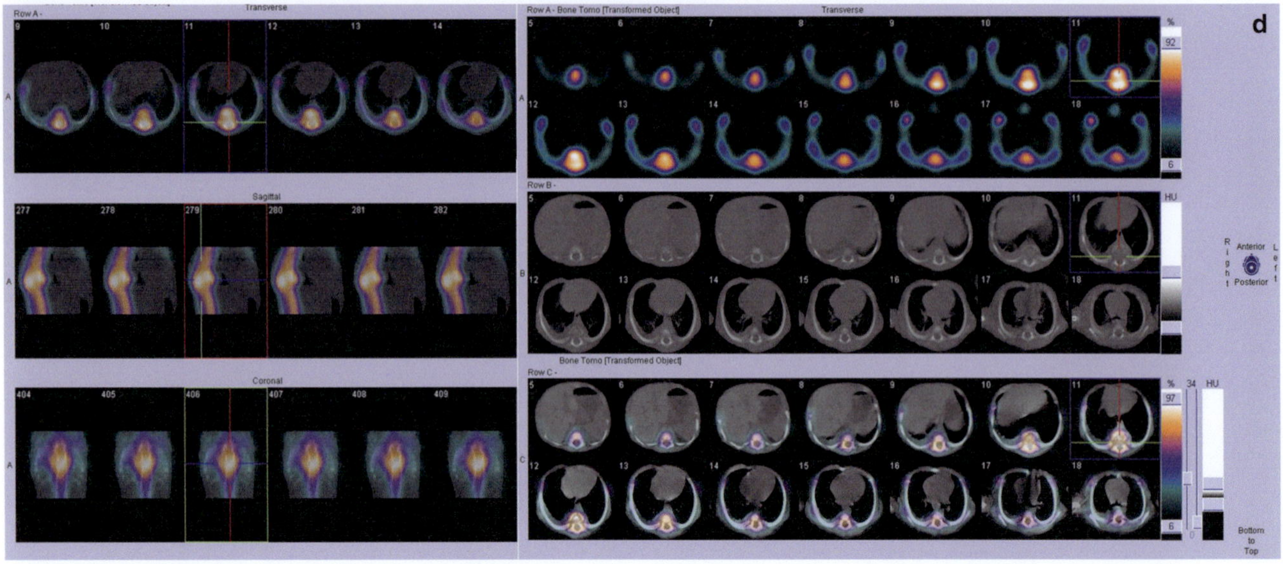

Fig. 21.7 (continued)

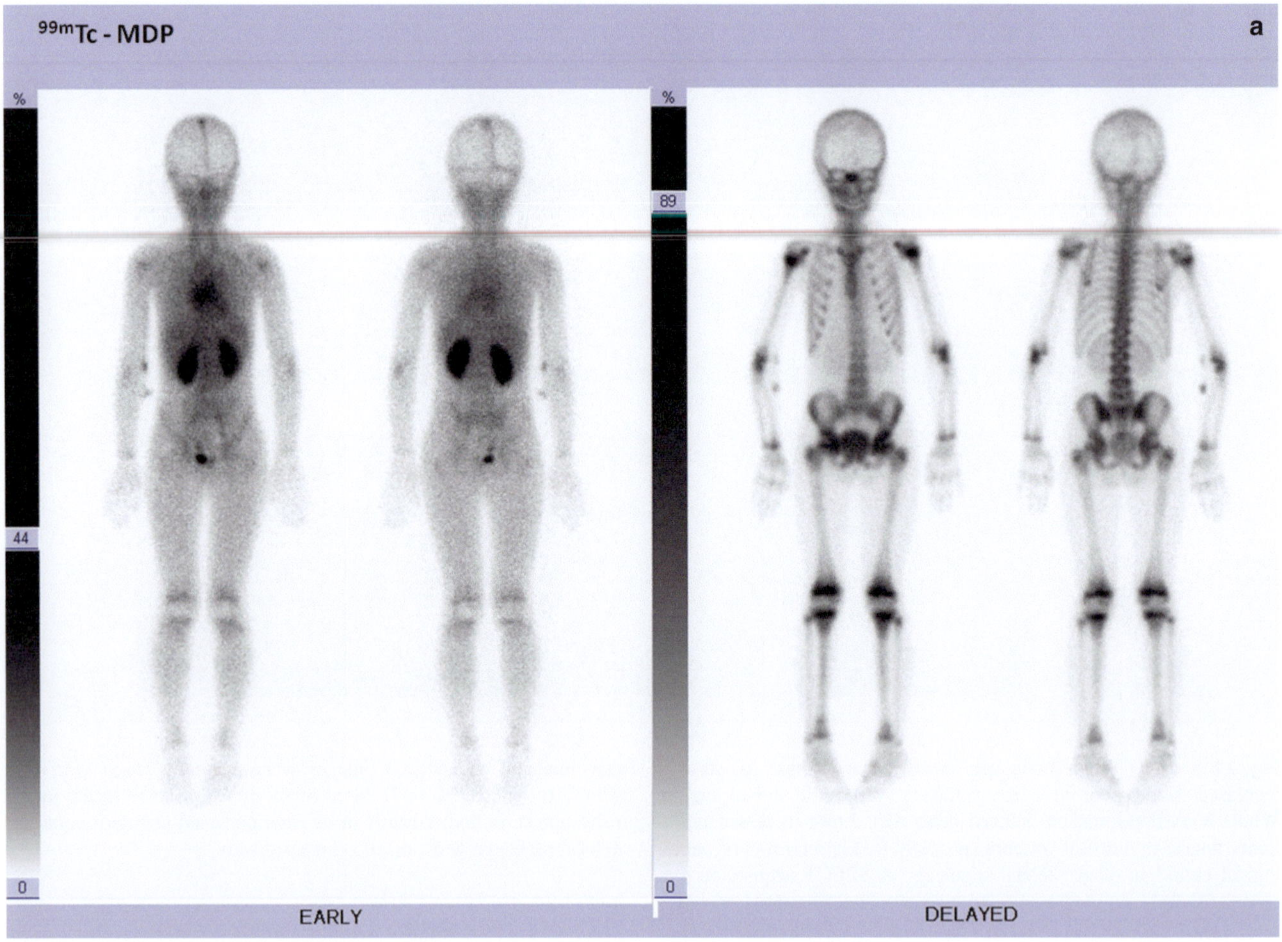

Fig. 21.8 (**a**, **b**) Diagnostic bone scintigraphy. Whole-body bone scan in early phase (**a**, *left image*) shows markedly increased blood pool in both knees and in distal tibiae; mild radiotracer uptake of radiotracer is also evident in both elbows and in right wrist. Whole-body bone scan in delayed phase (**a**, *right image* and **b**, *higher contrast image*, for better lesion detection) shows nonhomogeneous uptake in both femurs and both tibiae, with intense uptake in distal metaphyses of both femurs and in proximal and distal metaphyses of both tibiae. Intense uptake of radiotracer is also evident in both elbows and in distal right radius. Right emimandible shows a radiotracer uptake relatively higher than the left one.

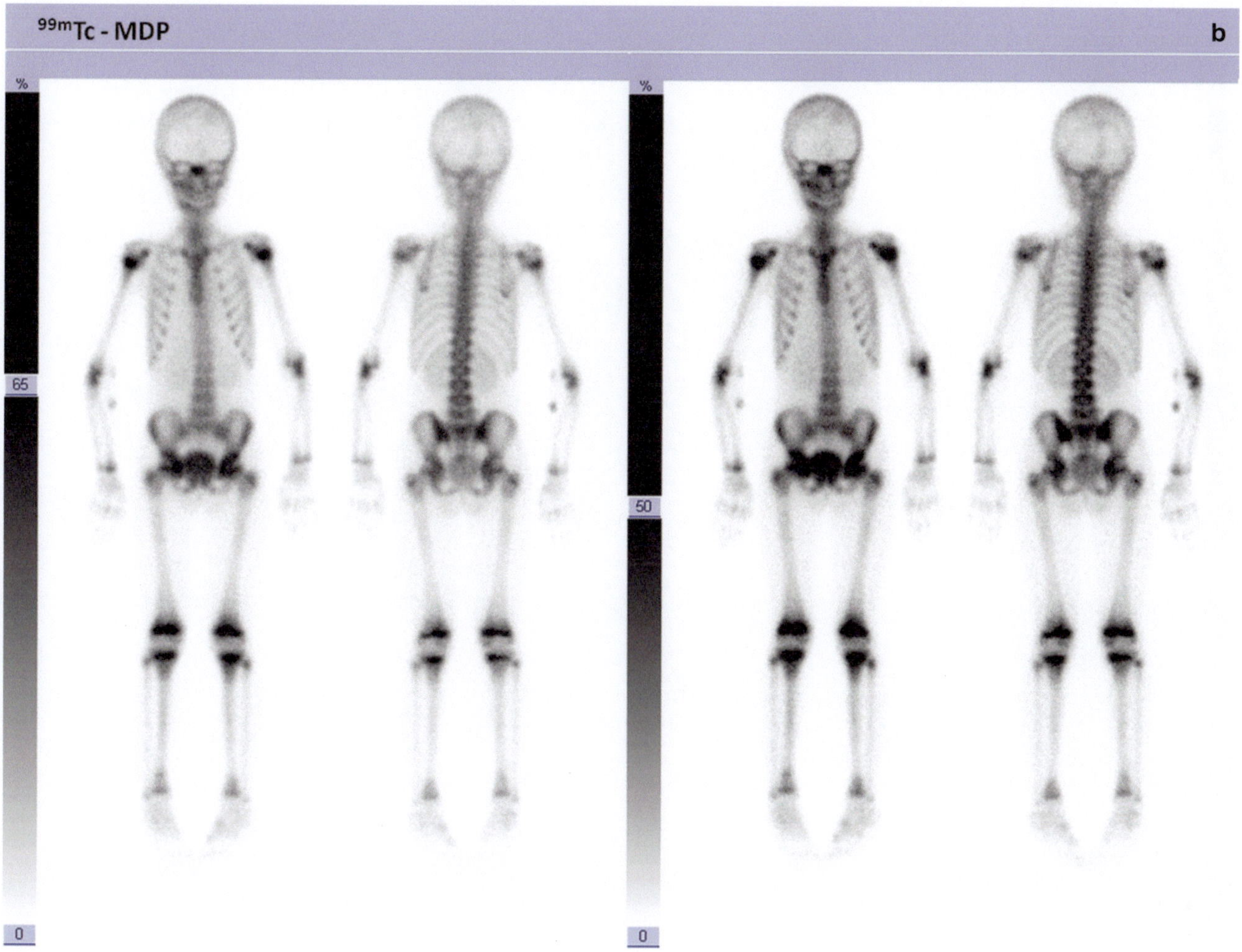

Fig. 21.8 (continued)

(**c**, **d**) Bone scintigraphy after therapy. Whole-body bone scan in early phase (**c**, *left image*) normal blood pool distribution. Whole-body bone scan in delayed phase (**c**, *right image* and **d**, *higher contrast image*, for better lesion detection), compared with the diagnostic study, shows a persistence of radiotracer uptake in distal right radius and of a focal uptake in mandible on median line. Radiotracer distribution is mildly altered in distal femurs (region above metaphyses), proximal (region below metaphyses), and distal tibiae (region above metaphyses) and elbows

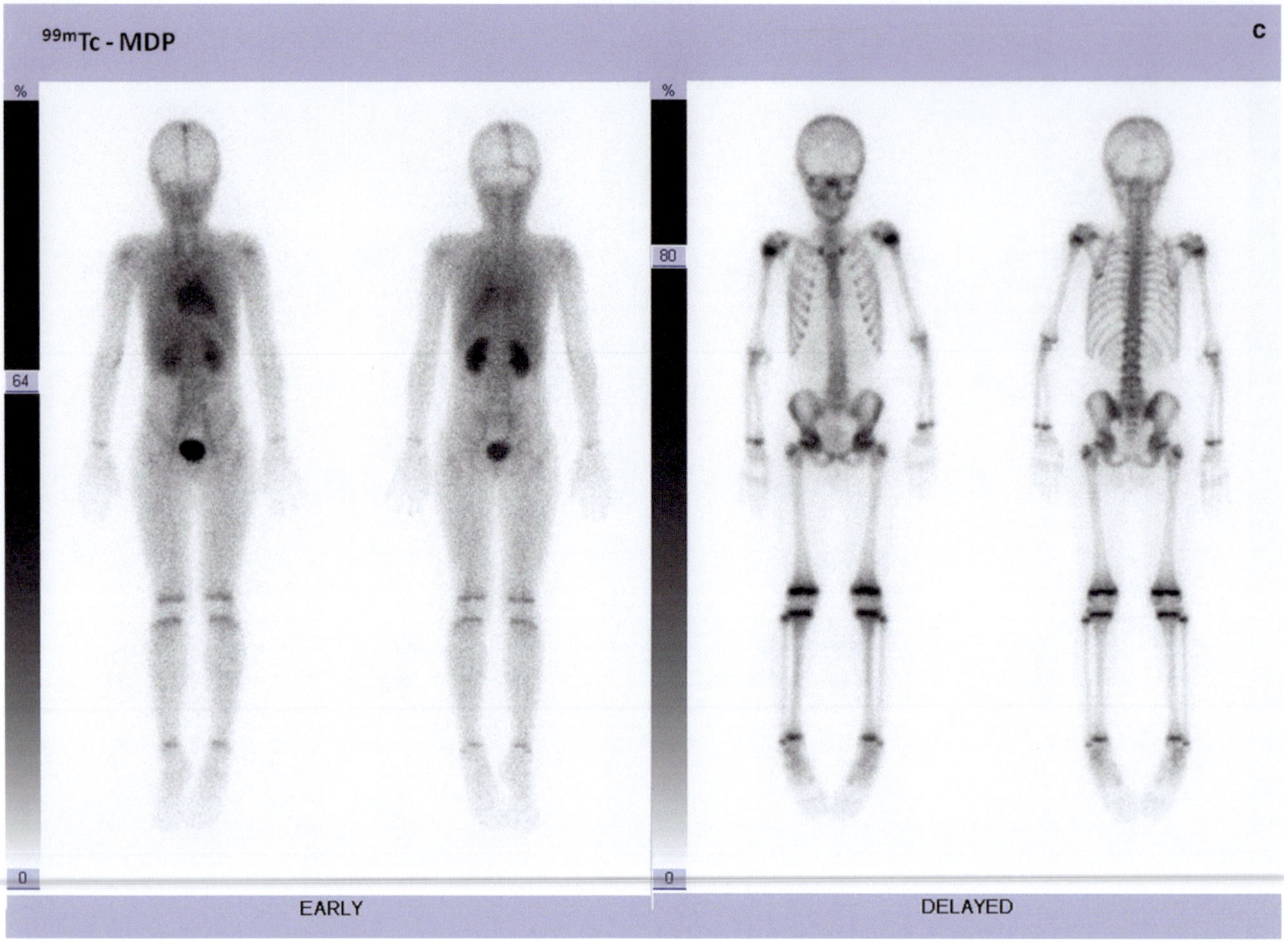

Fig. 21.8 (continued)

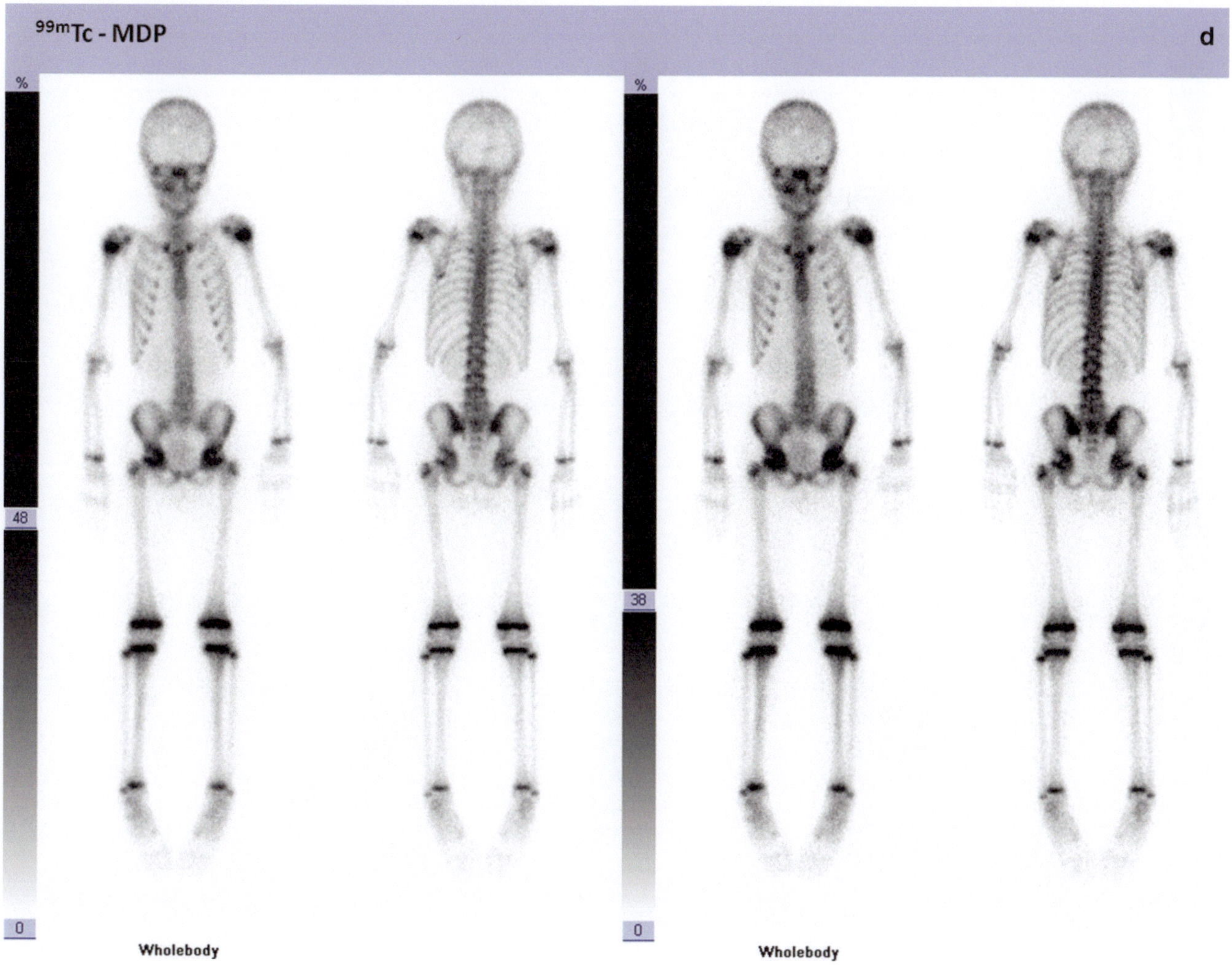

Fig. 21.8 (continued)

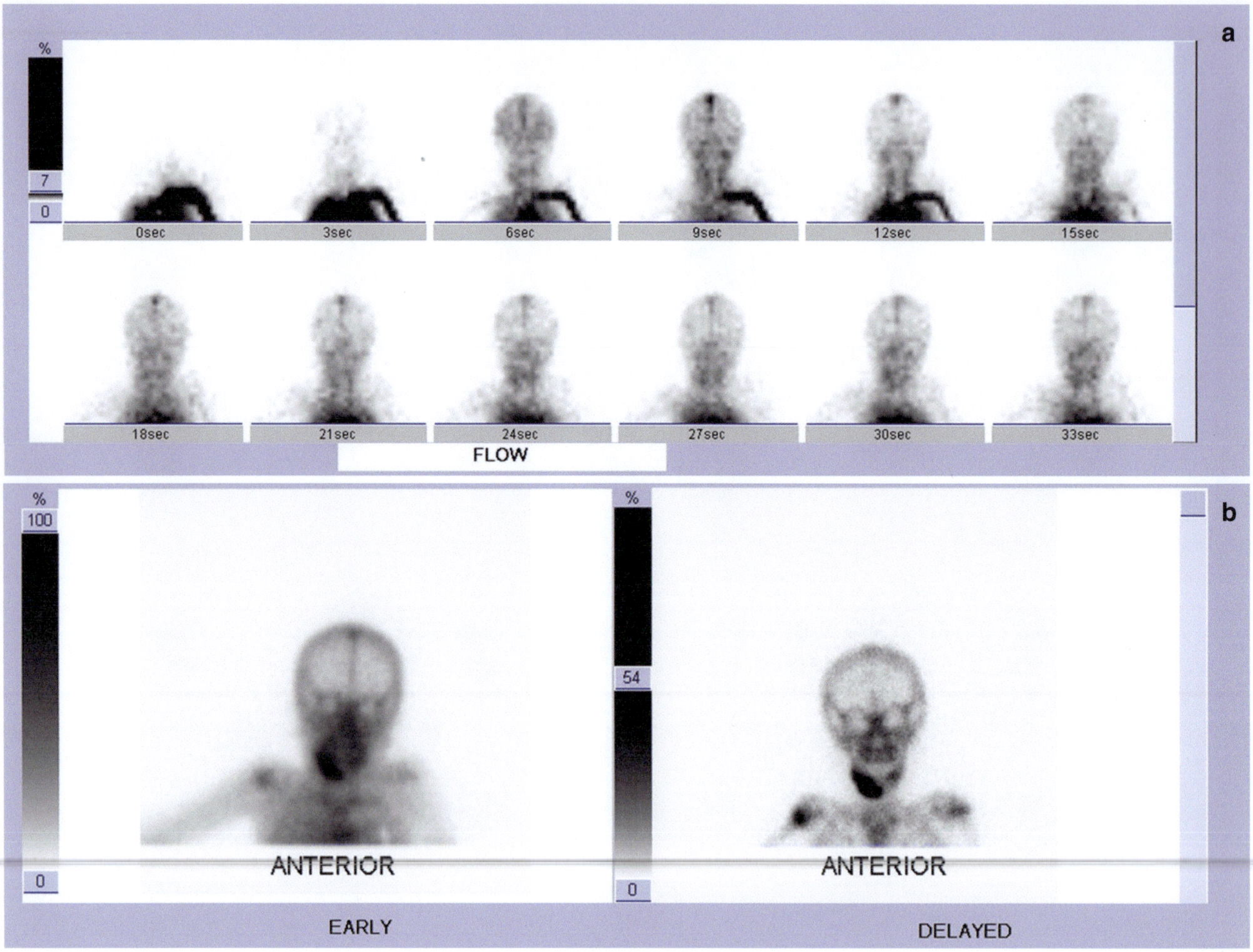

Fig. 21.9 (**a–c**) Diagnostic bone scintigraphy. Three-phase bone scintigraphy: Phase I (**a**) shows increased flow in right mandibular region; in phase II (early phase, **b**, *left image*), markedly increased blood pool is evident in the same site; phase III (delayed phase, **b**, *right image*) detects radiotracer uptake in right mandibular ramus, with a focal area in its distal segment. No pathological areas of radiotracer uptake are evident in other skeletal segments (Whole-body scan, **c**). (**d**, **e**) Bone scintigraphy after therapy. At early whole-body bone scan (**d**, *left image*), mild radiotracer uptake is still evident in mandible. Delayed whole-body bone scan (**d**, *right image* and **e**, *higher contrast image*, for better lesion detection) shows persistence of radiotracer uptake in mandible, markedly less intense than in the previous scintigraphy. No pathological areas of radiotracer uptake are evident in other skeletal segments

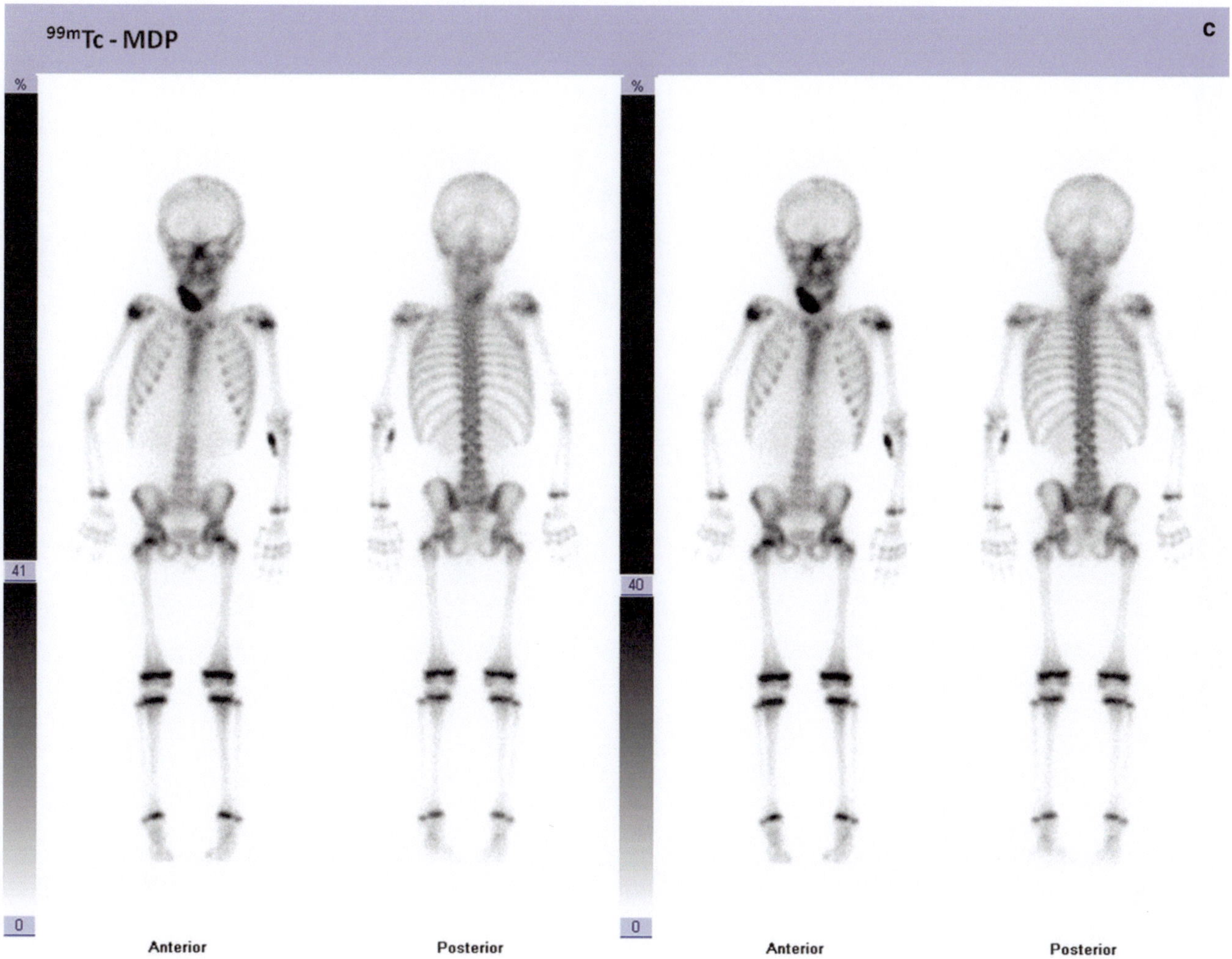

Fig. 21.9 (continued)

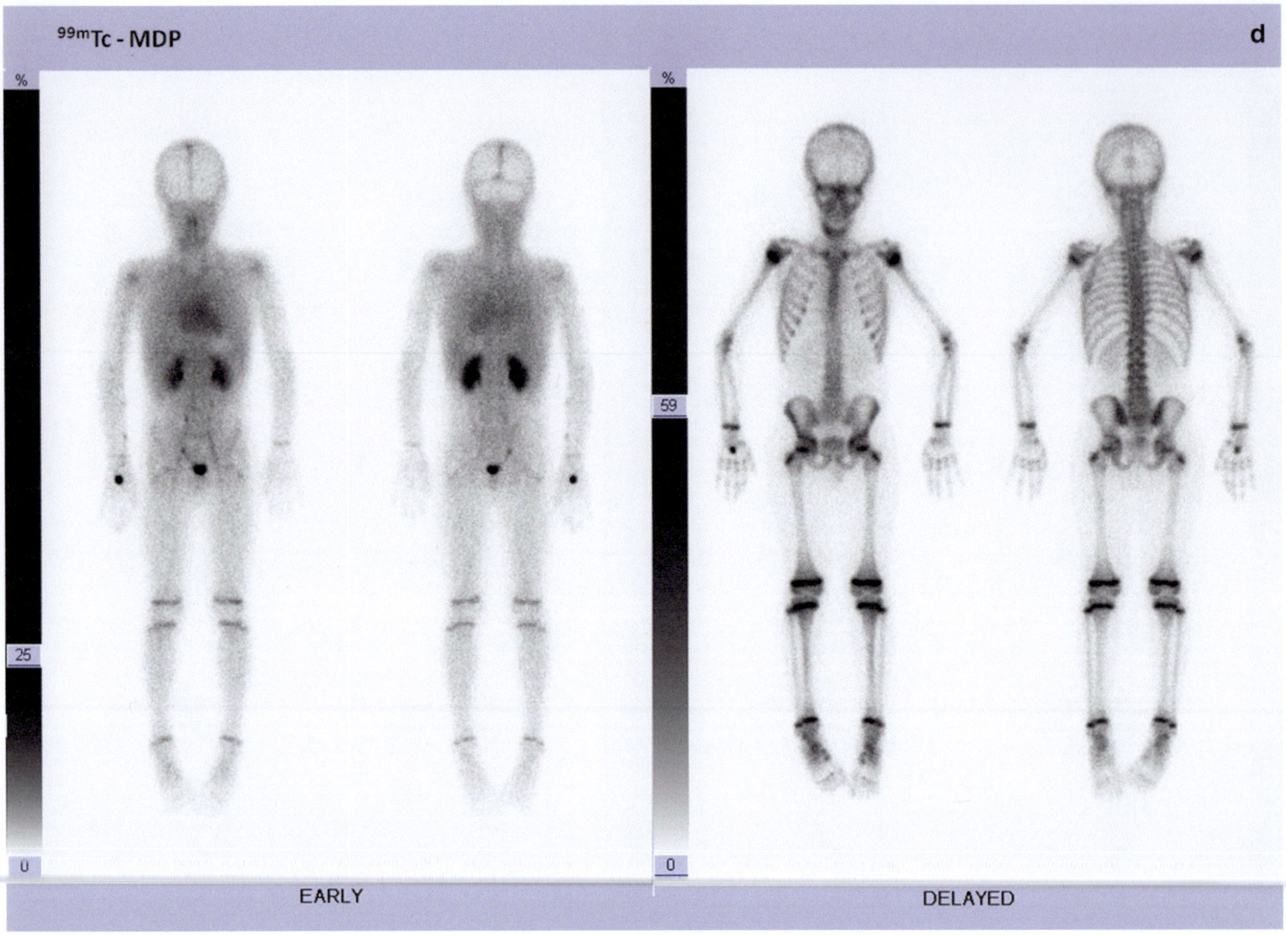

Fig. 21.9 (continued)

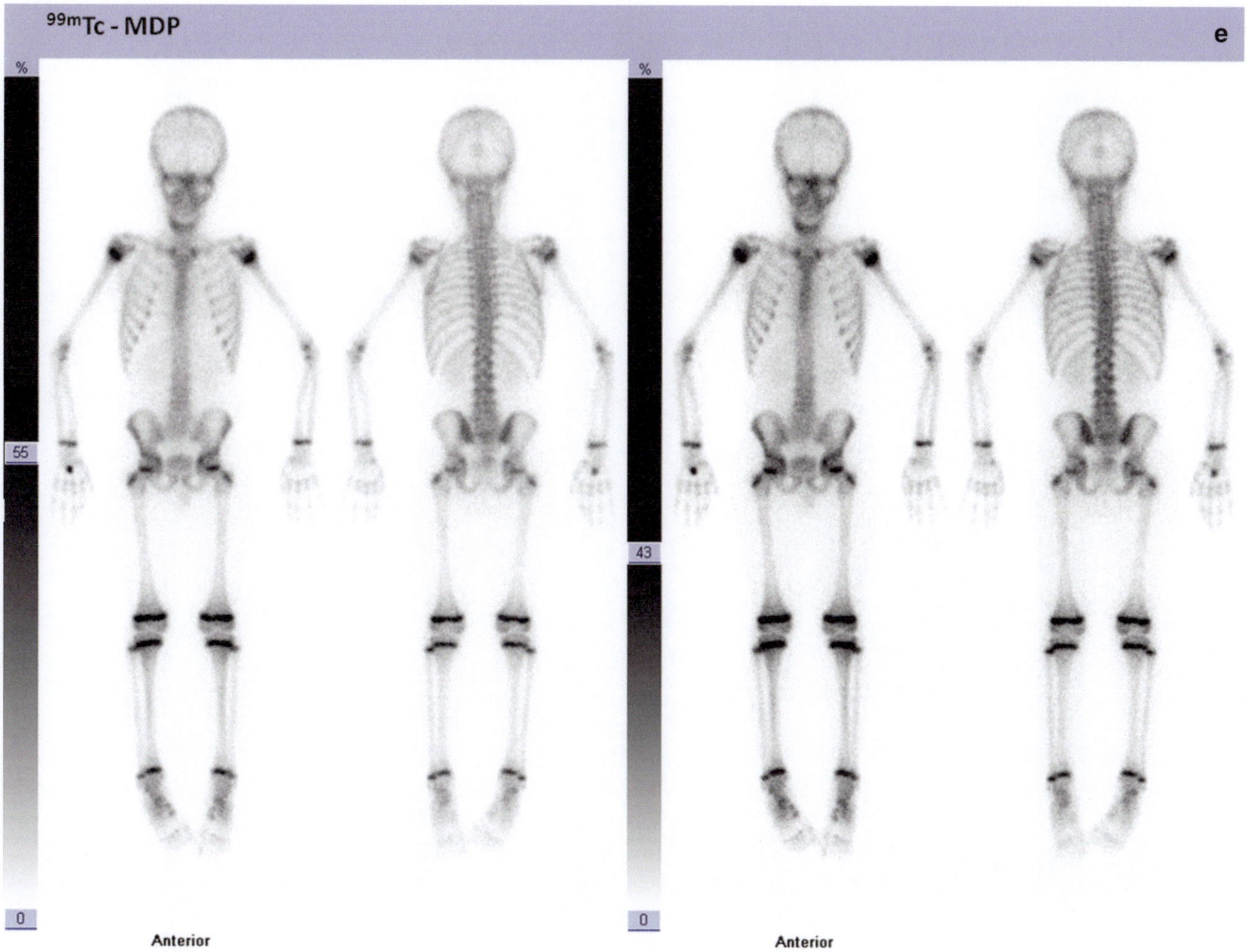

Fig. 21.9 (continued)

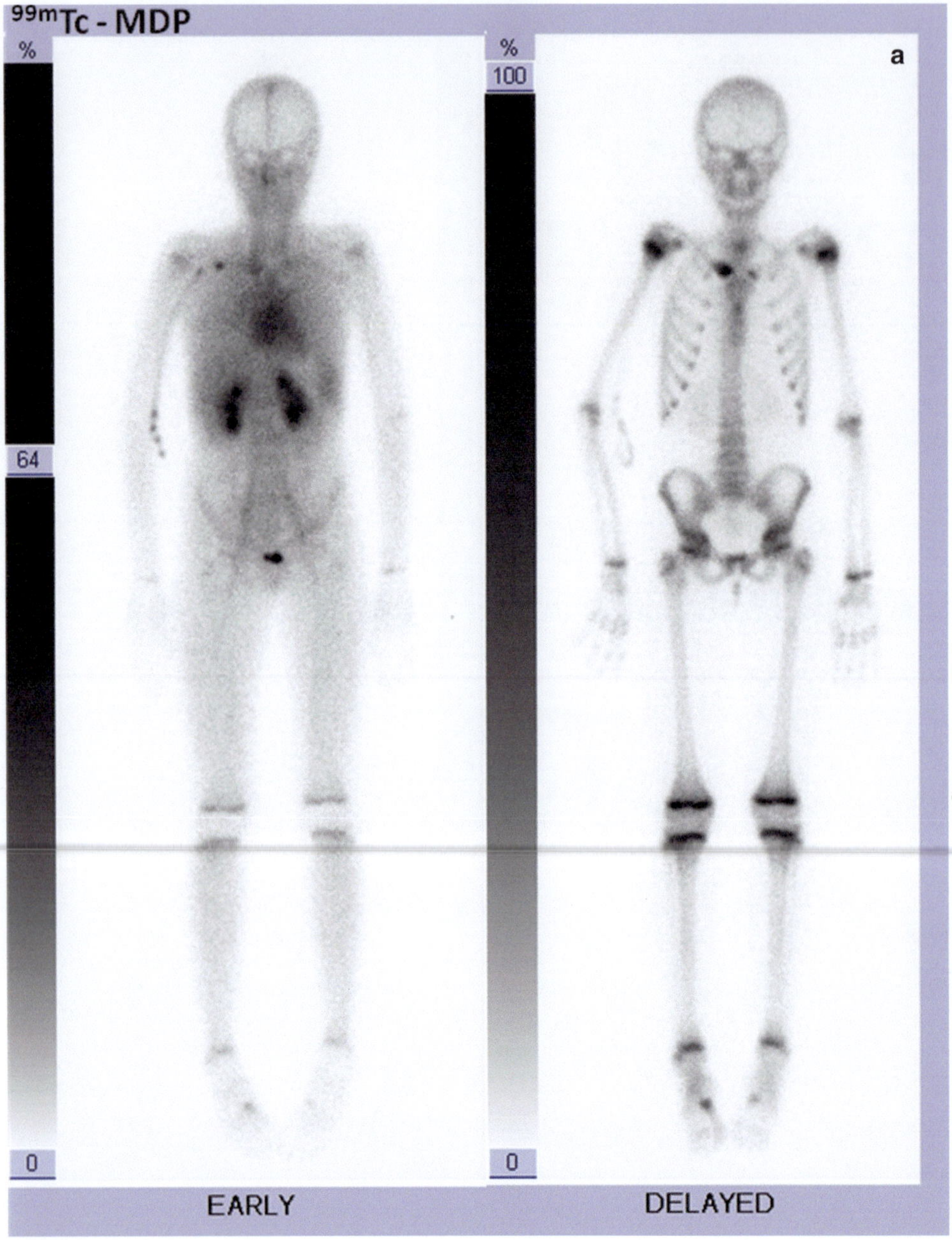

Fig. 21.10 (**a**–**e**) Diagnostic bone scintigraphy. Whole-body bone scan in early phase (**a**, *left image*) shows mild radiotracer uptake in right sternoclavicular joint. Whole-body bone scan in delayed phase (**a**, *right image* and **b**) shows focal radiotracer uptake in proximal sternum, on the basis of first metatarsal ray, in right sternoclavicular joint. Spot images of feet and ankles (in plantar, dorsal, and lateral view, **c**–**e**, respectively) detect radiotracer uptake in right tibioperoneal joint, in both tarsi, in several metatarsophalangeal joints and in proximal phalanx of fifth finger of right foot. (**f**, **g**) Bone scintigraphy after therapy. At early whole-body bone scan (**f**, *left image*), faint radiotracer uptake in right sternoclavicular joint region is still evident. Whole-body bone scan in delayed phase (**f**, *right image* and **g**, *higher contrast image*), for better lesion detection) shows focal radiotracer uptake in proximal sternum, in both sternoclavicular joints, in right proximal clavicle. Areas of uptake previously evident in feet are no longer detectable

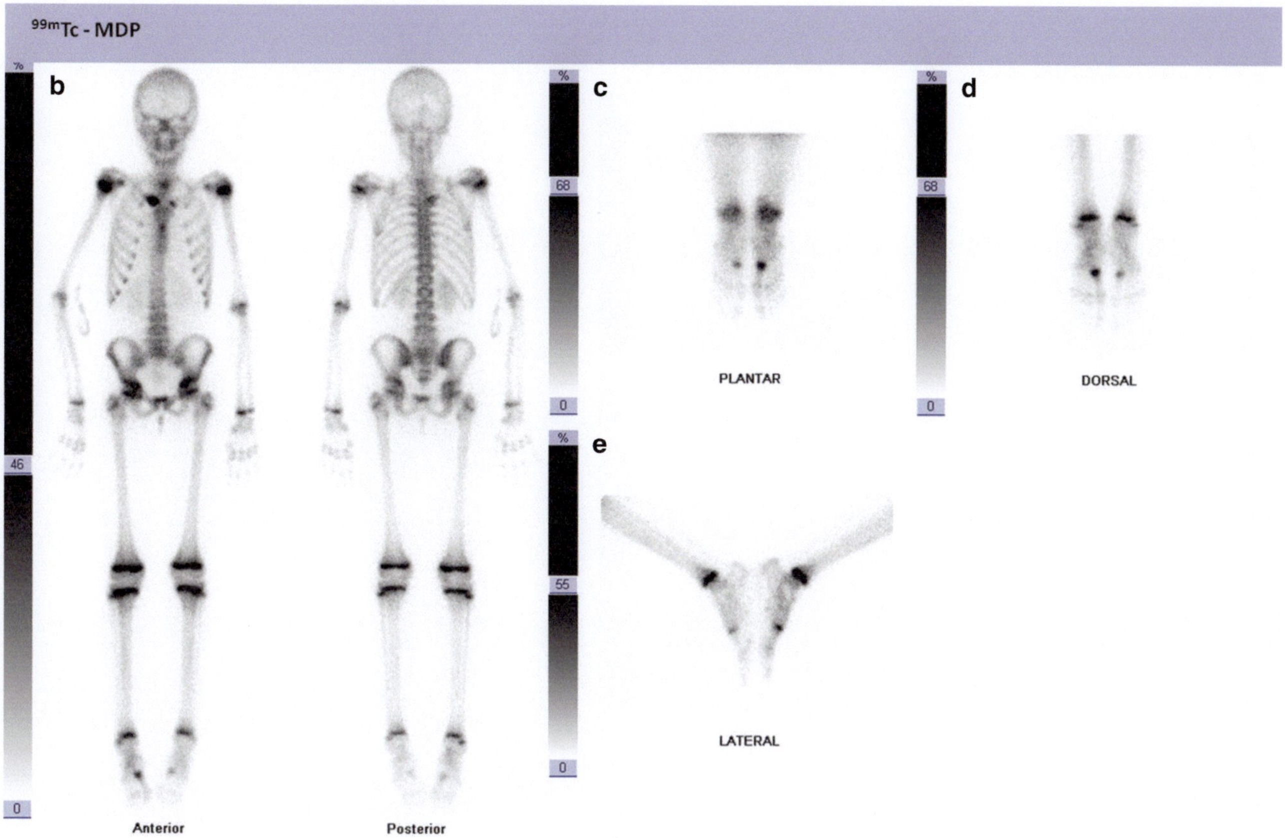

Fig. 21.10 (continued)

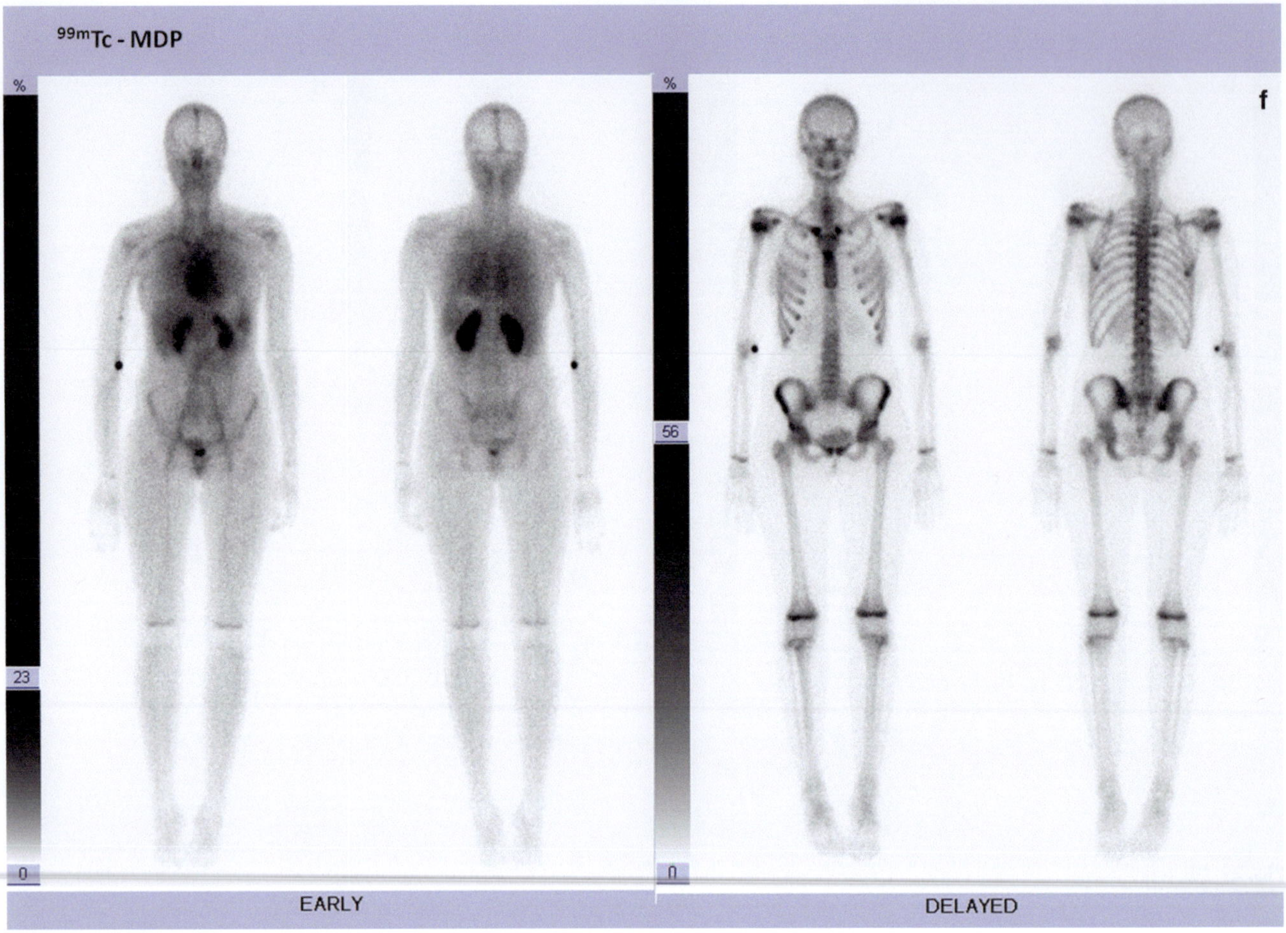

Fig. 21.10 (continued)

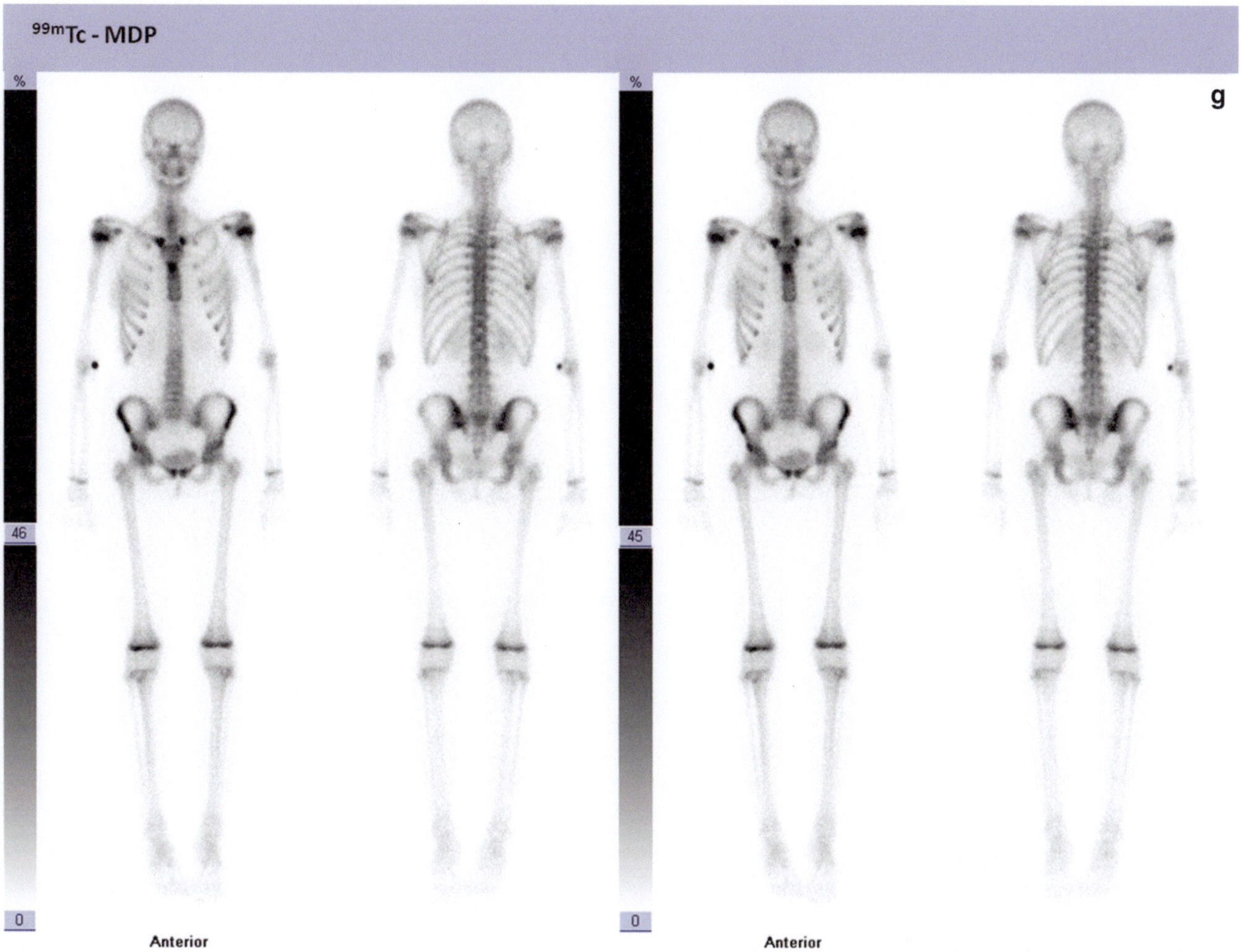

Fig. 21.10 (continued)

Endocrinology

22

Armando Grossi, Graziamaria Ubertini, and Milena Pizzoferro

22.1 Thyroid Nodules and Carcinoma

22.1.1 Introduction and Epidemiology

Thyroid nodules in children are much less common than in adults: a large study in 1975 estimated a 1.8 % prevalence in children by palpation and, more recently, 0.2–5.1 % by ultrasound. Because of their rarity, almost all the reports on thyroid nodules and cancer in pediatrics are retrospective. Conversely, nodule malignancy rate is estimated to be much higher in childhood than in adulthood: up to 25 % of pediatric thyroid nodules are malignant. A recent work on nodules ≥1 cm in the two populations statistically confirmed this data, reporting a 22 % cancer prevalence in children and 14 % in adults. Thyroid carcinoma is the commonest endocrine tumor in children: the U.S. National Institute of Health Surveillance, Epidemiology and End Results (SEER) Cancer Statistics Review Program reported across 1975–2006 an incidence of 1 per million for 5–9-year-old children, 5 per million in 10–14-year-olds, and 18 per million in 15–19-year-olds.

Pediatric thyroid cancer is almost invariably differentiated, DTC: among the histotypes those of follicular origin – follicular and papillary cancer (FTC, PTC) – prevails on the and medullary (MTC) ones, and the anaplastic and oxyphilic ones are exceptional.

Benign tumors account for approximately 10 % of all nodules and are mostly represented by toxic follicular adenomas, of prominent clinical relevance for its therapeutic implications.

Although differentiated thyroid cancer is usually slowly growing, a prompt diagnosis and accurate multistep workup are recommended in children, because greater tumor size, distant spread, and greater atypia are all factors associated with a worse prognosis and increased mortality.

22.1.2 Causes, Predisposing Factors, and Associated Disease

Preexisting thyroid diseases as congenital hypothyroidism or thyroiditis are usually considered as associated with nodules development; however, it is difficult to discern whether the disease itself represents a risk factor or if it only entails an increased detection of incidentalomas. Cases of malignant thyroid nodules have been described in patients with congenital hypothyroidism due to both dyshormonogenesis or dysgenesis and thyroglossal duct cysts as well.

Thyroid autoimmunity as a risk factor for thyroid cancer is a matter of some controversy. Very few studies evaluated this topic in the pediatric context, mostly viewing the issue from the opposite point of view by searching autoimmune disease among thyroid cancer patients. In a recent large series of children with autoimmune thyroiditis, thyroid cancer was diagnosed in 3 % of patients – 9.6 % of those with nodules with diameter >1 cm – providing a thyroid cancer prevalence of 20 %. Concerning the observations of associations between Hashimoto's thyroiditis and PTC in adults, it should be recognized that thyroiditis frequently leads to a hypothyroidism of variable degree and elevated serum TSH levels, leading some authors to hypothesize that serum TSH elevation itself is the real risk factor for the development of thyroid cancer, while thyroiditis may represent a confounder. TSH signaling via TSH–cAMP intrathyroidal pathway has a well-known growth-promoting effect on follicular-cell-derived cell and may hypothetically lead to cancer growth. Recent investigations in children indicated most cases with malignant nodules having serum TSH in the upper normal range (i.e. >2.6 mU/L) or mildly elevated (4.4–10 mU/l).

Ionizing radiations are well-known risk factors for thyroid cancer, and children are much more sensitive to their

A. Grossi (✉) • G. Ubertini
Unit of Endocrinoly, "Bambino Gesù" Children Hospital, Rome, Italy
e-mail: armando.grossi@opbg.net

M. Pizzoferro
Nuclear Medicine Unit, Imaging Departement – "Bambino Gesù" Children Hospital, Rome, Italy

© Springer International Publishing Switzerland 2017

M.C. Garganese, G.F.L. D'Errico (eds.), *Conventional Nuclear Medicine in Pediatrics*, DOI 10.1007/978-3-319-43181-9_22

carcinogenic action than adults. Thyroid cancer risk increases parallel to radiation dosages of up to 20–29 Gy, and then, for doses >30 Gy, decreases, probably because of cell killing and gland fibrosis. A great deal of our knowledge in this field has been achieved from observations on the high incidence of thyroid cancers following the widespread employment of radiotherapy for benign pathologies of the head, neck, and chest in the 1950s and 1960s, and the exposure to radioactive isotopes in the fallout from Chernobyl; almost exclusively, a papillary histotype developed in such cases. Currently, radiation is mostly employed in the treatment of childhood malignancies. Several observations evidenced that patients who underwent such treatments in childhood are prone to developing both cancerous and noncancerous thyroid diseases subsequently; the radiation-induced risk for thyroid cancer persisted elevated for 20 years after the primary cancer. Recently, data supporting a carcinogenetic role for radiations employed in the diagnostic phase of childhood cancer is accumulating. It has been observed that the increasing incidence of PTC observed in the last decades is paralleled by an increasing exposure to medical radiation: at present however, it is not clear whether PTC incidence is really increasing (or rather reflects improved detection of subclinical cases) nor which portion of PTC cases can be consequent to medical radiation exposure.

22.1.3 Genetics and Inheritance of Thyroid Neoplasms

22.1.3.1 Medullary Thyroid Carcinoma

Inheritance of thyroid neoplasms is well documented and studied from a genetic perspective for medullary thyroid carcinoma, which is derived from calcitonin-producing C cells and accounts for 5 % of all thyroid tumors. The familial form accounts for 20–25 % of cases, and belongs either to pure familial medullary thyroid carcinoma syndrome or to multiple endocrine neoplasia (MEN) type 2 syndromes, when associated with the development of pheochromocytoma. In MEN type 2A, further features are represented by hyperparathyroidism with parathyroid gland tumors. In MEN type 2B, the association includes mucosal neuromas, intestinal ganglioneuromatosis, and marfanoid habitus. Both Men syndromes are transmitted in an autosomal dominant mode of inheritance and are caused by specific gain-of-function mutations in the RET proto-oncogene detected in more than 95 % of cases. Aiming at detecting such cases, serum calcitonin is employed as a screening in thyroid nodules and as a disease marker in patients thyroidectomized for medullary thyroid cancer. As disease penetrance is almost complete and cancer development is nearly certain, in both MEN 2 syndromes, prophylactic thyroidectomy is advised, with a timing based on genotype–phenotype correlations.

22.1.3.2 Differentiated Thyroid Carcinoma

The mitogen-activated protein kinase (MAPK) signaling pathway is commonly overactivated in papillary thyroid cancer: rearrangements in genes implicated in this pathway have a pivotal role in pediatric thyroid cancer, while adult cases predominately harbor point mutations. Pediatric papillary carcinomas exhibit an increased rate of various RET/PTC (40–70 %, even more in cases following radiation exposure) or AKAP9–BRAF (11 %) rearrangements leading to the creation of fusion genes with increased signaling activity. Mutations in genes involved in the same signaling pathway and papillary cancer development occur in BRAF and RAS, the two oncogenes of the same pathway. Recently, the role of genes of the thyroid morphogenesis pathway (genes involved in thyroid gland formation, differentiation, function, and hormone synthesis implicated in congenital hypothyroidism) has been hypothesized as a player in modulating thyroid cancer risk.

Familiar nonmedullary thyroid cancer is mostly papillary, represents 3–6 % of all thyroid cancer cases, and has an autosomal dominant pattern of inheritance. No difference between sporadic and familial varieties of nonmedullary cancer is detectable in the type or number of mutations.

22.1.4 Fine Needle Aspiration Biopsy (FNAB)

FNAB is the most accurate and reliable test for nodule diagnosis and is recognized as the cornerstone and gold standard for the evaluation of solitary thyroid nodules. In spite of the lower occurrence of the disease in children, data on pediatric cases are consistent with those of adults and estimate its diagnostic accuracy as ranging from 75 to 95 %. In the last decades, FNAB has been imposed as the gold standard also in pediatric thyroid nodules demonstrating the highest sensitivity, specificity, and accuracy among other diagnostic investigations.

In spite of high diagnostic accuracy, since a few years ago, up to 20 % of thyroid nodules, FNAB cannot provide diagnostic indications: the large part of results of uncertain interpretation was defined "follicular lesion of undeterminate significance" or commonly referred to as having a "suspicious cytology." In 2007, the British Thyroid Association and the Italian Society of Pathology and Cytology (SIAPEC-IAP) introduced a new classification into five categories, respectively. In 2008, the Bethesda system for reporting thyroid FNAB specimens recommended that each report begin with one of six general diagnostic categories: I. Nondiagnostic or unsatisfactory; II. Benign; III. Atypia of undetermined significance or follicular lesion of undetermined significance; IV. Follicular neoplasm or suspicious for a follicular neoplasm specify if Hürthle cell (oncocytic) type; V. Suspicious for malignancy; VI. Malignant. Under this classification, the former "suspect" diagnostic category was further divided into "follicular lesion/suspected follicular neoplasm" (Thy 3) and "suspicious but not diagnostic for malignancy" (Thy 4). Cases belonging to the Thy 3 category, having an actual risk for malignancy\ reported to range from 15 to 34 %, were further defined into subcategories (thy 3a, 3b, and 3c) based on different risks of malignancy. The result of this novel classification system of follicular cytological specimens based on cytoarchitectural patterns is a reduction of superfluous or untimely thyroidectomies.

22.1.5 Management and Treatment of Benign Thyroid Nodules

Surgical intervention is required for an optimal management of toxic adenoma to resolve the hyperthyroid state. In this histologically benign tumor, which usually displays at scintigraphy with a "hot" pattern with silencing of the remnant thyroid tissue, FNAB does not offer much information and is considered superfluous: however, papillary carcinoma can be found in 1–5 % of these nodules [4]. Several options are available in other cytologically benign nodules: in asymptomatic cases, a conservative approach is largely employed, consisting in observation with yearly recheck or (sub-)suppressive medical treatment with levothyroxine aiming at reducing TSH stimulus and nodule shrinkage. When nodules are growing or are responsible for symptoms of local compression, several minimally invasive techniques allow to avoid the so-far employed (hemy-)thyroidectomies: percutaneous ethanol injection therapy (PEIT) is mostly employed in the treatment of prevalently cystic nodules; percutaneous thermal ablation by radiofrequency (RFA) or laser (LAT) or microwaves (MWA) or *high-intensity focused ultrasound (HIFU)* are employed in solid nodules. Further scientific data is needed to assess indications, limitations, and safety of these procedures in both adults and children. Surgery and radioiodine thyroid ablation remain the current standard in the treatment for benign/nodular disease.

22.1.6 Treatment of Thyroid Carcinoma

22.1.6.1 Surgery of DTC

Surgery is the primary therapy for pediatric patients with DTC. Recently developed pediatric guidelines indicated total thyroidectomy (TT) as the optimal surgical option.

Based on available data showing a better disease-free survival, total or near-total thyroidectomy in pediatric patients with DTC, rather than subtotal thyroidectomy, is the surgical approach generally preferred by most surgeons. The facilitation of radioiodine treatment and imaging and the use of serum Tg as a tumor marker for recurrent/residual disease are considered other practical advantages of extensive surgery. A primary procedure involving less than total thyroidectomy has been demonstrated to significantly increase the need for repeating surgery.

Since lymph node involvement at diagnosis is common, central neck dissection has been recommended, and modified neck dissection should be performed for clinically apparent and biopsy-proven lateral neck disease. Prophylactic lateral neck dissections are not recommended.

On the other hand, complications of total thyroidectomy and potential harms of the central compartment dissection such as hypoparathyroidism and injury to the recurrent laryngeal nerve should also be considered. Although these risks are minimized when surgery is performed by an experienced endocrine or pediatric surgeon, a high prevalence of hypoparathyroidism and both temporary and permanent recurrent laryngeal nerve palsies have to be taken into account. Recently, age (<16 years), familial history of thyroid cancer, preoperative gross neck lymph node diffusion, tumor diameter, and extrathyroidal invasion were identified as risk factors for disease-free survival (DFS) in children with PTC. Preoperative gross lymph node metastasis and distant metastasis at diagnosis were identified as significant factors for cause-specific survival (CSS), suggesting that routinary treatment of total thyroidectomy could not be performed in all childhood patients.

22.1.6.2 Surgery of MTC

MTC, as a sporadic cancer, is rare in childhood; and all cases in the pediatric population are considered inherited until proven otherwise. In general, treatment consists in total thyroidectomy for both sporadic and hereditary MTC associated with prophylactic central lymph node dissection (level VI), whereas lateral neck dissection (levels IIA, III, IV, V) is needed for patients with positive preoperative imaging. When distant metastatic disease is detected at diagnosis, less aggressive surgery might be appropriate in order to preserve speech and prevent morbidity.

The improved understanding of molecular basis of MEN2 and MTC heredity allows to define risk groups for development of MTC and, consequently, recommended time of prophylactic treatment. Prophylactic thyroidectomy is the standard of care in pediatrics, since patients with hereditary forms of MTC can develop metastases before the age of 5. RET mutation codon information indicates recommended age for prophylactic treatment.

22.1.6.3 Radioiodine Therapy

Radioactive iodine (Radioiodine, 131I-NaI) therapy is a mainstay of postsurgical treatment in DTC. 131I has been demonstrated to kill thyroid tumor cells several decades ago; moreover, a postsurgery 131I uptake by residual thyroid tissue is usually demonstrated. The frequent multifocal disease extension, nodal involvement, and distant metastases in pediatric patients with DTC together with a greater sodium iodine symporter expression than in adult DTC, possibly accounting for more successful treatment with 131I, are generally considered as factors making radioiodine as a therapeutic challenge. To date, it is generally suggested that most children should be treated with radioiodine in order to ablate residual disease, reduce the risk of disease recurrence, and positively affect progression-free survival rate (PFS) as recently reviewed.

In order to obtain 131I uptake by remnant and residual tissue, TSH elevation > 30 mU/l is needed. Levothyroxine administration should be discontinued 2–3 weeks in children and 4 weeks in adults before radioiodine ("thyroid hormone withdrawal", THW); alternatively, patients can be treated with 0.7 mcg/kg triiodothyronine for at least 1 month to be discontinued 2 weeks before 131I administration. TSH rise can also be achieved with recombinant human TSH (rhTSH) to be administered for two consecutive days. The use of rhTSH is approved in adults; however, it has to be emphasized that at present, rhTSH use is not approved for children by drug-regulatory agencies in the United States or Europe. Although it has the potential to reduce whole-body radiation exposure associated with it, 131I therapy and its clinical use have been reported in children with WDTC, data showing comparable efficacy to THW are lacking in pediatrics.

Main purposes of the use of radioiodine treatment include therapy of residual microscopic disease, metastatic or unresectable lesions, together with an accurate patient staging by means of 131I whole-body scanning, usually performed within 10 days of radioiodine therapy, for the detection of distant metastases. In addition, the postsurgery ablation of remaining thyroid tissue in the neck ("thyroid remnant ablation", RRA) allows the use of Tg as a tumor marker during the follow-up. There is no specific recommendation for the timing of 131I after total thyroidectomy; however, it is generally done within 3–6 weeks, till 3 months after surgery.

131I dosage strategies can be summarized in: administering fixed activities (eventually based on the patient's weight); dosaging based on the administered activity that is as high as safely administrable (AHASA), recently defined as the lowest safe limit administered activities up to 5 mCi/kg (200 MBq/kg) for treatment of distant metastases and DTC recurrence in children; and applying specific activities for tumor ablation, dosimetry, which is suggested to be mainly considered for individuals with lung metastases.

The use of pretherapy scans is limited because of its low impact on the decision to ablate, and because of 131I-induced stunning phenomenon, it is defined as a reduction in uptake of the radioioidine therapy dose induced by a pretreatment diagnostic activity. On the other hand, since it can be difficult to distinguish residual disease from thyroid remnant at post-therapy WBS, and when the extent of the thyroid remnant cannot be accurately ascertained from the surgical report or neck ultrasonography, 123I (1.5–3 mCi) or low-activity 131I (1–3 mCi) pretherapy scans may provide additional informations in order to distinguish residual disease from thyroid remnant, and then to plan more adequate therapeutic strategies. This procedure including the use of 123I is considered in recent ATA pediatric guidelines.

22.1.6.4 Levothyroxine Therapy

Levothyroxine (LT4) therapy is a fundamental part of the treatment of thyroid carcinoma; it is well recognized that TSH suppression (TST) can reduce rates of recurrence for DTC, whereas there is no role for TST in MTC, and LT4 replacement should be undertaken in these patients.

The ATA pediatric guidelines recommends in low-risk DTC patients to obtain TSH values between 0.5–1 mU/l, and a more aggressive suppression is suggested for intermediate (0.1–0.5 mU/l TSH values) and high-risk (TSH values below 0.1 mU/l) patients.

22.1.6.5 Other Therapies

External beam radiation does not have a clear role in the treatment of WDTC, its use being beneficial as a palliative measure in advanced disease stages. Chemotherapy is not considered in the initial therapy of DTC; newer agents are being evaluated for patients with metastatic or recurrent disease.

Treatment of anaplastic cancer (ATC), the most aggressive thyroid tumor and one of the most aggressive cancers in humans, has not been standardized, and unfortunately there is not yet an efficient treatment; surgery, chemotherapy, radiotherapy, alone or in combination, are used with no impact on survival rate. Most used cytotoxic agents include doxorubicin, cisplatin, and bleomycin.

In advanced MTC, mono- or poly-chemotherapy has not shown significant clinical benefit. Radiation may be used in the presence of local invasion, or in the setting of bone (with bisphosphonates to control symptoms) or CNS metastasis, although there are no strong data indicating an effect on long-term survival. New compounds of the family of RET kinase inhibitor may have important clinical benefits. The FDA-approved vandetanib, a RET kinase inhibitor, has been shown to lengthen progression-free survival This compound has been demonstrated to also inhibit the epidermal and vascular endothelial growth factor receptors. Prognosis of MTC, however, has been most closely related to the extent of disease at presentation and to the extent of first surgery.

22.2 Congenital Hypothyroidisms

The incidence of primary congenital hypothyroidism (CH) ranges from 1:3000 to 1:4000 newborn infants. Any infant with low T4 concentration and TSH > 40 mUI/l is considered to have primary hypothyroidism. CH is one of the most common cause of mental retardation, because thyroid hormones are fundamental in the development of brain.

The initial recommendation of American Academy of Pediatrics for newborn screening for CH was published in 1993. Early detection and treatment of congenital hypothyroidism by neonatal screening prevents neurodevelopment disability.

Congenital hypothyroidism can be "primary" for thyroid abnormalities or "secondary" for hypothalamic pituitary thyroid axis damage.

In most cases, this disorder is "permanent" and results from an abnormality in thyroid gland development (dysgenesis or agenesis) or a defect in thyroid hormonogenesis. Less commonly, the alteration of thyroid hormones is "transient" due to transplacental passage of maternal medication, maternal blocking antibodies, or iodine deficiency or excess.

22.2.1 Screening Test

Three possible screening strategies for detection of CH are possible:

1. A primary TSH measurement supplemented by T4 determination only in infants with elevated TSH
2. A primary T4 measurement supplemented by TSH determination only in infants with low T4
3. A combined TSH plus T4 method.

Every infant should be tested before discharge from the nursery optimally by 48 h to 4 days of age.

1. In the first case (screening programs in Europe, Japan, Canada, and Mexico), primary TSH measurements are supplemented by T4 determination for infants with elevated TSH value. The first screening specimen commonly is obtained before 48 h of age. With this approach, delayed TSH elevation in infants with thyroid-binding globulin (TBG) deficiency, central hypothyroidism, and isolated reduced level of T4 (hypothyroxinemia) can be missed.
2. The primary T4 approach can identify primary CH in infants with low and very low T4 levels and elevated TSH (1:3000–1:4000 newborn infants). Otherwise, this approach can also identify infants with TBG deficiency (1:5000–1:10,000 newborn infants) and central hypothyroidism (low levels of T4 with normal or low levels of TSH) that is a very rare cause of hypothyroidism (1:50,000 newborn infants). However, this approach will miss the conditions with initial normal T4 and delayed elevated TSH levels (patient with low and very low birth weight).
3. The combined approach represents the ideal screening test.

22.2.2 Definition

Any infant with a low T4 concentration and TSH > 40 is considered affected by primary hypothyroidism. These infants should be examined immediately to confirm the diagnosis with a new serum test, and therapy with LT4 should be initiated. The patients with TSH between 20 and 40 should be submitted to another filter-paper screening test (10 % of patients with confirmed CH have TSH value in this range).

Hyperthyrotropinemia is characterized by elevated TSH concentration with T4 or FT4 in the normal range. The etiologies of these clinical conditions are different and can be either transient of permanent thyroid abnormality such as TSH receptor mutation or delayed maturation of hypothalamic–pituitary axis.

TSH concentration is the most sensitive indicator that the hypothalamic pituitary axis is sensing a circulating T4 level less than optimal. Most physicians consider a persistent TSH value superior than 10 mUI/L after 2 weeks of live to be abnormal and treat these infants. In case of no initial therapy, FT4 and TSH should be repeated in 2–4 weeks, and treatment with LT4 should be initiated in case of subsequent FT4 and TSH abnormal levels.

Low T4 and Normal TSH Value

Infants with normal TSH but low T4 value may have thyroid insufficiency. This pattern is seen in 3–5 % of neonates and can be transient and caused by hypothalamic immaturity (particularly in preterm infants). Low T4 but normal TSH levels are also present during illness or as the result of infusion of dopamine or high dose of glucocorticoids. The same pattern may be present in permanent clinical condition such as central hypothyroidism (since 1:25,000 to 1:50,000 newborn infants) or in primary hypothyroidism with delayed TSH elevation (1:100,000 newborn infants). Many infants with low T4 concentration and normal TSH value on initial screening, with subsequent elevated TSH concentration, are of low birth and very low birth or critically ill preterm and term neonates. Serum TSH levels increase in these infants in the first few weeks of life.

The infants with this delayed TSH elevation have abnormalities of pituitary thyroid feedback or transient hypothyroidism or mild form of permanent CH. It is important to consider that also in the absence of human error, 5–10 % of LBW and VLBW infants with CH may have normal hormone concentration at screening. So, in these patients, the repetition of serum control of TSH and FT4 is fundamental in 2–6 weeks of age.

22.2.3 Transient Hypothyroidism

A small number of infants with abnormal screening value will have transient hypothyroidism (1:50,000). Transient hypothyroidism may result from intrauterine exposure to maternal antithyroid drugs, maternal TRB antibodies, mutation of TSH receptor, endemic iodine deficiency, or prenatal and postnatal exposure to excess of iodine. The transplacental passage of maternal TRSAbs (1:180,000) should be suspected if there is a maternal clinical history of autoimmune thyroid disease.

22.2.4 Clinical Management

The infants with low T4 and elevated TSH concentration have primary CH and should be treated as soon as possible. It is important to perform a confirmatory serum measurement of TSH and FT4 levels.

An elevated level of thyroglobulin suggests dyshormonogenesis. When there is a history of maternal autoimmune thyroid disorder, measurement of TRBAbs in the infants may identify a transient form of neonatal hypothyroidism.

22.2.5 Optional Diagnostic Studies

The use of imaging studies such as ultrasound and scintigraphy should be considered in neonates with high TSH concentration in order to clarify the diagnosis.

Imaging should never determine the dilation of the treatment that should be initiated as soon as possible and no later than 2 weeks of life. The goal of therapy is to normalize FT4 within 2 weeks and TSH within 1 month of therapy. Scintigraphy should be carried out within 7 days of starting LT4 treatment.

Scintigraphy may be carried out with either 10–20 MBq of technetium 99 m or 1–2 MBq of iodine 123. Technetium 99 m is more widely available, less expensive, and quicker to use than 123 I. 123 I is specifically taken by thyroid gland and gives a clear scan.

Scintigraphy is very useful in identifying the different causes of primary CH (Table 22.1). It can identify:

- Athyreosis (absence of uptake)
- Hypoplasia of gland in situ (with or without hemithyroid)
- A normal or large gland in situ (with or without high levels of uptake)
- An ectopic gland at any point along the normal embryological descent from the base of the tongue to the thyroid cartilage

The scintigraphy may show no uptake despite the presence of a eutopic thyroid gland (ultrasound) in:

- Exposure to excess of iodine (antiseptic preparation)
- Maternal TSH receptor blocking antibodies
- TSH suppression from LT4 treatment
- Inactivating mutation of TSH receptor and/or the sodium/iodide symporter (NIS)

To avoid unnecessary radiation and for the less difficulties of the method, some investigators prefer ultrasonography as the initial imaging procedure. But the use of ultrasonography without scintigraphy in the diagnosis of the different etiologies in primary CH could be incomplete. This image method cannot always detect lingual and sublingual thyroid ectopy and is highly observer-dependent.

Combining scintigraphy and thyroid ultrasound in CH patients helps to:

- Improve diagnostic accuracy
- Identify a eutopic gland which may be normal, enlarged, or hypoplastic, guiding other investigation exams such as molecular studies
- Prevent the incorrect diagnosis of athyreosis in the presence of no uptake on scintigraphy when ultrasound shows normal gland in situ
- Detect thyroid ectopy reliably

Table 22.1 Ultrasound, scintigraphic patterns and Thyroglobuline values in different forms of primary Congenital Hypothyroidism (CH)

Defect	Thyroid ultrasound	Thyroid scintigraphy	Serum thyroglobulin concentration
Thyroid dysgenesis			
Apparent athyreosis	No thyroid tissue seen	No uptake	Detectable (>2 mcg/L)
True athyreosis	No thyroid tissue seen	No uptake	Undetectable
Ectopy	Either no thyroid tissue seen or ectopic tissue seen	Uptake into ectopic gland	Usually ↑ bau may be N or ↓
Hypoplasia in situ	Small ectopic gland	Low level of uptake in a normally sited gland	N or ↓
Hemiagenesis	Hemithyroid	Hemithyroid	N
Dyshormonogenesis			
NIS/SCL5A5	Enlarged gland	Uptake absent or ↓↓	↑
Thyroid peroxidase, TPO (iodide organification defects)	Enlarged gland	High level of uptake; positive perchlorate discharge test	↑↑
Dual oxidase 2 (DUOX2); dual oxidase 2 maturation factor (DUOXA2) (iodide organification defects)	Enlarged gland	High level of uptake; positive perchlorate discharge test	↑
Pendred syndrome; pendrin PDS	Normal/enlarged gland	High level of uptake; positive perchlorate discharge test	↑
Thyroglobulin	Enlarged gland	Avid uptake; normal perchlorate discharge test	↓↓ or undetectable
Transient CH			
Acute iodine excess	Normal gland in situ	No uptake	N or ↓
Chronic iodine deficiency	Large gland	Avid uptake	↑
Maternal blocking antibodies	Normal or small gland	Uptake absent or ↓	N or ↓
TSH receptor	Normal or small gland	Uptake absent or ↓	N or ↓

Modified from European Society for Pediatric Endocrinology [6]

22.3 Hyperparathyroidism

Hyperparathyroidism exists in three different forms: primary, secondary, and tertiary.

Diagnosis of *primary hyperparathyroidism (PHPT)* is characterized by suggestive clinical presentation and laboratory investigations (hypercalcemia and elevated serum concentrations of intact PTH). PHPT is a rare disease in adolescents, and limited data exist on pediatric and adolescent patients with primary hyperparathyroidism.

The causes of PHPT in the adolescent population include parathyroid adenomas, multiglandular disease (MGD), and parathyroid carcinoma. Neonatal hyperparathyroidism is a rare disorder, and it has been classified as a distinct disease entity; it is caused by inactivating calcium-sensing receptor (CASR) mutations that result in life-threatening hypercalcemia and metabolic bone disease.

PHPT in the majority of adolescents is due to a single adenoma, just as in adults. Symptoms of PHPT in children are often more severe and more common than in adults. One potential explanation for this difference is due to the delay in diagnosis with consequent progression of disease. PHPT is usually identified in younger patients only when they become symptomatic, because routine biochemical screening is common in adults but not in youth. Alternatively, it has been hypothesized that juvenile PHPT is a pathophysiological different and more aggressive disease than adult PHPT. In fact, it has been observed that juvenile PHPT presents greater hypercalcemia and hypercalciuria than adult PHPT at similar concentrations of serum intact PTH, reflecting an apparent decrease in the sensitivity of the parathyroid adenoma to negative feedback by calcium and increased sensitivity of target tissues to the effects of PTH.

MGD in younger patients is generally due to hereditary family disorders including multiple endocrine neoplasia type1 (MEN1), MEN2a, or familial isolated hyperparathyroidism.

In adults, PHPT is usually an asymptomatic disorder that presents as incidentally discovered hypercalcemia.

Secondary hyperparathyroidism (SHPT) is consequent to a chronic hypocalcemic condition that can be caused by renal failure, gastrointestinal malabsorption, and dietary rickets which generate a decreased intestinal absorption of calcium. SHPT is a severe disease of patients who undergo hemodialysis, causing substantial morbidity and mortality consequent to progressive osteodystrophy and vascular and soft tissue calcification. The continuous stimulus (hypocalcemia, hyperphosphatemia, and low calcitriol concentrations) to produce and to secrete PTH results in parathyroid cell hypertrophy, determining initially diffuse and reversible and successively nodular and irreversible hyperplasia of parathyroid glands.

Tertiary hyperparathyroidism is a condition where parathyroid hyperplasia, secondary to chronic hypocalcemia, becomes autonomous with the development of hypercalcemia.

Establishing the diagnosis of hyperparathyroidism, the clinical question is to locate hyperfunctioning parathyroid gland or glands.

As in adults, in pediatric population study, approaches of parathyroid function must consider the anatomy and the embryogenic origin of parathyroid glands.

Parathyroid glands are generally four in number (even if five or more glands can be present), are subdivided into two upper and two lower, and their most probable location is behind the thyroid gland. In relation to the longer embryogenetic pathway and the difficult migration process, the location of parathyroid glands can vary and presence of ectopic glands must be ruled out (very high in the neck or within the thyrothymic ligament, the thymus, or in the mediastinum).

Ultrasonography and 99mTc-sestamibi scintigraphy are the dominant imaging techniques for hyperfunctioning location of parathyroid. However, intrathyroid parathyroid gland (even if rare) is difficult to distinguish sonographically from a thyroid nodule, and ultrasound scan has poor sensitivity for detecting ectopic glands in retrotracheal region or in the mediastinum.

In case of parathyroid adenomas, contrast-enhanced CT and MRI can be helpful when findings at sonography and 99 m Tc-sestamibi scintigraphy are discordant or in the setting of failed parathyroidectomy for the detection of suspected ectopic (often mediastinal) glands.

Bibliography

1. Bargren AE, Meyer-Rochow GY, Delbridge LW, Sidhu SB, Chen H. Outcomes of surgically managed pediatric thyroid cancer. J Surg Res. 2009;156:70–3.
2. Chao M. Management of differentiated thyroid cancer with rising thyroglobulin and negative diagnostic radioiodine whole body scan. Clin Oncol (R Coll Radiol). 2010;22:438–47.
3. Cooper DS, Doherty GM, Haugen BR, Kloos RT, Lee SL, Mandel SJ, Mazzaferri EL, McIver B, Pacini F, Schlumberger M, Sherman SI, Steward DL, Tuttle RM; American Thyroid Association (ATA) Guidelines Taskforce on Thyroid Nodules and Differentiated Thyroid Cancer. Revised American Thyroid Association management guidelines for patients with thyroid nodules and differentiated thyroid cancer. Thyroid. 2009;19(11):1167–214.
4. Diesen DL, Skinner MA. Pediatric thyroid cancer. Semin Pediatr Surg. 2012;21:44–50.
5. European Society for Pediatric Endocrinology. Consensus guidelines on screening, diagnosis and management of congenital hypothyroidism. Horm Res Pediatr. 2014;81:80–103.
6. Gupta A, Ly S, Castroneves LA, Frates MC, Benson CB, Feldman HA, Wassner AJ, Smith JR, Marqusee E, Alexander EK, Barletta J, Doubilet PM, Peters HE, Webb S, Modi BP, Paltiel HJ, Kozakewich H, Cibas ES, Moore Jr FD, Shamberger RC, Larsen PR, Huang SA. A standardized assessment of thyroid nodules in children confirms higher cancer prevalence than in adults. J Clin Endocrinol Metab. 2013;98(8):3238–45.
7. Kloos RT, Eng C, Evans DB, et al. Medullary thyroid cancer: management guidelines of the American Thyroid Association. Thyroid. 2009;19:565–612.
8. Lugo-Vicente H, Romero-Estremera NJ. Thyroid nodules in children: what should be a minimal work-up preceding surgery? Bol Asoc Med P R. 2012;104(4):33–6.

9. Luster M, Handkiewicz-Junak D, Grossi A, et al. Recombinant tyrotropin use in children and adolescents with differentiated thyroid cancer. J Clin Endocrinol Metab. 2009;94:3948–53.
10. Markovina S, Grigsby PW, Schwarz, JK, DeWees T, Moley JF, Siegel BA, Perkins S. Treatment approach, surveillance and outcome of well-differentiated thyroid cancer in childhood and adolescence. Thyroid. 2013. doi:10.1089/thy.2013.0297.
11. Niedziela M. Thyroid nodules. Best Pract Res Clin Endocrinol Metab. 2014;28(2):245–77.
12. O'Gorman CS, Hamilton J, Rachmiel M, Gupta A, Ngan BY, Daneman D. Thyroid cancer in childhood: a retrospective review of childhood course. Thyroid. 2010;20(4):375–80.
13. Pacini F, Castagna MG, Brilli L, Pentheroudakis G, et al. Thyroid cancer: ESMO Clinical Practice Guidelines for diagnosis, treatment and follow-up. Ann Oncol. 2010;21 Suppl 5:v214–9. doi:10.1093/annonc/mdq190.
14. Pawelczak M, David R, Franklin B, Kessler M, Lam L, Shah B. Outcomes of children and adolescents with well-differentiated thyroid carcinoma and pulmonary metastases following 131I treatment: a systematic review. Thyroid. 2010;20(10):1095–101. doi:10.1089/thy.2009.0446.
15. Rivkees SA, Mazzaferri EL, Verburg FA, Reiners C, Luster M, Breuer CK, Dinauer CA, Udelsman R. The treatment of differentiated thyroid cancer in children: emphasis on surgical approach and radioactive iodine therapy. Endocr Rev. 2011;32(6):798–826. doi:10.1210/er.2011-0011. Epub 2011 Aug 31.
16. Rose SR, Brown RS, Foley T, Kaplowitz PB, Kaye CI, Sundararajan S, Varma SK. Update of newborn screening and therapy for congenital hypothyroidism. Pediatrics. 2006;117(6):229–303.
17. Spencer C, Fatemi S, Singer P, Nicoloff J, Lopresti J. Serum Basal thyroglobulin measured by a second-generation assay correlates with the recombinant human thyrotropin-stimulated thyroglobulin response in patients treated for differentiated thyroid cancer. Thyroid. 2010;20:587–95.
18. Verburg FA, Biko J, Diessl S, Demidchik Y, Drozd V, Rivkees S, Reiners C, Hanscheid H. I-131 activities as high as safely administrable (AHASA) for the treatment of children and adolescents with advanced differentiated thyroid cancer. J Clin Endocrinol Metab. 2011;96:E1268–71.
19. Wells Jr SA, Pacini F, Robinson BG, Santoro M. Multiple endocrine neoplasia type 2 and familial medullary thyroid carcinoma: an update. J Clin Endocrinol Metab. 2013;98(8):3149–64.
20. Xing M, Haugen BR, Schlumberger M. Progress in molecular-based management of differentiated thyroid cancer. Lancet. 2013;381(9871):1058–69.

Endocrinology: Thyroid Carcinoma

23

Milena Pizzoferro, Maria Felicia Villani, Armando Grossi, Debora De Pasquale, and Maria Carmen Garganese

23.1 Study Technique and Interpretation

23.1.1 Diagnostic Whole-Body Scan: ^{123}I WBS After rh-TSH Stimulation

Differentiated thyroid carcinoma (DTC) is rare in childhood, but is the most frequent tumor of endocrine glands in children and adolescents (0.2–0.5/100,000/year), and is more aggressive with regard to clinical course. Total thyroidectomy, followed by ablative radioiodine therapy, is recommended; on the other hand, less aggressive treatment modalities should be taken into consideration, due to the high life expectancy of these patients and the potential impairment of quality of life.

For more accurate staging and therapy strategies, avoiding L-T4 withdrawal effect and stunning phenomenon, the combined use of recombinant human TSH (rh-TSH) and radioiodine imaging has been proven to be safe and useful in adults. On the basis of more recent experiences, it has been pointed out that usefulness of rh-TSH use in pediatrics can be considered similar to that of adults.

In our department, standard schedule for rh-TSH administration resulted in intramuscular injections of 0.9 mg for two consecutive days followed by 185 MBq of 123I-Na (day 3). Thyroglobulin (Tg) and TSH are evaluated at baseline and 5 days after rh-TSH administration. 123I-WBS was obtained on day 4. All parents provided an informed consent for their children, according to local ethical committee. No side effects have been recorded after rh-TSH administration, and 123I-WBS imaging and Tg levels after rh-TSH have been concordant with TxWBS imaging and Tg levels in hypothyroidism.

23.1.2 Therapeutic Whole-Body Scan

All patients were submitted to radioiodine treatment (RAI) in hypothyroidism condition after an adequate low iodine content diet preparation. A TSH peak was observed in all patients, and posttherapy WBS (TxWBS) was obtained 3 days after ^{131}I administration.

M. Pizzoferro • M.F. Villani
Nuclear Medicine Unit, Imaging Department–"Bambino Gesù" Children Hospital, Rome, Italy

A. Grossi (✉)
Unit of Endocrinology, "Bambino Gesù" Children Hospital, Rome, Italy
e-mail: armando.grossi@opbg.net

D. De Pasquale
Oncohematology Department, "Bambino Gesù" Children Hospital, Rome, Italy

M.C. Garganese
Diagnostic Imaging Department of Nuclear Medicine, IRCCS Bambino Gesù Paediatric Hospital, Rome, Italy

© Springer International Publishing Switzerland 2017

M.C. Garganese, G.F.L. D'Errico (eds.), *Conventional Nuclear Medicine in Pediatrics*, DOI 10.1007/978-3-319-43181-9_23

23.1.3 Teaching Cases

Case 23.1 Diagnostic ^{123}I WBS in DTC: Staging and Therapeutic Efficacy Assessment in Remnant Ablation (Fig. 23.1)

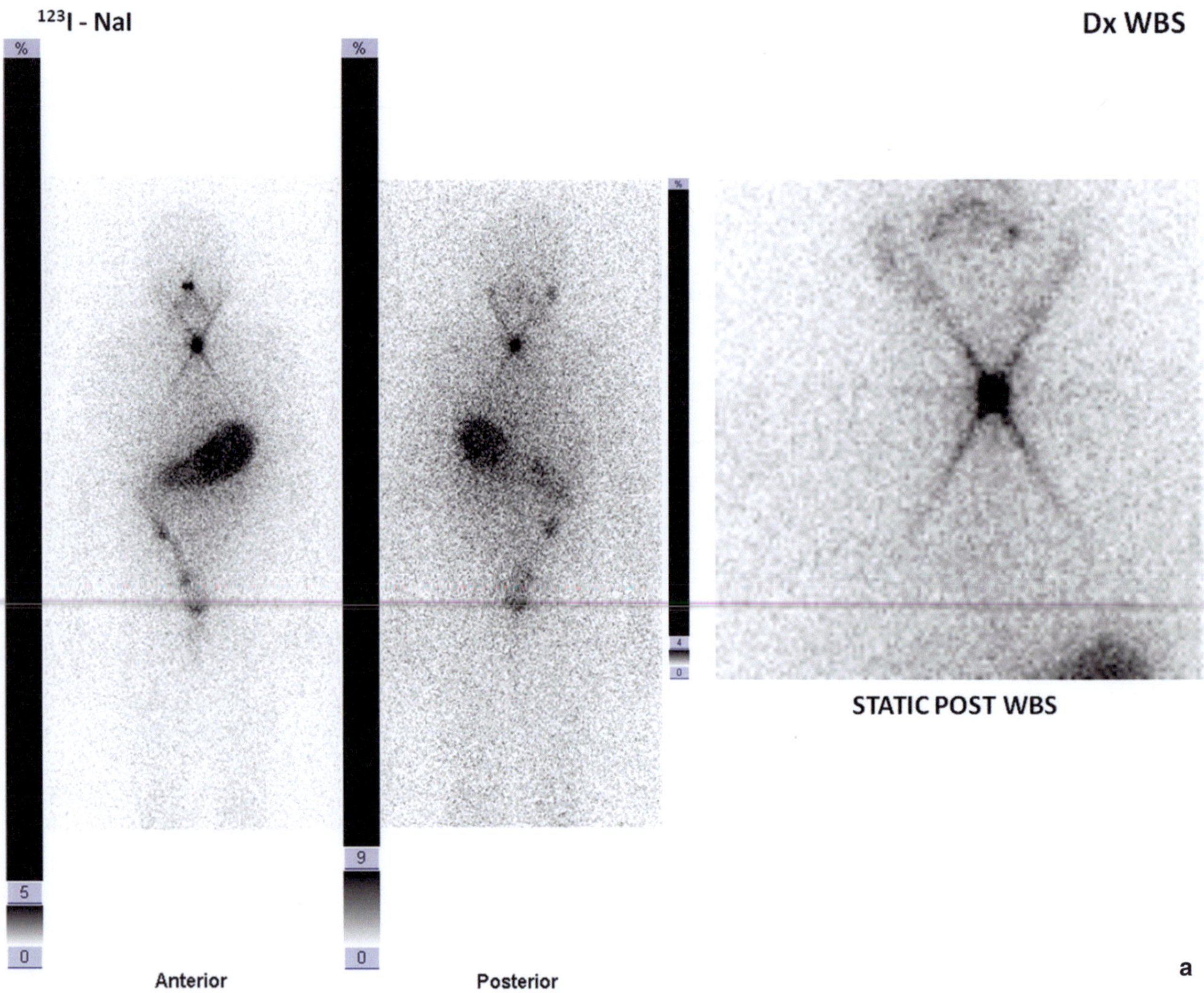

Fig. 23.1 (**a–b**) A 12-year-old boy affected by papillary thyroid carcinoma (pT3 pN0 pMx). After total thyroidectomy, diagnostic ^{123}I WBS shows radioiodine uptake in thyroid remnants (**a**). After RAI assessment, any focus of radioiodine uptake is evident in thyroid bed, as for complete metabolic RAI response (**b**)

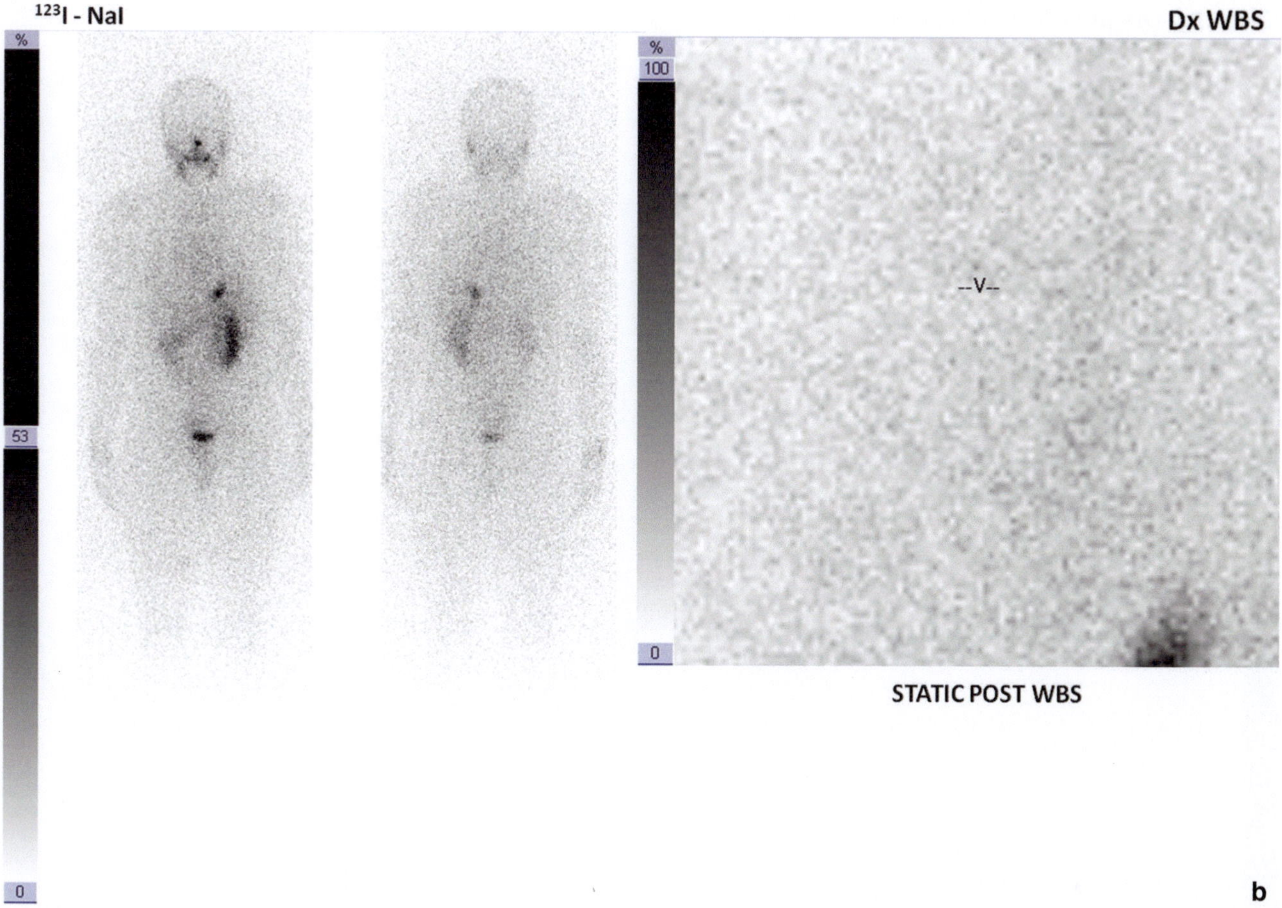

Fig. 23.1 (continued)

Case 23.2 Diagnostic ^{123}I WBS in DTC Staging: Remnant and Lymph Node Involvement (**Fig.** 23.2)

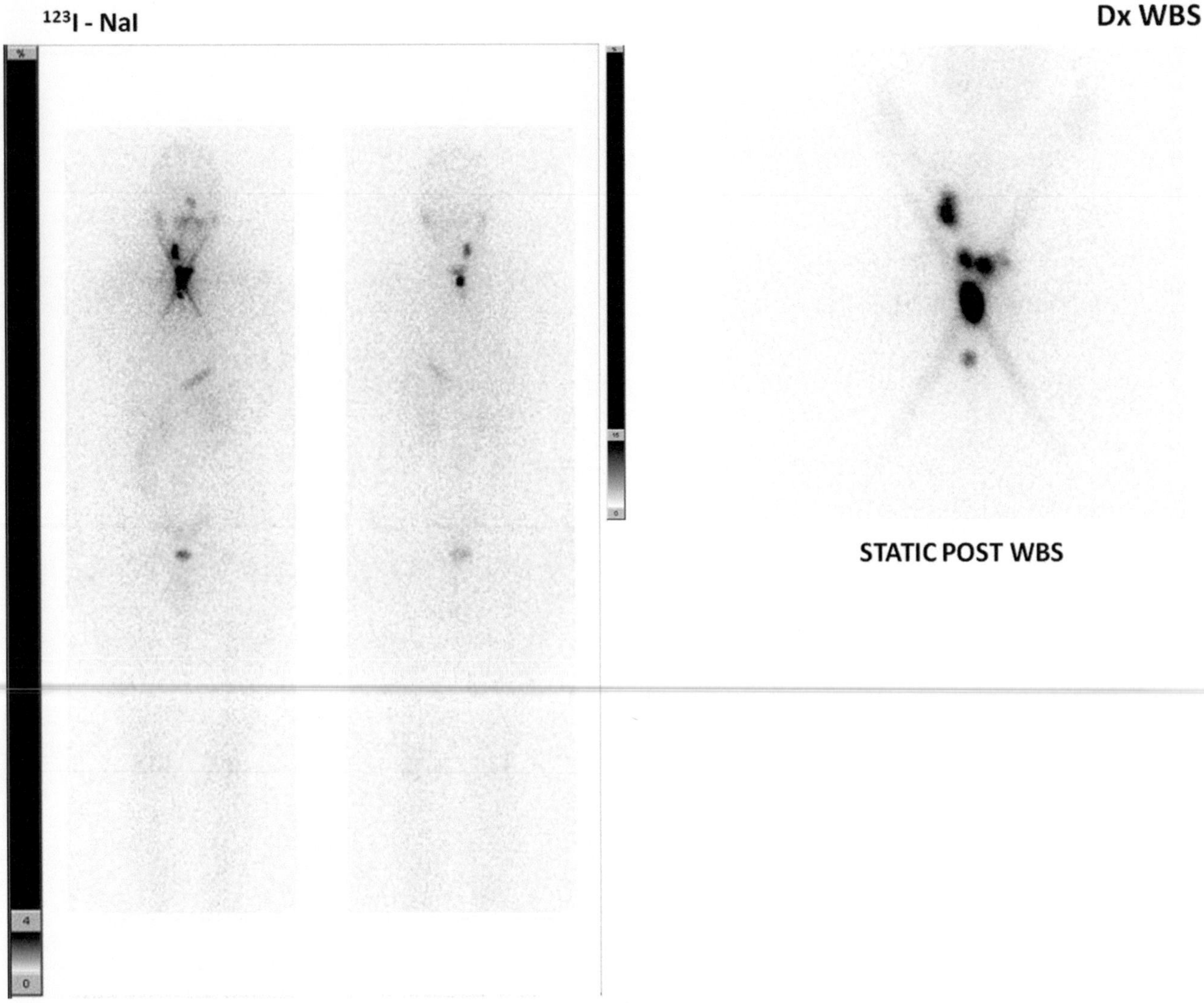

Fig. 23.2 A 15-year-old boy with diagnosis of papillary thyroid carcinoma underwent total thyroidectomy (pT2 pN+ pMx). After total thyroidectomy, diagnostic 123I WBS shows radioiodine uptake in thyroid bed with evidence of neck lymph node uptake

Case 23.3 Diagnostic ^{123}I WBS in DTC Restaging: Relapse of Disease in Lymph Nodes and Lungs (Focal Pattern) (Fig. 23.3)

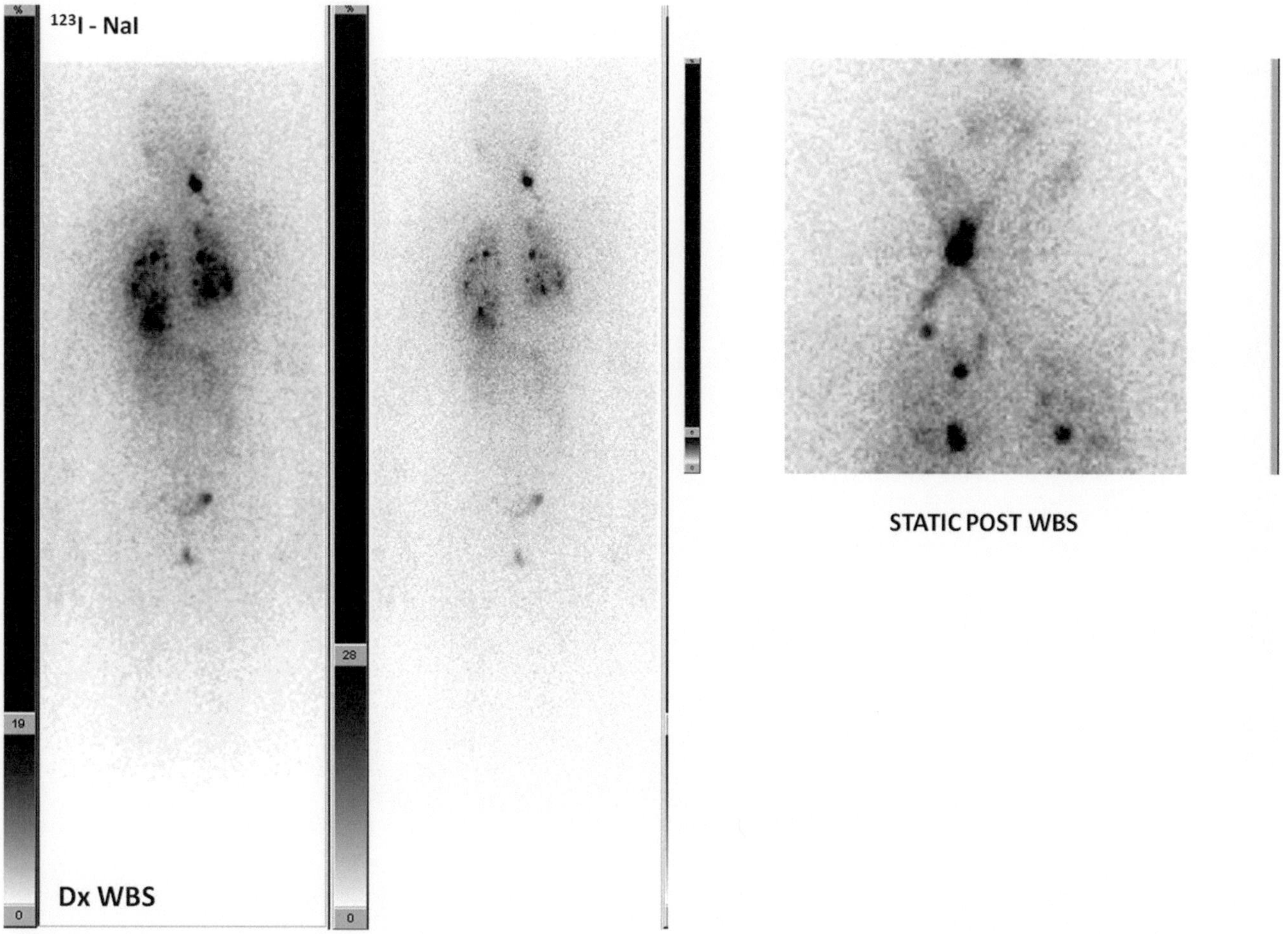

Fig. 23.3 A 16-year-old girl affected by papillary thyroid carcinoma underwent total thyroidectomy (pT3 pN+ pMx) at the age of 14 years, followed by RAI therapy with complete metabolic response. Follow-up was negative up to 2 years later when thyroglobulin level increased, and restaging by ^{123}I WBS was performed showing radioiodine uptake in neck lymph node (on right side) and in both lungs (focal pattern)

Case 23.4 Diagnostic ^{123}I WBS IN DTC Staging: Lymph Nodes and Lungs (Diffuse Pattern) (Fig. 23.4)

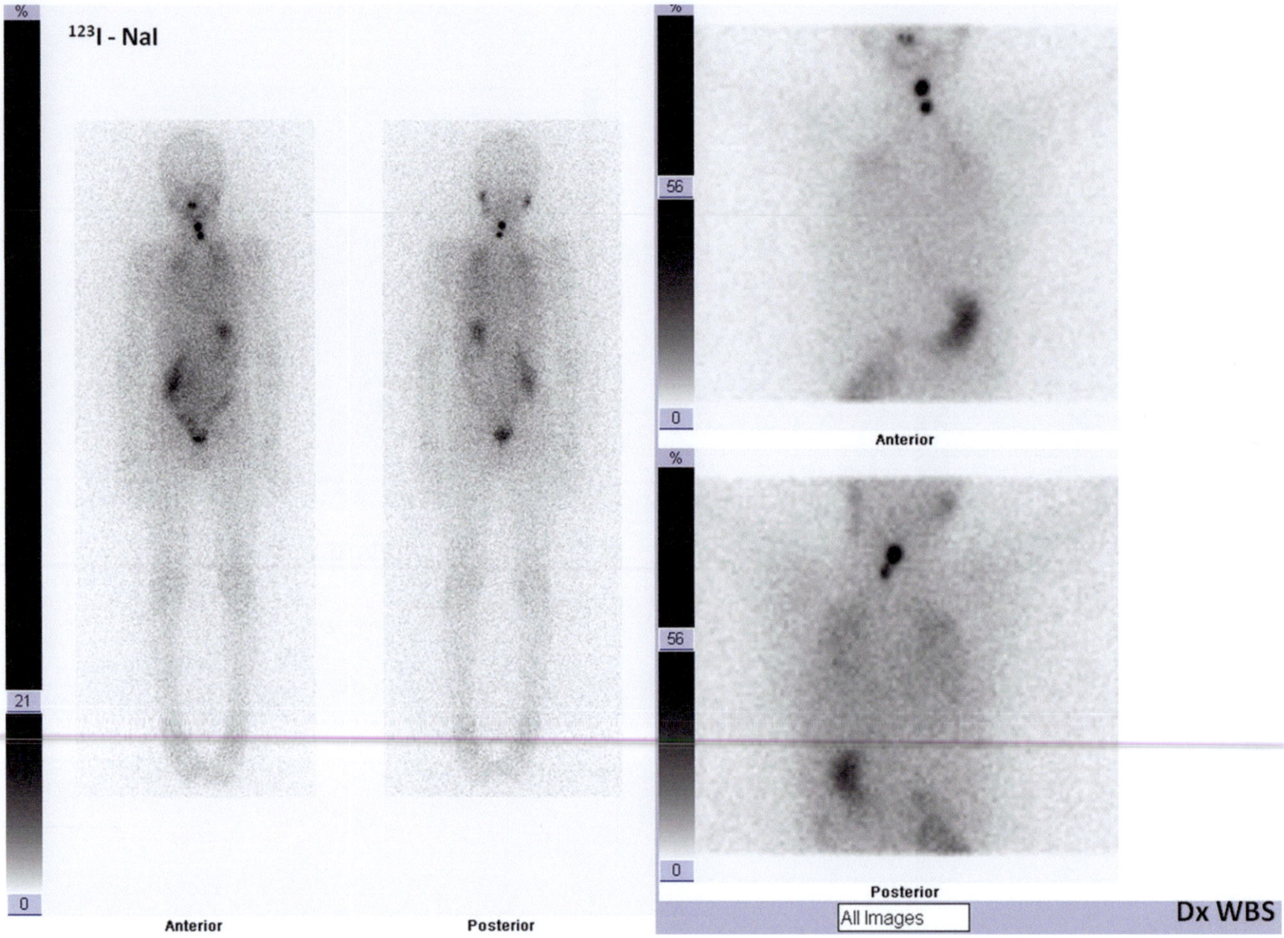

Fig. 23.4 A 7-year-old boy with diagnosis of papillary thyroid carcinoma underwent total thyroidectomy (pT4 pN+ pMx). After total thyroidectomy, diagnostic ^{123}I WBS shows radioiodine uptake in the neck (two areas of focal uptake in upper jugular and upper cervical region, as for remnant and thyroglossal duct, respectively) with evidence of mild and diffuse radioiodine uptake (miliary pulmonary involvement is a frequent pattern in young patients affected by DTC)

Case 23.5 Planar and SPECT/CT Evaluation in Therapeutic ^{131}I WBS: Lymph node and Lung Involvement (Diffuse vs. Focal Pattern) (Fig. 23.5)

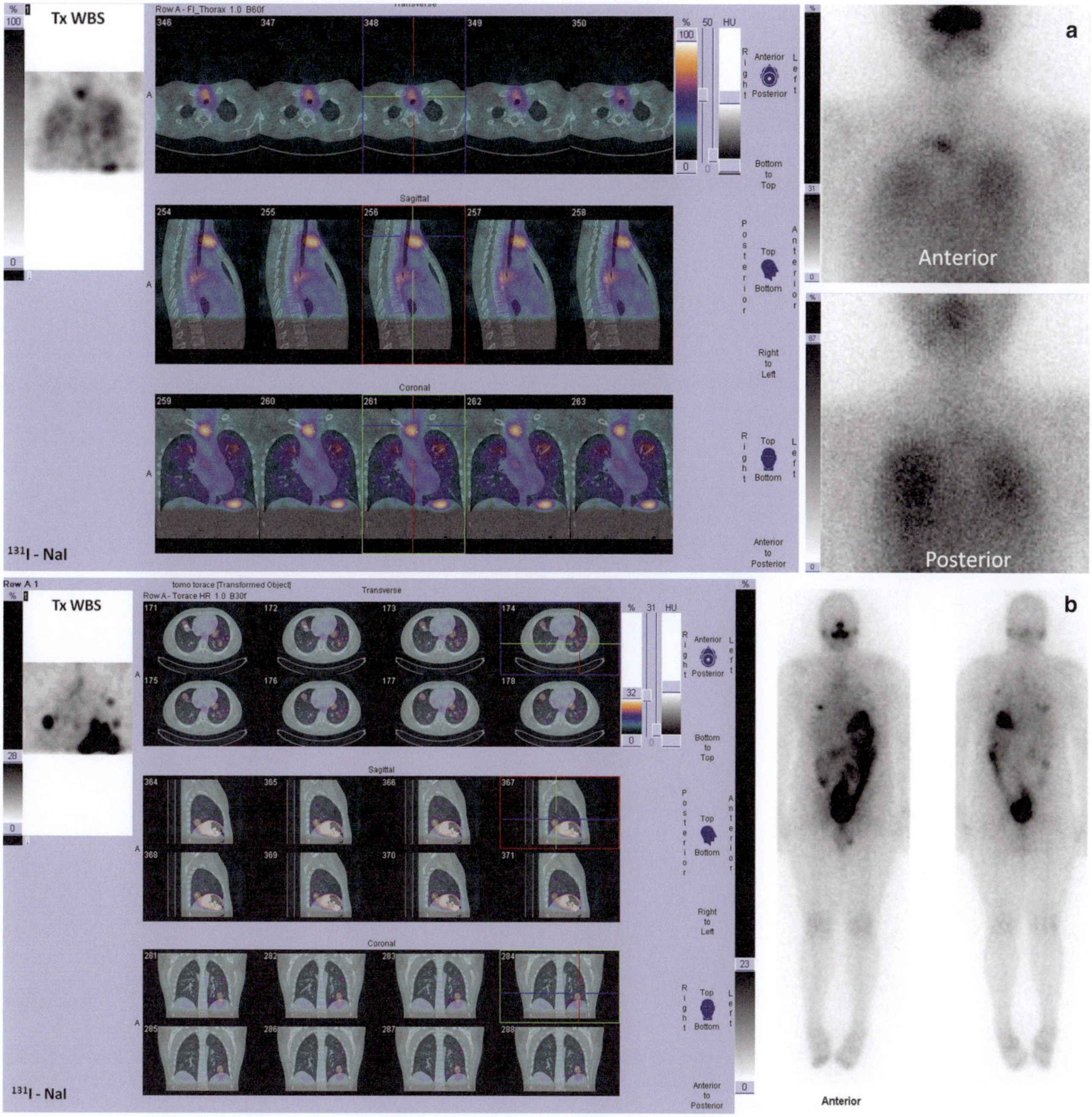

Fig. 23.5 When radioiodine uptake is detected in the thoracic region at whole-body scan, spot image acquisition is performed for a better imaging evaluation. SPECT acquisition and SPECT/CT fused images are useful for a precise localization of pathological findings and improvement of diagnostic accuracy. (**a**) Planar imaging (*right side*): a focal radioiodine uptake is evident in the superior mediastinum region associated with diffuse bilateral lung uptake. Fused images (**a** *left*) confirm miliary lung pattern; mediastinal lymph node involvement is also detected, and a precise localization and characterization by anatomical and metabolic features are allowed. (**b**) WBS (*right side*) shows focal areas of radioiodine uptake in both lungs associated with moderate uptake corresponding to mediastinum region. Fused images (**b**, *left side*) confirm focal pulmonary involvement and show further pulmonary lesions; lymph node involvement (in upper and inferior mediastinum) is also clearly evident

Case 23.6 Diagnostic and Therapeutic $^{123}I/^{131}I$ WBS in DCT Restaging: Relapse of Disease with Bone Metastases

A 16-year-old girl affected by secondary thyroid carcinoma (after a previous total body irradiation for T-cell leukemia at 20 months of life) underwent total thyroidectomy (papillary thyroid carcinoma, pT4 pN+ pMx)) followed by ablative radioiodine therapy at 10 years of life. Follow-up was negative up to 3 years later when thyrooglobulin level increased (with negative anti-Tg antibodies), and restaging by ^{123}I WBS was performed showing two areas of radioiodine uptake corresponding to the proximal region of both femurs (Fig. 23.6a). The girl was submitted to 131I-NaI therapy. ^{18}F-FDG PET scan pretherapy was negative for metastasis with high glucose metabolic activity (as for a disease still well-differentiated). ^{131}I WBS post therapy (Fig. 23.6b) revealed a progression of disease.

Secondary thyroid carcinoma is more aggressive with regard to clinical course, and the prognosis is poor when metastatic cancer occurs. Close monitoring is required in these patients, and $^{123I/131}$I whole-body scan has a central role in the diagnostic and therapeutic workup of relapsed disease.

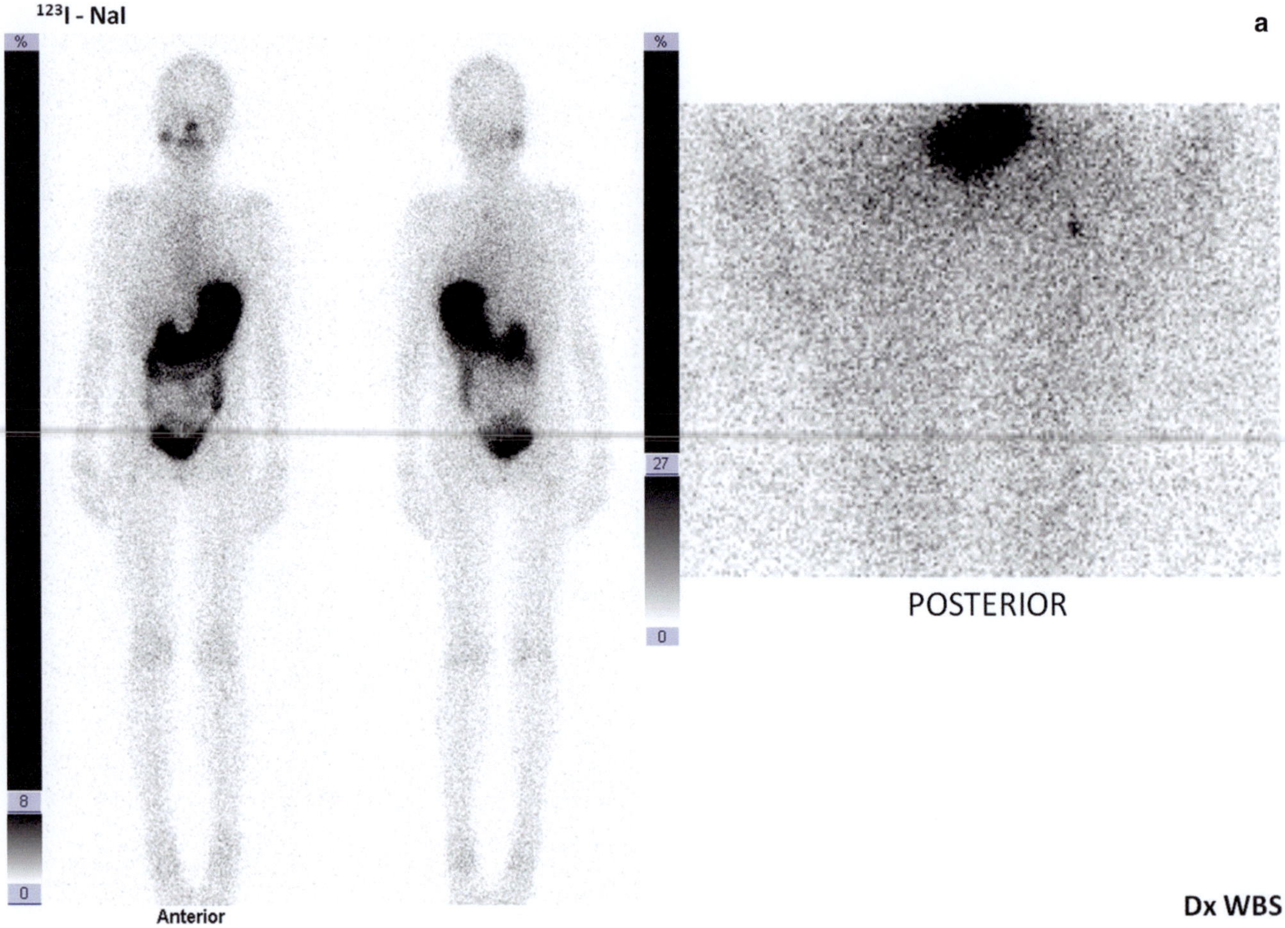

Fig. 23.6 (**a**) Diagnostic whole-body scan after rh-TSH stimulation (Tg of 78.4 ng/ml with TSH of 73 microIU/mL and negative anti-Tg antibodies) shows an area of mild radioiodine uptake corresponding to proximal region of right femur. Planar imaging in posterior view confirms this finding showing a further area of uptake in contralateral femur. (**b**) Posttherapy ^{131} I WBS (after two high-dose RAI therapy) reveals the persistence of disease in the femoral bones, showing further localization of metastatic disease in other skeletal sites (skull, vertebrae of the dorsal and lumbar spine). (**c**) SPECT acquisition followed by fusion SPECT/CT imaging is helpful to split intestinal activity from pathological radioiodine uptake, allowing a precise finding localization (skeletal and nonabdominal lymph node as evident in figure)

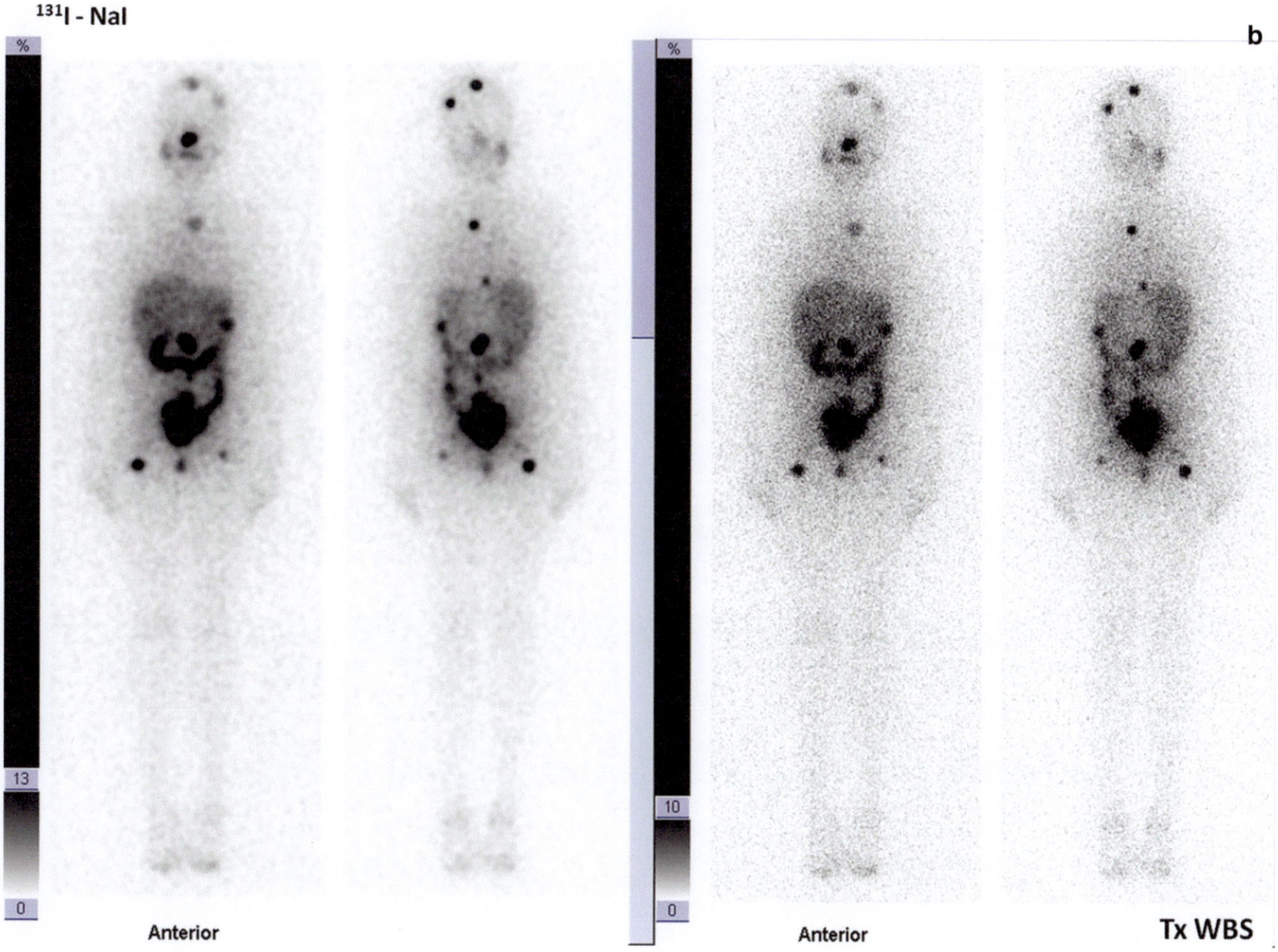

Fig. 23.6 (continued)

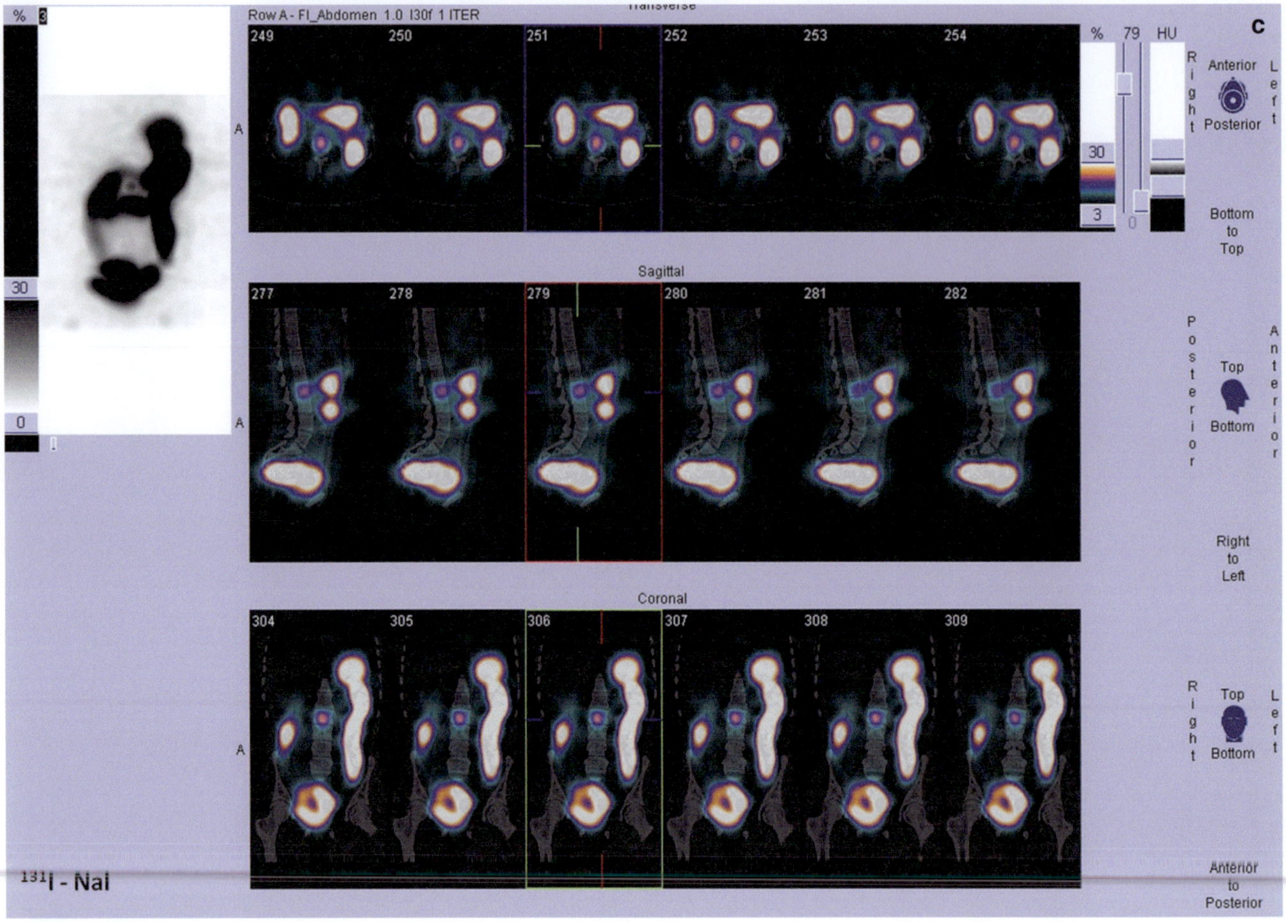

Fig. 23.6 (continued)

Bibliography

1. Alzahrani AS, AlShaikh OA, Tuli M, Al-Sugair A, Alamawi R, Al-Rasheed MM. Diagnostic value of recombinant human thyrotropin–stimulated 123I whole-body scintigraphy in the follow-up of patients with differentiated thyroid cancer. Clin Nucl Med. 2012;37(3):229–34.
2. Luster M, Handkiewicz-Junak D, Grossi A, Zacharin M, Taïeb D, Cruz O, Hitzel A, Casas JA, Mäder U, Dottorini ME, Pediatric rhTSH Investigators Group. Recombinant *thyrotropin* use in children and adolescents with differentiated thyroid cancer: a multicenter retrospective study. J Clin Endocrinol Metab. 2009;94(10):3948–53.
3. Luster M, Lippi F, Jarzab B, Perros P, Lassmann M, Reiners C, Pacini F. rhTSH-aided radioiodine ablation and treatment of differentiated thyroid carcinoma: a comprehensive review. Endocr Relat Cancer. 2005;12:49–64.

24 Endocrinology: Congenital Hypothyroidism

Milena Pizzoferro, Maria Felicia Villani, Graziamaria Ubertini, and Maria Carmen Garganese

24.1 Study Technique and Interpretation

Thyroid scintigraphy in evaluation of congenital hypothyroidism is acquired with gamma camera rotated in posterior view and the newborn in prone position with the neck extended. Administered activity of radiotracer is very low (adjusted to the patient's weight, according to EANM dosage card and to the national regulations). Thyroid uptake measurements are performed at 2, 10, and 15 min after an intravenous injection of ^{99m}Tc-pertechnetate. Lateral image has to be performed when an ectopic sublingual thyroid uptake is detected. Thyroid uptake is determined using a dedicated software by calculating syringe counts (before and after radiopharmaceutical injection) and counts present in the thyroid (drawing regions of interest around the gland borders and just below the gland for background subtraction).

M. Pizzoferro • M.F. Villani
Nuclear Medicine Unit, Imaging Departement – "Bambino Gesù" Children Hospital, Rome, Italy

G. Ubertini (✉)
Unit of Endocrinoly, "Bambino Gesù" Children Hospital, Rome, Italy
e-mail: graziamaria.ubertini@opbg.net

M.C. Garganese
Diagnostic Imaging Department of Nuclear Medicine, IRCCS Bambino Gesù Paediatric Hospital, Rome, Italy

© Springer International Publishing Switzerland 2017

M.C. Garganese, G.F.L. D'Errico (eds.), *Conventional Nuclear Medicine in Pediatrics*, DOI 10.1007/978-3-319-43181-9_24

24.1.1 Teaching Cases

Case 24.1 Differential Diagnosis of Congenital Hypothyroidism: Scintigraphic Thyroid Uptake Pattern (Fig. 24.1)

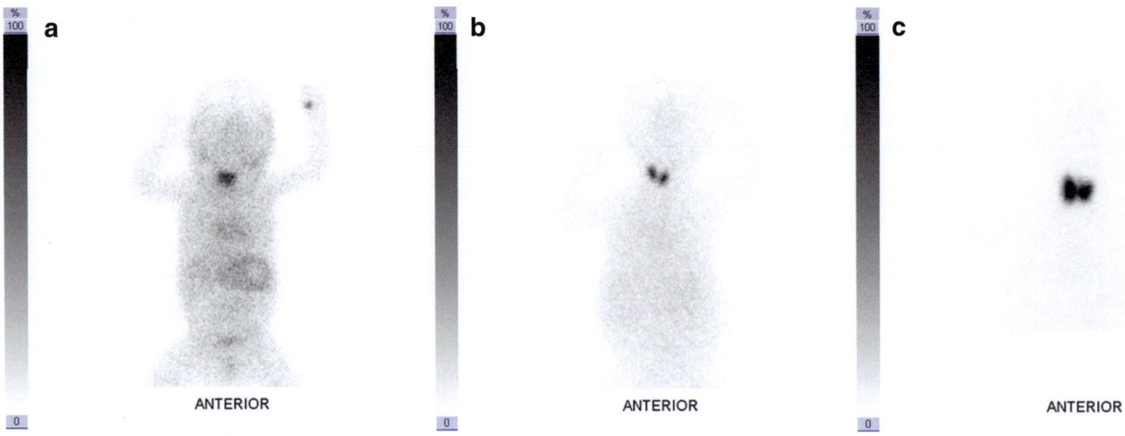

Fig. 24.1 In these figures three thyroid scans showing normal bilobed gland in proper side with moderately low (**a**), normal (**b**), and high (**c**) tracer uptake are displayed, respectively. Qualitative and quantitative analyses reveal different levels of organ/background activity ratio. Using the dedicated method of calculation, thyroid uptake can be evaluated comparing to normal range value (i.e., Sue Clark's normal value: 0.4–4 %)

Case 24.2 Scintigraphic Detection of Unilateral Thyroid Agenesis (Fig. 24.2)

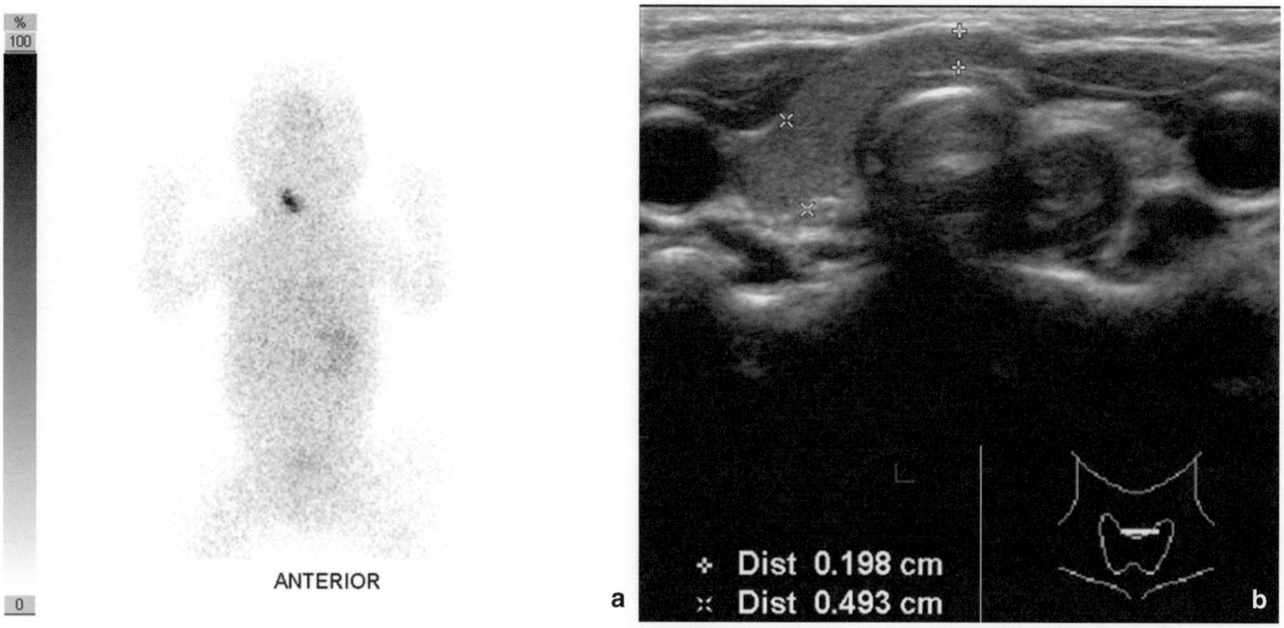

Fig. 24.2 (**a**) Thyroid scintigraphy with 99mTc-pertechnetate reveals nonvisualization of right lobe (suggesting the absence of right thyroid lobe). Left lobe shows homogeneous tracer uptake; a slightly enlarged shape of the left lobe and isthmus is evident (known as characteristic "hockey stick sign" pattern). (**b**) Thyroid hemiagenesis is a rare form of thyroid dysgenesis; ultrasonography scan confirms functional finding detected by scintigraphy

Case 24.3 Diagnosis of Thyroid Dysgenesis by Scintigraphy with 99mTc-Pertechnetate: Ectopic Pattern (Fig. 24.3)

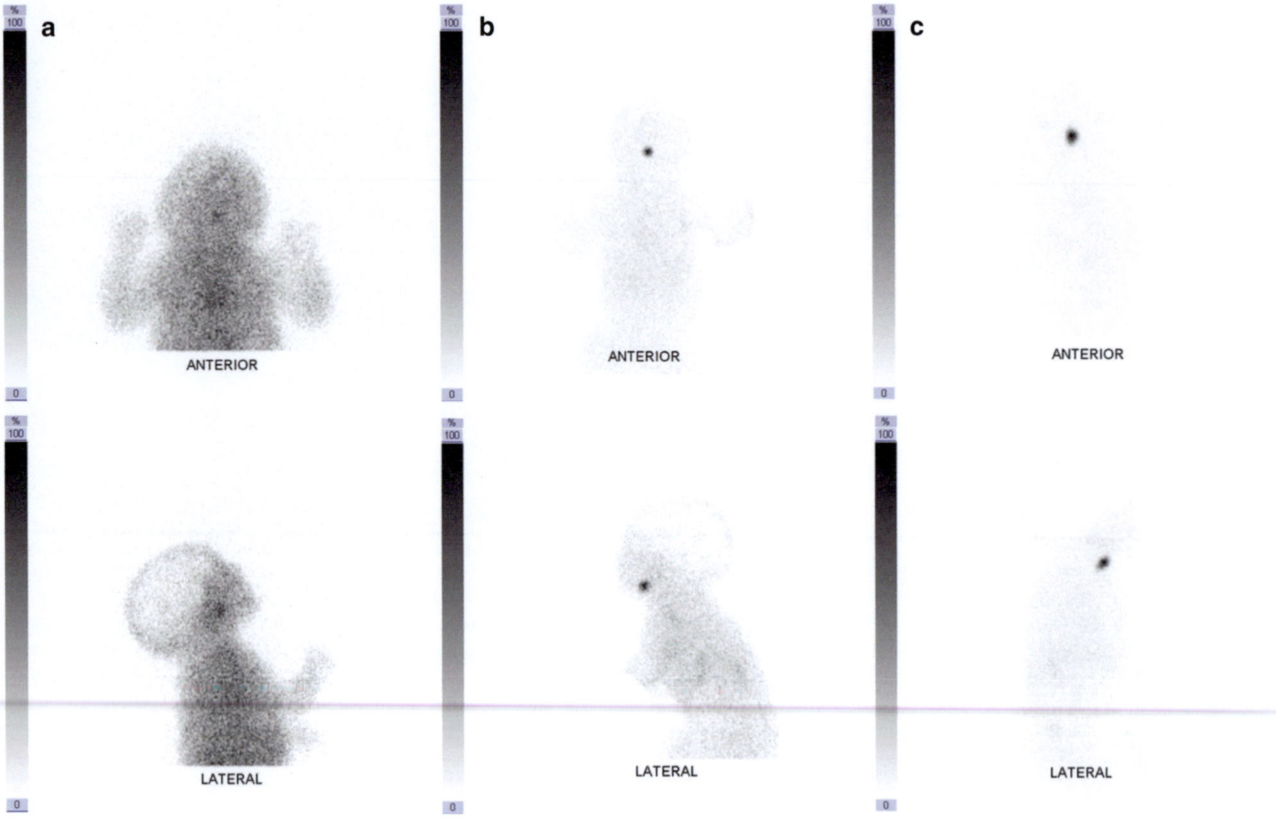

Fig. 24.3 In these figures are displayed three thyroid scans showing ectopic sublingual thyroid pattern with different tracer uptake intensity: low (**a**), quite normal (**b**), and high uptake (**c**), respectively. Anterior and lateral views are necessary for a clear evaluation of uptake localization

Case 24.4 Diagnosis of Thyroid Dysgenesis by Scintigraphy with 99mTc-Pertechnetate: Agenesis Pattern (Fig. 24.4)

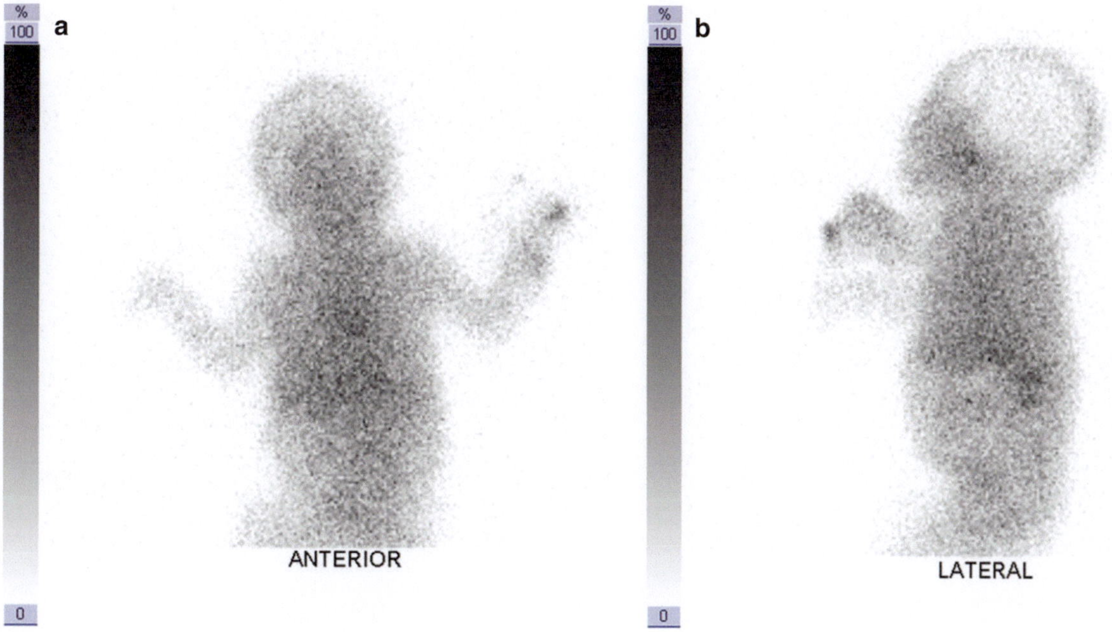

Fig. 24.4 (**a**) In thyroid dysgenesis, absence of thyroid is easily detected by thyroid scintigraphy. No tracer uptake is evident in the neck or in ectopic side. (**b**) Lateral image confirms this finding, ruling out the presence of small ectopic sublingual uptake. It is important to perform a technically correct lateral view, avoiding that salivary gland activity (seen as slight tracer activity evident in Fig. 24.2b) could be misinterpreted as thyroid uptake in the upper neck region

Bibliography

1. Treves ST, Grand RJ. Pediatric nuclear medicine, Chapter 3, 3rd ed. In: Thyroid. Springer-Verlag, New York; 2007. p. 192–208.
2. Volkan-Salancı B, Kıratlı PO. Nuclear medicine in thyroid diseases in pediatric and adolescent. patients. Mol Imag Radionuclide Ther. 2015 (Review);24(2):47–59.

25 Endocrinology: Hyperparathyroidism

Milena Pizzoferro, Maria Felicia Villani, Armando Grossi, Graziamaria Ubertini, and Maria Carmen Garganese

25.1 Study Technique and Interpretation: Parathyroid Scintigraphy

Parathyroid scintigraphy is useful to localize hyperfunctioning parathyroid gland(s) in the presurgical diagnostic workup and to detect recurrent or persistent disease, both in case of primary and secondary hyperparathyroidism.

Specific tracer with selective parathyroid tissue uptake does not exist, and various parathyroid scintigraphy protocols (using single or dual-tracer) have been developed.

99mTc sestamibi is the most commonly used radiotracer for imaging the parathyroid glands and represents the agent of choice for dual-phase parathyroid scintigraphy. The administered activity of radiotracer is adjusted to the patient's weight, according to EANM dosage card and to the national regulations. This protocol is based on the different uptake and washout timing of this tracer in the hyperfunctioning parathyroid gland(s) rather than in thyroid and normal parathyroid tissues. No particular patient preparation is necessary for this examination, but calcimimetics should be interrupted for at least 2 weeks before the parathyroid imaging.

99mTc sestamibi is taken up by both the thyroid and parathyroid glands, and planar images obtained in early phase (full anterior views of the neck and thorax and magnified view of the neck acquired with the patient in the supine position at 10 min after intravenous administration) show both thyroid and parathyroid tissues. Focal areas of increased radiotracer uptake represent abnormal parathyroid tissue superimposed on the normal thyroid. Delayed planar image, performed approximately 2 h after radiotracer administration, detects the presence of foci of retained radiotracer, characteristic of hyperfunctioning parathyroid tissue.

However, concomitant thyroid disease can lead to imaging pitfalls, and a thyroid scan by 99mTc-pertechnetate administration (shortly after delayed planar image with gamma camera setting identical to MIBI neck scintigraphy) is useful to rule out the presence of thyroid nodules and to aid in the interpretation of parathyroid images.

By subtraction (visual or computed) techniques, a second radiotracer is administered and taken up only by the thyroid gland; the MIBI scan is considered positive for hyperfunctioning parathyroid gland when there is a focal area of increased uptake in the early MIBI phase, showing a relative increase over time and not detectable in thyroid scintigraphy.

For patient preparation in case of 99mTc-pertechnetate administration, previous radiological studies with iodine-containing contrast media should be avoided during 4–6 weeks, hormone replacement should be withheld for 2–3 weeks before the investigation, and treatment with methimazole or propylthiouracil should be stopped for 1 week.

Planar scintigraphic images can be obtained over 15 min with a parallel-hole, low-energy, high-resolution collimator, or using a pinhole collimator. SPECT of the neck can help to differentiate parathyroid activity (located in posterior position) from the overlying thyroid in early MIBI phase, showing an increase in the sensitivity of scintigraphic parathyroid imaging.

25.2 Teaching Cases

25.2.1 Case 25.1 "Negative Pattern of Parathyroid Scintigraphy in Clinical Suspicion of Primary Hyperparathyroidism"

A 9-year-old boy with familiar history of parathyroid adenoma, incidental finding of mild hypercalcemia, and elevated

M. Pizzoferro • M.F. Villani
Nuclear Medicine Unit, Imaging Departement – "Bambino Gesù" Children Hospital, Rome, Italy

A. Grossi • G. Ubertini (✉)
Unit of Endocrinology, "Bambino Gesù" Children Hospital, Rome, Italy
e-mail: graziamaria.ubertini@opbg.net

M.C. Garganese
Diagnostic Imaging Department of Nuclear Medicine, IRCCS Bambino Gesù Paediatric Hospital, Rome, Italy

© Springer International Publishing Switzerland 2017

M.C. Garganese, G.F.L. D'Errico (eds.), *Conventional Nuclear Medicine in Pediatrics*, DOI 10.1007/978-3-319-43181-9_25

serum concentrations of intact PTH. Renal and thyroid ultrasound scans were negative for pathological findings, and laboratory investigations showed a normal renal function (Fig. 25.1).

25.2.2 Case 25.2 "Negative Pattern of Parathyroid Scintigraphy in Clinical Suspicion of Secondary Hyperparathyroidism"

Accentuated hyperparathyroidism in a 12-year-old boy affected by type II Bartter syndrome (hypokalemia, metabolic alkalosis, hypercalciuria, and nephrocalcinosis caused by homozygous mutation in *c.277 T > G KCNJ1* gene). After 3 years of persistent detection of increased level of serum concentrations of intact PTH, a parathyroid scintigraphy was required in the clinical suspicion of secondary hyperparathyroidism (Fig. 25.2).

25.2.3 Case 25.3 "Parathyroid Adenoma Detected by Parathyroid Scintigraphy"

A 14-year-old boy with renal colic episode and consequent finding of hypercalcemia and increased serum PTH level (11.7 mg/dl and 240 pg/ml, respectively). Ultrasonography of the neck revealed a homogeneously hypoechoic, oval, and vascularized image corresponding to postero-inferior region of left thyroid lobe. Parathyroid scintigraphy was required for a preoperative integrated approach that combines both the anatomical information of sonography and the physiological information of scintigraphy. Minimally invasive surgery was successfully performed, and solitary adenomas were histologically confirmed (Fig. 25.3).

25.2.4 Case 25.4 "Parathyroid Adenoma with a Markedly Increased 99mTc Sestamibi Uptake Detected by Parathyroid Scintigraphy"

A 13-year-old girl affected by cardiomyopathy was surgically corrected by Fontan procedure. At 12 years of life, during follow-up biochemical examination, hypercalcemia and hyperphosphatemia were detected associated with increased PTH (454 pg/ml) and reduced vitamin D level (14.7 ng/ml). An ultrasonography of cervical region was performed showing a hypoechoic and vascularized image corresponding to right thyroid lobe compatible with hyperplastic parathyroid. Parathyroid scintigraphy showed intense uptake and slow washout of radiotracer in the middle third of the right thyroid lobe. Therefore, it carried out targeted parathyroid surgery with histological diagnosis of parathyroid adenoma (Fig. 25.4).

25.2.5 Case 25.5 "Parathyroid Hyperplasia Secondary to Hypophosphatemic Rickets"

Patient with diagnosis of rickets not due to vitamin D deficiency at 1 year of age. Finding of progressive increase in PTH levels was detected at last clinical controls. An ultrasonography of cervical region was performed with the evidence of parathyroid in the right lower thyroid lobe (1.5 cm in diameter). Parathyroid scintigraphy was required to complete diagnostic preoperative workup confirming hyperfunctioning parathyroid gland sonographically detected and revealing another suspicious finding below left lower thyroid lobe. Hyperplastic parathyroid glands were surgically removed, and postoperative follow-up was uneventful with PTH and calcium level normalization (Fig. 25.5).

25.2.6 Case 25.6 "Severe Secondary Hyperparathyroidism in Patient with Transplanted Kidney"

A 17-year-old boy with transplanted kidney (for chronic renal failure in relation to nephrotic syndrome secondary to focal and segmental glomerulosclerosis). In the period after transplantation, recurrence of nephrotic syndrome occurred with markedly increased calcium and PTH levels. Ultrasound scan and parathyroid scintigraphy detected multiple hyperfunctioning parathyroid glands (Fig. 25.6).

25.2.7 Case 25.7 "Tertiary Hyperparathyroidism in Dialysis Patients"

A 12-year-old boy with chronic renal failure in dialysis therapy. Parathyroid scintigraphy was performed after detection of severe increased PTH level, showing a hyperfunctioning lesion of primary hyperplasia of parathyroid gland in the middle third of the right thyroid lobe. The child was treated with medical therapy with partial decrease of PTH level. A parathyroid scintigraphy revealed a persistence of hyperfunctioning parathyroid gland, with mildly reduced tracer concentration in the parathyroid lesion compared with the previous study. This result is suggestive of tertiary hyperparathyroidism pattern, and surgical parathyroid removal was performed with clinical improvement (Fig. 25.7).

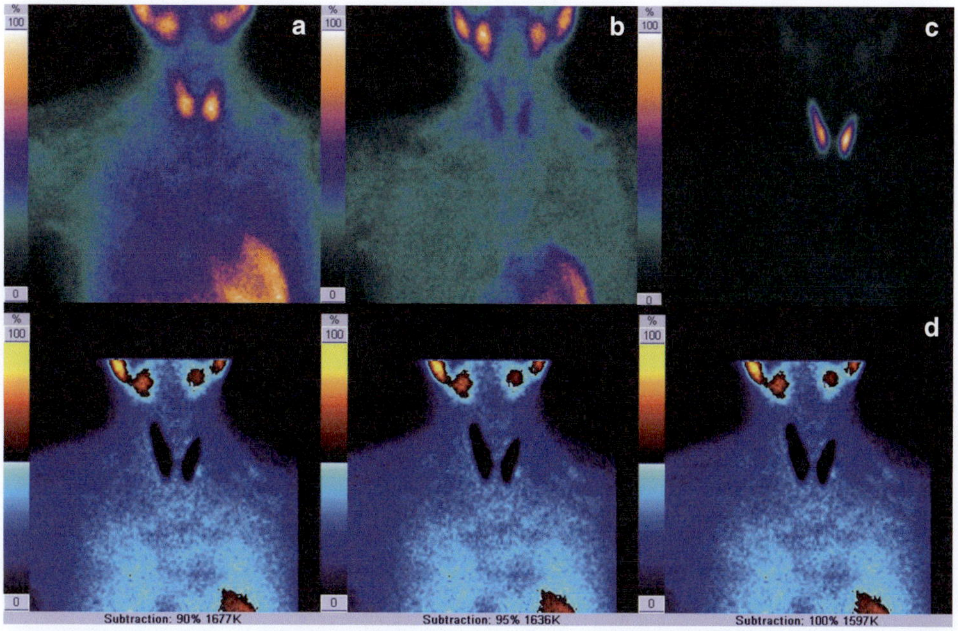

Fig. 25.1 (**a–d**) Parathyroid scintigraphy. (**a**) Planar image in early phase shows normal uptake of 99mTc sestamibi in the thyroid, submandibular glands, and heart. No abnormal uptake in the thoracic region is evident. The image acquired 2 h after intravenous administration (**b**) shows normal clearance of sestamibi from the thyroid without focus of radiotracer retention to suggest parathyroid disease. Thyroid scan (**c**), acquired after 99mTc-pertechnetate administration, does not reveal focal uptake or other abnormal findings. Progressive incremental subtraction scanning (**d**) performed by dedicated software confirmed absence of focal MIBI uptake suspicious for hyperfunctioning parathyroid gland(s)

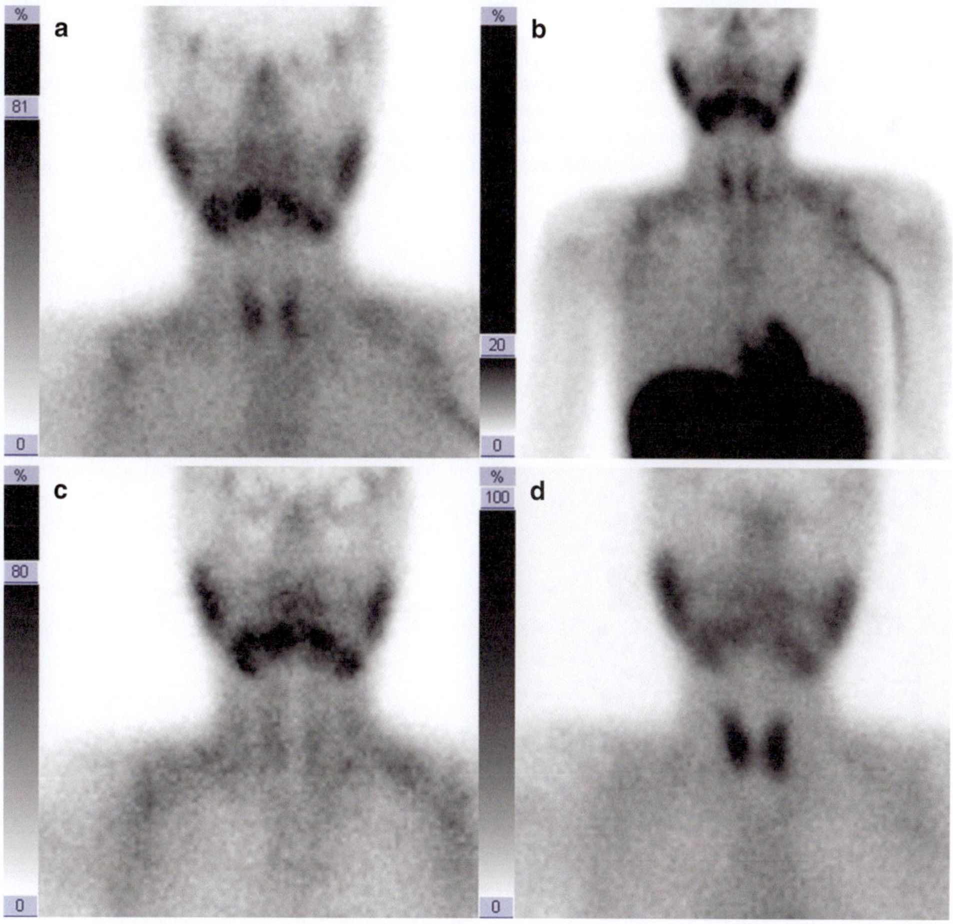

Fig. 25.2 (**a–d**) Parathyroid scintigraphy. (**a**) In early phase, 99mTc-MIBI uptake is homogeneous within the thyroid gland that shows normal size and shape. Brown fat uptake is evident as physiological finding in pediatric patient. No abnormal uptake in the thoracic region is evident (**b**). Delayed image (**c**) shows regular washout of the tracer from the thyroid. Thyroid scan (**d**), acquired after 99mTc-pertechnetate administration, does not reveal focal uptake or other abnormal findings. Negative scintigraphic result rules out parathyroid hyperplasia

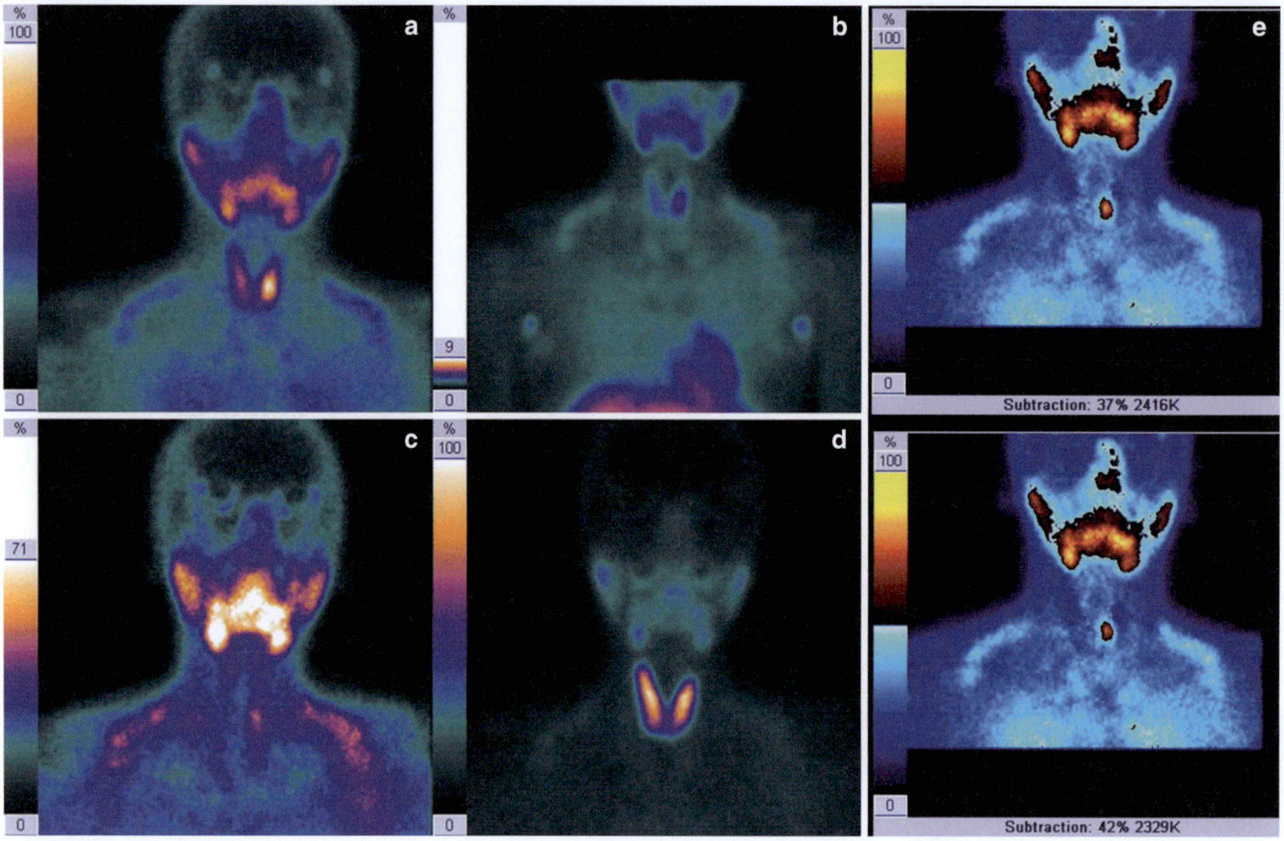

Fig. 25.3 (a–e) Parathyroid scintigraphy. (**a**) Early-phase 99mTc sestamibi image shows physiological uptake in salivary glands and thyroid gland, with focus of more intense uptake overlying inferior pole of left thyroid lobe. No other foci of abnormal uptake are evident in the thoracic region (**b**). Two-hour delayed image (**c**) shows regular washout of the tracer from thyroid parenchyma, but radiotracer retention in the area of focal uptake detected in the early image and not detectable in thyroid scintigraphy (**d**). Computed subtraction scanning performed by dedicated software (**e**) confirmed the presence of focal MIBI uptake suspicious for hyperfunctioning parathyroid gland

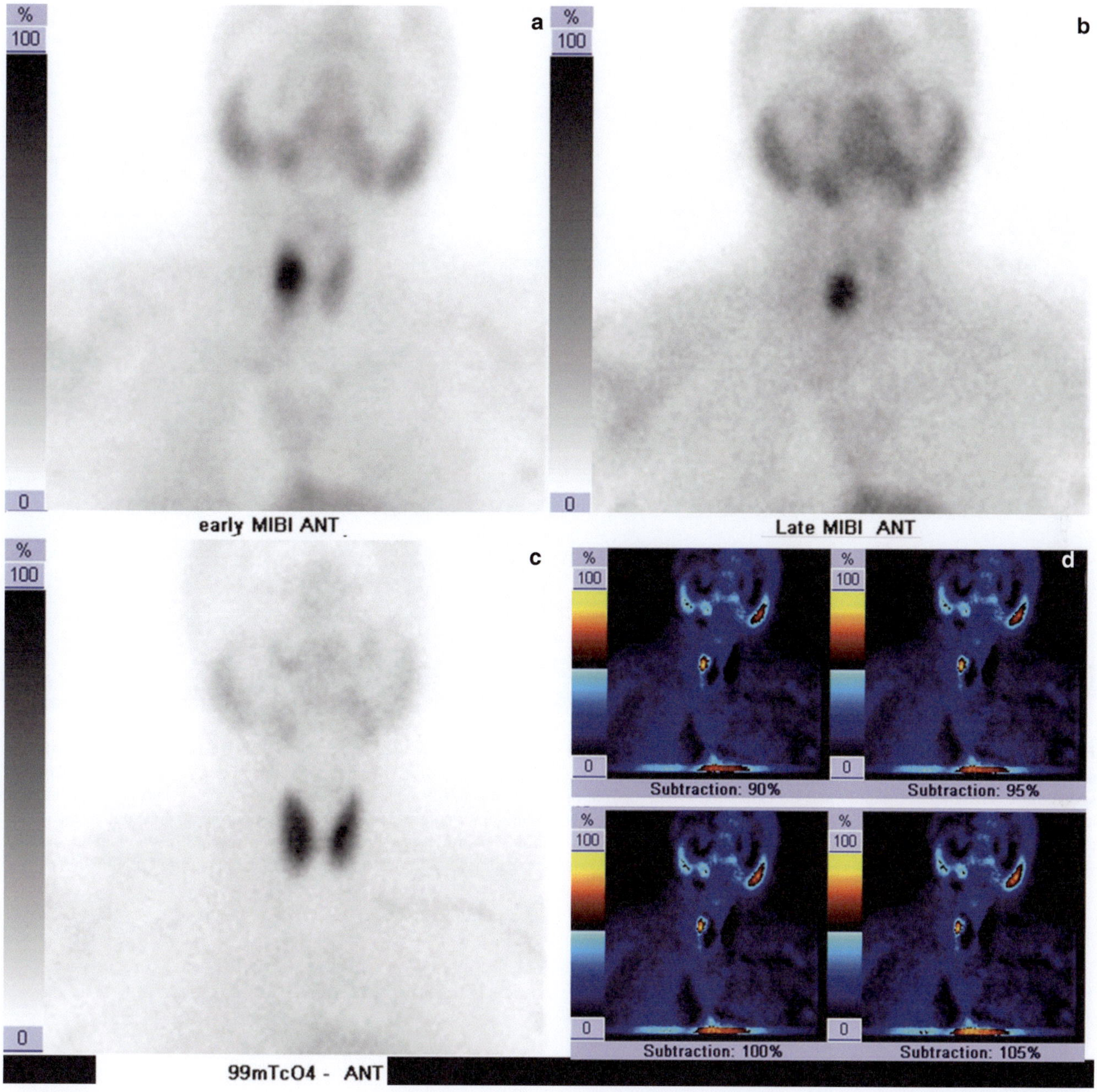

Fig. 25.4 (**a**–**d**) Parathyroid scintigraphy. (**a**) Early-phase 99mTc sestamibi image shows a large area of markedly intense and focal uptake in the middle third of the right thyroid lobe. Tracer uptake in the thyroid gland is reduced in relation to higher uptake in focal lesion. No other foci of abnormal uptake are evident in the thoracic region. Two-hour delayed image (**b**) shows regular washout of the tracer from thyroid parenchyma, but an intense radiotracer retention in the area of focal uptake is detected in the early image. No abnormal area of focal uptake is detectable in thyroid scintigraphy (**c**). Computed subtraction scanning performed by dedicated software (**d**) clearly confirmed the presence of focal MIBI uptake suspicious for hyperfunctioning parathyroid gland

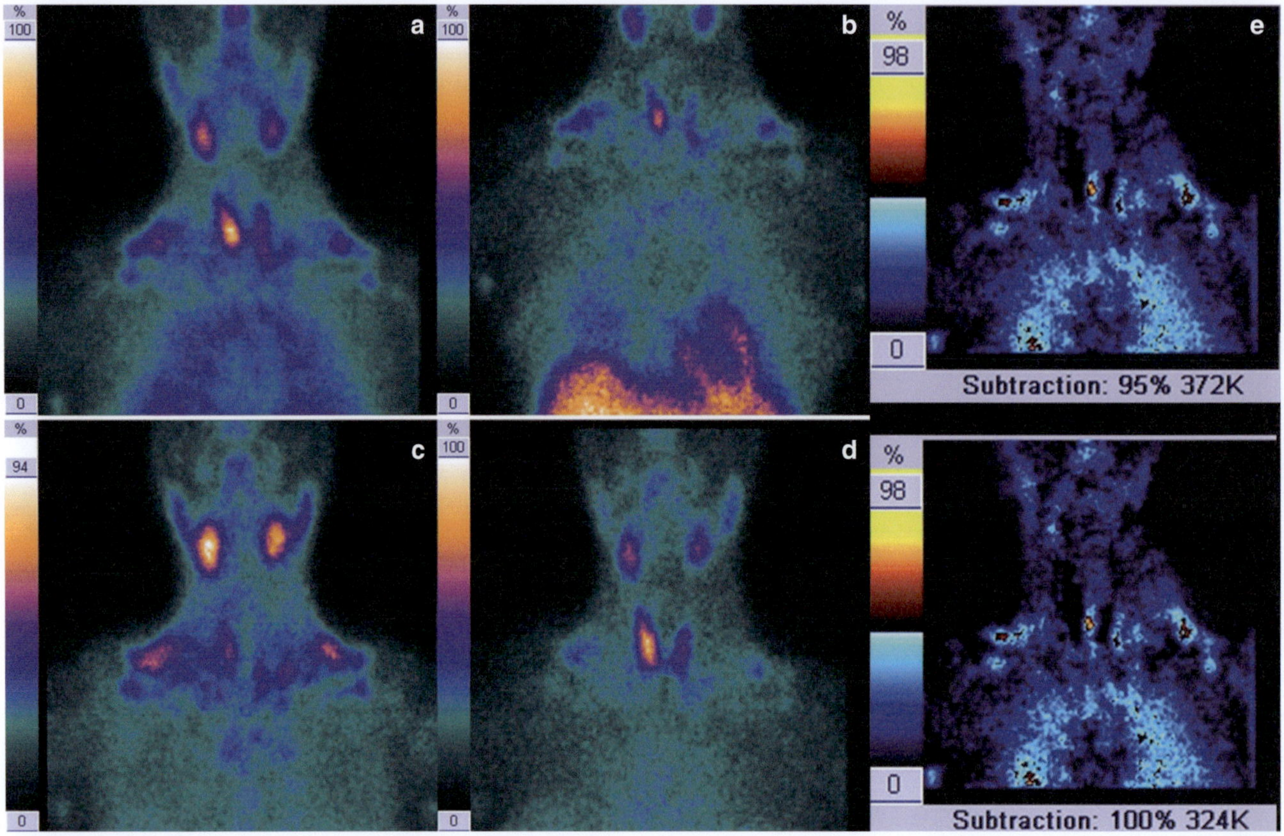

Fig. 25.5 (a–e) Parathyroid scintigraphy. (**a**) In early imaging, an area of increased MIBI uptake is evident in right lower thyroid lobe, corresponding to sonographic finding, and no extinction of the uptake in delayed imaging (**c**). However, another small area of mild uptake is detectable below left lower thyroid lobe in early phase with slow washout in delayed image (**c**). No abnormal uptake in the thoracic region is evident (**b**). By visual and computed subtraction comparison with thyroid images (**d**, **e**), the two areas with relative increased uptake over time are not detectable in thyroid scintigraphy and are confirmed as abnormal findings. By integration of dual-phase and subtraction protocols, parathyroid scintigraphy confirms ultrasonographic finding revealing furthermore another hyperplastic parathyroid gland

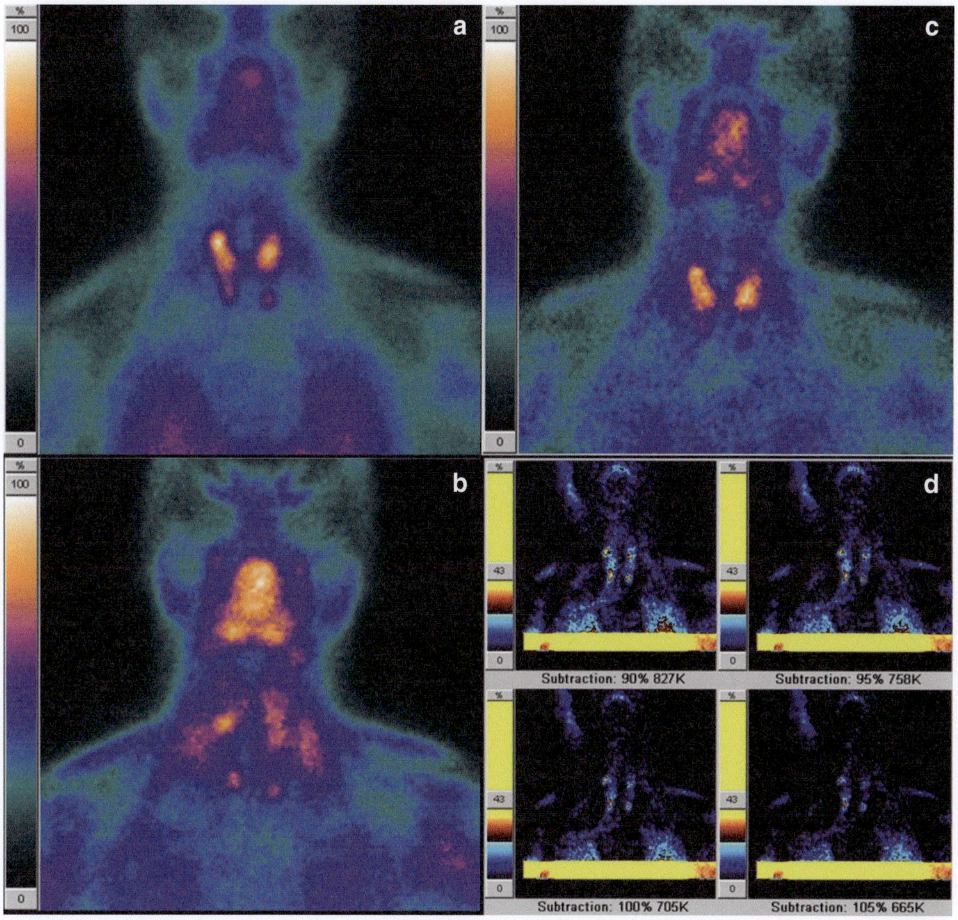

Fig. 25.6 (**a**–**d**) Early-phase 99mTc sestamibi image shows foci of more intense uptake overlying superior pole of right thyroid lobe and below bilateral inferior thyroid poles (**a**) and slow clearance over time (**b**). These focal areas are not detectable on thyroid scan (**c**) and confirmed as abnormal findings by progressive incremental subtraction scanning (**d**)

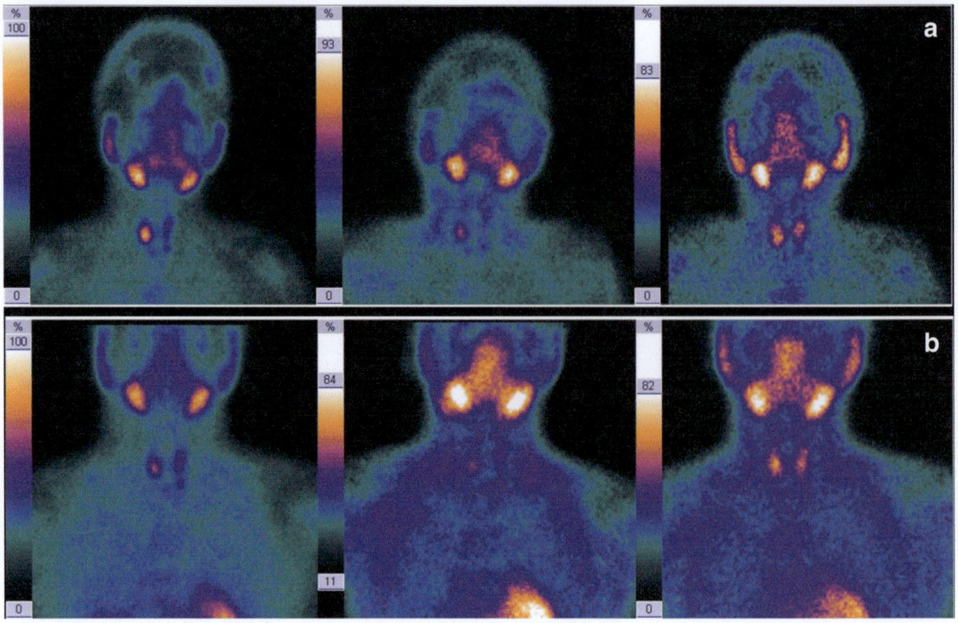

Fig. 25.7 (**a**–**b**) In the upper row (**a**) is evident a focal area of increased uptake in the early MIBI phase showing a relative increase over time and not detectable in thyroid scintigraphy, as for hyperfunctioning parathyroid. In the lower row (**b**), parathyroid scintigraphy revealed persistence of hyperfunctioning parathyroid gland, with mildly reduced tracer concentration compared with previous study

Bibliography

1. Belcher R, Metrailer AM, Bodenner DL, Stack BD. Characterization of hyperparathyroidism in youth and adolescents: a literature review. Int J Pediatr Otorhinolaryngol. 2013;77(3):318–22.
2. Hindié E, Ugur O, Fuster D, O'Doherty M, Grassetto G, Ureña P, Kettle A, Gulec SA, Pons F, Rubello D, Parathyroid Task Group of the EANM. EANM parathyroid guidelines. Eur J Nucl Med Mol Imaging. 2009;36(7):1201–16.
3. Johnson NA, Tublin ME, Ogilvie JB. Parathyroid imaging: technique and role in the preoperative evaluation of primary hyperparathyroidism. Head Neck Imag Rev. 2007;188(6):1706–15.
4. Roizen J, Levine MA. Meta-analysis comparing the biochemistry of primary hyperparathyroidism in youths to the biochemistry of primary hyperparathyroidism in adults. J Clin Endocrinol Metab. 2014;99(12):4555–64.

Benign Skeletal Disease

26

Milena Pizzoferro, Maria Felicia Villani, Domenico Barbuti, Gian Luigi Natali, and Maria Carmen Garganese

This chapter is a focus on benign skeletal disease. We present a series of children and adolescents affected by rare or unusual conditions, showing characteristic bone scintigraphy patterns.

Each case is well documented by several radiological findings, which clarify the site or the morphological aspect of the scintigraphic framework.

26.1 Case 26.1

A 6-year-old girl with McCune Albright syndrome (Fig. 26.1)

26.2 Case 26.2

A 2-year-old child with McCune Albright syndrome (Fig. 26.2)

26.3 Case 26.3

A 2-year-old child with Gorham-Stout syndrome (Fig. 26.3)

26.4 Case 26.4

A 9-year-old girl with drepanocytosis (Fig. 26.4)

M. Pizzoferro • M.F. Villani
Nuclear Medicine Unit, Imaging Departement – "Bambino Gesù" Children Hospital, Rome, Italy

D. Barbuti (✉) • G.L. Natali
Imaging Department, "Bambino Gesù" Children Hospital, Rome, Italy
e-mail: domenico.barbuti@opbg.net

M.C. Garganese
Diagnostic Imaging Department of Nuclear Medicine, IRCCS Bambino Gesù Paediatric Hospital, Rome, Italy

26.5 Case 26.5

A 10-year-old girl with Ollier disease (Fig. 26.5)

26.6 Case 26.6

An 8-year-old boy with Ollier disease (Fig. 26.6)

26.7 Case 26.7

A 12-year-old boy with fibrous dysplasia of the skull (Fig. 26.7)

26.8 Case 26.8

An 11-month-old infant with fibrous dysplasia of the tibia (Fig. 26.8)

26.9 Case 26.9

A 14-year-old boy with multiple sites of fibrous dysplasia (Fig. 26.9)

26.10 Case 26.10

A 2-year-old child with incidental finding of spiroid fracture of the left tibia (Fig. 26.10)

26.11 Case 26.11

A 6-year-old child with Perthes disease, stage I (Fig. 26.11)

© Springer International Publishing Switzerland 2017

M.C. Garganese, G.F.L. D'Errico (eds.), *Conventional Nuclear Medicine in Pediatrics*, DOI 10.1007/978-3-319-43181-9_26

26.12 Case 26.12

A 5-year-old child with Perthes disease, stage IIA (Fig. 26.12)

26.13 Case 26.13

A 4-year-old child with Perthes disease, stage III (Fig. 26.13)

26.14 Case 26.14

Two children compared affected by osteoid osteoma of the left humerus (Fig. 26.14)

26.15 Case 26.15

A 9-year-old boy with referred pain in the right hip: osteoid osteoma of the neck of right femur (Fig. 26.15)

26.16 Case 26.16

A 10-year-old girl with referred pain in the left hip: bone scintigraphy detected osteoid osteoma in the spine (Fig. 26.16)

26.17 Case 26.17

A 16-year-old girl with referred pain in the left hip: bone scintigraphy detected intramedullary osteoid osteoma in left acetabulum (Fig. 26.17)

26.18 Case 26.18

A 3-year-old child with limping and pain generically referred in the whole left lower limb: bone scintigraphy detected intramedullary osteoid osteoma in left tibia (Fig. 26.18)

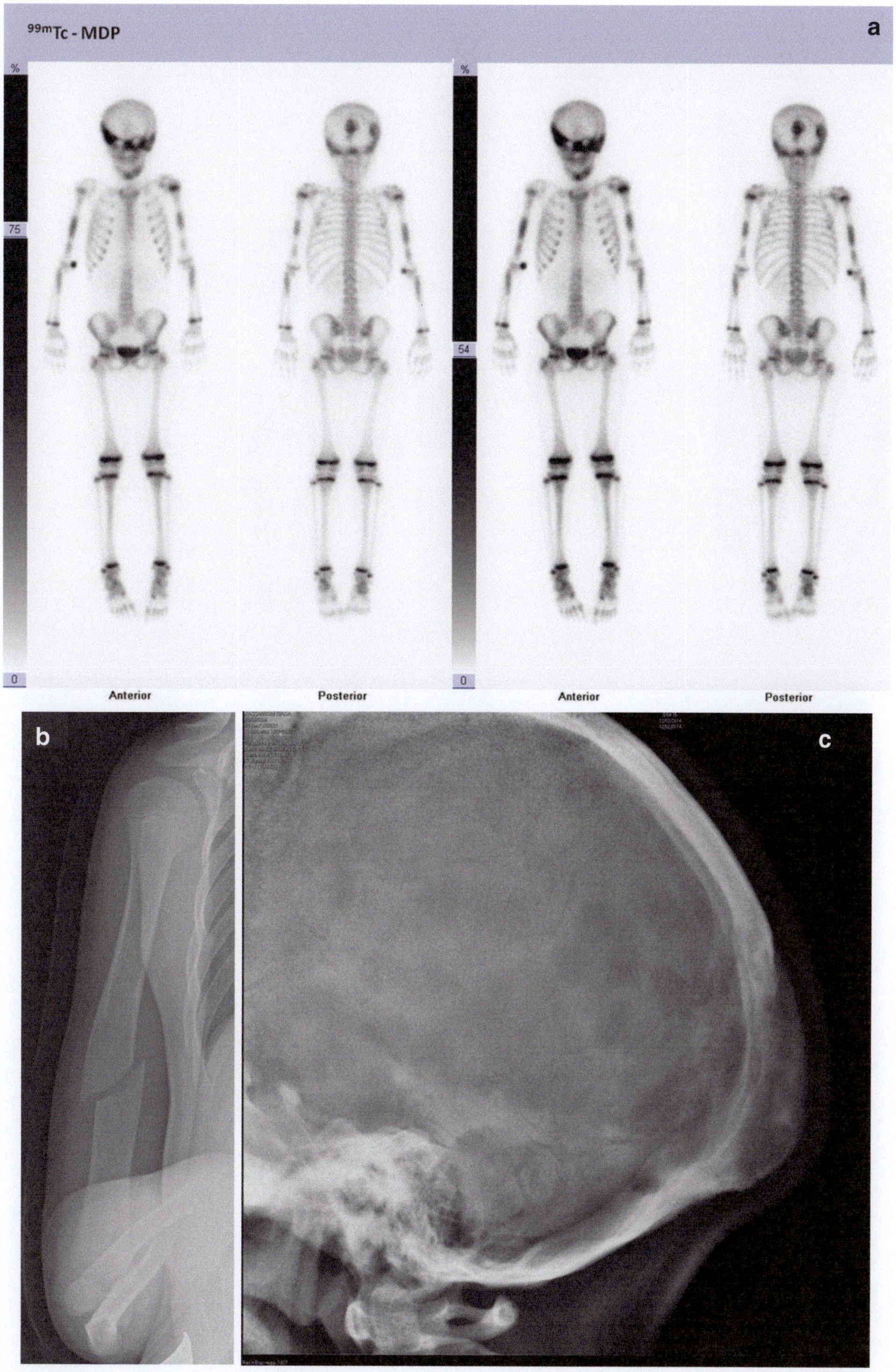

Fig. 26.1 (**a**) Bone scan shows multiple areas of intense uptake in the skull, bilateral humeral shafts, and proximal radii. (**b–c**) The right humerus plain film shows an oblique diaphyseal pathological fracture: the medullary channel is enlarged and the cortical is thinned with reduced bone density (**b**); lateral skull radiograph (**c**): enlargement of the occipital diploe with inhomogeneous reduced bone density

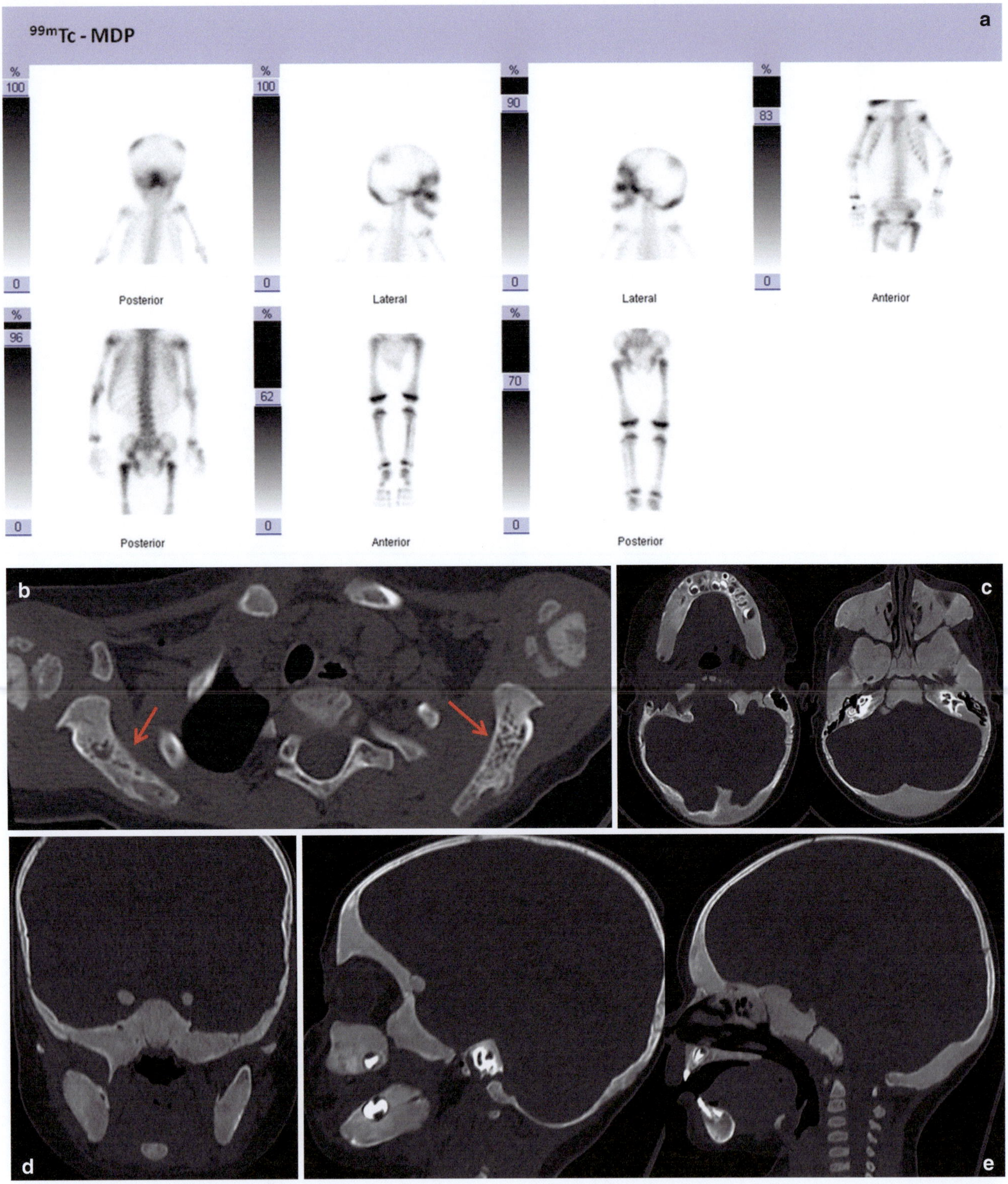

Fig. 26.2 (**a**) Bone scan shows multiple areas of intense uptake in the skull, facial bones, left humerus, proximal radii, pelvis, femurs, tibiae. (**b–e**): CT (b) shows a widening of both shoulder blades with diffuse moth eating of cancellous bone (*red arrows*). Axial cranial CT (**c**) widening of the bones of the skull base, of the mandible, and maxilla with a "ground glass" density. Cranial CT (**d**) in coronal and sagittal (**e**) plane: thickening of the frontal bones, of the lower part of the occiput, of the bones of the skull base, of the mandible, and maxilla with ground glass density. Normal appearance of the bones of the vault. (**f–h**) X-rays of the upper limbs (f): osteoporosis, flaring of the bone marrow channel and thinning of corticals. X-ray of the lower limbs (**g**): osteoporosis, flaring of the bone marrow channel and thinning of corticals. Plain film of the pelvis (**h**) shows left coxa vara with multiple radiolucent areas (*white arrows*). In the internal part of the right femoral neck, radiolucent areas are seen with associated vertical rhyme of pathological fracture of the femoral neck without displacement (*black arrow*)

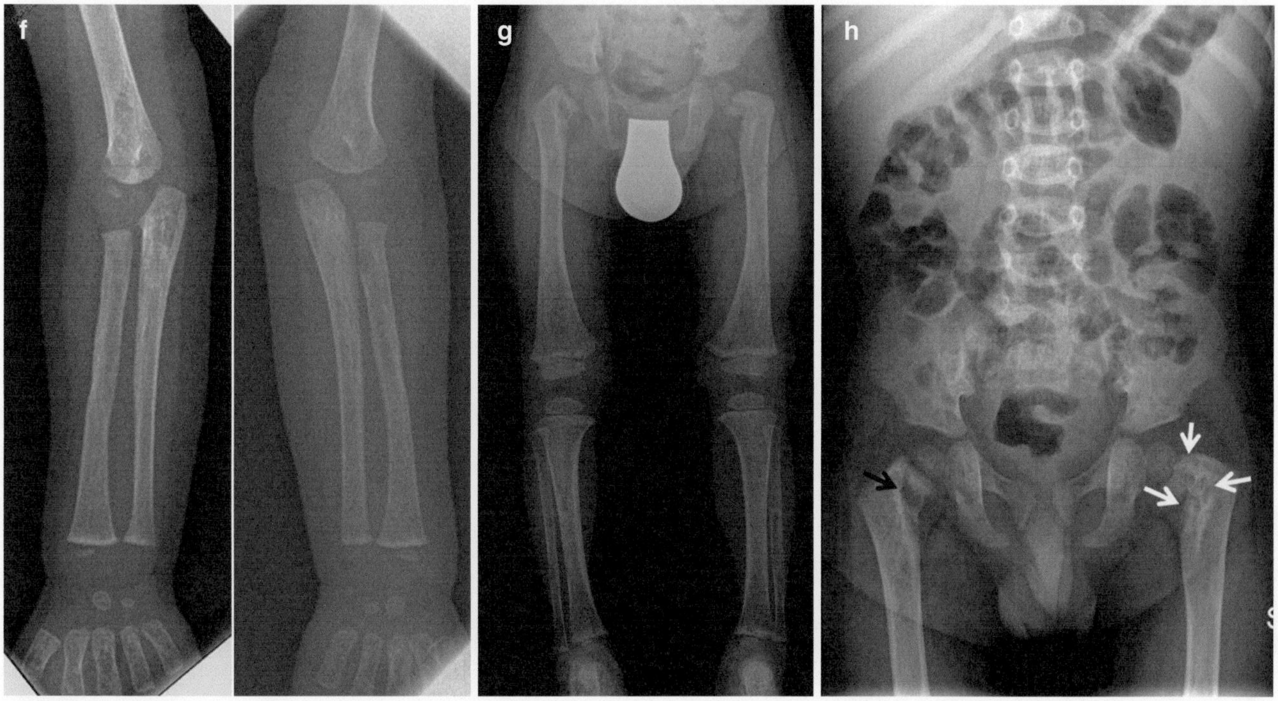

Fig. 26.2 (continued)

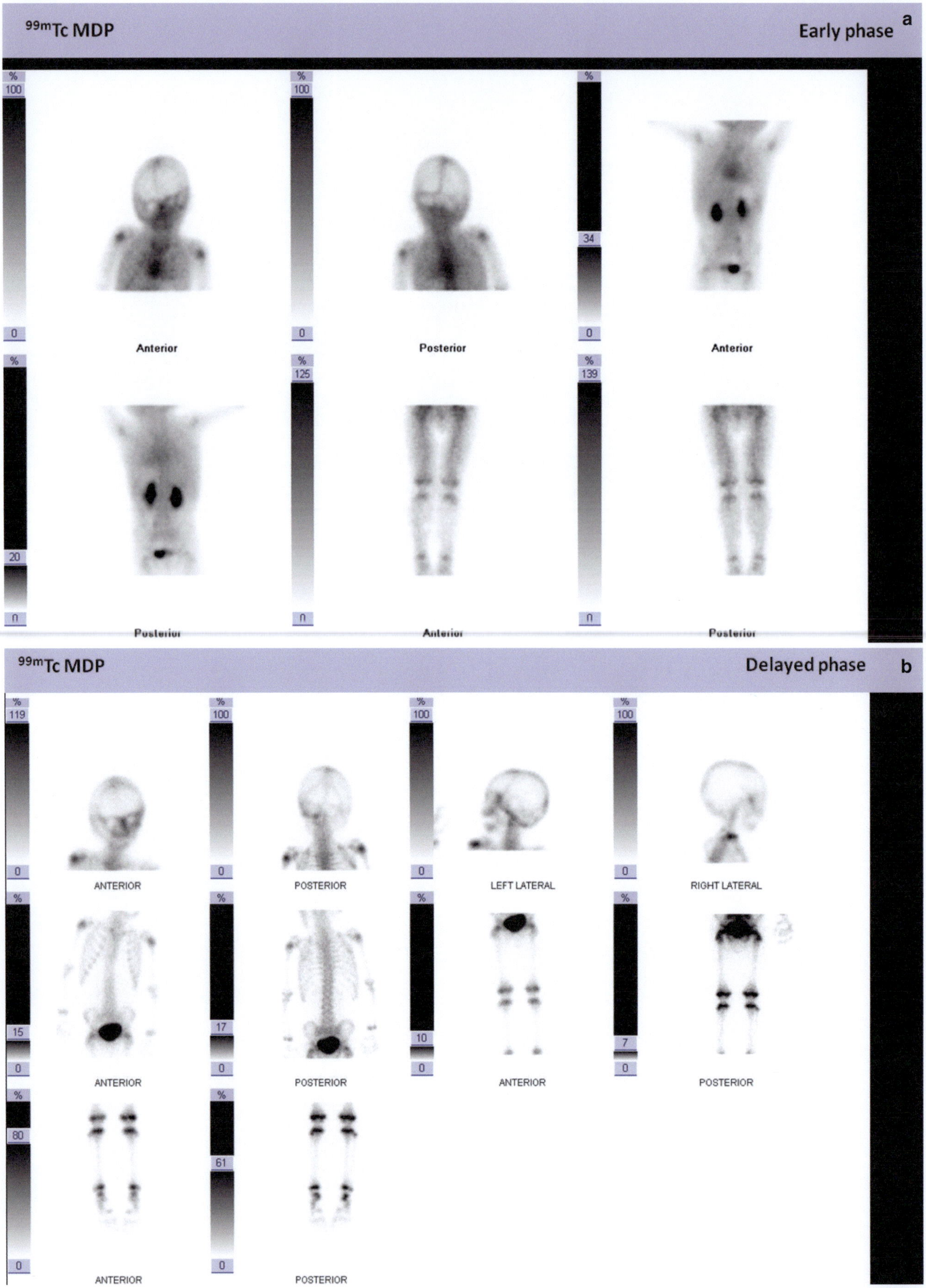

99mTc MDP
Early phase
a
Anterior
Posterior
Anterior
Posterior
Anterior
Posterior
99mTc MDP
Delayed phase
b
ANTERIOR
POSTERIOR
LEFT LATERAL
RIGHT LATERAL
ANTERIOR
POSTERIOR
ANTERIOR
POSTERIOR
ANTERIOR
POSTERIOR

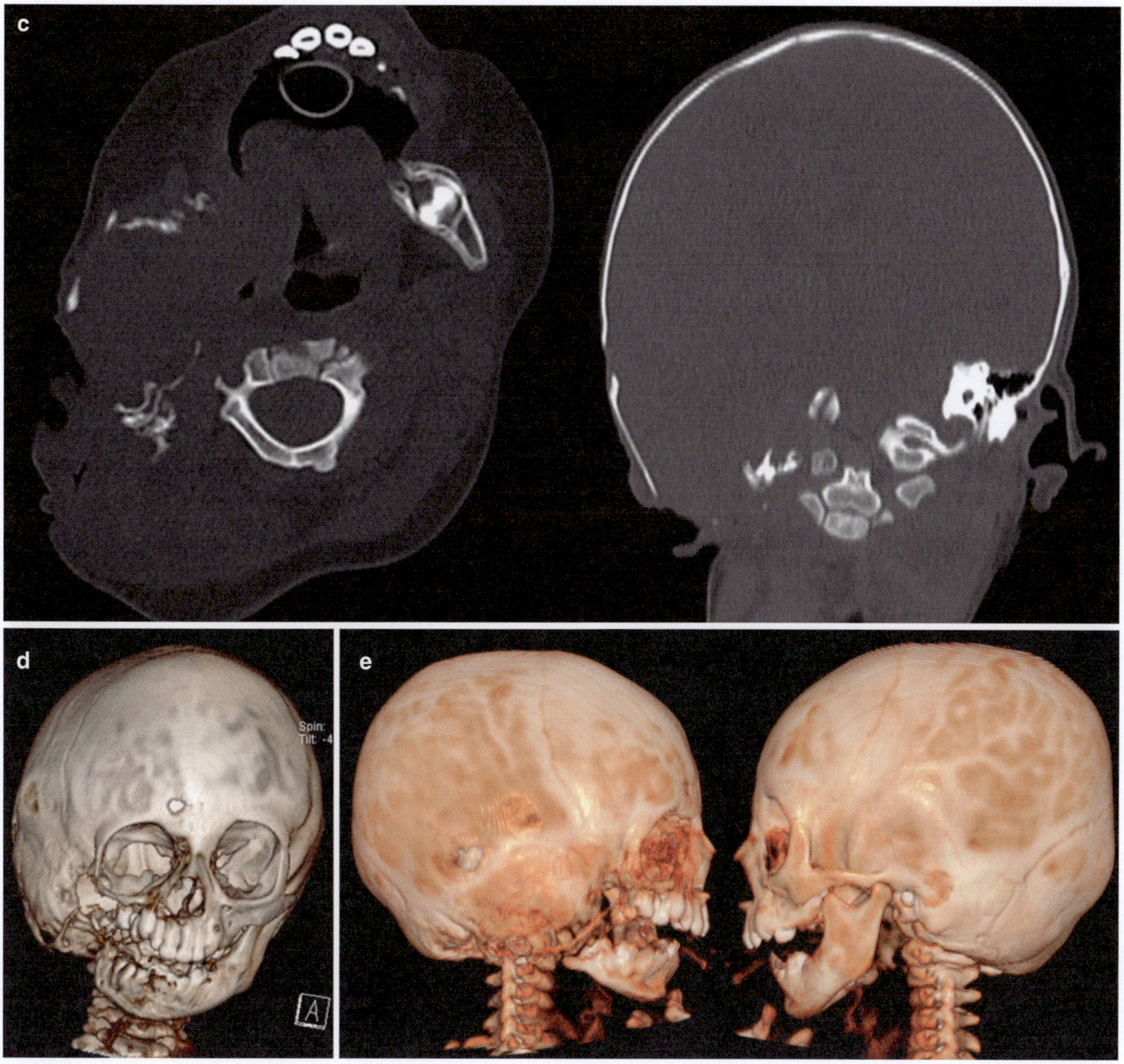

Fig. 26.3 (continued)

Fig. 26.3 (**a**-**b**) Three-phase bone scan shows normal blood-pool images (**a**) and diffuse reduced radiotracer uptake into the right skull and of the right skull base (**b**). (**c**–**e**) Axial and coronal CT (**c**) show right extensive osteolysis of the temporal bone, of the zygomatic arch, of the ramus, and condyloid process of the mandible; three-dimensional CT (**d**) in frontal view confirms the above findings with marked facial asymmetry; (**e**) The three-dimensional CT in the *right* side view shows the above alterations in comparison with the normal appearance of the *left* side

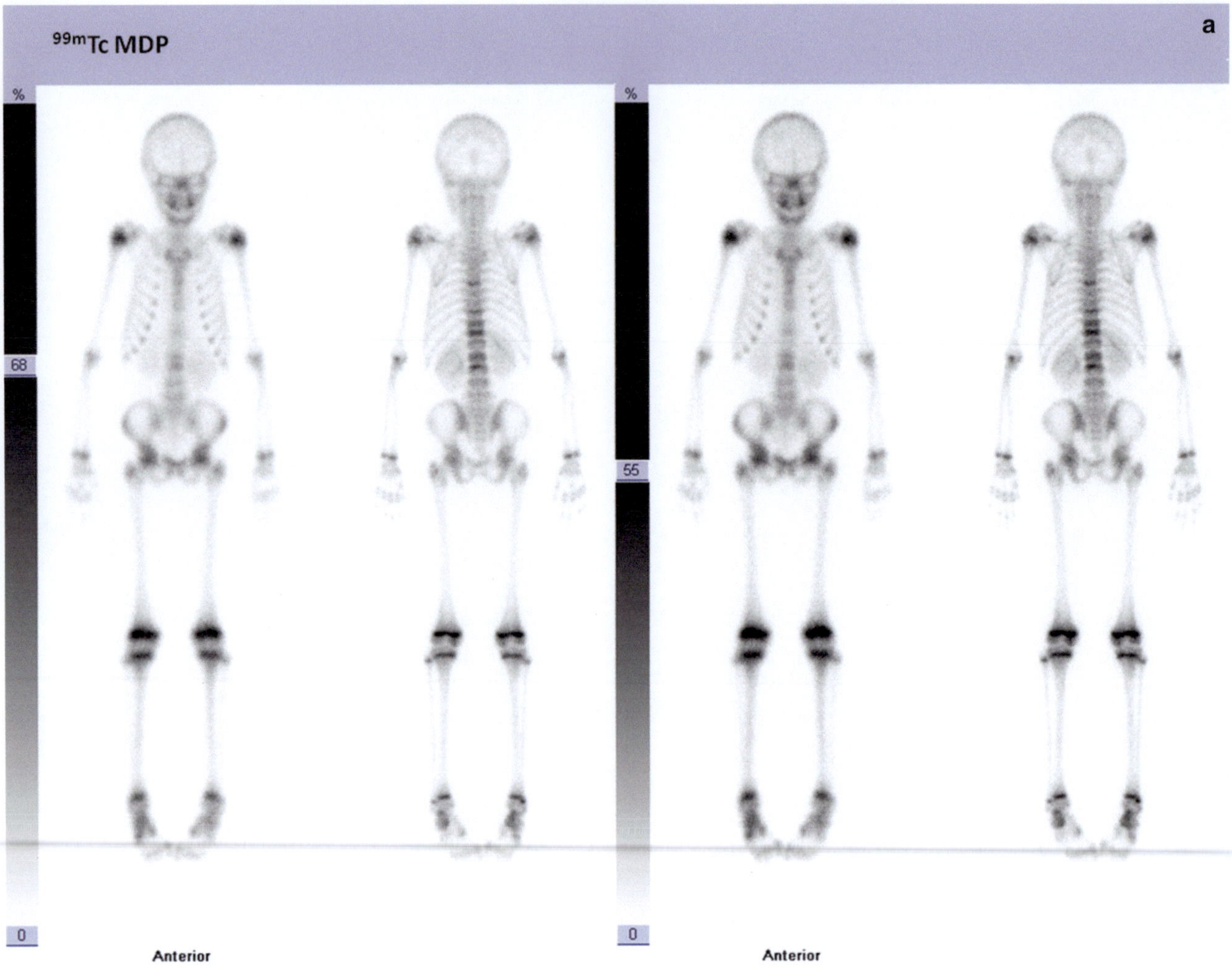

Fig. 26.4 (**a**–**c**) Bone scan (WBS and SPECT fused images) shows multiple areas of linear intense uptake in the dorsal (T6–T9–T10–T11) and in the lumbar spine (L1–L2–L3). (**d**–**e**) Frontal and lateral plain film (**d**) of the thoracic and lumbar spine shows rarefaction of cancellous bone design with "spider web" appearance and multiple vertebral collapses (*black arrows*). Sagittal T2-weighted MRI of the spine (**e**) confirms multiple somatic collapses (*black arrows*), some with increased signal due to edema of the bone marrow (*white arrows*). The intervertebral disks have a regular signal, and they are slightly expanded near somatic major collapses seats (*white oval*). The posterior somatic walls are intact, and spinal cord is normal

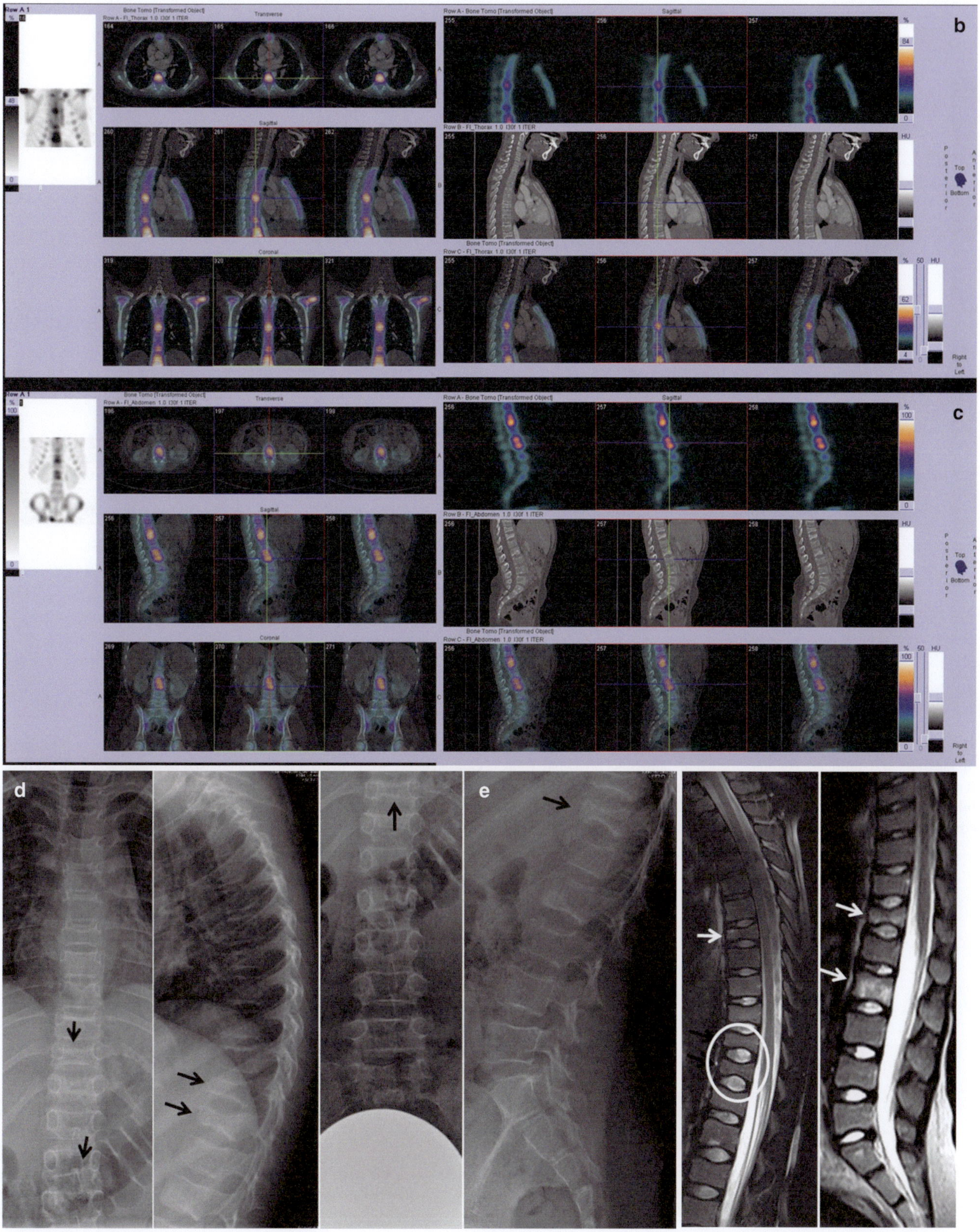

Fig. 26.4 (continued)

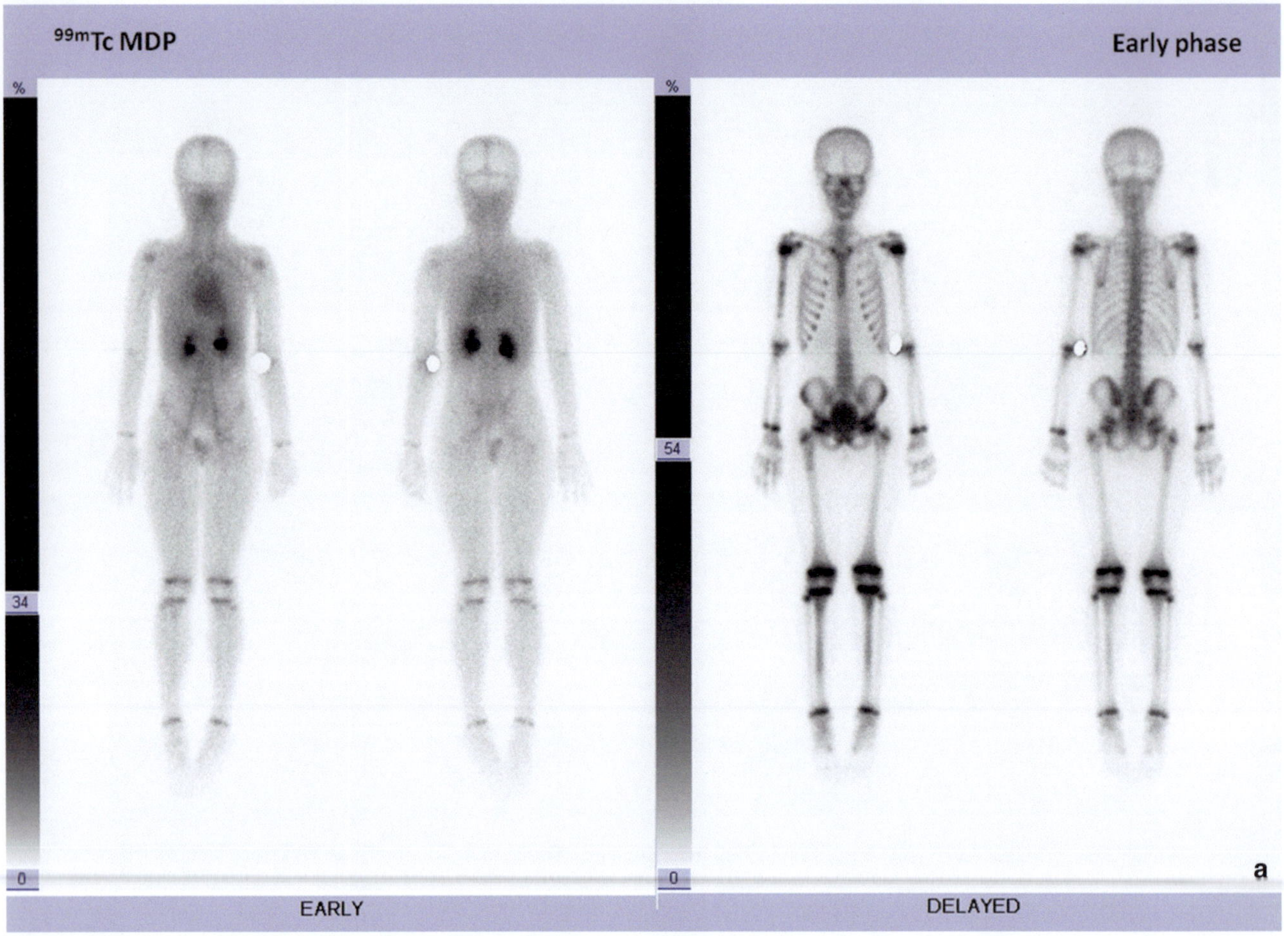

Fig. 26.5 (**a**–**c**) Three-phase bone scan shows normal blood-pool images (**a**) and mild uptake into the right humerus, proximal right femur, distal radius, and distal ulnae bilaterally, into metacarpal bones bilaterally, several foci of uptake in the phalanges of both hands (**b**–**c**) corresponding to the radiological findings. (**d**–**e**) Plain radiography: the humeral shaft is slightly flared with thinned cortical and small radiolucent areas (**d**, *white oval*). Flaring, increased radiolucency with cortical bulging, and thinning at the level of the metacarpals and proximal phalanges of the second and third fingers and middle phalanges of the third and fourth fingers (**e**, *white arrows*)

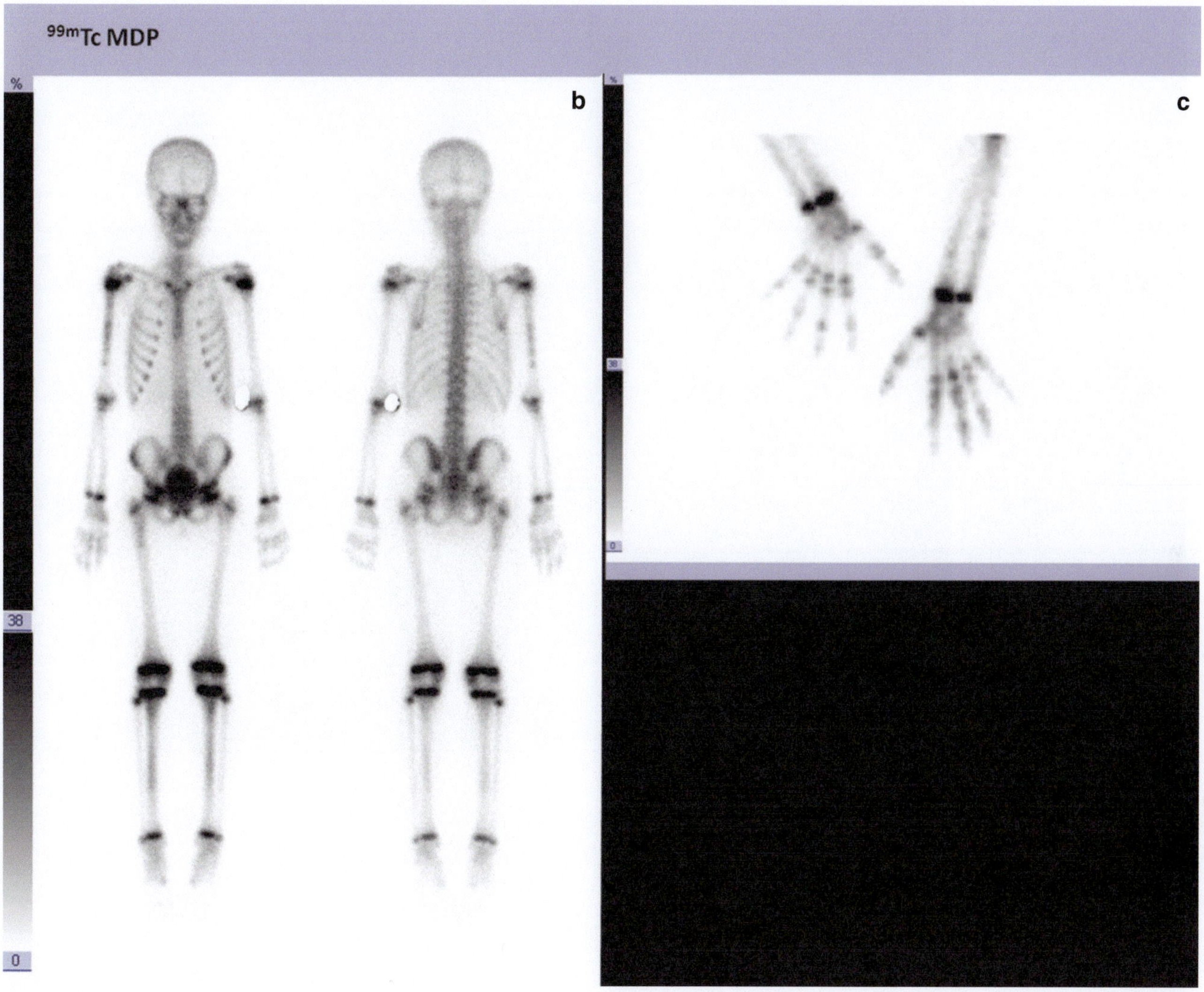

Fig. 26.5 (continued)

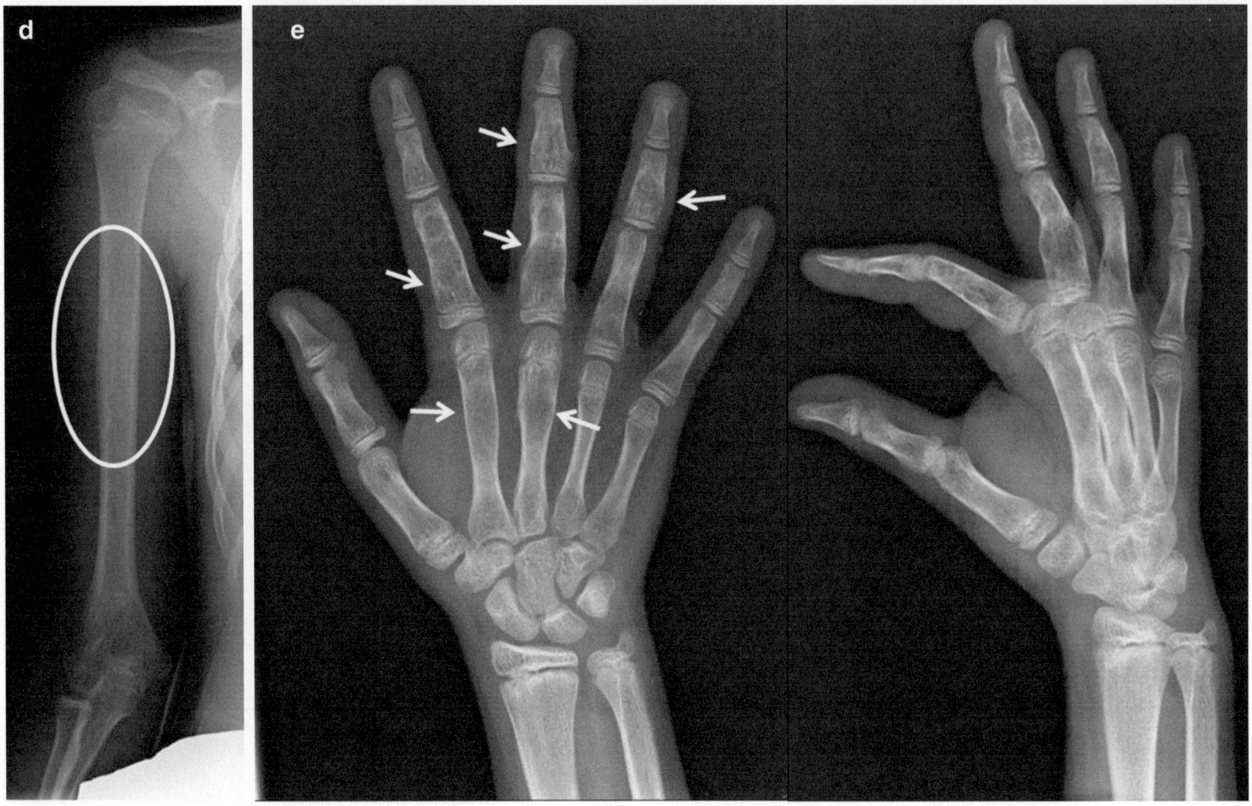

Fig. 26.5 (continued)

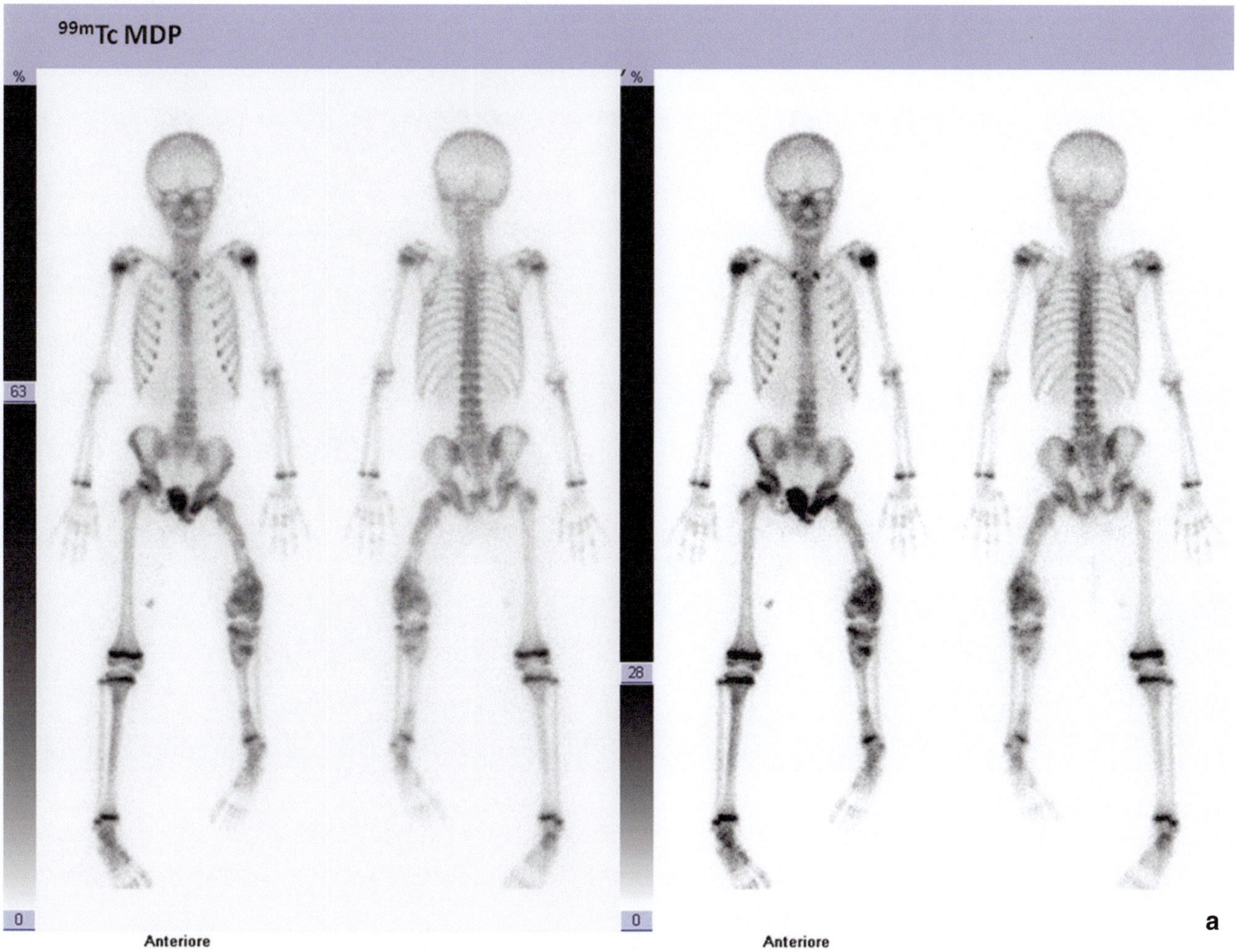

Fig. 26.6 (**a**) Bone scan shows short left lower limb, which appears deformed and with multiple areolas of increased uptake inside, in a context of widespread maldistribution, extensively in the femur and tibia. Mild and widespread increase in the left iliac bone, with maldistribution and poor definition of the iliac crest, is also noted. (**b–e**) AP telemetry with grid of the lower limbs (**b**): shortening of the left lower limb. Radiographs of the femur and tibia (**c**): marked femoral diaphyseal and metaphyseal flaring with large areas of osteolysis and multiple small calcifications. Coronal MRI T2 * (**d**): metaphyseal flaring with hypersignal in the context of which are present multiple hypointense nodules due to calcifications in chondroid tissue. MRI axial T2 fat/sat of pelvis (**e**): flaring and hypersignal of left ileum due to chondroid tissue with microcalcifications in the context

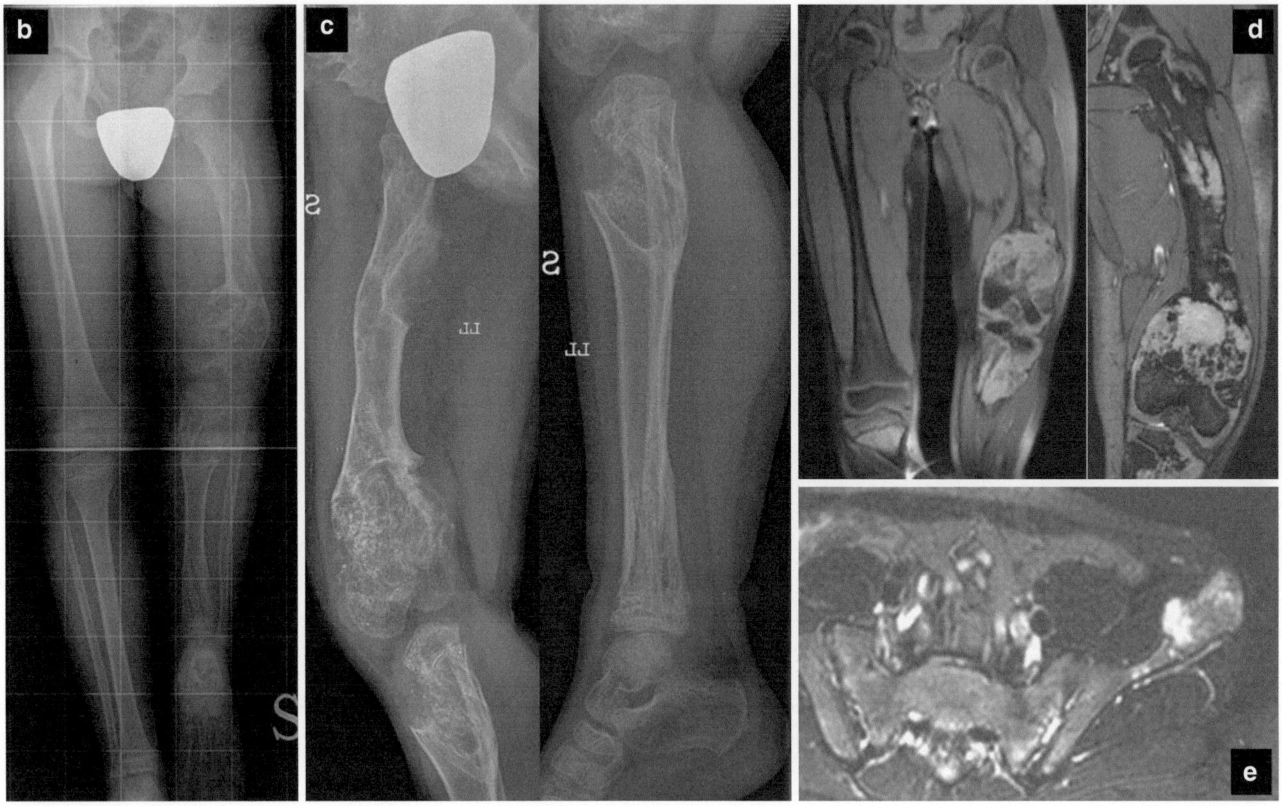

Fig. 26.6 (continued)

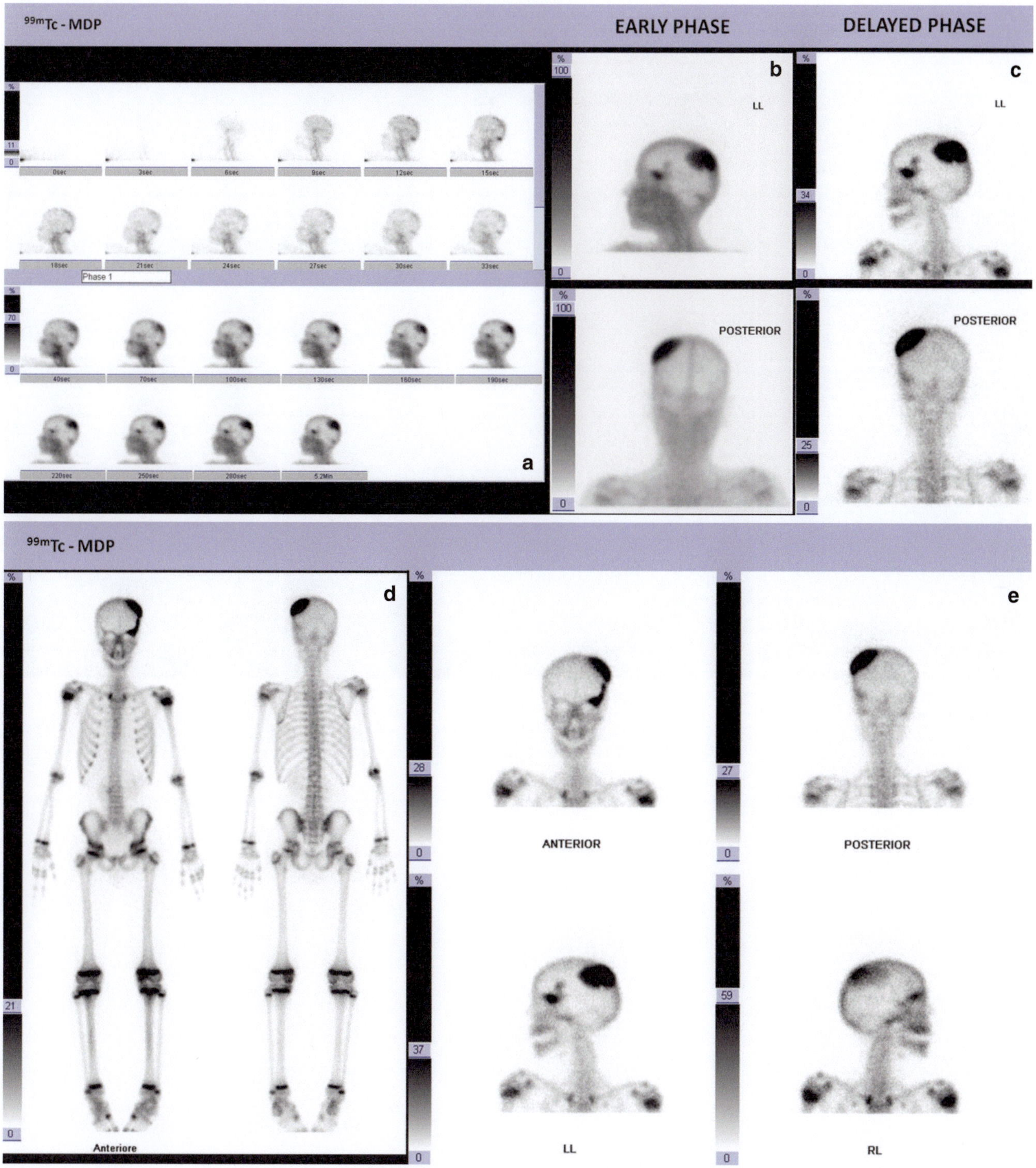

Fig. 26.7 (**a–e**) Three-phase bone scan shows: Phase I (a): moderate increase of flow in the posterior parietal region and in the temporal region. Phase II (early phase) (b): intense radiotracer uptake in the same regions. Phase III (delayed phase) (**c–e**): large intense uptake in the parietal bone and in the ipsilateral temporal bone extending to the upper and lateral orbital wall. (**f**) Axial and coronal CT scan of the skull with "bone window": enlargement and reduced density of diploe of left parietal and frontal bones which reaches the left orbital roof with "ground glass" aspect

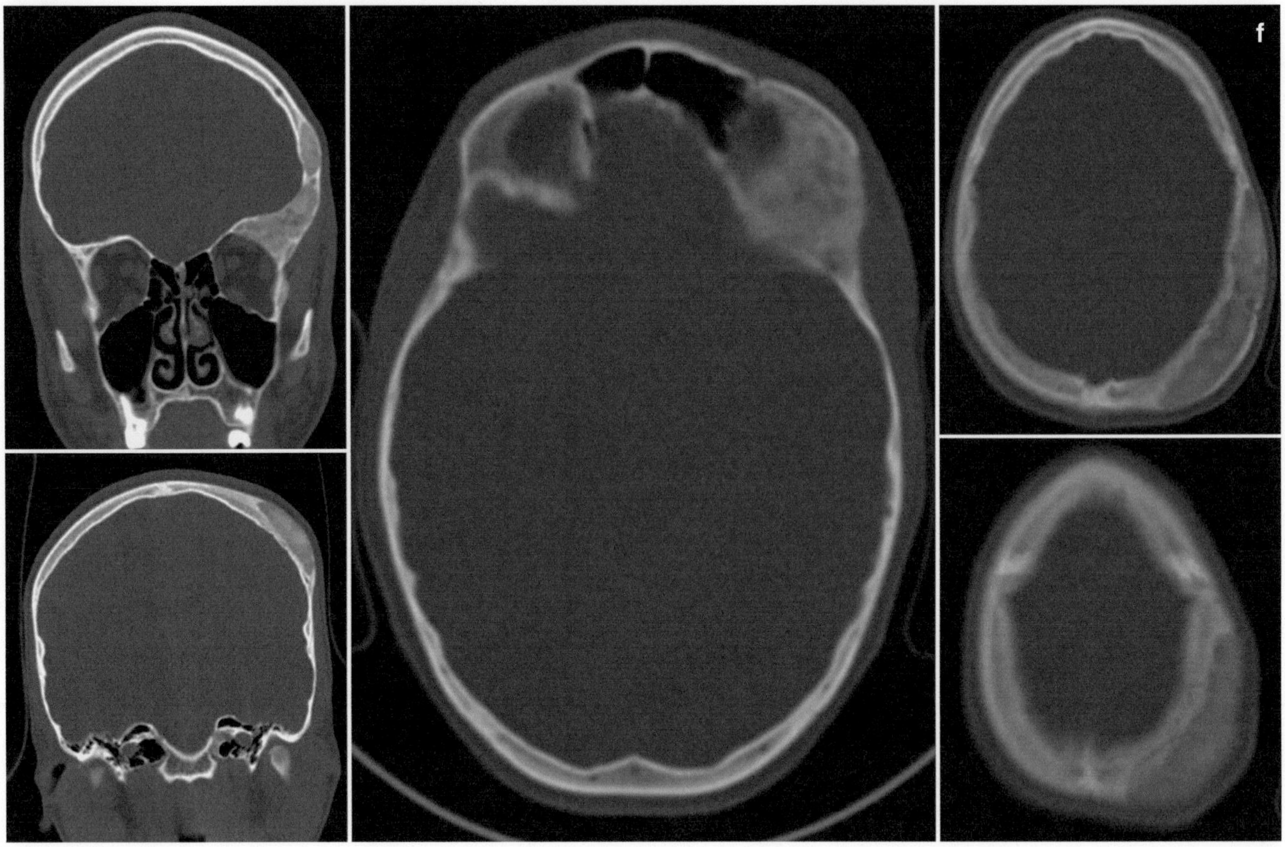

Fig. 26.7 (continued)

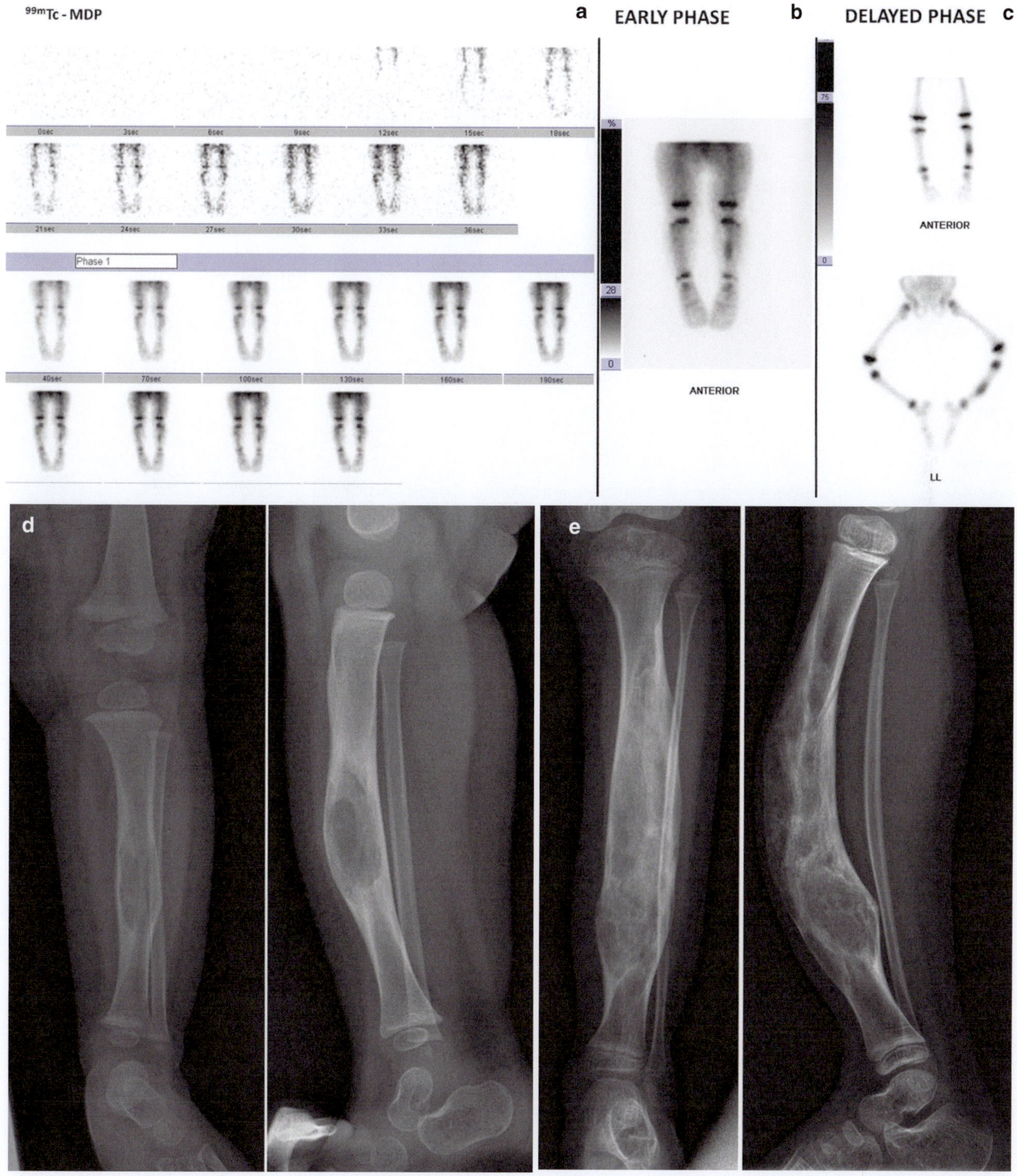

Fig. 26.8 (**a–c**) Three-phase bone scan shows: first phase (blood flow): normal distribution of the flow (**a**); second phase (blood-pool): moderate increase of the blood volume in the left tibia, middle third (**b**); third phase (skeletal accumulation): focal uptake of the radiotracer in the middle third of the left tibia (**c**), corresponding to the swelling clinically evaluable and described in the MRI study. (**d–e**) Frontal and lateral X-ray of the right leg at the diagnosis (**d**): tibial osteolysis with cortical bulging and thinning and slight procurvatum. Frontal and lateral X-ray of the right leg at 5 years of age (**e**): the osteolysis is polycyclic and much more extensive, with the cortical more swollen and thinned; worsened procurvatum. (**f–g**) Sagittal MRI of the tibia T1, T2 fat/sat, and T2-weighted at the diagnosis (**f**): oval area of low signal on T1 and increased in T2, with the cortical swollen and thin. Axial MRI T2 fat/sat shows widening and hypersignal of the medullary canal with thinning of cortical bone (**g**)

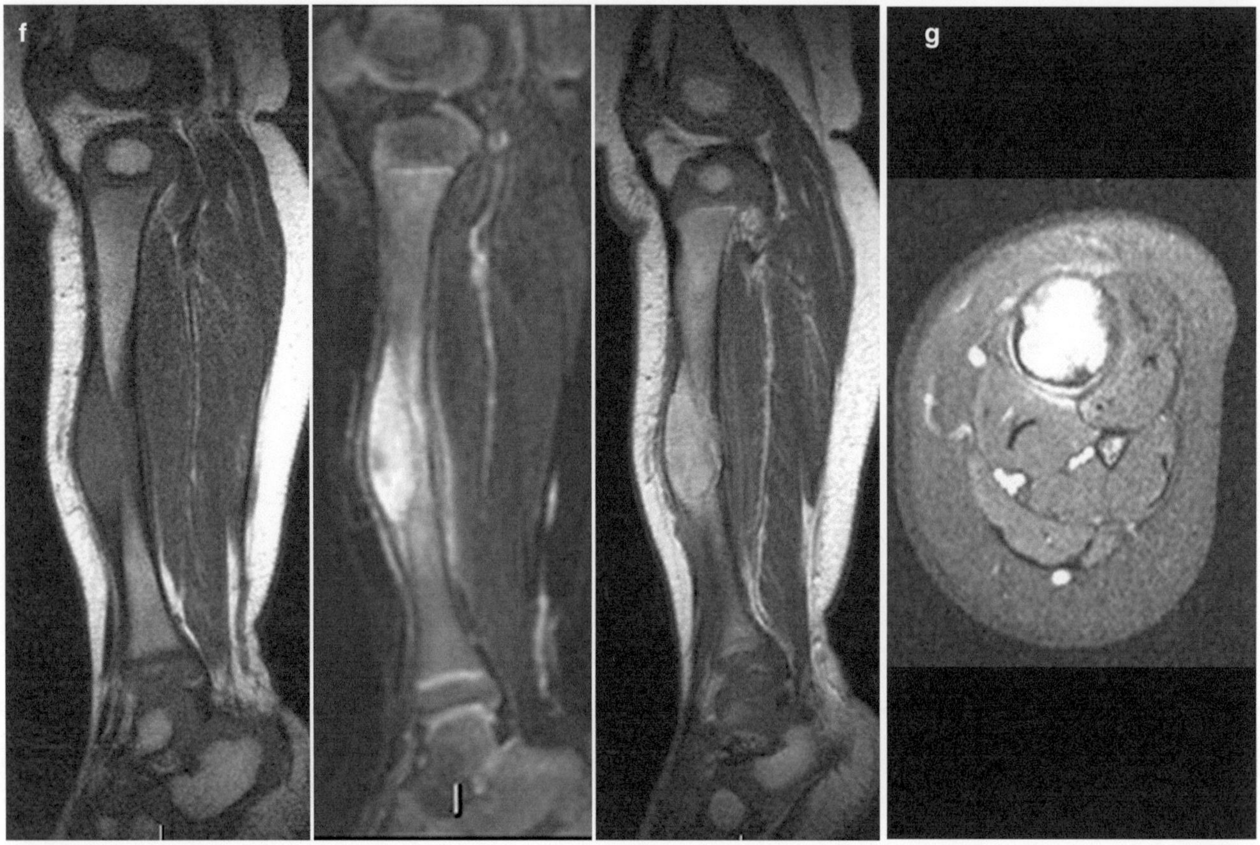

Fig. 26.8 (continued)

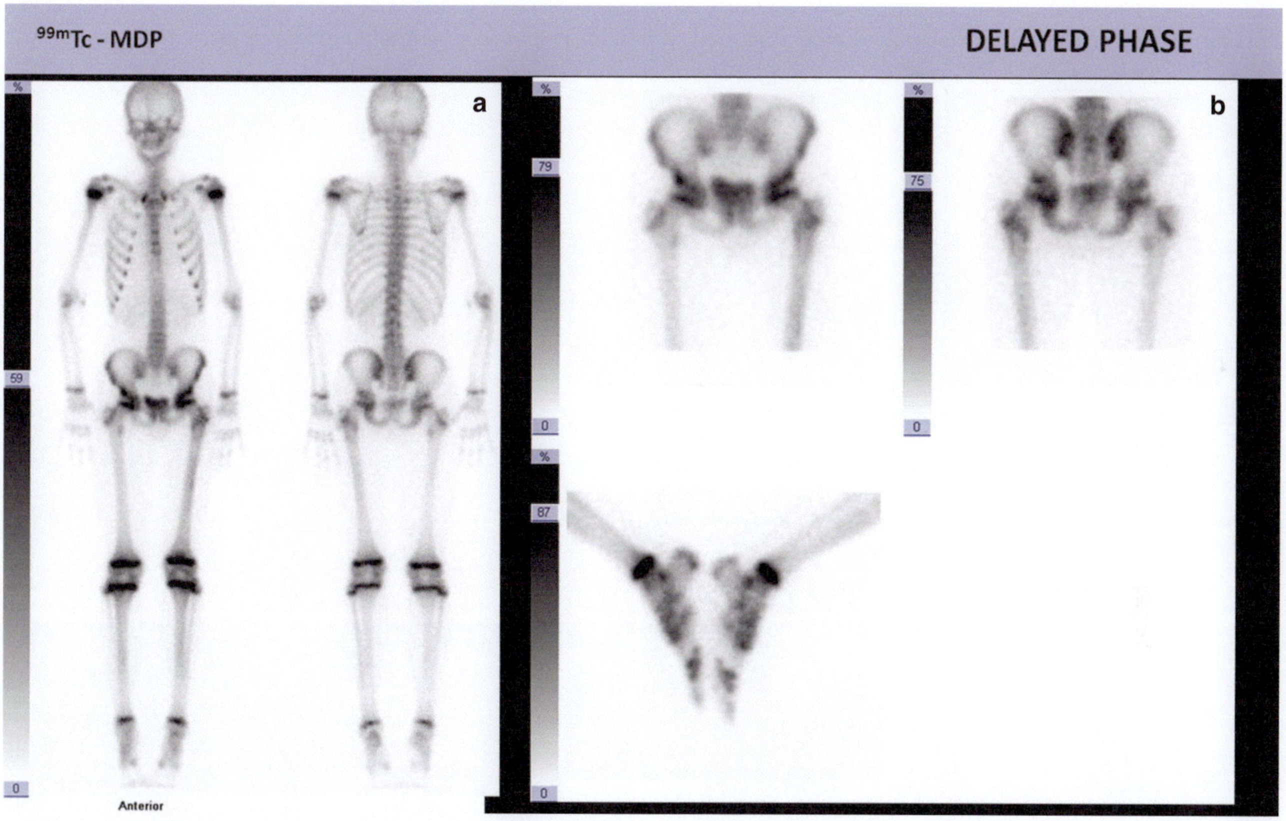

Fig. 26.9 (**a–b**) Bone scan shows: increased uptake in the proximal left femur, into ischiatic bone (posterior column of the left acetabulum), in the ipsilateral iliac wing. Mild uptake is also evident in left ischiopubic branch and in the posterior region of the left heel. (**c**) MRI of the pelvis coronal T1, T2, and T2 * fat/sat weighted (**c**): oval area of reduced signal in T1 and increased signal in T2 in the left femoral neck with sharp margins without perilesional edema (*red arrows*); oval area of reduced signal in T1 in the left ischium (*white arrows*). (**d–e**) Coronal CT (d) of the left femoral neck shows an oval osteolytic area with net nonthickened margins (*black arrows*). Axial CT of the left hip (**e**): oval osteolytic area with well-defined margins of the left ischium and the ischiopubic branch (*red arrows*). The top of the osteolytic lesion of the left femoral neck (*yellow arrow*) is also visible. (**f**) Lateral and axial X-rays of the calcaneus (**f**): area of reduced bone density with cortical bulging and thinning in the lower internal side of the heel bone (*black arrows*)

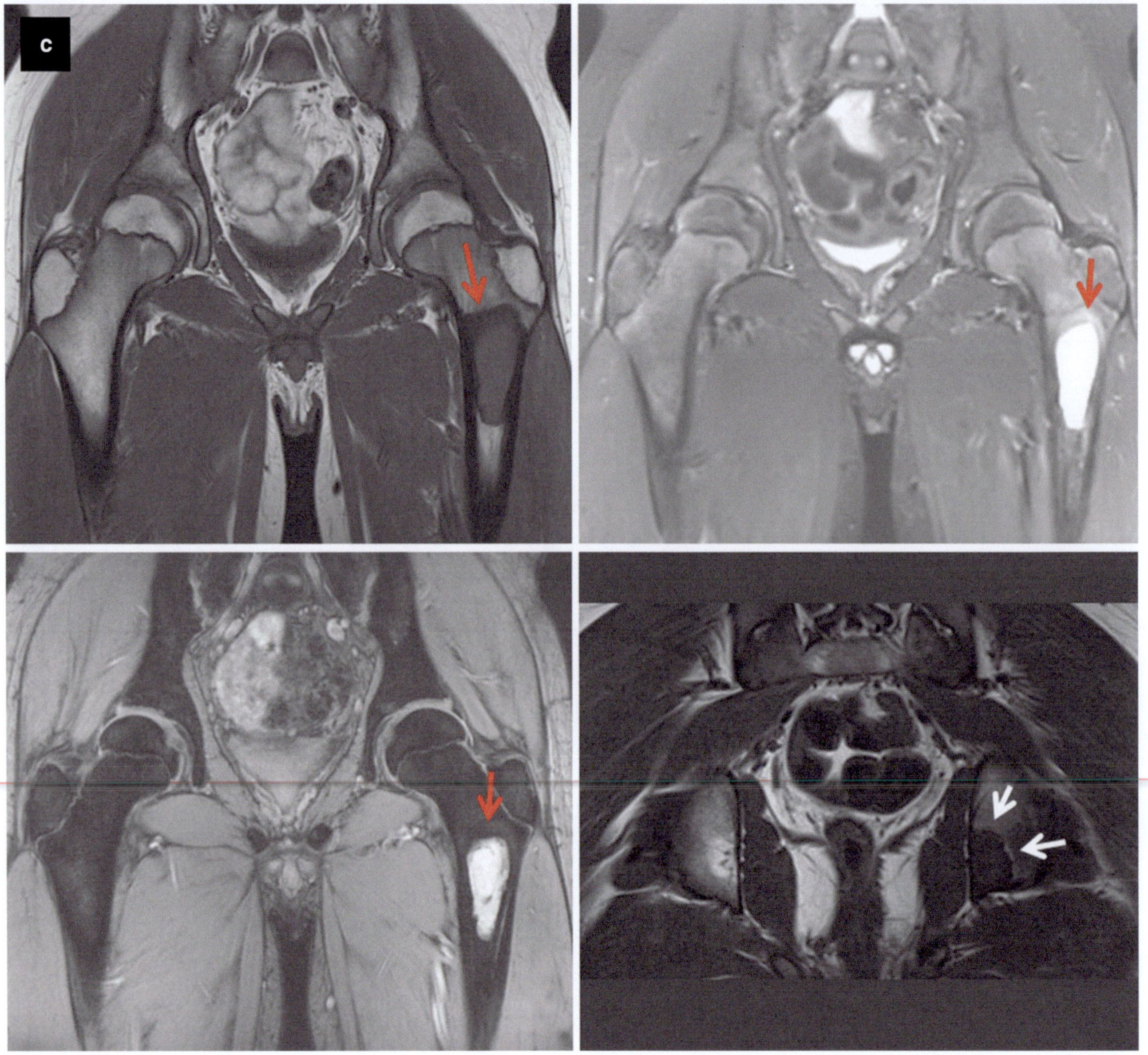

Fig. 26.9 (continued)

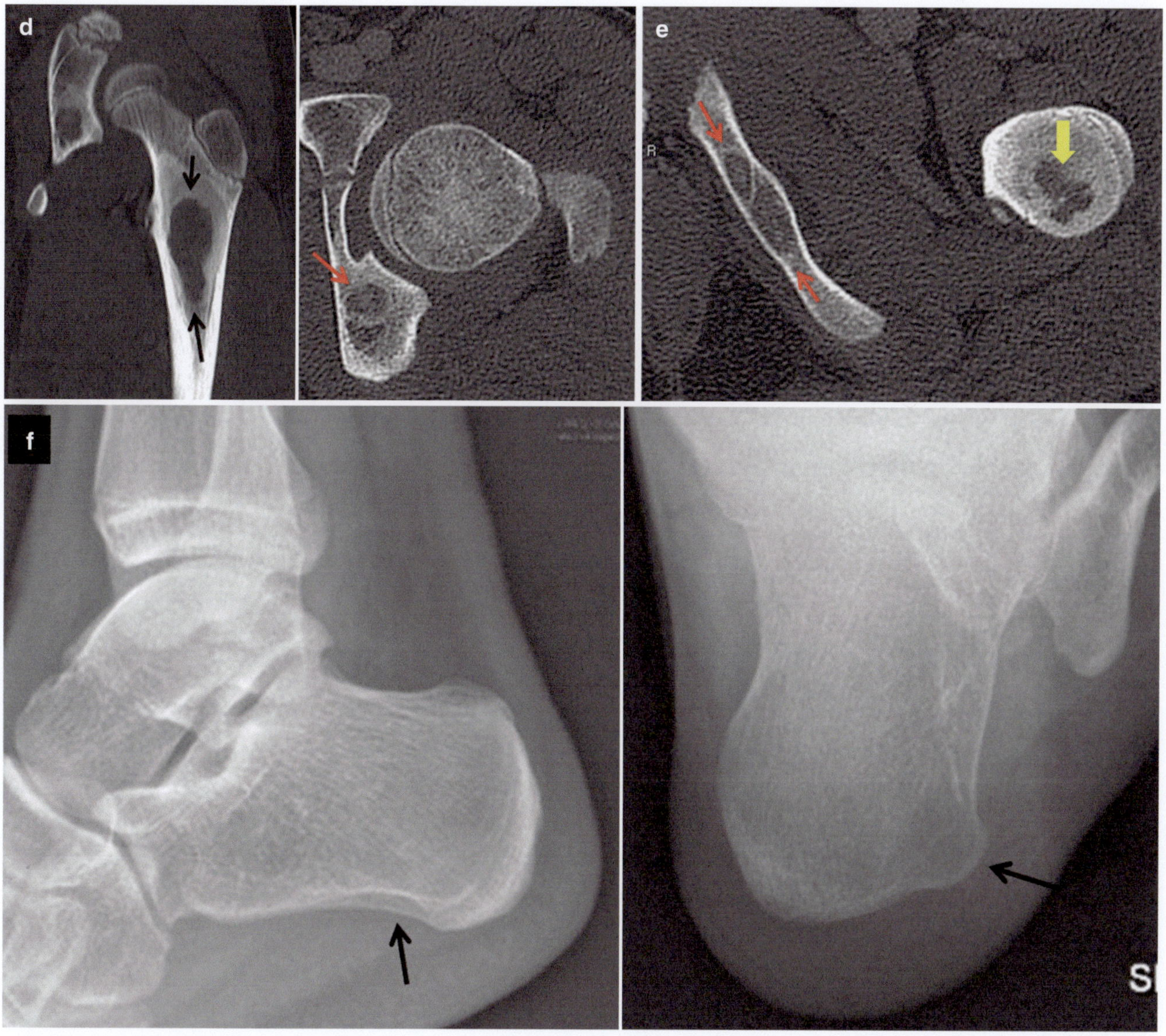

Fig. 26.9 (continued)

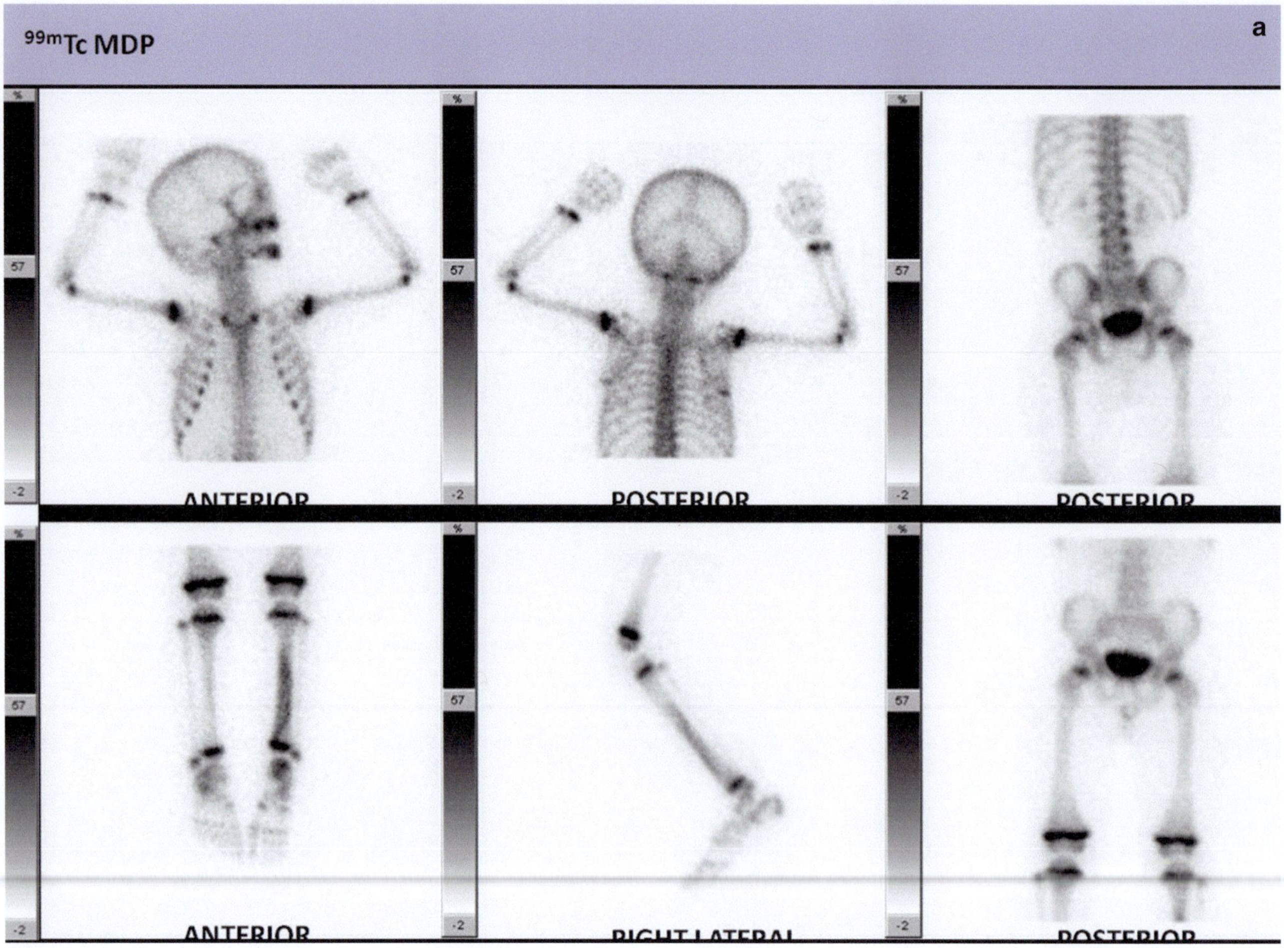

Fig. 26.10 (**a**) Bone scan shows: linear increased uptake in the left tibia with a typical "spiroid" aspect confirmed by radiological imaging. (**b**) Frontal and lateral X-rays of the left leg: prolonged spiroid thin fracture line in the distal shaft of the tibia without dislocation (*white arrows*). This is the classic "toddler fracture," typical of the uncertain gait of children 2–3 years old who fall with twist mechanism

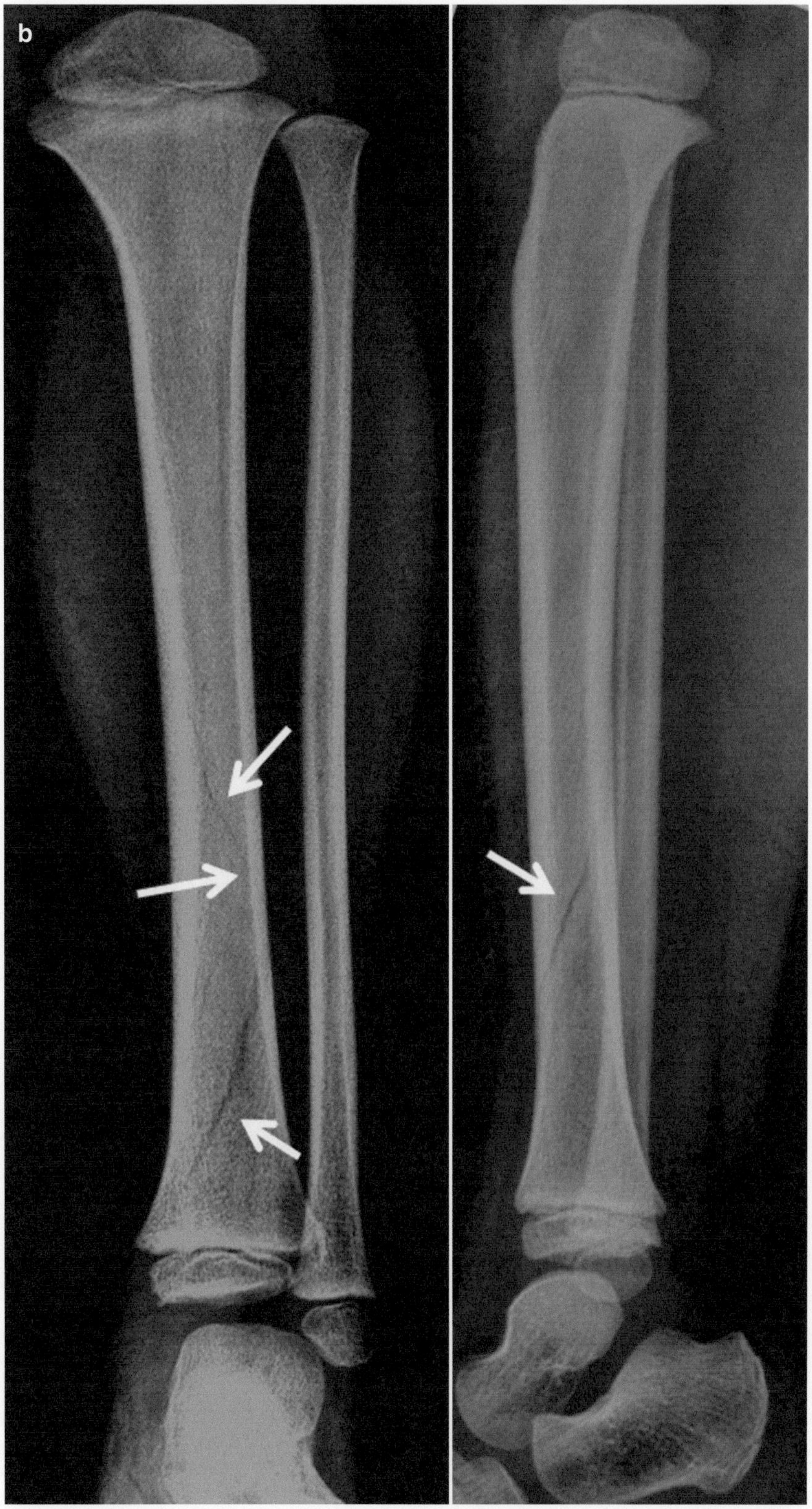

Fig. 26.10 (continued)

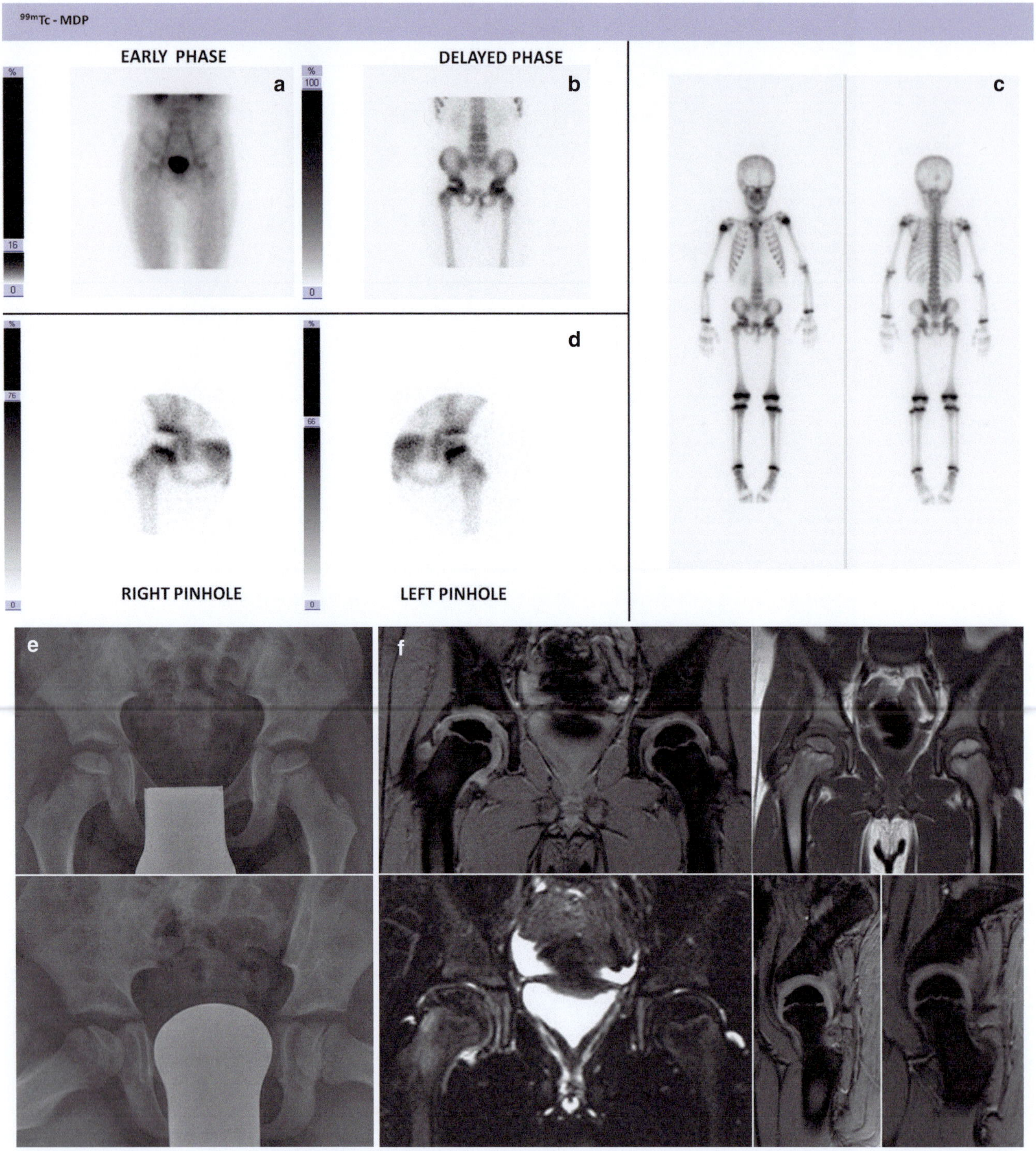

Fig. 26.11 (**a–d**) Bone scan shows absence of metabolic activity in the lateral columns of the right femoral head. Early phase, Perthes disease, stage I (J. Conway). (**e–f**) Hip X-ray (**e**) in frontal and "frog-legs" projection: the right femoral head shows slight thickness reduction and sclerosis compatible with an early form of Legg-Calvé-Perthes disease. MRI in coronal and sagittal T1, T2*, and T2 fat/sat (**f**): slightly reduced signal of femoral head in T1 and moderately increased in T2 fat/ sat. Slight joint effusion on the right: MRI confirms an early form of Legg-Calvé-Perthes disease

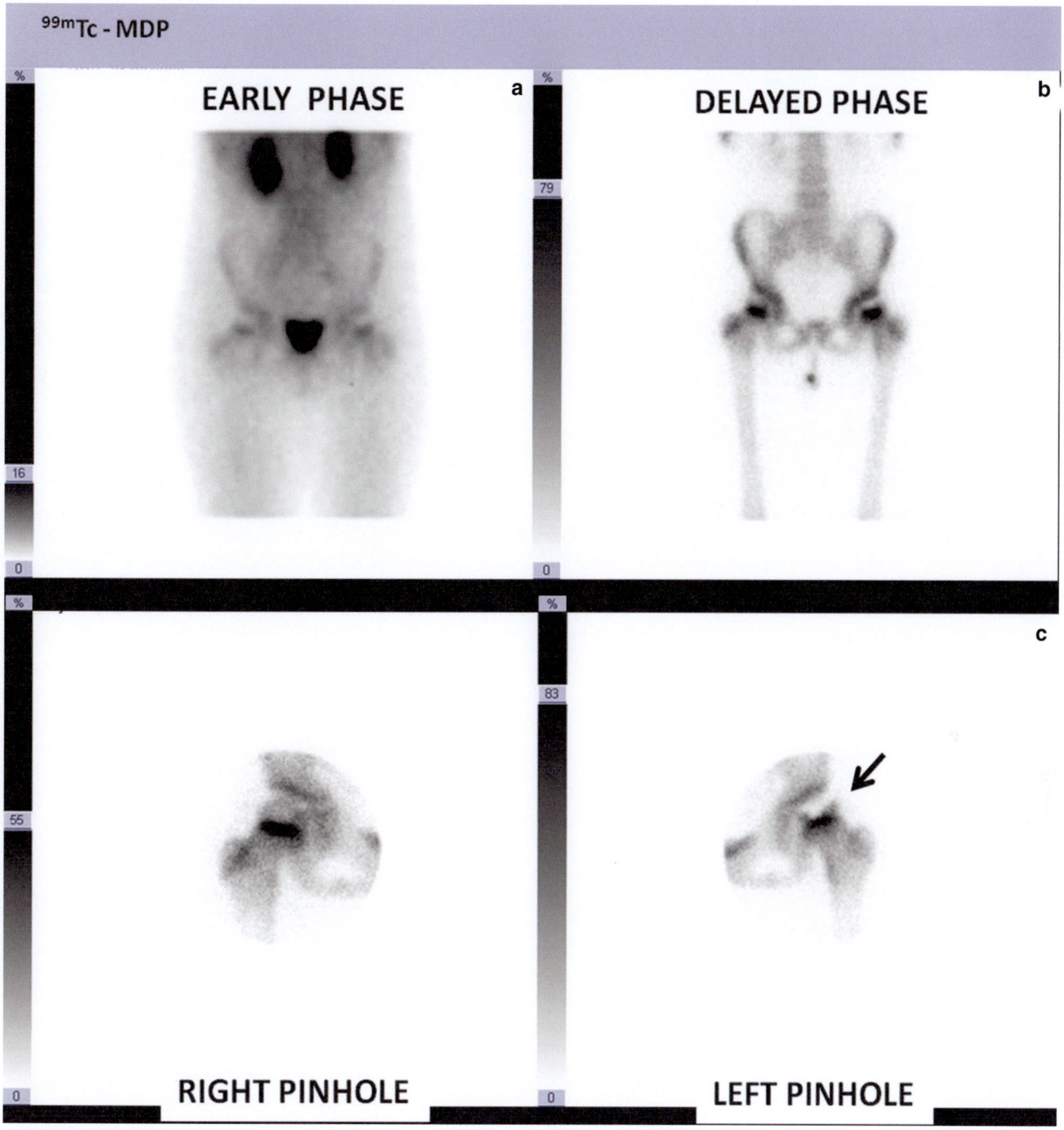

Fig. 26.12 (**a–c**) Bone scan shows presence of metabolic activity in the lateral columns of the left femoral head (*black arrow* in **c**). A pathway, stage II (J. Conway), with a good prognosis. X-ray of the pelvis in frontal and "frog-legs" projection (**d**): the left femoral head has a reduced thickness with sclerosis and subchondral radiolucent fissure (*crescent sign, black arrow*). MRI in coronal T1, T2, and T2* fat/sat (**e**): reduced thickness of left femoral head with a reduced signal in T1 and heterogeneously increased signal in T2 fat/sat. Cephalic cartilagine is slightly thickened; joint effusion on the left. Pseudocyst of the femoral neck (*red arrow*)

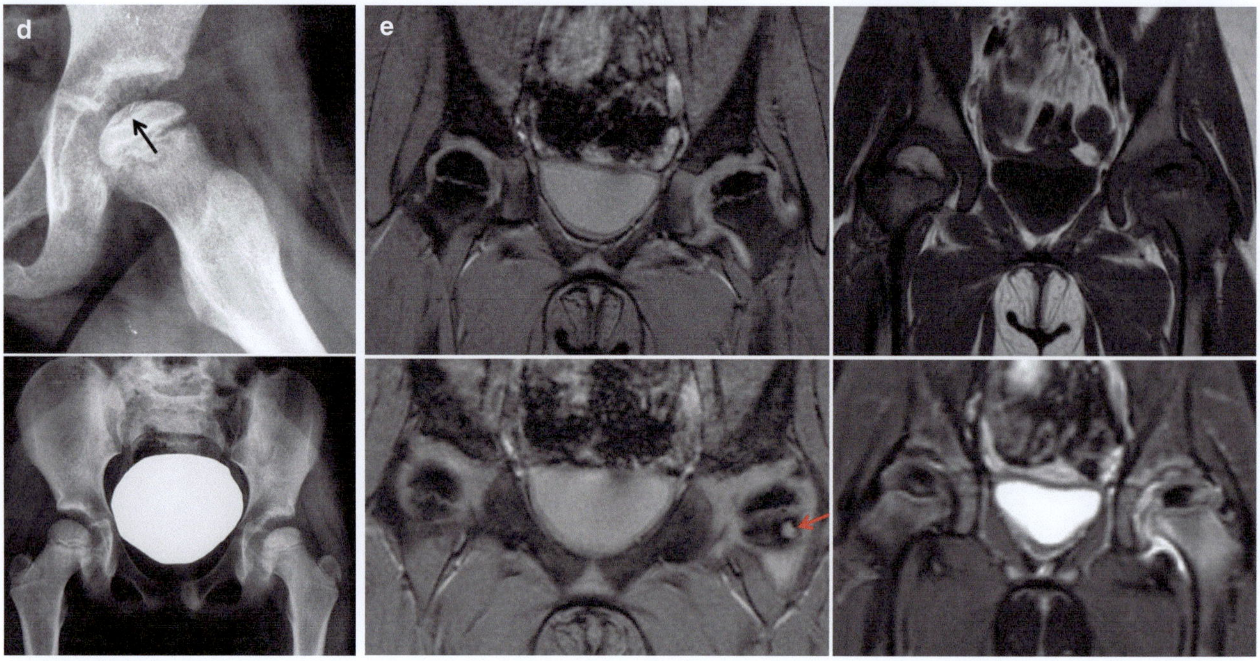

Fig. 26.12 (continued)

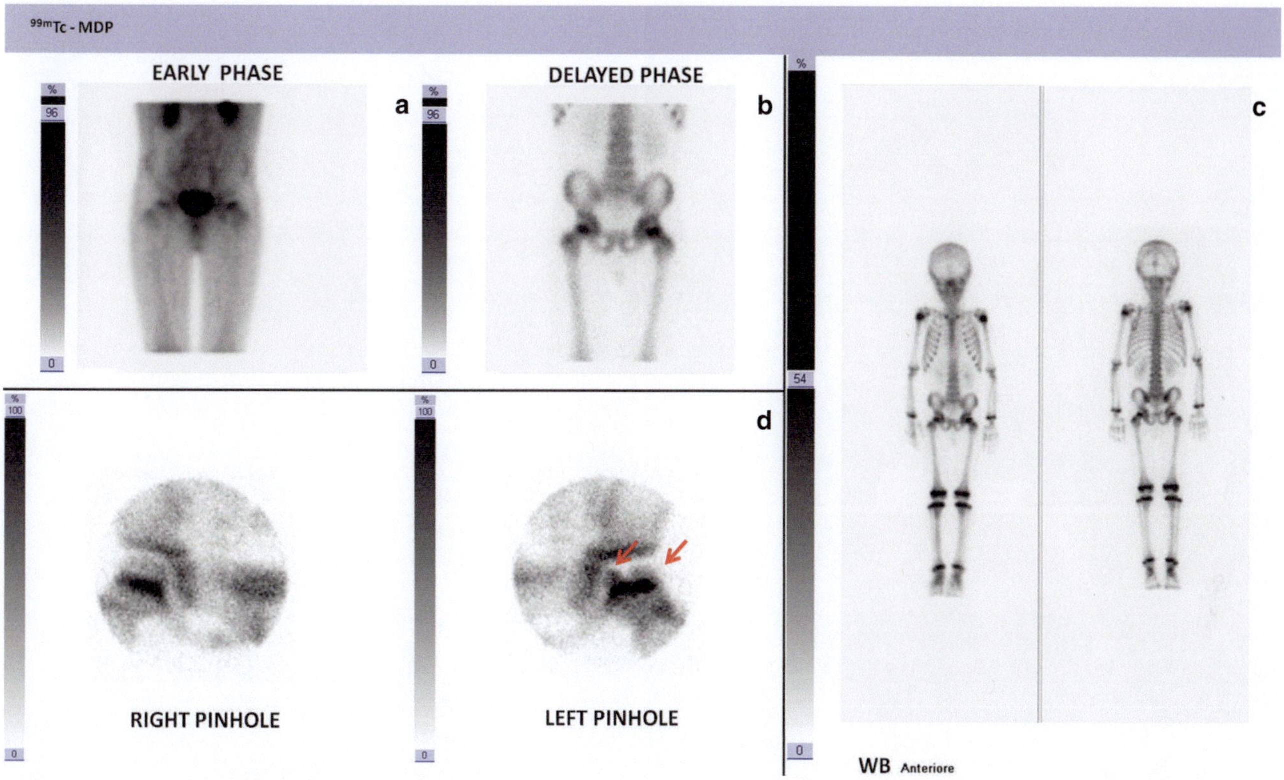

Fig. 26.13 (**a**–**d**) Bone scan shows presence of metabolic activity in the lateral columns of the left femoral head (*red arrows* in figure **d**), strongly evident. A pathway, III Stage (J. Conway), with a good prognosis. (**e**–**f**) Hip X-ray in the frontal and lateral view (**e**): reduced thickness of left femoral head which is flared and fragmented. MRI in coronal T1, T2, T2* d T1 fat/sat after contrast medium (**f**): reduced signal in T1 and heterogeneously increased in T2 fat/sat of the left femoral head. Cephalic cartilage is thickened; minimal joint effusion on the left. After contrast reduced signal in the central part of the left avascular femoral head (*black arrow*)

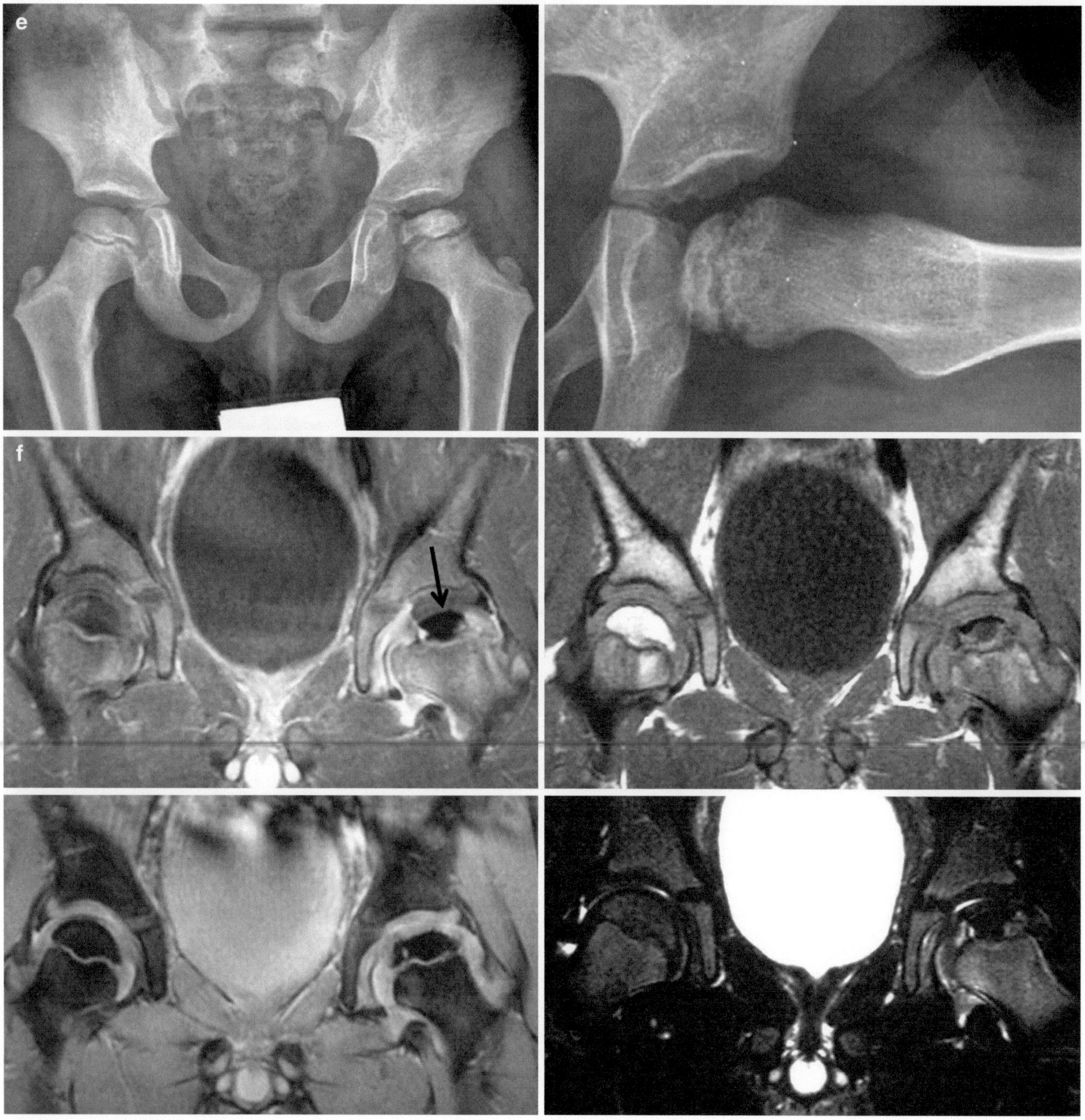

Fig. 26.13 (continued)

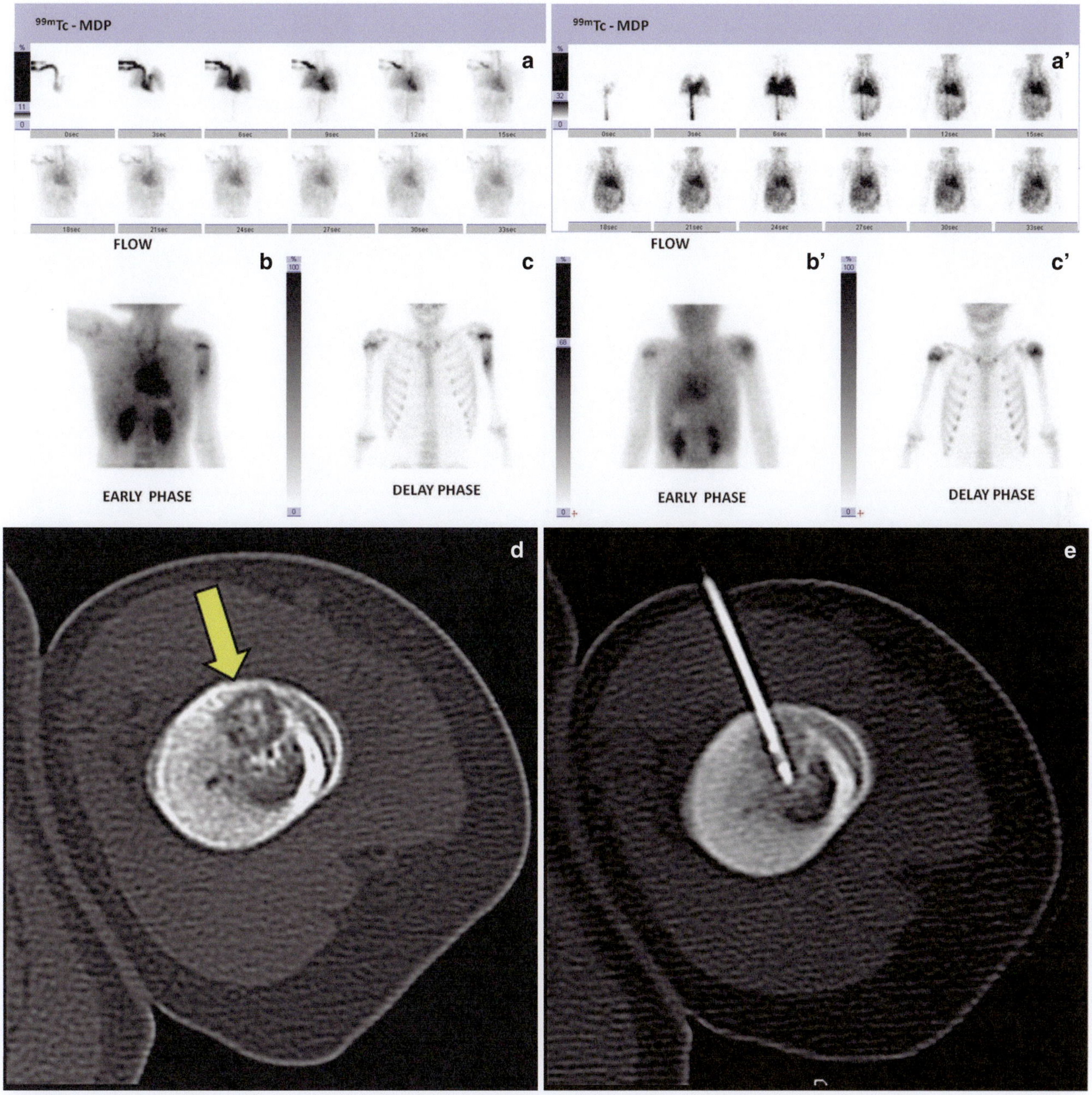

Fig. 26.14 (**a**-**b**-**c**–**a'**-**b'**-**c'**) Bone scan clearly shows presence of focal increased uptake in the diaphyseal of left humerus (**c**) in the image on the left. A very small area of focal increased uptake is evident in the head of the left humerus (**c'**) closely to metaphysis, in the image on the *right*. (**d**–**e**) TC cortical lesion with calcified nidus (*yellow arrow*) and sclerotic reaction of the periosteum (**d**); RF thermal ablation (**e**). (**d'**–**e'**) Axial CT nodule subperiosteal calcified nidus (*white arrow*) with nuanced sclerotic reaction peripheral (**d'**) sagittal CT reconstruction (**e'**)

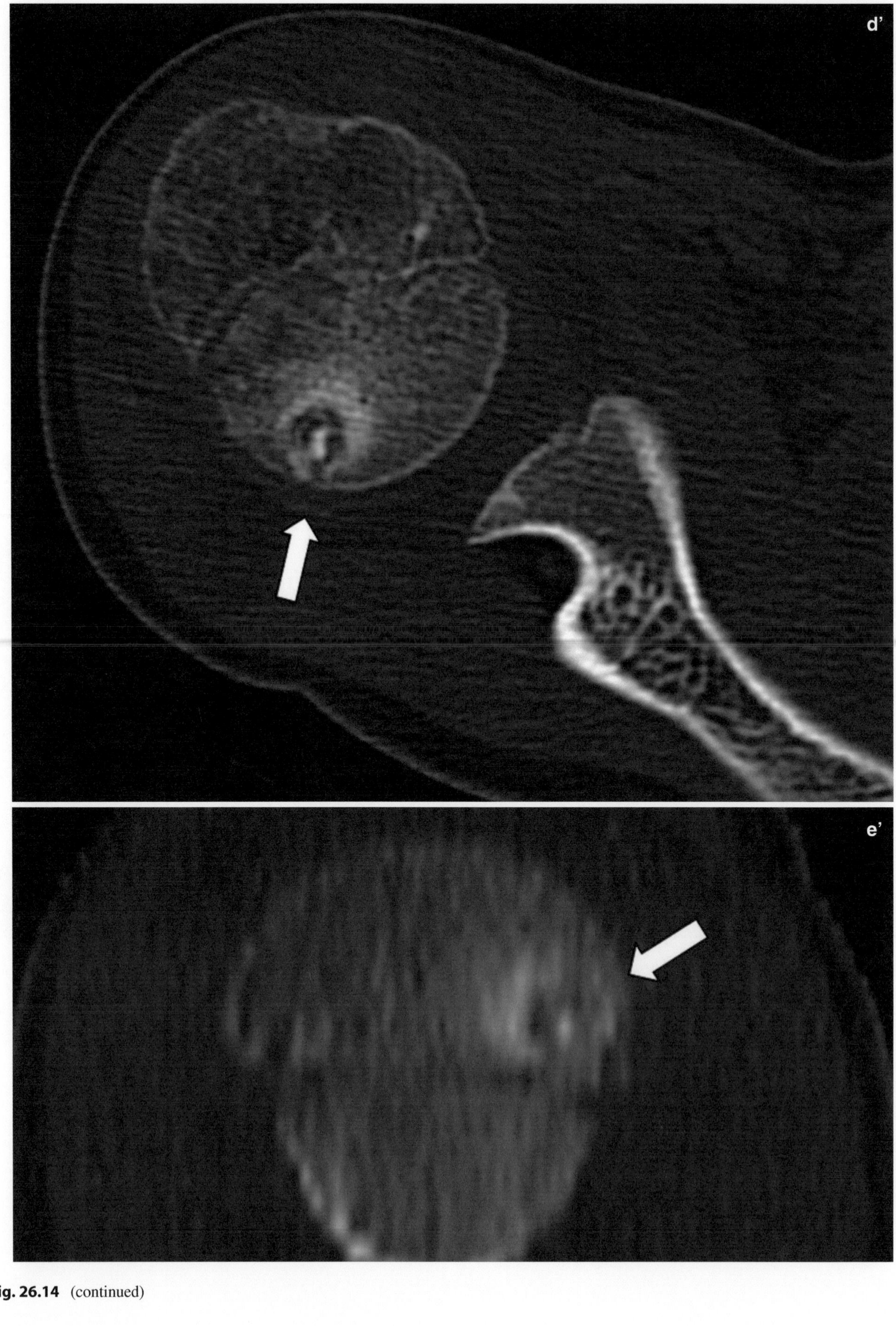

Fig. 26.14 (continued)

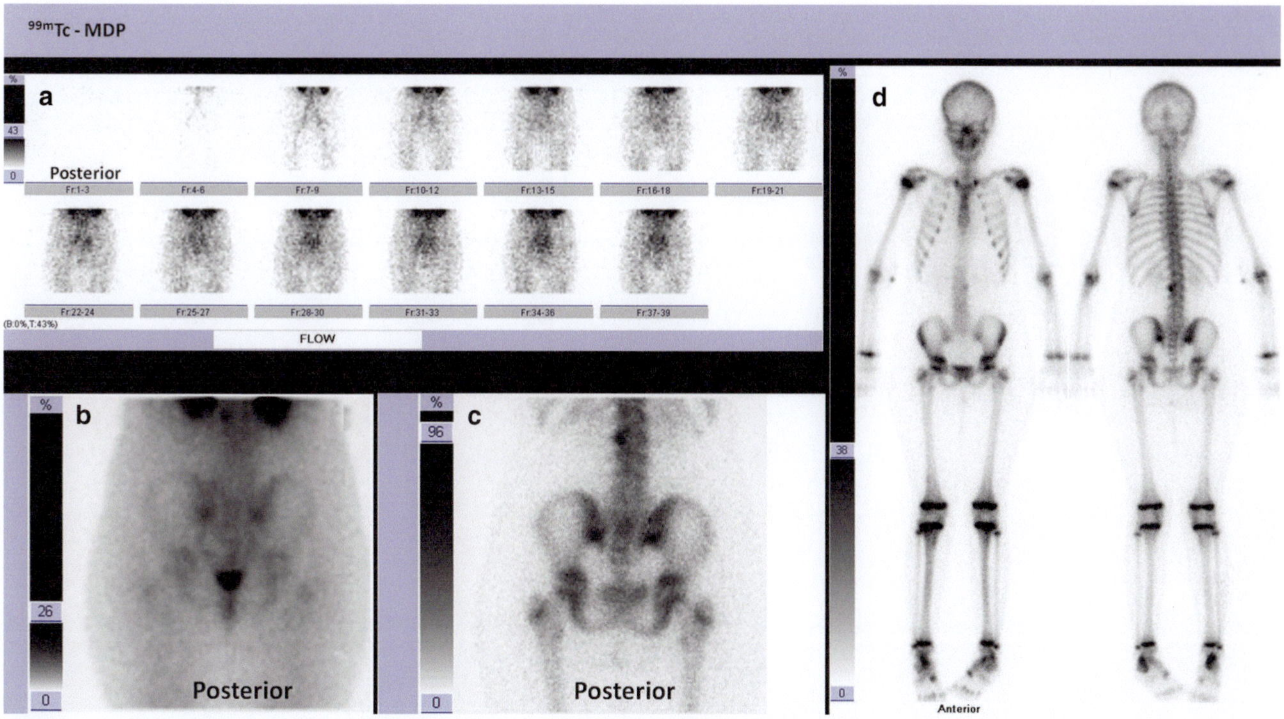

Fig. 26.15 (**a**–**d**) Bone scan reveals presence of a small area of focal increased uptake in the right femoral neck (**c**), well-defined by pinhole acquisition (**d**). A diffuse mild uptake is also evident in the intertrochanteric region of right femur. (**e**–**h**) Osteoid osteoma right femur. MRI T2 STIR (**e**–**f**): hypointense lesion (*white arrow*) with hyperintense edema of the contiguous spongy bone. Axial CT (**g**): periosteal lesion with thin sclerotic rim (*yellow arrow*). RF thermal ablation (**h**)

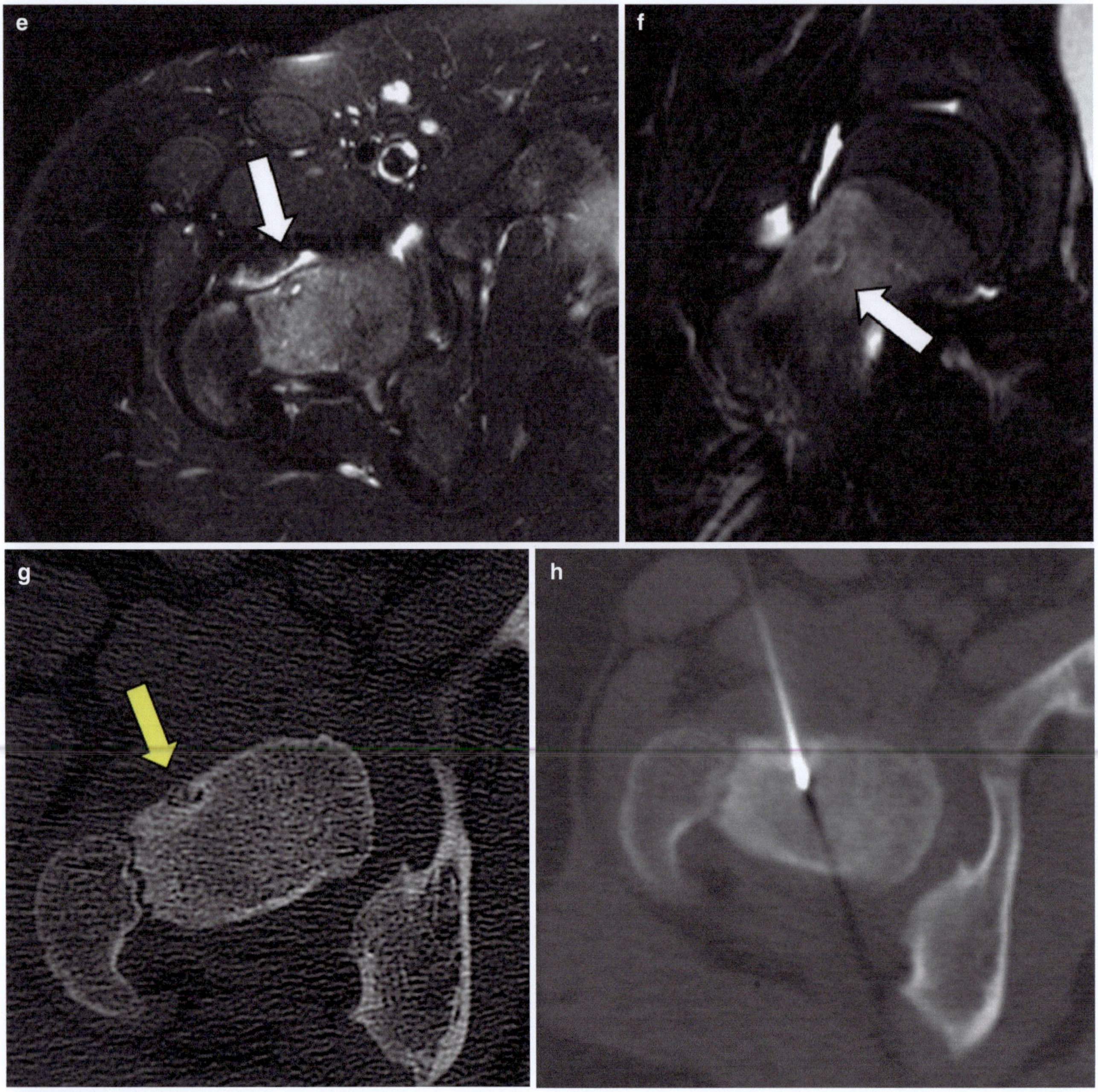

Fig. 26.15 (continued)

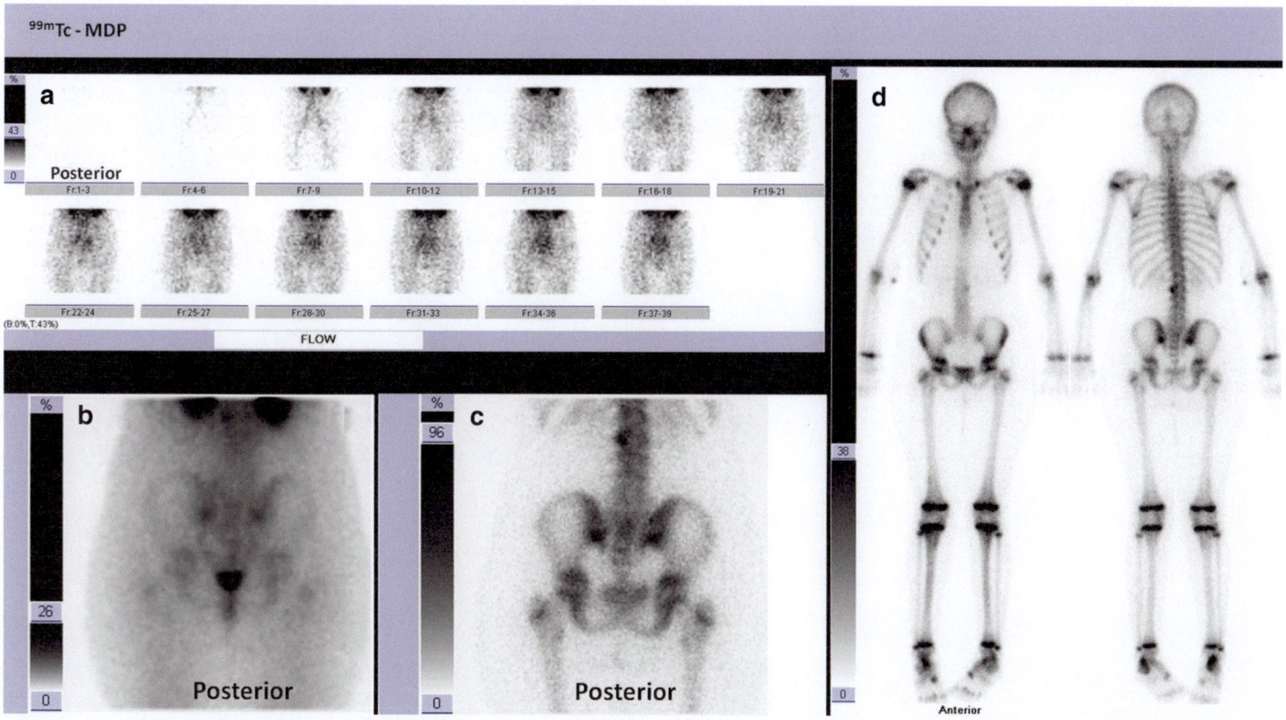

Fig. 26.16 (**a–d**) Bone scan (**a–d**) shows normal radiotracer uptake in pelvis and coxofemoral regions; presence of focal increased uptake in a vertebra of lumbar spine is evident; eSPECT-MRI fused images localize the focus of uptake in left hemisoma of L2. (**f–i**) Axial and coronal CT images (**f–g**) nodular lesion with calcified nidus and minimum contiguous sclerotic reaction (*white arrows*). MRI T2 (**h–i**): hypointense lesion with mild edema reaction of the adjacent spongy bone

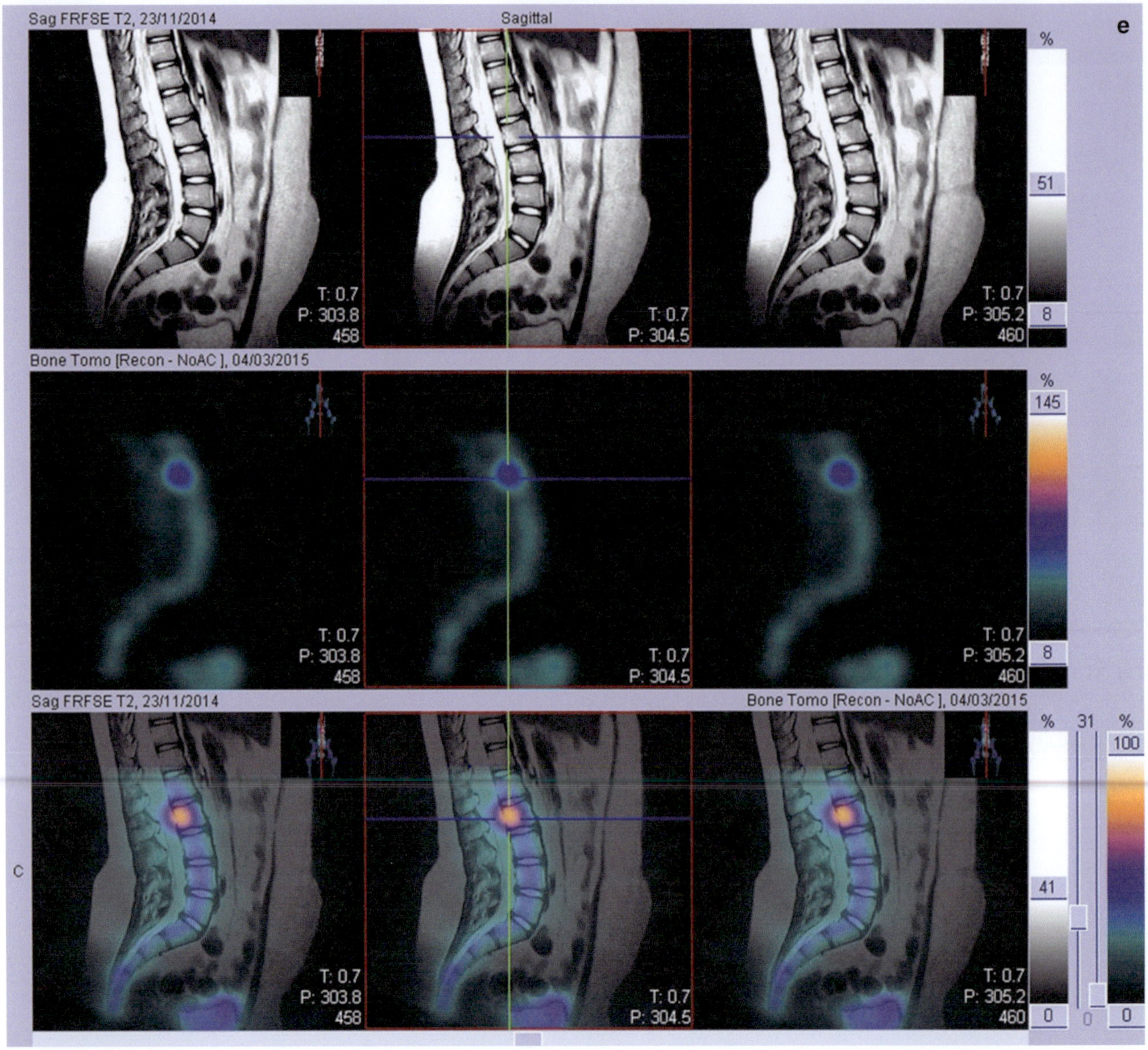

Fig. 26.16 (continued)

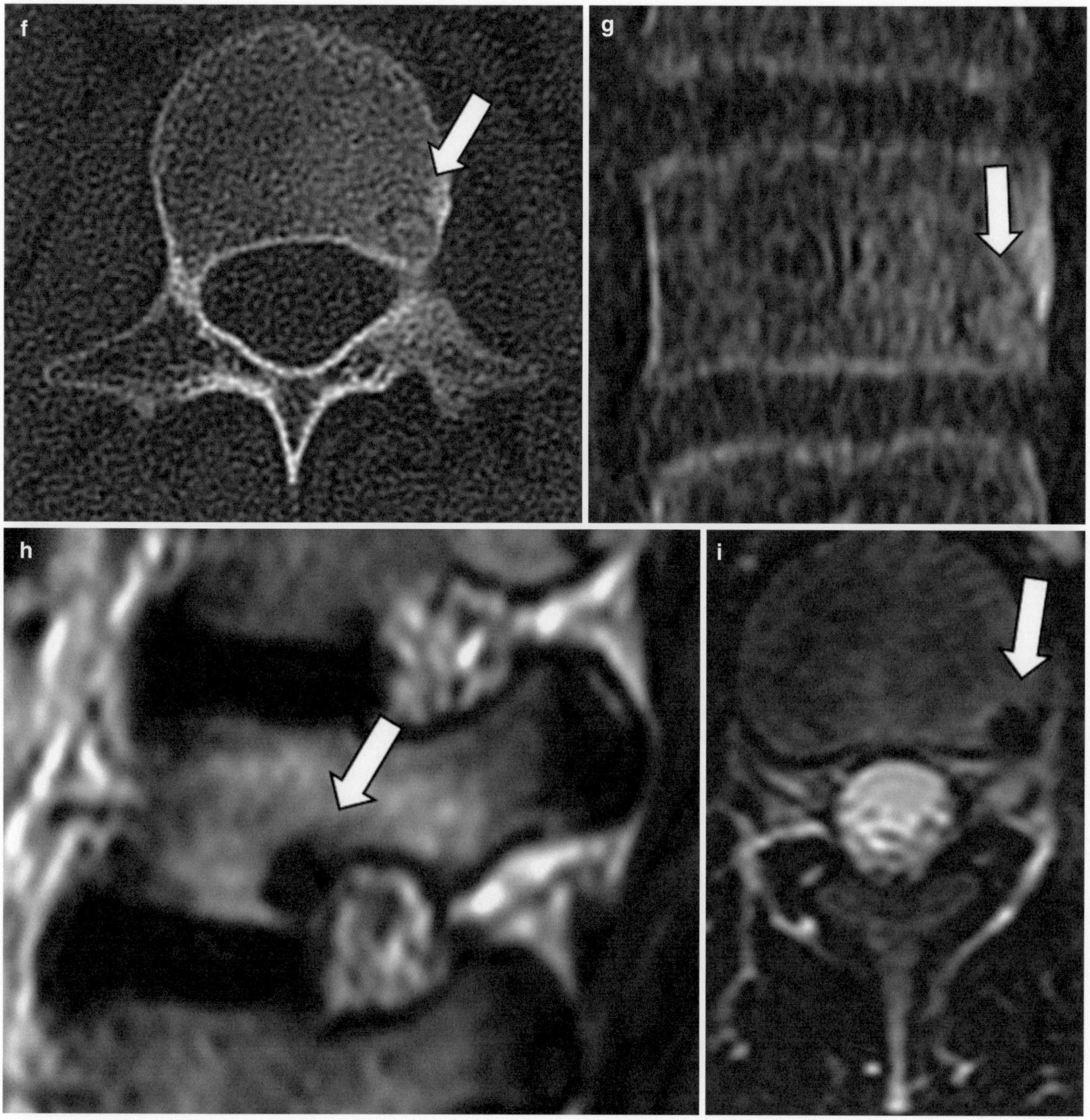

Fig. 26.16 (continued)

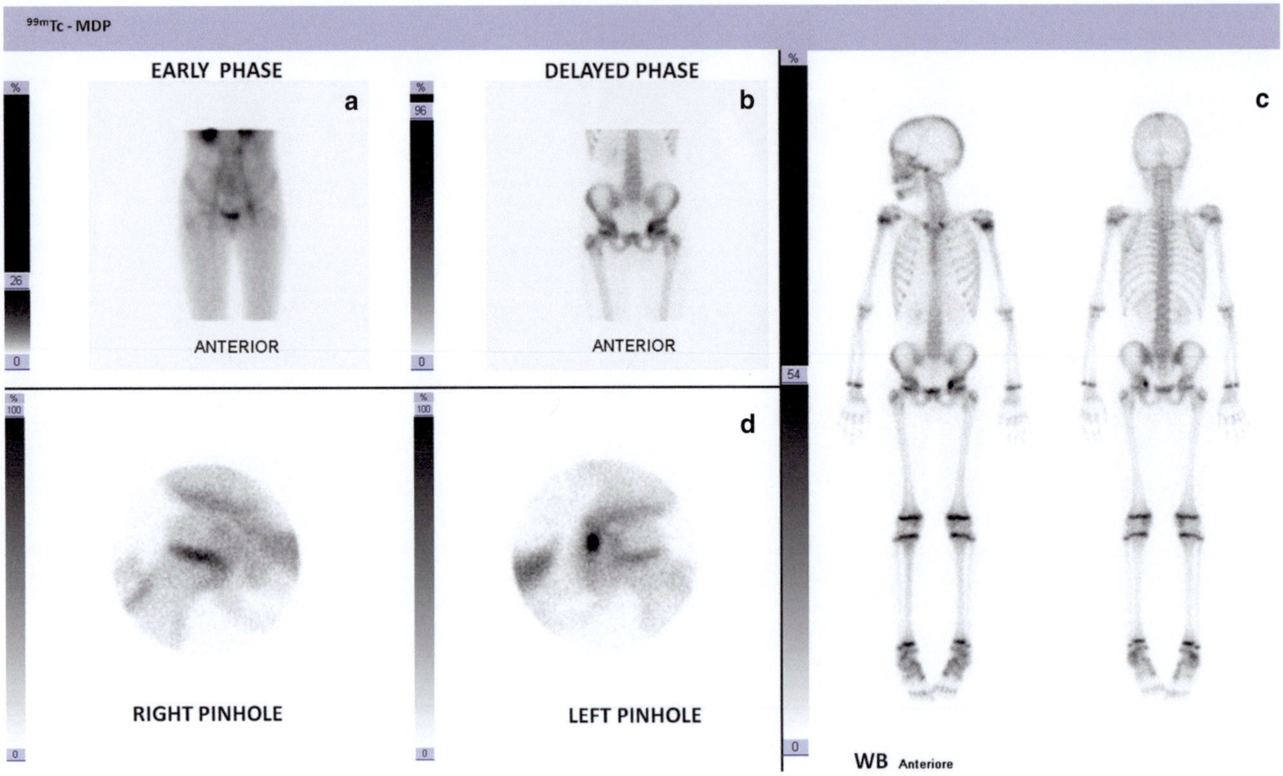

Fig. 26.17 (**a–d**) Bone scan (**a–d**) shows presence of a focal area of increased radiotracer uptake in left acetabulum. (**e–f**) MRI (**e**) and axial CT (**f**) images: intramedullary lesion of the left ischial bone with edema of spongy bone and of adjacent soft tissues. (**g**): RF thermal ablation procedure

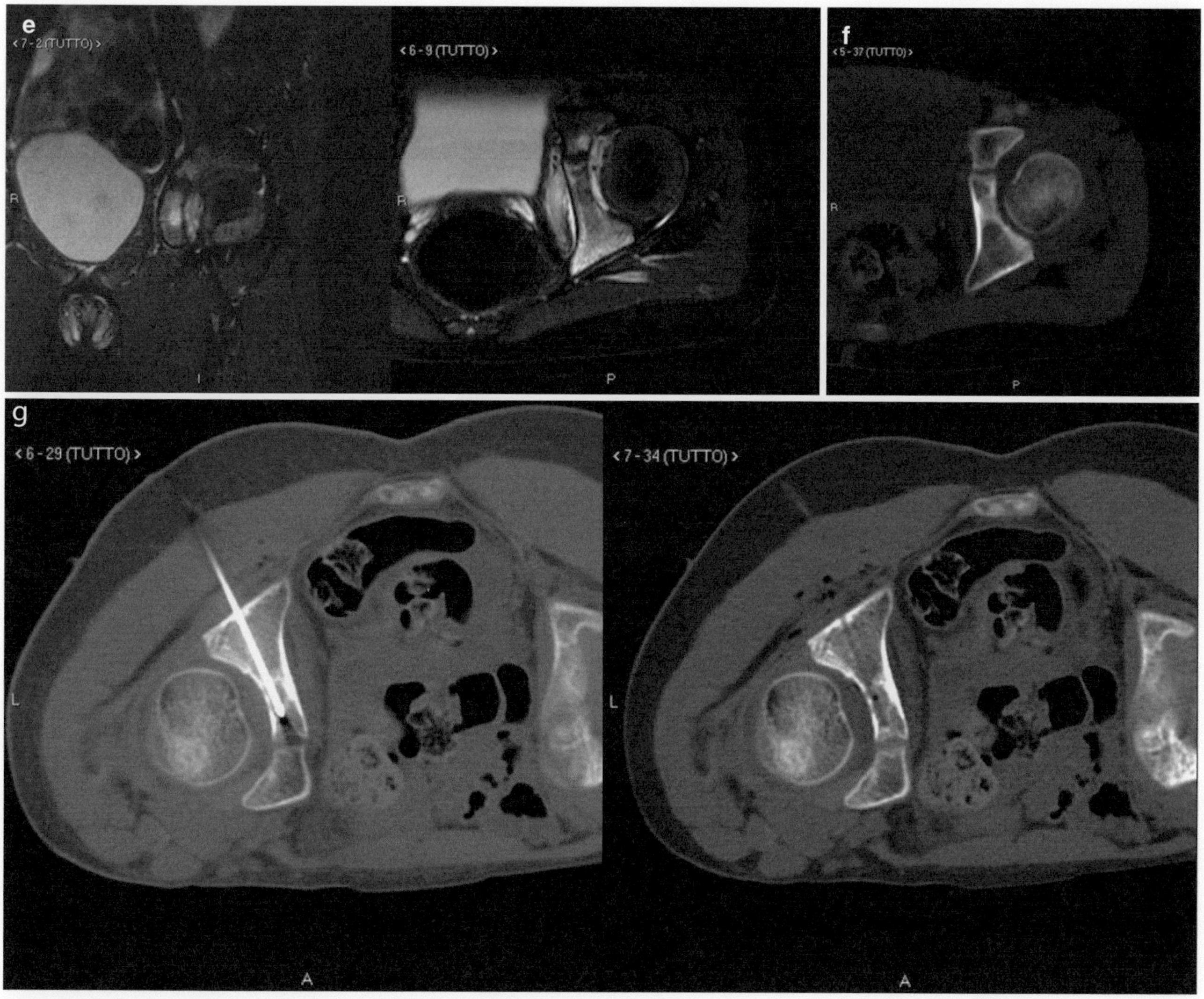

Fig. 26.17 (continued)

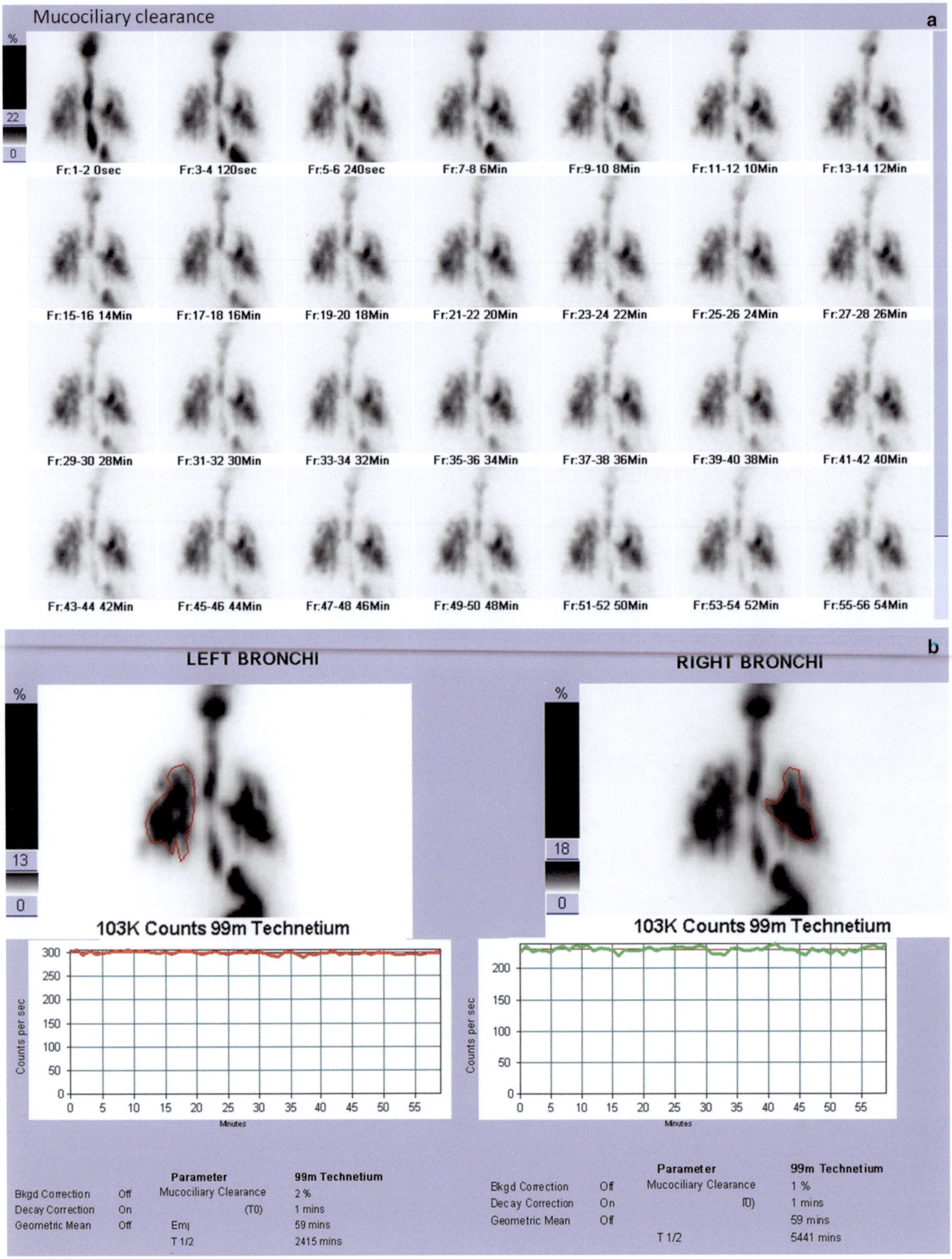

Fig. 26.18 (**a–d**) Bone scan (**a–d**) shows presence of a focal area of increased radiotracer uptake in left tibia. As in this case, rarely babies are able to define the exact site of bone pain. (**e–f**) Axial CT (**e**) images intramedullary lesion of the left tibia with thin sclerotic rim; RF thermal ablation procedure (**f**)

26.19 Other Localization of Osteoid Osteoma (Fig. 26.19)

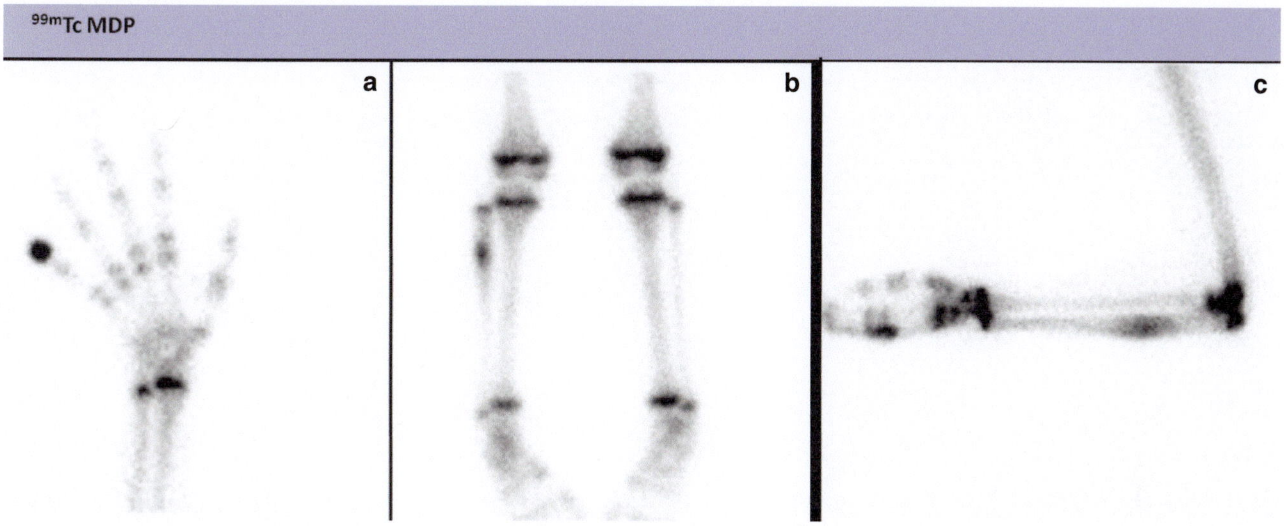

Fig. 26.19 (**a**–**c**) Bone scan shows presence of a focal area of increased radiotracer uptake in distal phalanx of fifth finger of right hand (**a**), right fibula (**b**), and right ulna (**c**), respectively

27 Bronchopneumology

Milena Pizzoferro, Maria Felicia Villani, Laura Menchini, and Maria Carmen Garganese

27.1 Introduction

Perfusion lung scan is usually performed in order to verify the presence of anomalies of the blood flow in the lungs, as in the case of pulmonary thromboembolism, although the gold standard for this pathology is now computed tomography. In patients with pulmonary embolism exist, in fact, at the level of the areas affected by the event embolism, blood perfusion deficits which are not associated by changes in ventilation.

The perfusion lung scan can also be performed in case of breathing disease such as COPD or in pneumonia, as analysis of lung function pre- and post-lobectomy, with or without the ventilation study.

Furthermore, in children, lung perfusion scan is often used during follow-up of congenital disease after or before surgery for assessing lung function.

Ventilation lung scan studies include measurements of ventilation, mucus, and cough clearance. Clearance measurements have been used to assess therapeutic response in conditions such as cystic fibrosis.

27.2 Study Technique and Interpretation: Lung Perfusion Scan

Lung perfusion scan is a simple study performed by acquisition planar images. No fasting is required. In children, four images in anterior, posterior, left posterior oblique, and right posterior oblique are enough. In case of study during post-surgery follow-up administration both in the upper limb and in inferior limb must be considered. The administered activity of radiotracer (99mTc-MAA) is adjusted to the patient's weight, according to EANM dosage card and to the national regulations.

In children, we must remember that the dose administered is the result of the reduction of activity, like in other procedures, and of the correct dilution of MAA according to the child's weight.

27.3 Study Technique and Interpretation: Lung Ventilation Scan

Ventilation lung scan is performed by acquisition planar images. No fasting is required. In children, four images in anterior, posterior, left posterior oblique, and right posterior oblique are enough in case of using 99mTc-DTPA.

Ventilation lung scan using 99mTc-colloids for measuring mucociliary clearance is acquired subsequently to a radioaerosol, in dynamic modality (60 min study, 60 s per frame).

Immediately following the radioaerosol inhalation, the patients must rinse their mouth by gargling, when the child is able. Then, the patient is placed in the supine position, and a gamma camera detector is posteriorly positioned for acquiring lung radioactivity.

M. Pizzoferro (✉) • M.F. Villani
Nuclear Medicine Unit, Imaging Department – "Bambino Gesù" Children Hospital, Rome, Italy
e-mail: milena.pizzoferro@opbg.net

L. Menchini
Imaging Department, "Bambino Gesù" Children Hospital, Rome, Italy

M.C. Garganese
Diagnostic Imaging Department of Nuclear Medicine, IRCCS Bambino Gesù Paediatric Hospital, Rome, Italy

© Springer International Publishing Switzerland 2017
M.C. Garganese, G.F.L. D'Errico (eds.), *Conventional Nuclear Medicine in Pediatrics*, DOI 10.1007/978-3-319-43181-9_27

27.4 Teaching Cases

27.4.1 Case 27.1: Lung Perfusion Scan – Normal Pattern

A 10-year-old boy affected by ALS treated by immunosuppressant therapy. Radiological investigations were performed for dyspnea and fatigue, showing negative results. D-dimer level was mildly increased, and lung perfusion scintigraphy was requested in suspicion of pulmonary embolism (Fig. 27.1).

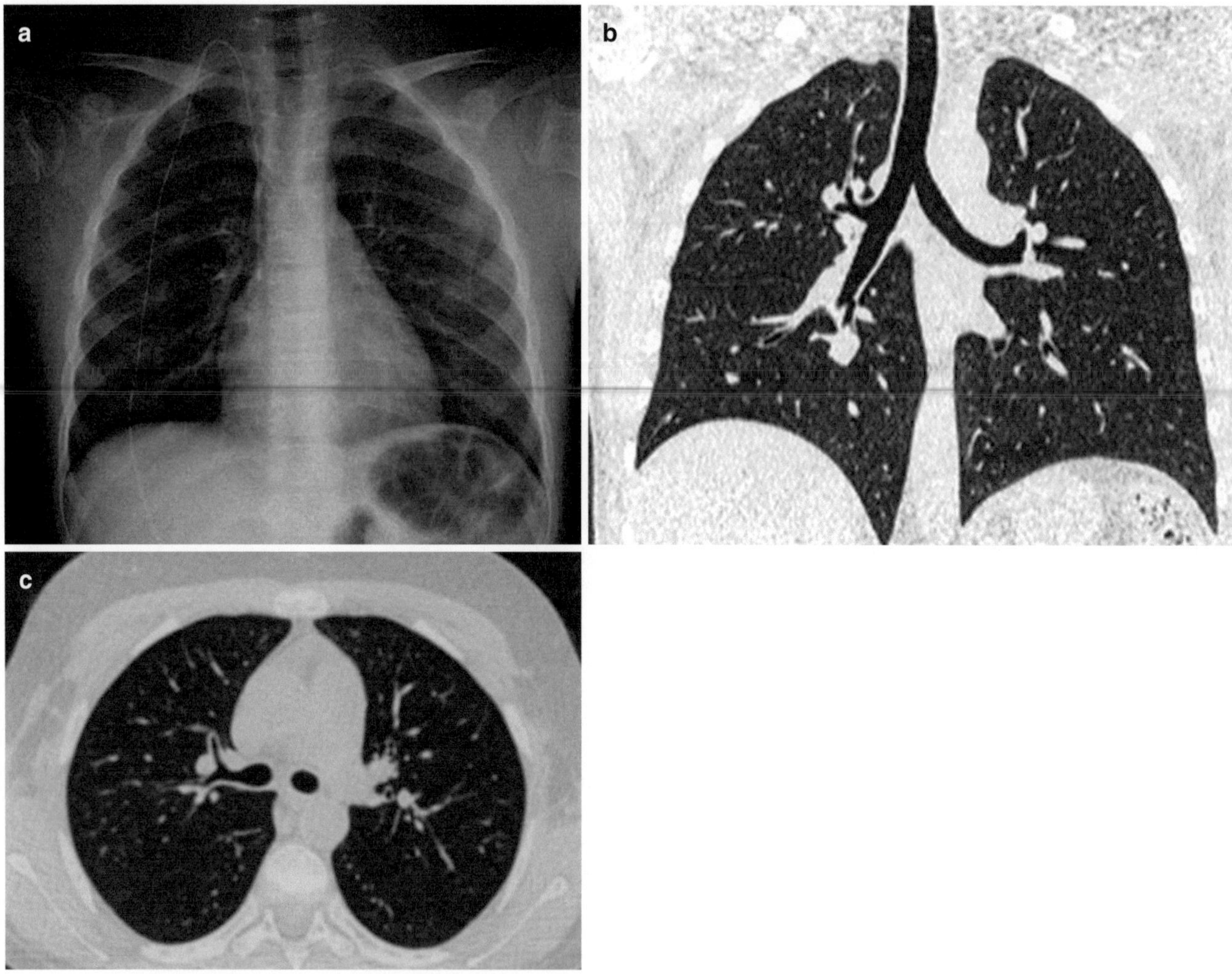

Fig. 27.1 (**a–c**) Chest X-ray (**a**) and coronal (**b**) and axial (**c**) CT scan of the chest show normal findings, the absence of parenchymal or pleural abnormalities, regular airway. (**d–e**) Lung perfusion scan: normal tracer uptake and normal distribution are evident in both lungs showing symmetrical function. Lung perfusion scan ruled out pulmonary embolism

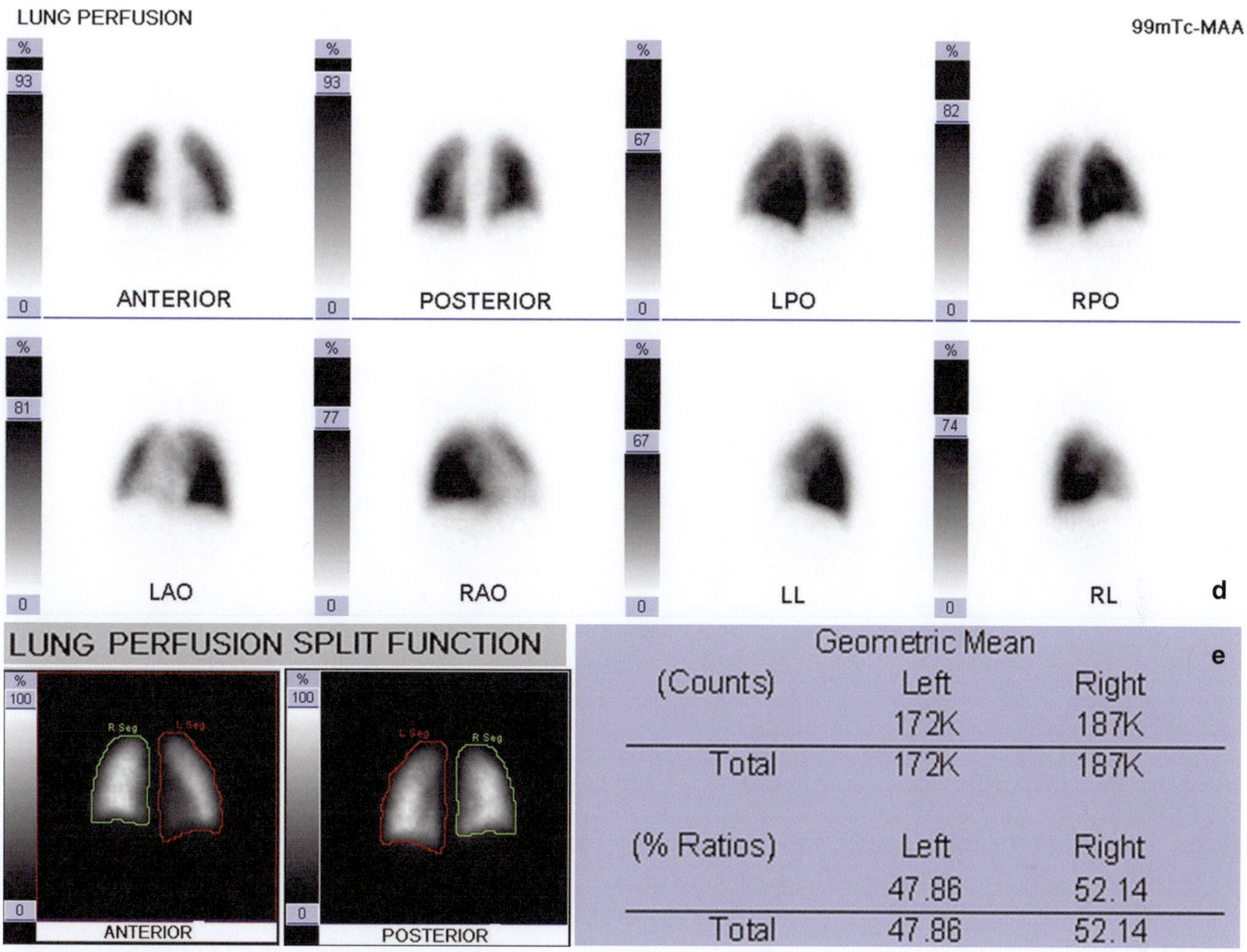

Geometric Mean (Counts)	Left	Right
	172K	187K
Total	172K	187K
(% Ratios)	Left	Right
	47.86	52.14
Total	47.86	52.14

Fig. 27.1 (continued)

27.4.2 Case 27.2: Lung Perfusion and Ventilation Scan – Normal Pattern in Newborn

A 9-month-old infant presenting persistent wheezing since the first month of life, treated by asthma therapy and leukotriene. Negative sweat test on two occasions. At 9 months of life, a worsening dyspnea and bronchospasm episode occurred, and chest X-ray showed atelectatic areas with air trapping and bilateral consolidations, especially in the right hemithorax.

A further examination of the chest by CT angiography showed tracheal bronchus (upper right of lobar bronchus that departs from the right edge of the lower third of the trachea), while lung perfusion and ventilation scan revealed a normal perfusion and pulmonary ventilation. Respiratory physiotherapy has been associated to medical therapy, and the child no longer had episodes of bronchospasm (Fig. 27.2).

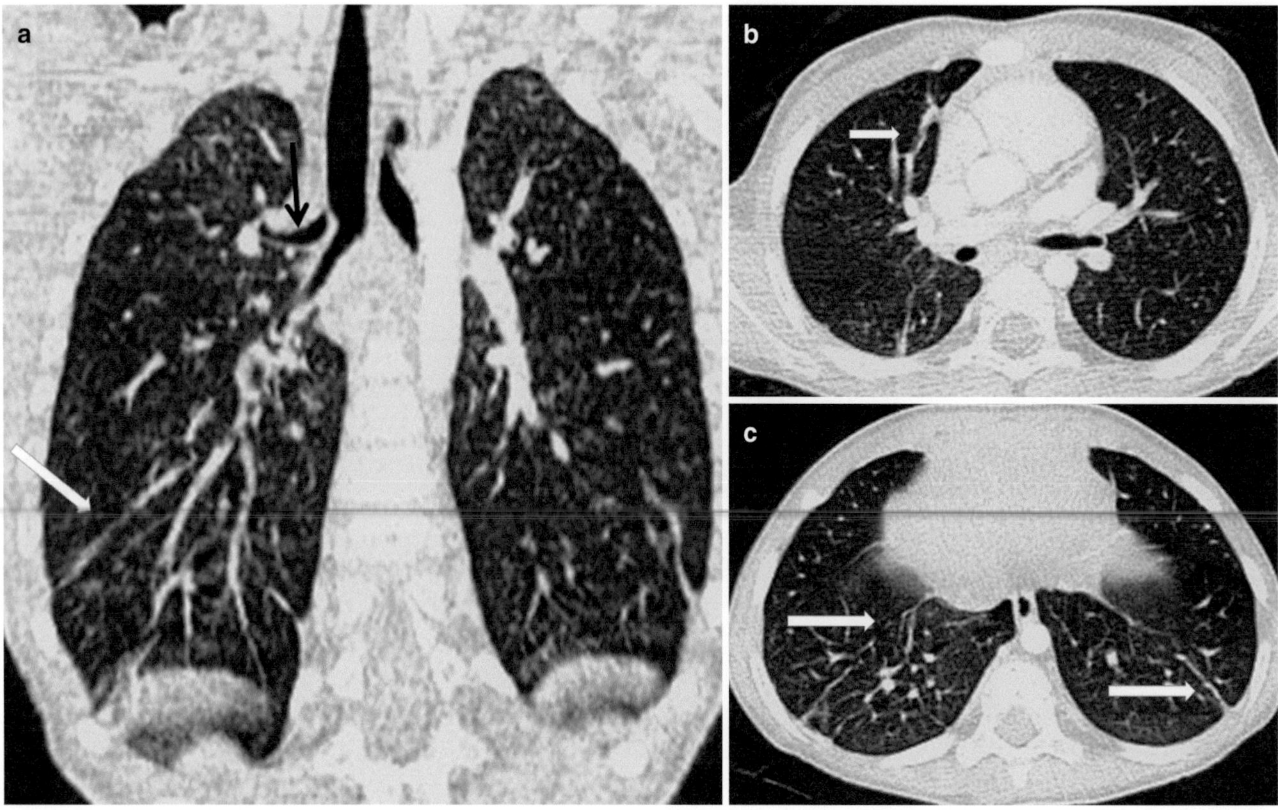

Fig. 27.2 (**a**–**c**) CT coronal view image of the chest (**a**) shows upper right lobar bronchus that departs from the right edge of the lower third of the trachea (tracheal bronchus, *black arrow*). Images in the axial view (**b**) show streaks of laminar atelectasis in the front segments of the right upper lobe and apical right lower lobe and in the basal segments of the posterior side of the lower lobes bilaterally (**c**) (*white arrows*). (**d**–**e**) In the first row (**d**) is evident normal tracer uptake and distribution in both lungs showing symmetrical function. In newborn, lung perfusion scan can be performed by only four views (anterior, posterior, left, and right posterior obliques). In the second row (**e**), normal distribution of ventilation is evident in both lungs. To perform a good ventilation scan in newborn, an adequate mask is necessary eliciting infant crying

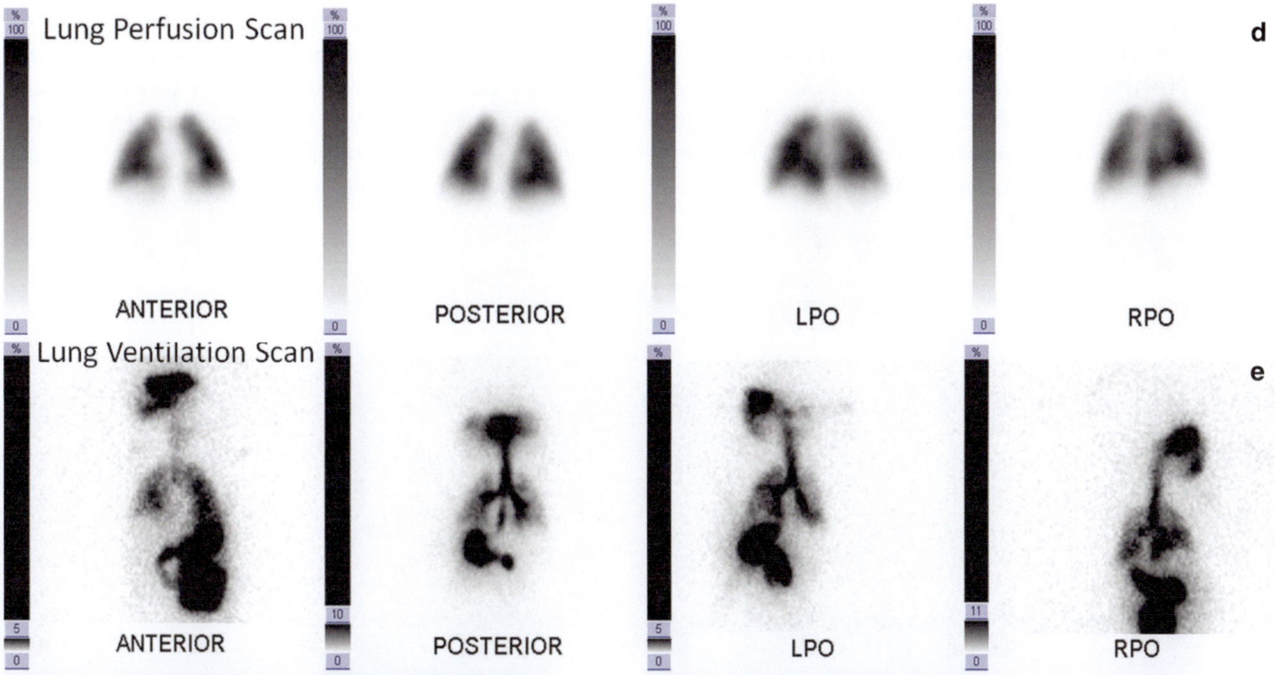

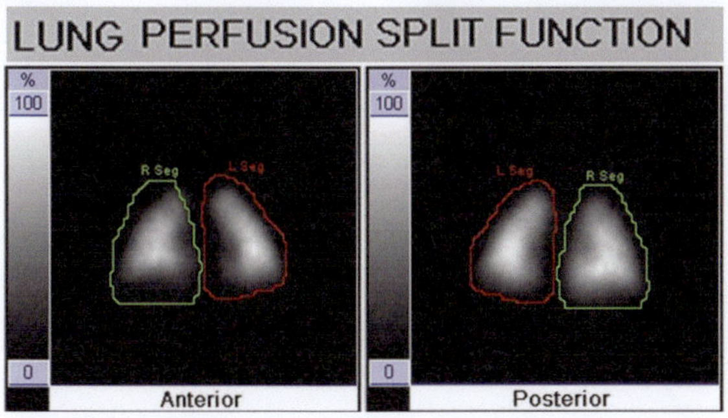

Geometric Mean		
(Counts)	Left	Right
	196K	208K
Total	196K	208K
(% Ratios)	Left	Right
	48.43	51.57
Total	48.43	51.57

Fig. 27.2 (continued)

27.4.3 Case 27.3: Lung Ventilation Scan for Measuring Mucociliary Clearance – Normal Pattern

An 8-year-old girl with frequent respiratory infection. Chest X-ray was performed showing diffuse thickening of the bronchial walls bilaterally with lung hyperinflation in the absence of areas of parenchymal consolidation. In suspicion of primary ciliary dyskinesia, the child underwent nasal brushing which showed a nondiagnostic result. Lung ventilation scan for measuring mucociliary clearance was required, revealing a normal pattern (Fig. 27.3).

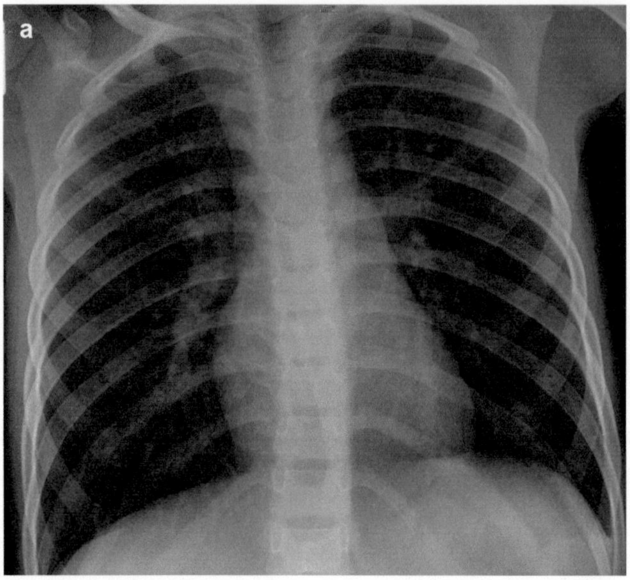

Fig. 27.3 (**a**). Chest X-ray image in the front projection shows diffuse thickening of the bronchial walls bilaterally with lung hyperinflation in the absence of areas of parenchymal consolidation. (**b**) By visual assessment, normal distribution of ventilation is evident in both lungs. Regular particle deposition and normal mucociliary clearance from the respiratory airways are evident in both lungs. (**c**) A/T curve analysis shows a bilaterally rapid decrement of activity, resulting in normal quantitative clearance parameters in 60 min

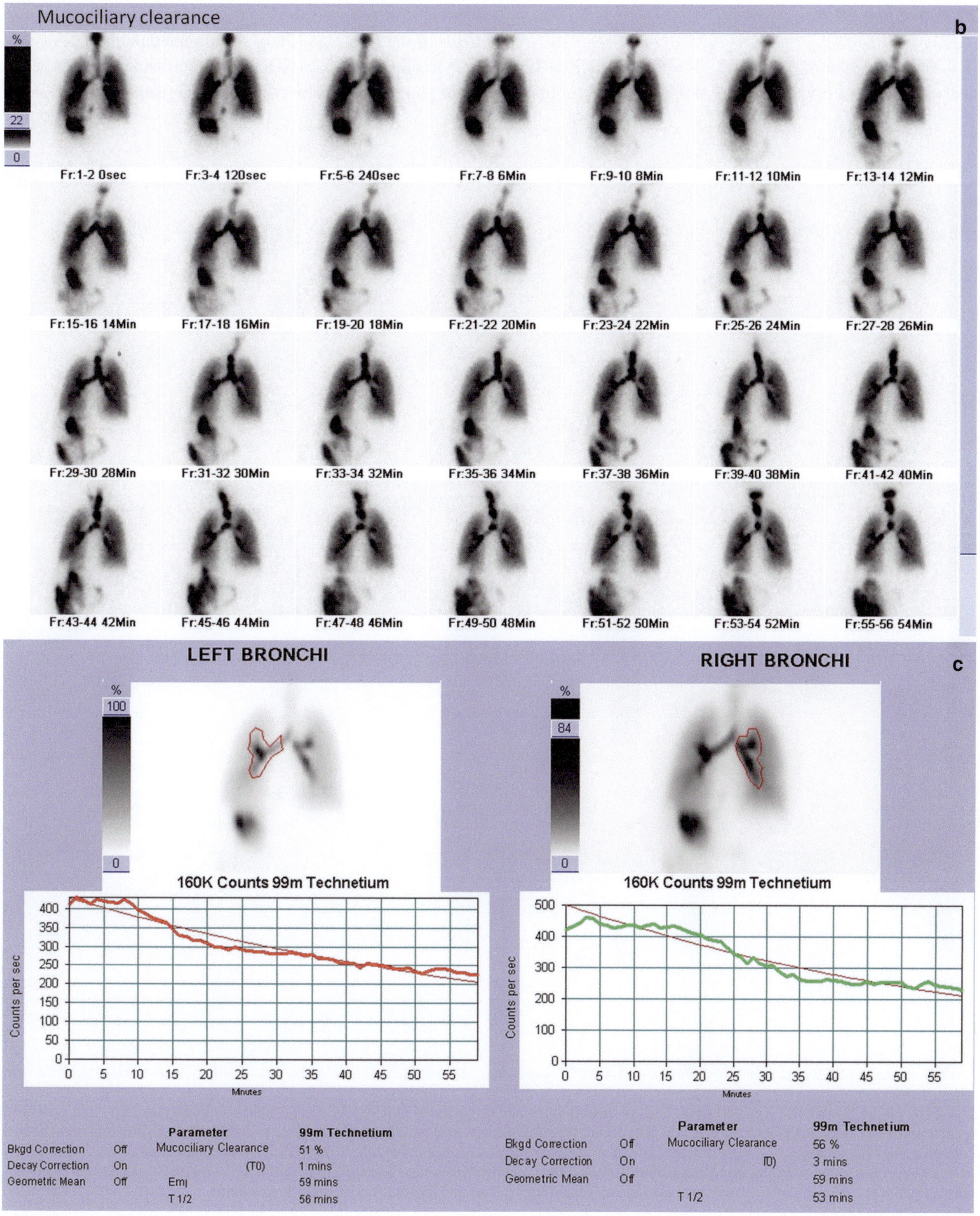

Fig. 27.3 (continued)

27.4.4 Case 27.4

A 9-day-old newborn with good general condition at birth and cardiorespiratory parameters within normal limits. At clinical skill, reduced air penetration at the upper and middle fields of the right lung. He was submitted to chest X-rays at first and then to chest-CT and lung perfusion scan for better definition of the clinical condition and therapy (Fig. 27.4).

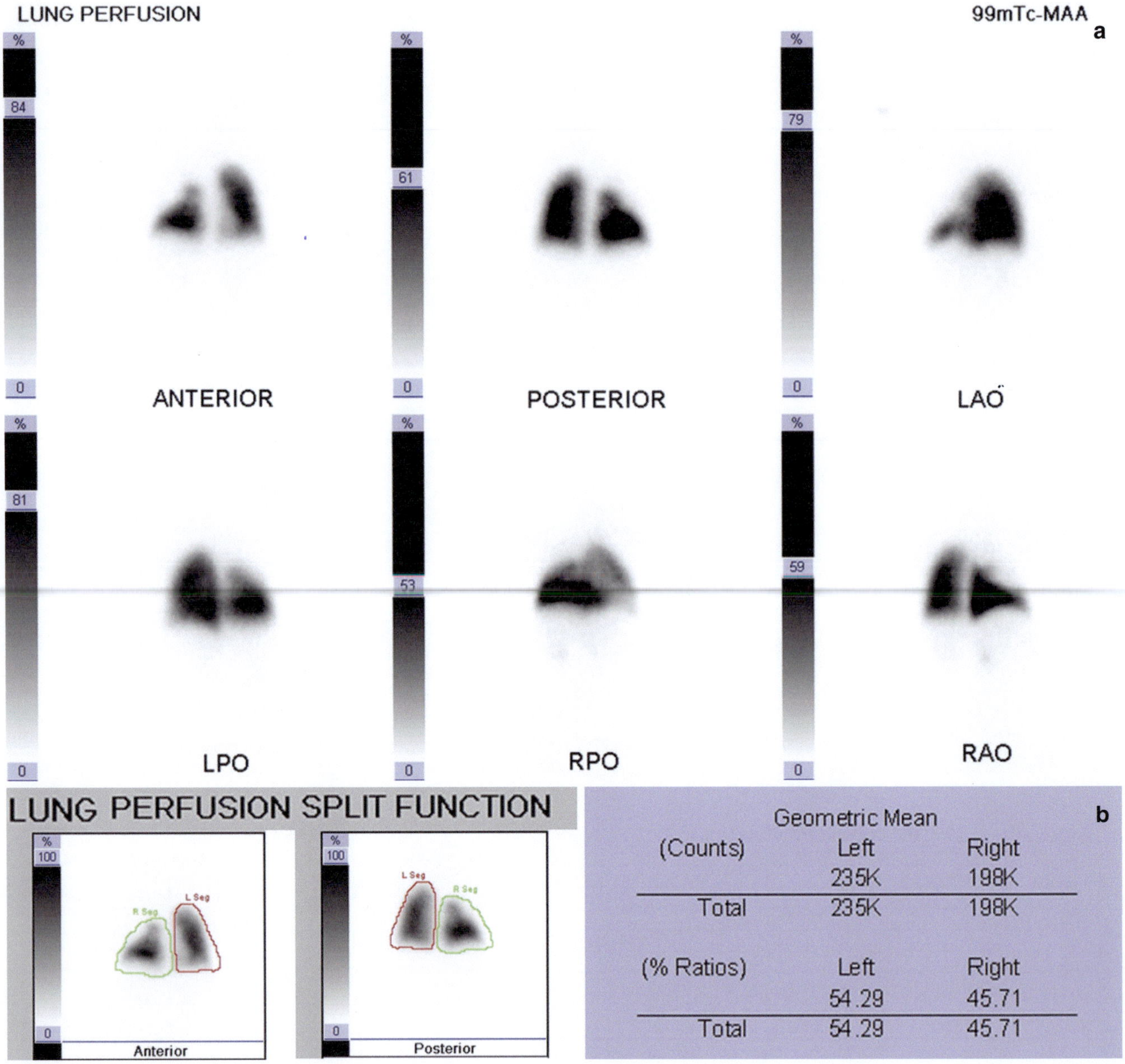

Fig. 27.4 (**a**–**b**) Normal left lung perfusion. Hypoperfusion in the entire upper and middle lobe of the right lung due to the hypoventilation and regular perfusion of the lower lobe. (**c**–**f**). Chest X-ray front view (**c**) displays extensive hyperlucency area in right lung, with thinning bronchovascular markings (*black arrow*) and bundling in lung plot in the baseline paracardiac (*asterisk*). Chest CT image in coronal reconstructions MIP (**d**) shows right upper lobar bronchus originating from the distal third of the trachea (tracheal bronchus, *white arrow*) with hypodense parenchymal lung's right upper lobe due to air trapping, as also shown in the TC axial (**e**) and coronal (**f**) images (*black arrows*)

27.4.5 Case 27.5: Lung Embolism in Child Affected by LES

A 13-year-old girl affected by SLE treated by steroid therapy. She had more hospitalizations for pain in the anterior chest region during which echocardiographic controls resulted normal. After several months, she showed left lower limb thrombophlebitis associated with dyspnea. During hospitalization, in suspicion of lung thromboembolism, a chest CT and a lung perfusion scan were performed. He was hospitalized once again in spite of crisis characterized by "air hunger," which was interpreted as panic attack (chest CT and lung scan performed during hospitalization were normal) (Fig. 27.5).

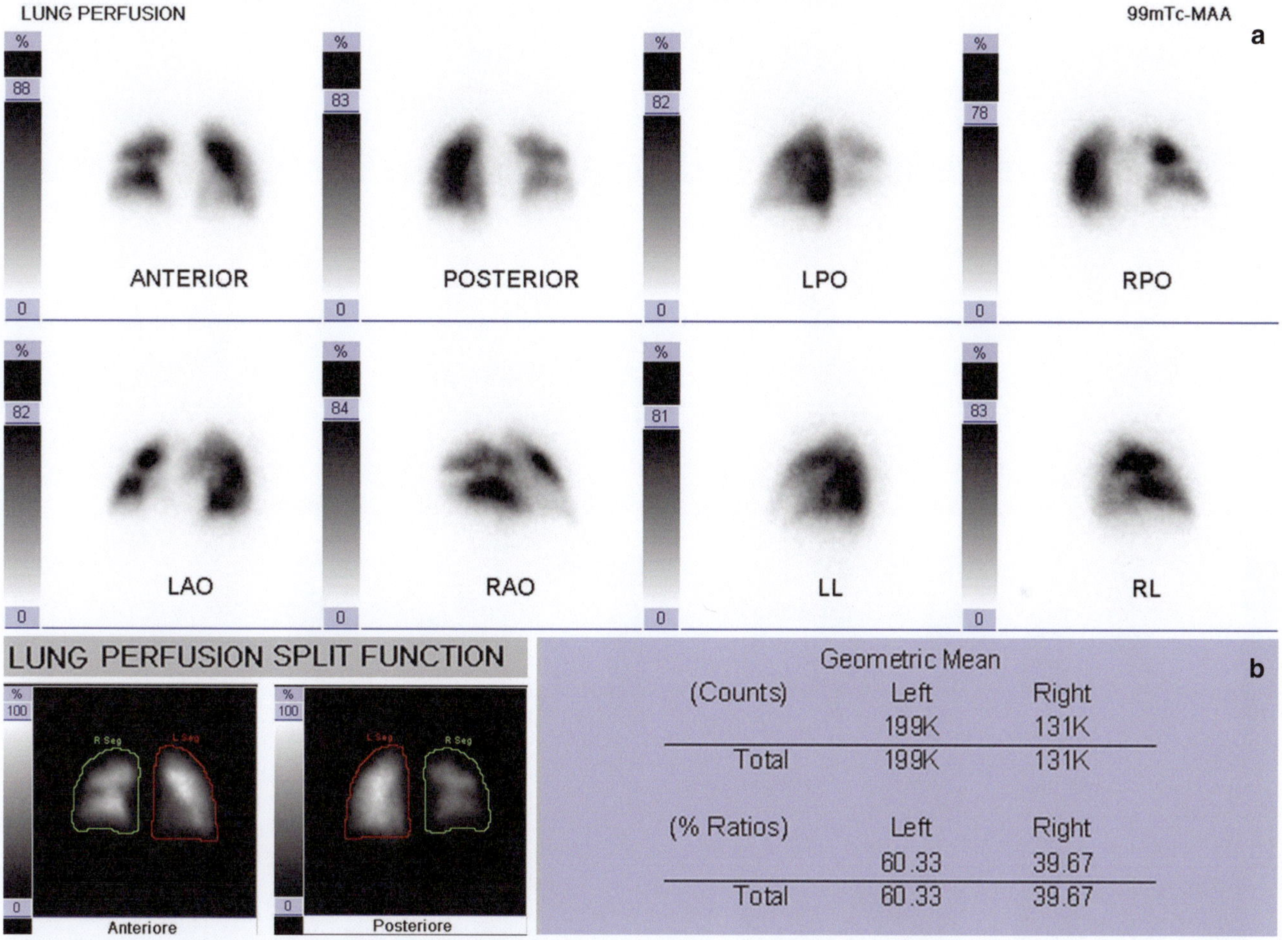

Fig. 27.5 (**a–b**) Lung perfusion scan in the course of embolism showed multiple segmental perfusion deficits in the right lung which showed associated reduced uptake (quantitative perfusion parameters: 60.33 % left lung and 39.67 % right lung). Axial CT image (**c**) shows mild heterogeneity of parenchymal density with relative hyperdensity of the apical segment of the right lower lobe and striations dense front subppleuriche left fibro-disventilative (*black arrow*). Axial CT image (**d**) of distant examination performed 2 years later shows substantial stability of the finds with increasingly evident parenchymal inhomogeneous density and areas of low attenuation lobular air trapping. (**e–f**) Lung perfusion scan showed increased perfusion in the right lung with better distribution of the radiopharmaceutical uptake (quantitative perfusion parameters: 55.70 % left lung and 44.30 % right lung)

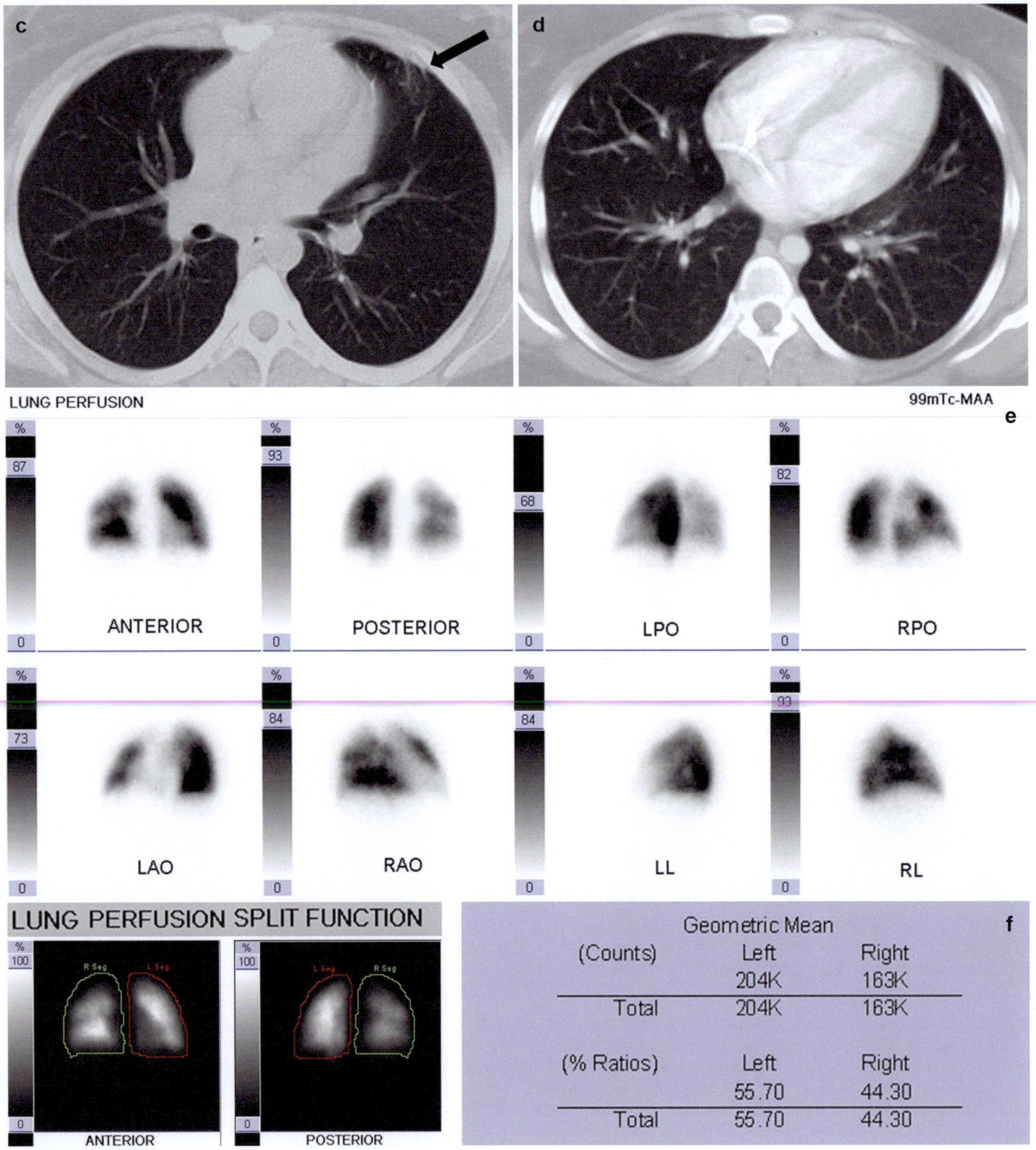

Fig. 27.5 (continued)

27.4.6 Case 27.6: A Case of Acute Respiratory Distress at Birth

A 4-month-old baby who presented at birth cyanosis and cardiorespiratory depression. She needed resuscitation in the delivery room. The diagnosis was hyaline membrane disease, tracheomalacia, and suspected ciliary dyskinesia. At 2 months of life, she was intubated for 45 days. O_2 therapy has been required.

The child reached our hospital for a sudden worsening of respiratory symptoms, and she was admitted into the intensive care unit. The patient was placed on mechanical ventilation. During mechanical ventilation, sudden worsening of the general conditions with dyspnea and cyanosis crisis occurred. She was submitted to chest CT and lung perfusion scan for clarifying the pulmonary framework (Fig. 27.6).

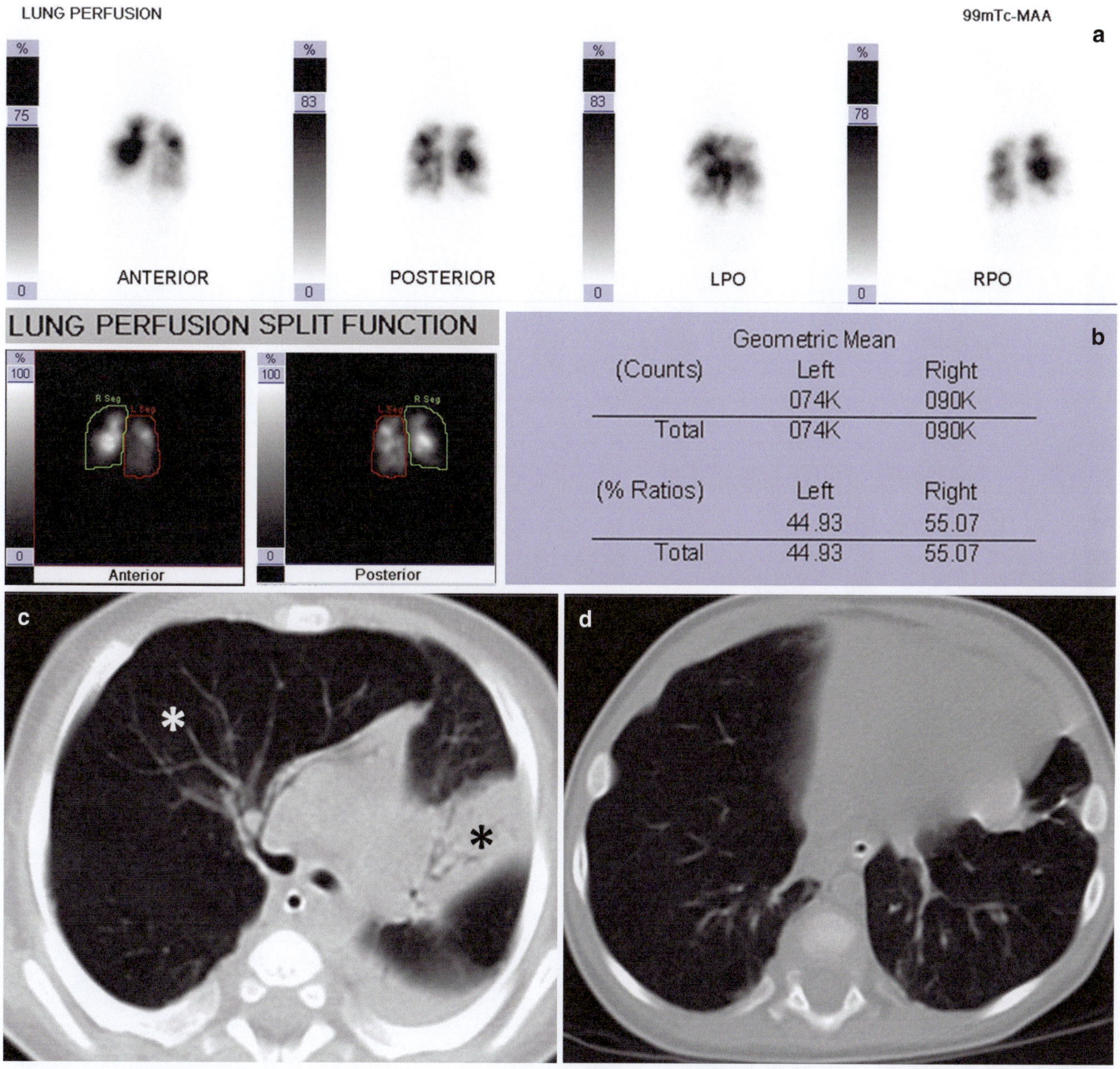

Fig. 27.6 (**a–b**) Lung perfusion scan shows multiple areas of reduced or absent perfusion signal in both lungs, extending from the apical zones to the pulmonary bases; only few defects had segmental shape. The quantitative evaluation of pulmonary perfusion is symmetrical as follows: Left lung = 44.9 %; Right lung Dx = 55.1 %. This scintigraphic framework suggested widespread disease of lung parenchyma as often observed in patients with bronchodysplasia. (**c–d**) Axial CT images of the thorax (**c**) show widespread disease of lung parenchyma with hypodiafania due to hyperinflation of the middle lobe (white asterisk), partial atelectasis of left upper lobe (*black asterisk*), and of right upper lobe with mediastinal shift to the left, and evidence of striae, consolidations, and parenchymal distortion (**d**)

27.4.7 Case 27.7: A Child with Recurrent Bronchitis

A 4-year-old child comes to our hospital for further investigations in spite of many episodes of recurrent bronchitis and evidence of bronchiectasis and suspicion of panlobular unilateral emphysema to a previous radiological examination. The sweat test resulted negative, and screening for hepatitis and HIV were negative. Mantoux test resulted negative. In clinical history, her parents reported many episodes of foreign bodies inhalation and a case in which it was necessary removing foreign body with bronchoscope (Fig. 27.7).

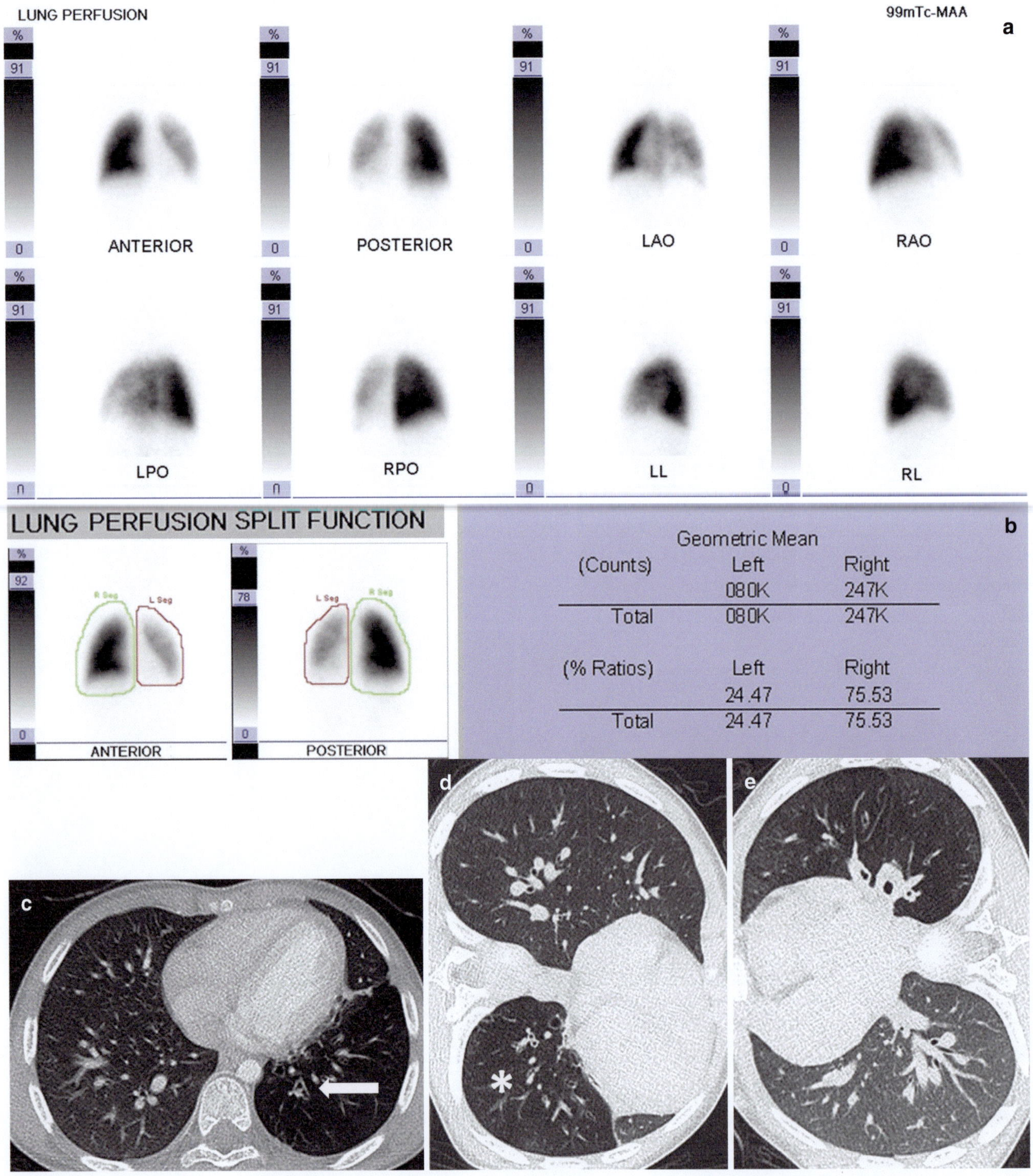

Fig. 27.7 (**a–b**) Lung perfusion scan shows no abnormalities in the right lung. In the left lung, parenchymal uptake is widely reduced, and no segmental defects are documented. The rate of uptake, calculated based on the geometric mean, is asymmetric and equal to 24.5 % for the left lung and to 75.5 % for the right lung. (**c–e**) Axial CT image in supine (**c**) shows cylindrical bronchiectasis basal pyramid of the lower left lobe (*white arrow*) with diffuse hypodense parenchyma adjacent to the left as for air trapping, as demonstrated in acquisitions in the left decubitus (**d**) and right (**e**), where the portion sloping seat air trapping (*left side*, *white asterisk*) does not change the density and remains markedly hypodense

27.4.8 Case 27.8: A Child with Lobar Emphysema

A 2-year-old child arrived to our hospital with allergic rhinitis treated with antipyretics. The day before admission, because of coughing, aerosol was administered. In the next days, he became pale and lost appetite. At clinical skill, he had chest gasps with medium bubbles in the bases of both lungs and hyperemic pharynx. He underwent chest X-ray and lung perfusion scan in the suspicion of lobar emphysema (Fig. 27.8).

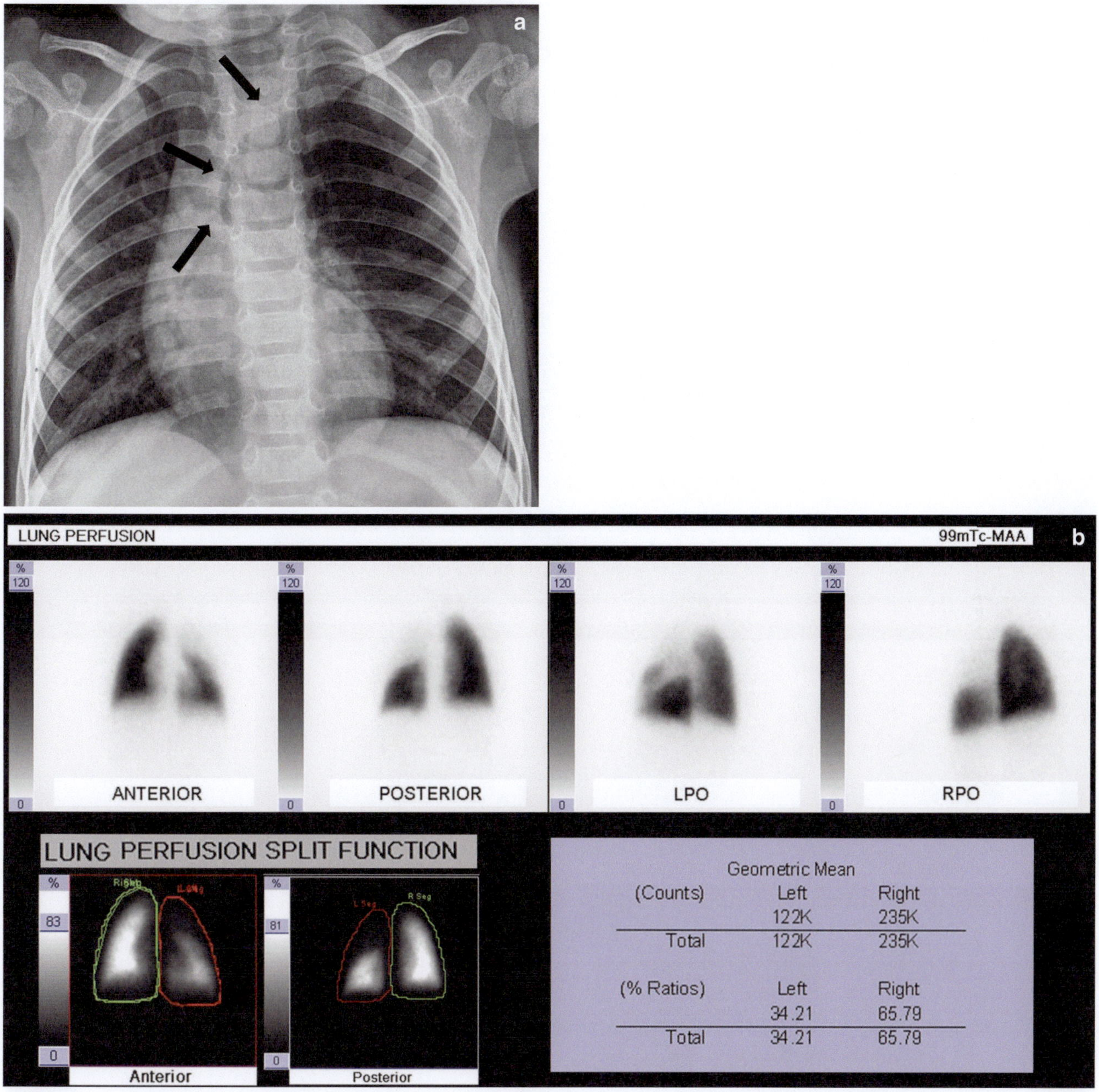

Fig. 27.8 (**a**) Chest X-rays in the front projection documents extended hyperlucency in the upper left lobe, with herniation trans-mediastinum in the contralateral left lung, due to hyperinflation (lobar emphysema, *black arrows*). (**b–c**) Lung perfusion scan shows deficit of the perfusion in the upper lobe of the left lung, confirming lobar emphysema. Normal perfusion of the right lung. Rate of uptake: 34 % for the left lung and 66 % for the right lung

27.4.9 Case 27.9: A Child with Diaphragmatic Hernia

A 1-month-old infant reached our hospital with a previous diagnosis of lung hypoplasia and a rib malformation associated. He was in good clinical condition (Fig. 27.9).

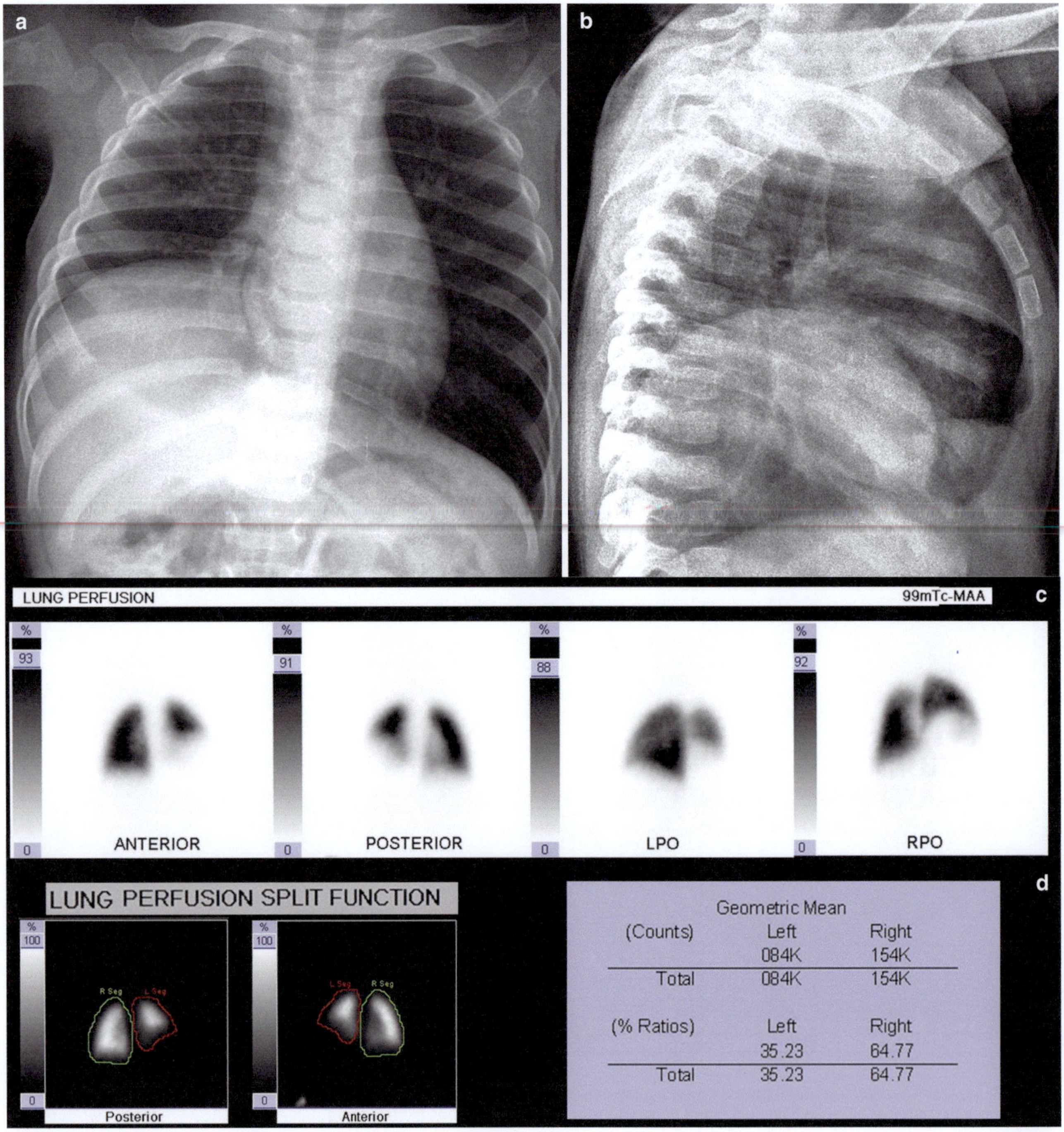

Fig. 27.9 (**a–b**) Chest X-ray in AP and LL projections shows volumetrical asymmetry of the lungs with lifting the right hemidiaphragm and ipsilateral lung hypoplasia. (**c–d**) Perfusion lung scan: left lung is normal; right lung is small, but shows normal uptake and intraparenchymal distribution of the radiocompound as in the scintigraphic framework of hypoplasia. The rate of uptake is asymmetric and equal to 35 % for the left lung and 65 % for the right lung, confirming the visual data

27.4.10 Case 27.10: A Case of Congenital Left Diaphragmatic Hernia Associated with PNX

A 2-month-old infant operated at birth for congenital left diaphragmatic hernia. In the immediate postoperative phase, evidence of left PNX that was drained by a pleurotomic probe. The infant was then submitted to additional surgery for local recurrence, gastropleuric fistula, and bronchial fistula.

The general conditions of the infant have gradually improved, but occasional episodes of vomiting occurred. New diagnostic examinations were performed to assess the chest conditions (Fig. 27.10).

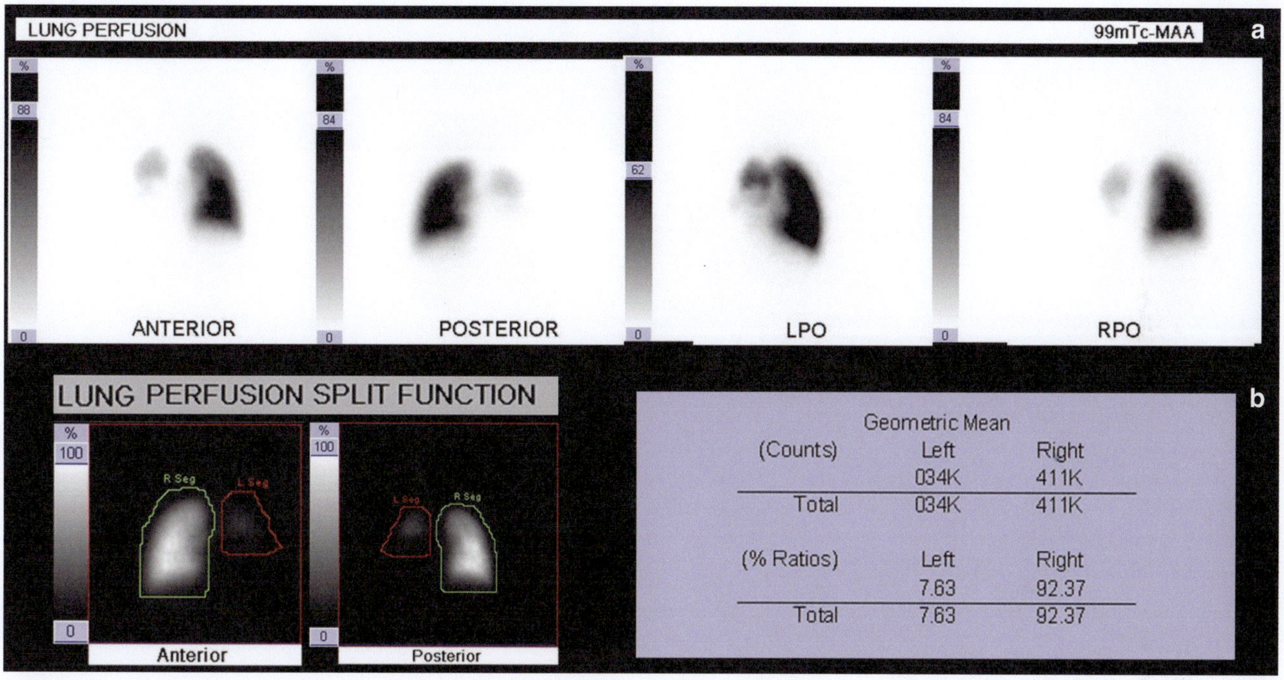

Fig. 27.10 (**a**, **b**) Lung perfusion scan shows severe hypoperfusion of left lung which appears significantly reduced in size. Right lung is normal. The rate of uptake is asymmetrical (Left lung : 8 %, right lung: 92 %). Coronal and axial view CT images show extended consolidation of the lung parenchyma in upper and lower left lobes with excavation areas in the context (*black arrows*) as for cavitary necrosis (**c**) and of hypodensity areas for colliquative necrosis phenomena (**d**, **e**, *black asterisks*).

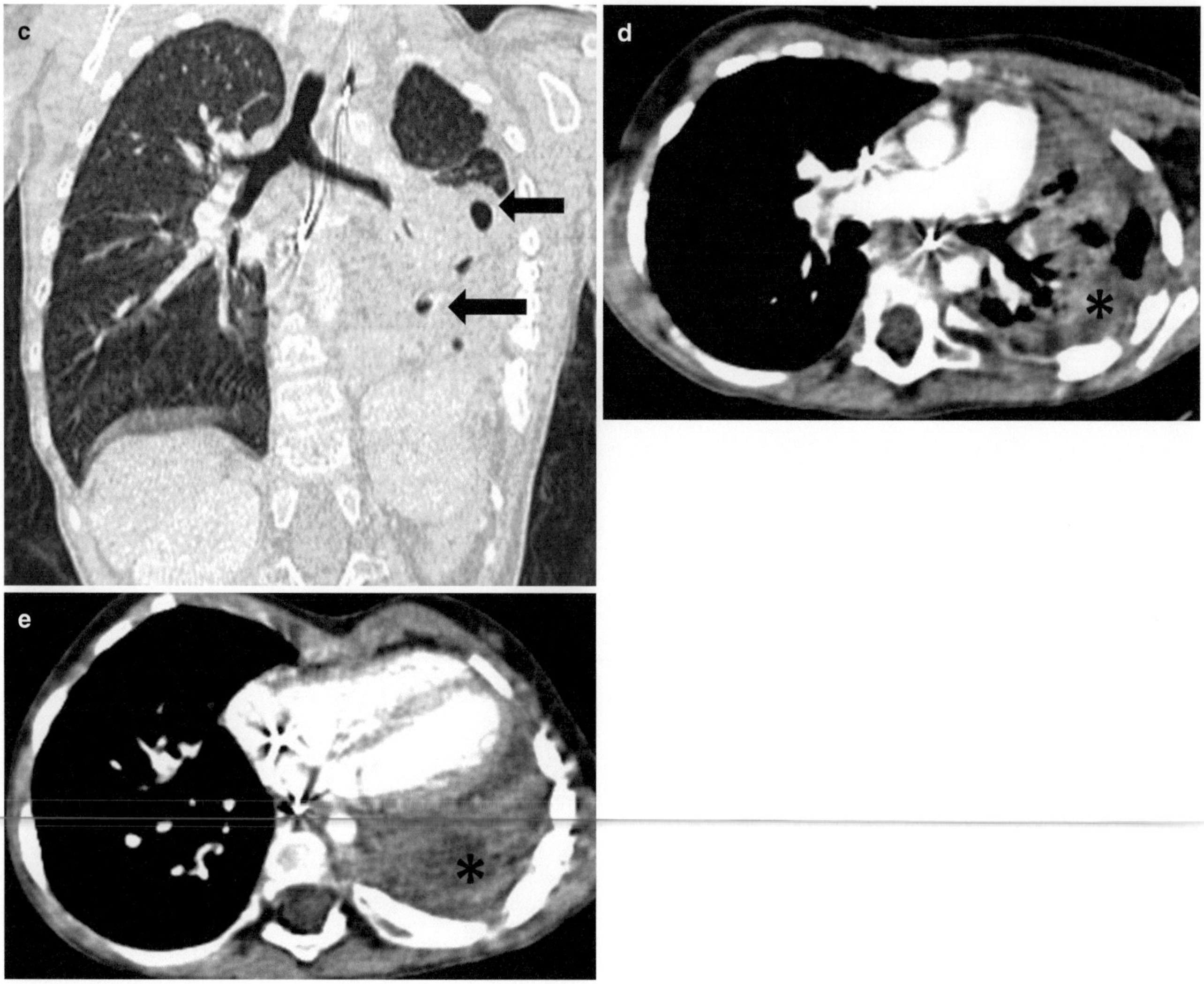

Fig. 27.10 (continued)

27.4.11 Cases 27.11 and 27.12: Pulmonary Deformations Secondary to Skeletal Abnormalities (Figs. 27.11 and 27.12)

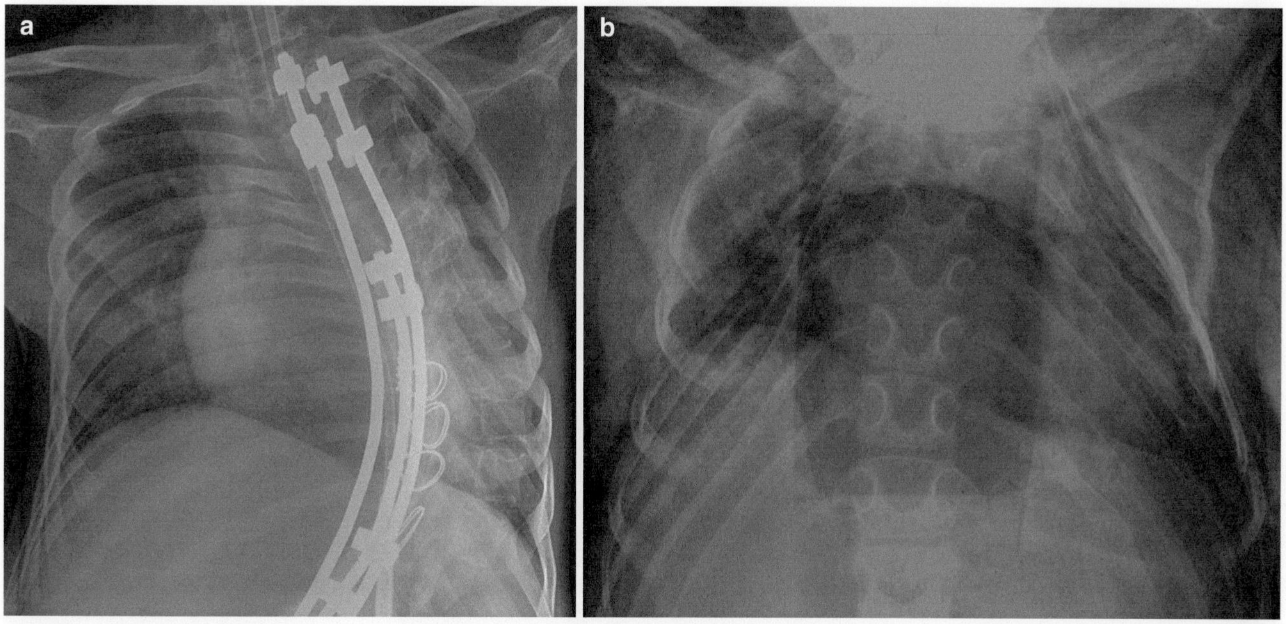

Figs. 27.11 and 27.12 (**a**) Front projection chest X-ray shows severe left-convex scoliosis of the thoracic spine associated with left lung hypoplasia. (**b**) Chest X-ray shows severe chest deformity with narrowing of the pulmonary space. (**c–f**) Lung perfusion scans show normal perfusion of both lungs but irregular pulmonary shape due to the skeletal abnormalities. In these cases, lung perfusion scan rules out functional lung impairment despite the severity of radiological framework

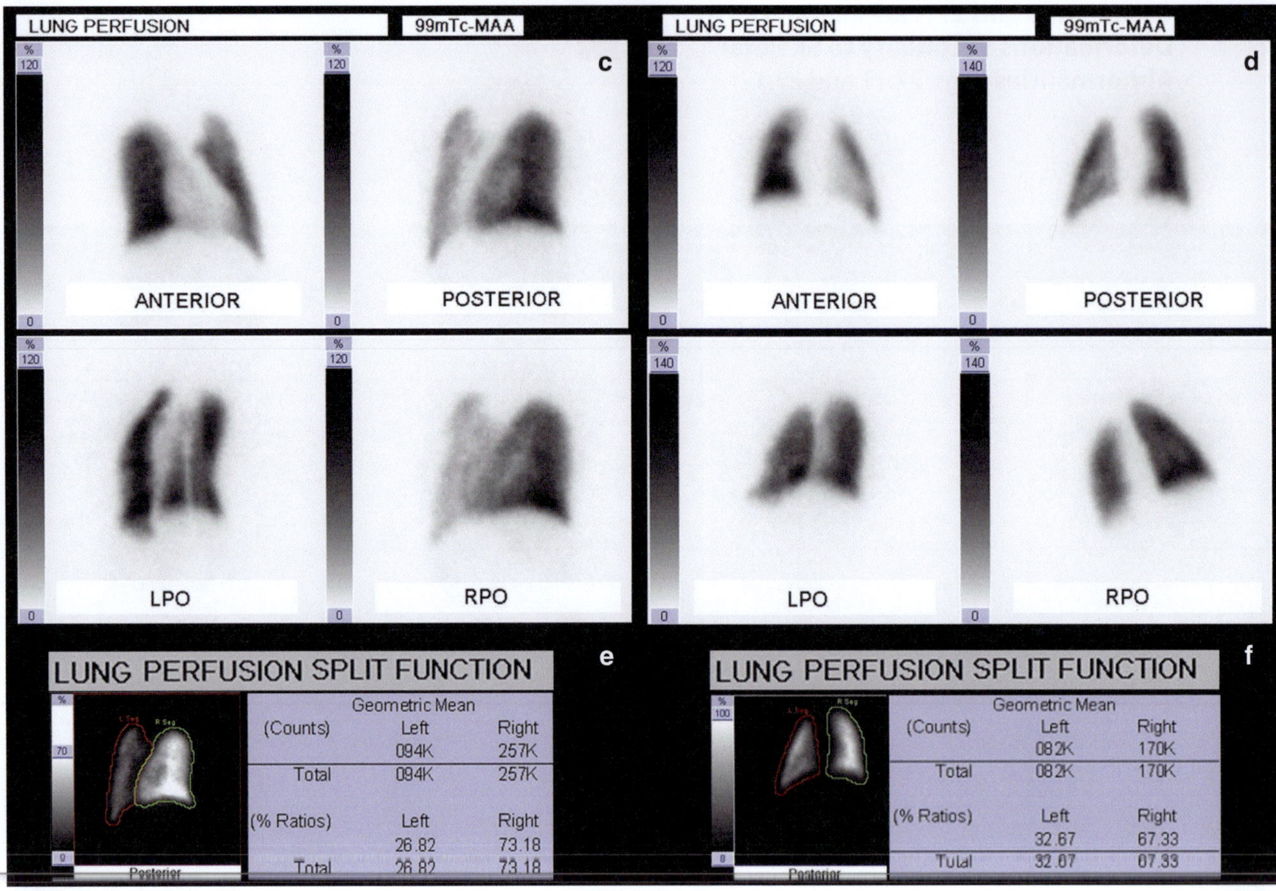

Figs. 27.11 and 27.12 (continued)

27.4.12 Case 27.13: A Child with Acute Dyspnea due to Angiomatosis

A 4-month-old infant. Several episodes of acute dyspnea, some of them with apnea and cyanosis. At clinical skill, reduced air penetration into left hemithorax and prolonged expiration (Fig. 27.13).

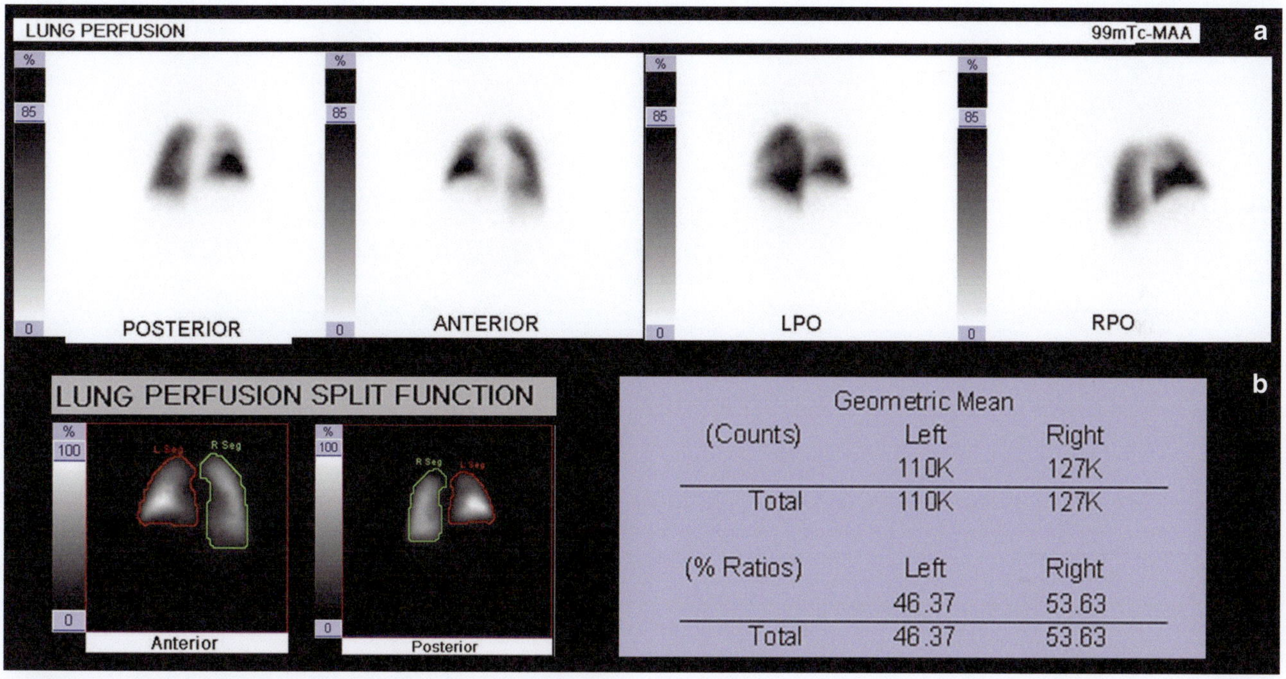

Fig. 27.13 (**a**-**b**) Lung perfusion scan shows small right lung with hypoperfusion in the upper lobe. Normal perfusion signal in left lung. Rate of uptake of perfusion: left lung=46 %; right lung =54 %. (**c**–**e**) Chest X-ray image (**c**) shows extended right hilar and ipsilateral upper lobar hypodiafania (*arrow*). Axial CT images (**d, e**) show areas of parenchymal consolidation and increased density ("ground glass") in the right lung with evidence of right hilar dense tissue that partially obliterates the lumen of the bronchus (**e**, *asterisk*)

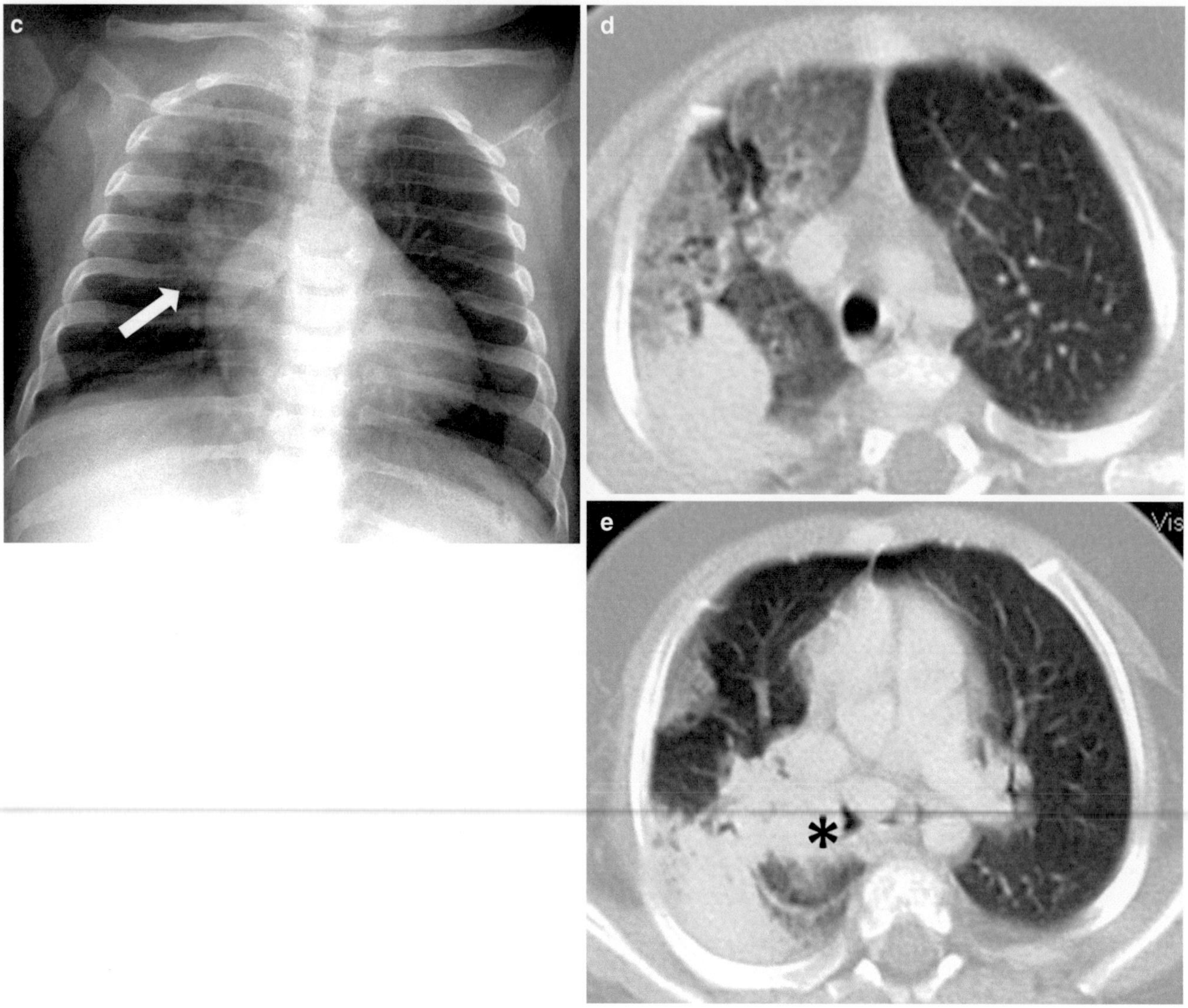

Fig. 27.13 (continued)

27.4.13 Case 27.14: A Girl with Cystic Fibrosis

A 16-year-old girl affected by cystic fibrosis with full expression of disease. Positive newborn screening test. Sweat test positive at birth: Cl 114 mmol/L. Chronic lung colonization by *Pseudomonas aeruginosa* and *Staphylococcus aureus*. Lung perfusion and ventilation scan were required in the diagnostic workup for lung transplantation (Fig. 27.14).

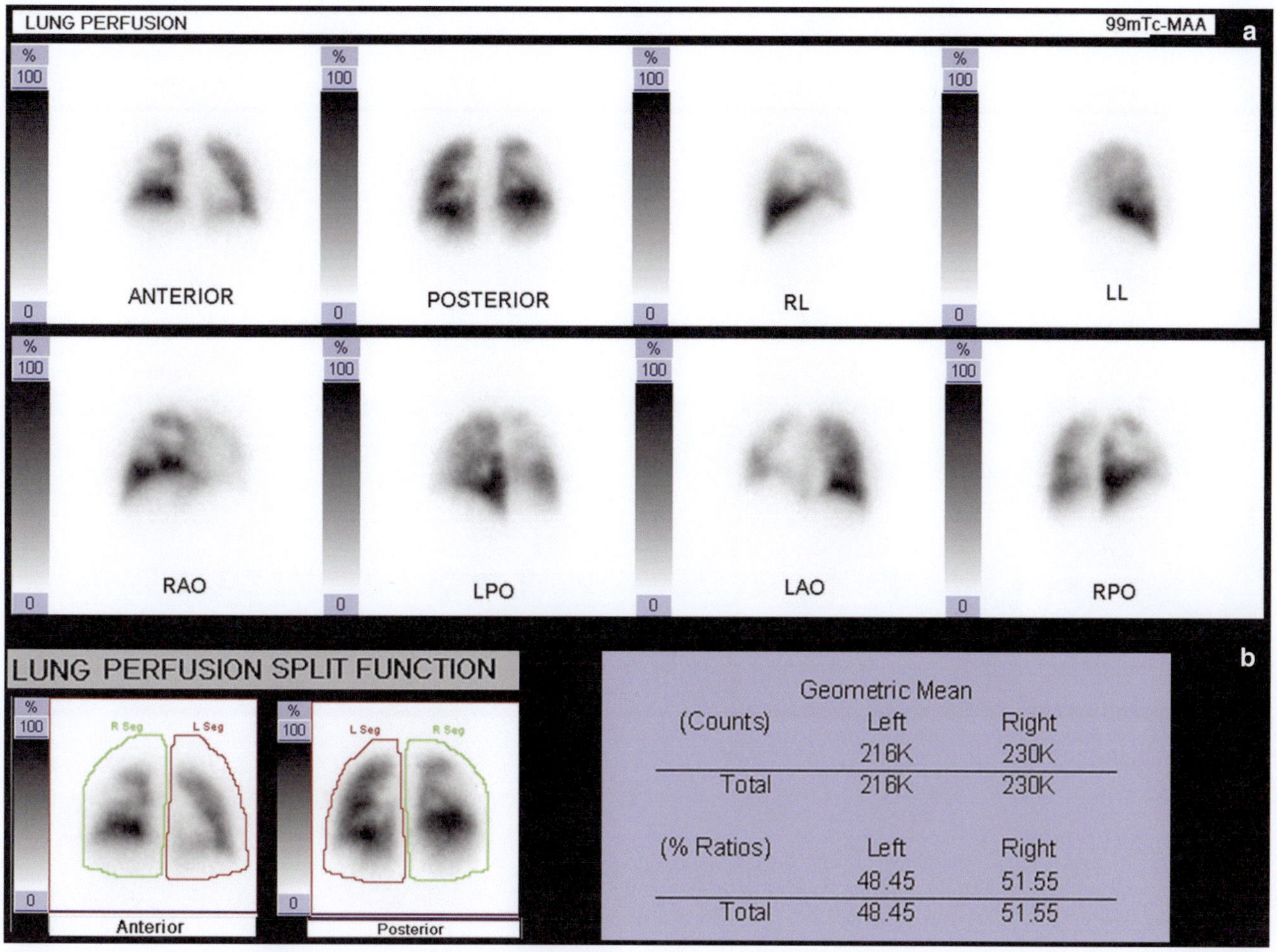

Fig. 27.14 (**a**–**d**). Lung perfusion and ventilation scan show multiple abnormalities of perfusion in both lungs. These altered perfusion areas correspond to which that are hypoventilated. In this case, the hypoperfusion is due to reduced ventilation. (**e**–**g**) Axial (**e**, **f**) and coronal (**g**) view CT images show bronchiectasis in the right upper lobe (**e**, *red arrows*), associated with CAP endobronchial inflammation and mucus of the distal airway (*white arrows*), and bronchiectasis at the basal pyramid of the left lower lobe (**f**, *red arrow*), associated with bronchial wall thickening in patients with cystic fibrosis

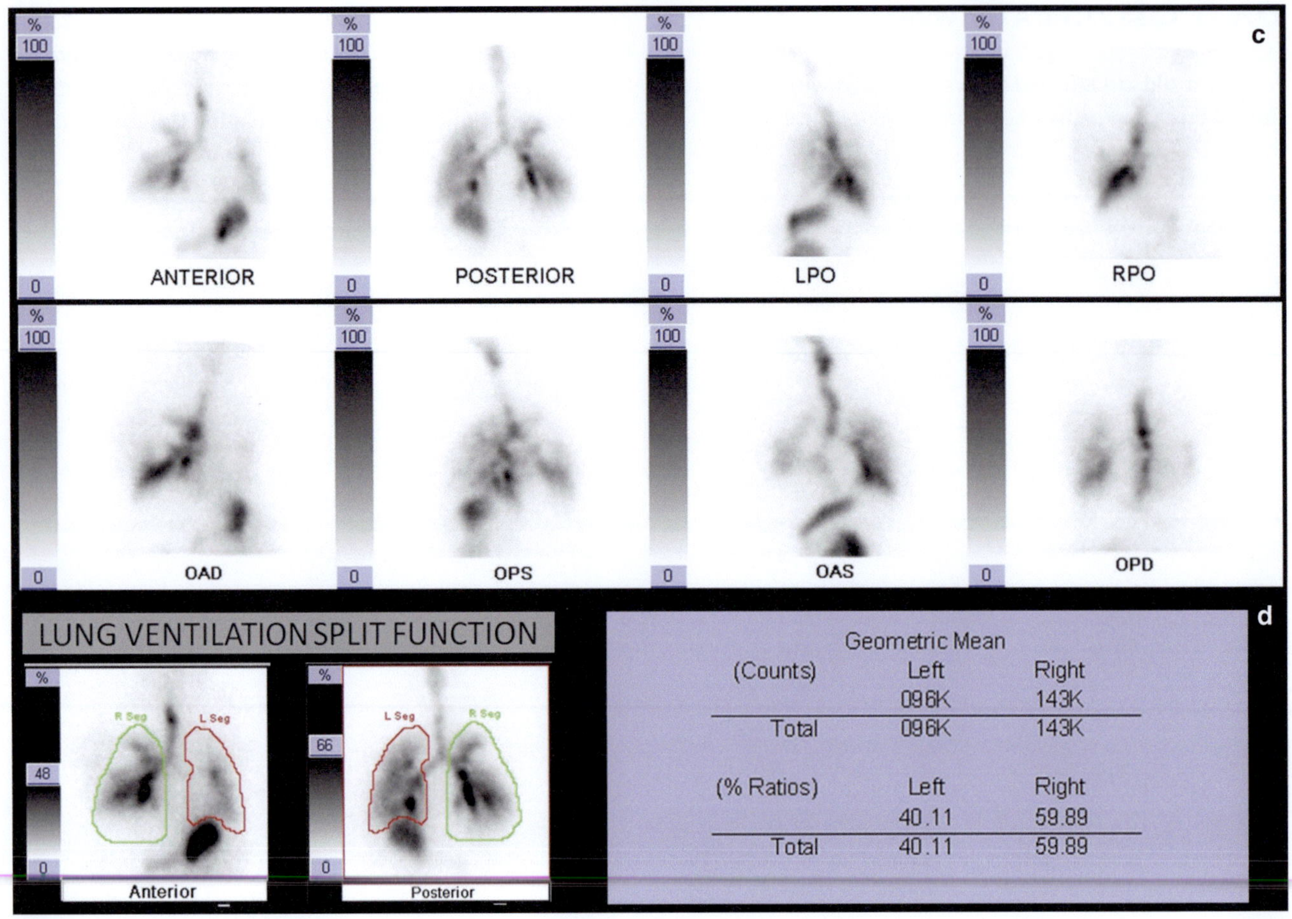

Fig. 27.14 (continued)

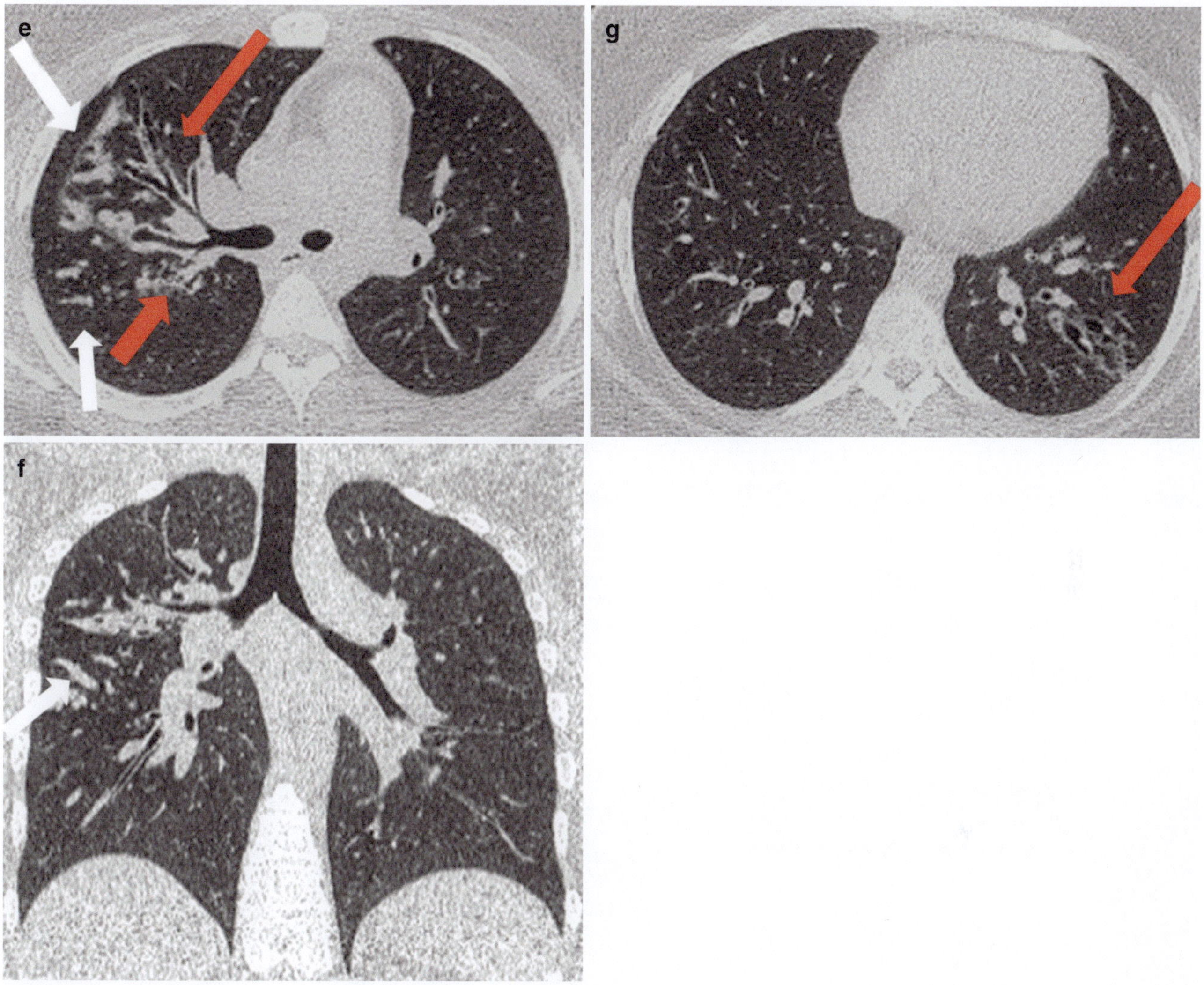

Fig. 27.14 (continued)

27.4.14 Case 27.15: Vascular and Pulmonary Malformation

A 14-year-old girl affected by ingravescent chronic respiratory failure treated by O_2 therapy (Fig. 27.15).

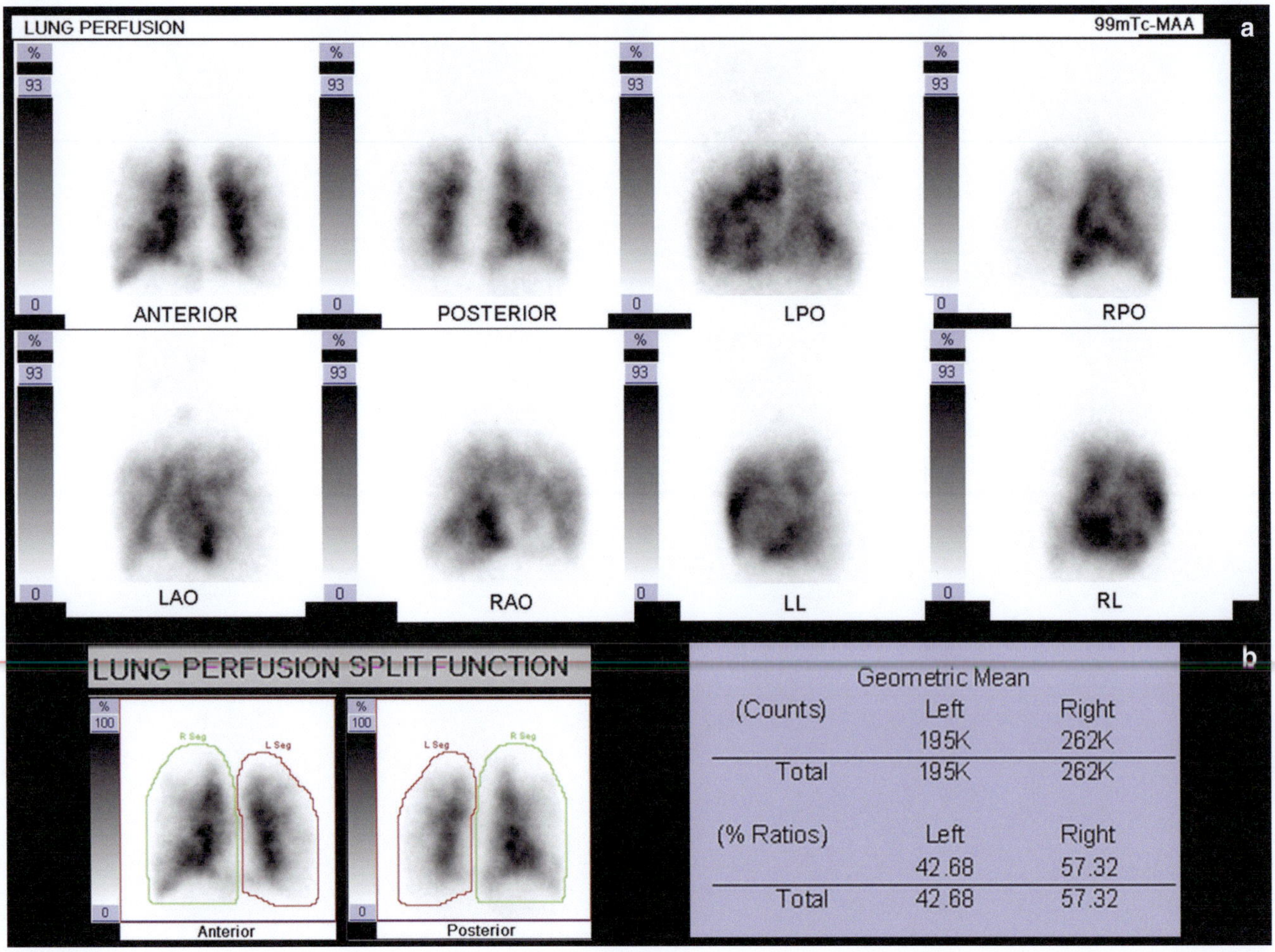

Fig. 27.15 (**a–b**) Lung perfusion scan shows multiple abnormalities of perfusion in both lungs, corresponding to multiple areas of subversion of the structure evident in the CT study. Left lung is slightly smaller than the contralateral. (**c–e**) Chest X-ray (**c**) and coronal (**d**) and axial (**e**) CT images show increased lung volumes, with extended area of hypodense parenchyma and paucity of the interstitial and vascular pattern secondary to hyperexpansion; such alterations are due to panlobularis emphysema

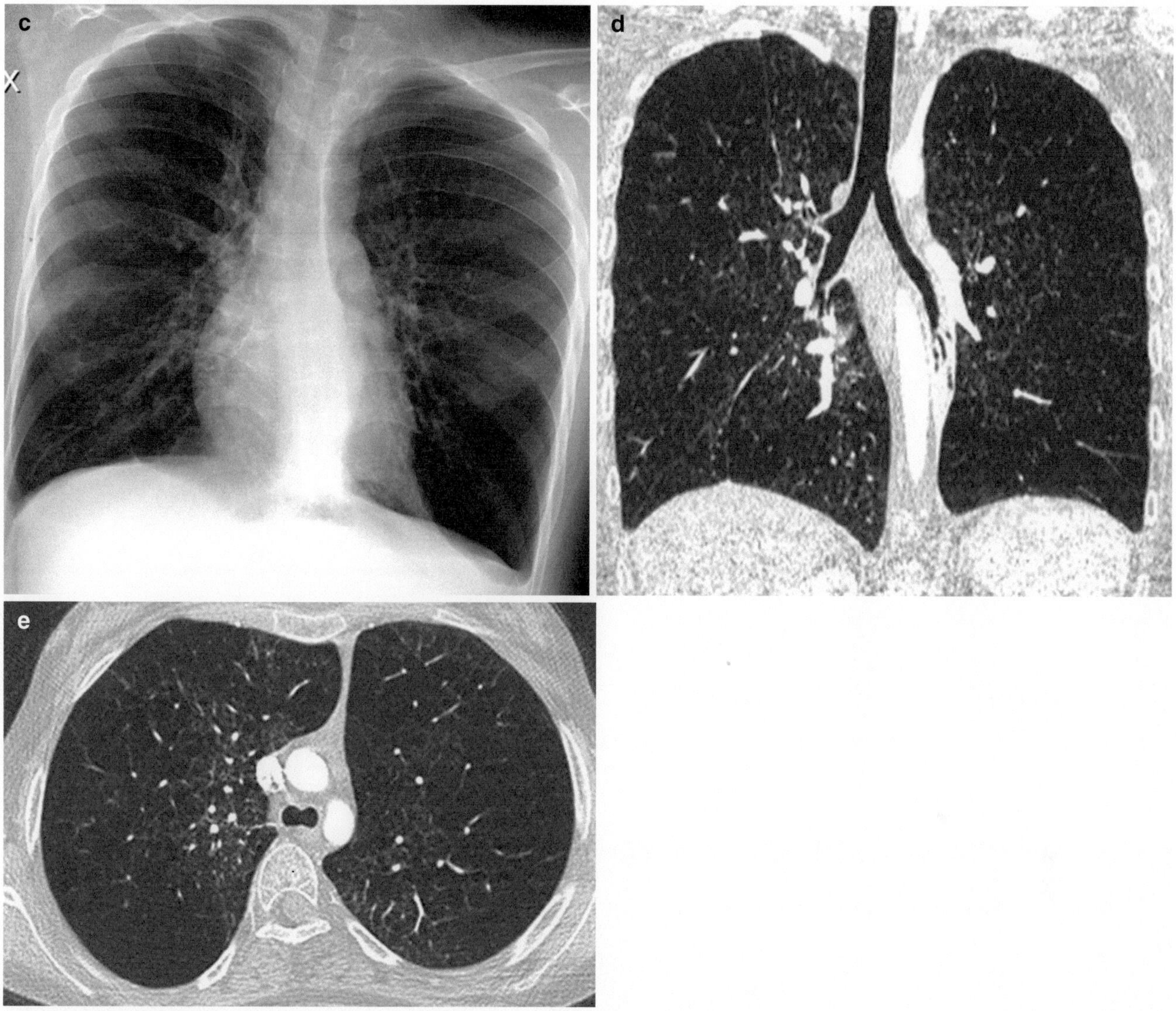

Fig. 27.15 (continued)

27.4.15 Case 27.16: Pulmonary Infection in Nephrotic Syndrome

A 13-year-old girl affected by nephrotic syndrome. During follow-up, asthenia, lumbosacral pain, and persistent cough occurred. Laboratory tests revealed fungal infections (Fig. 27.16).

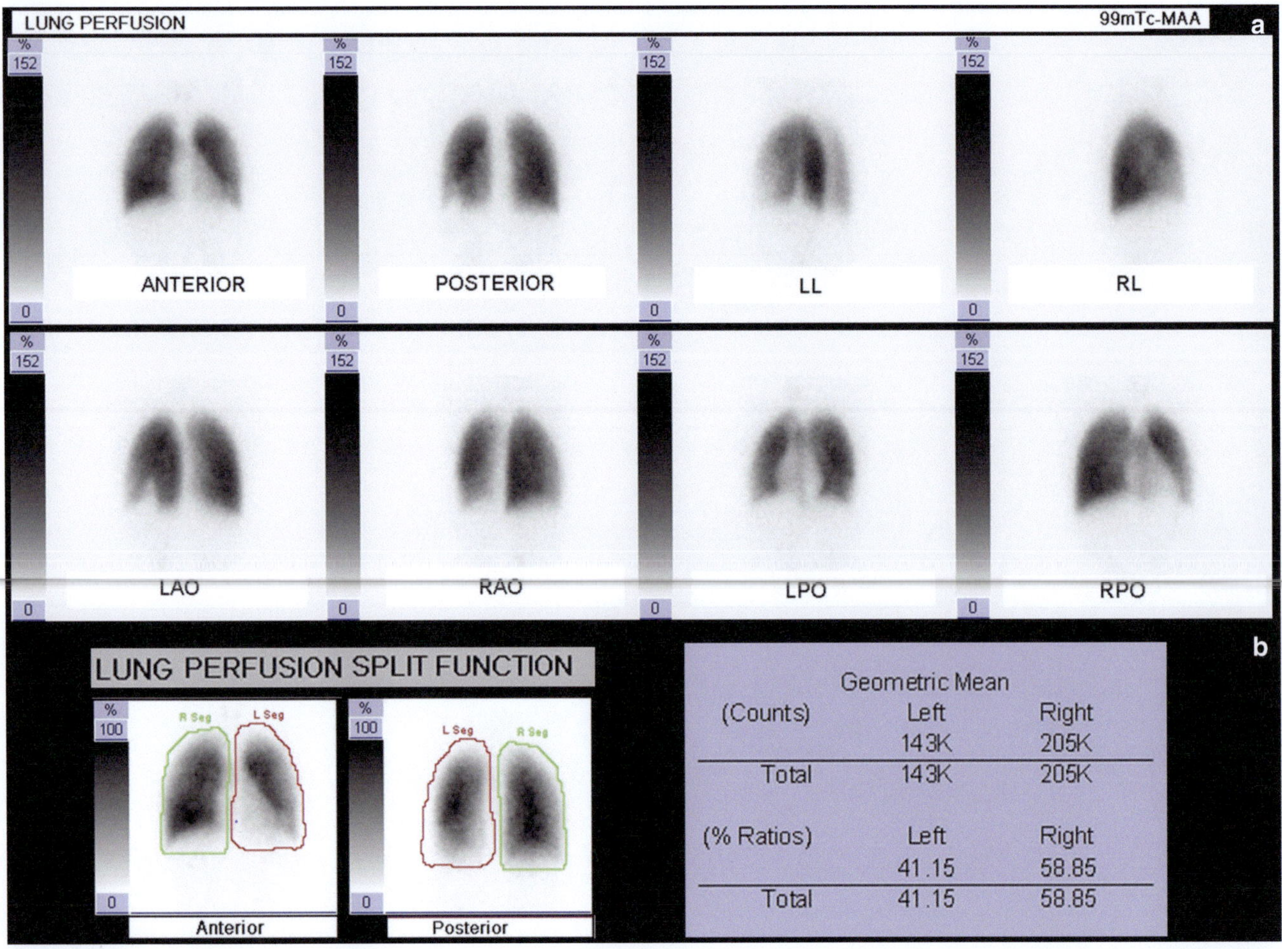

Fig. 27.16 (**a–d**) Lung perfusion scan (**a**, **b**) shows segmental perfusion defect in the posterior basal segment of the left lung and normal perfusion in the remaining parenchyma; in SPECT–CT fused images (**c**, **d**), the absence of perfusion corresponds to the area of parenchymal consolidation showed by CT, excluding lung embolism. (**e–h**) Chest x-ray (**e**) shows the left basal consolidation with hyperdiafania antideclive as possible cavitation (*red arrow*). Coronal CE-CT images (**f**, **g**) show filling defect in left lobar branch of the pulmonary artery as for embolism (*white arrow*). Axial CT image (**h**) shows excavated parenchymal consolidation in left lower lobe (bronchopneumonia)

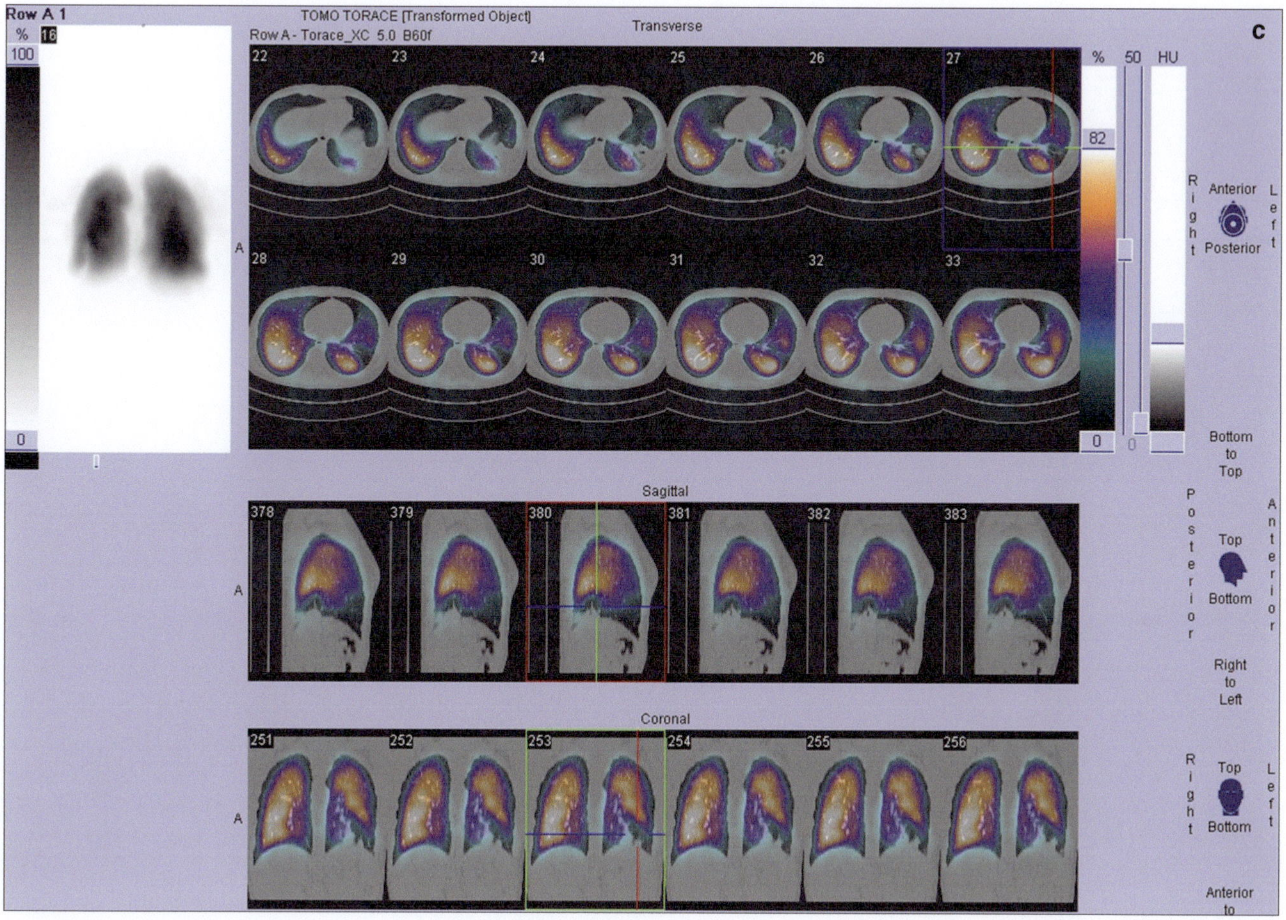

Fig. 27.16 (continued)

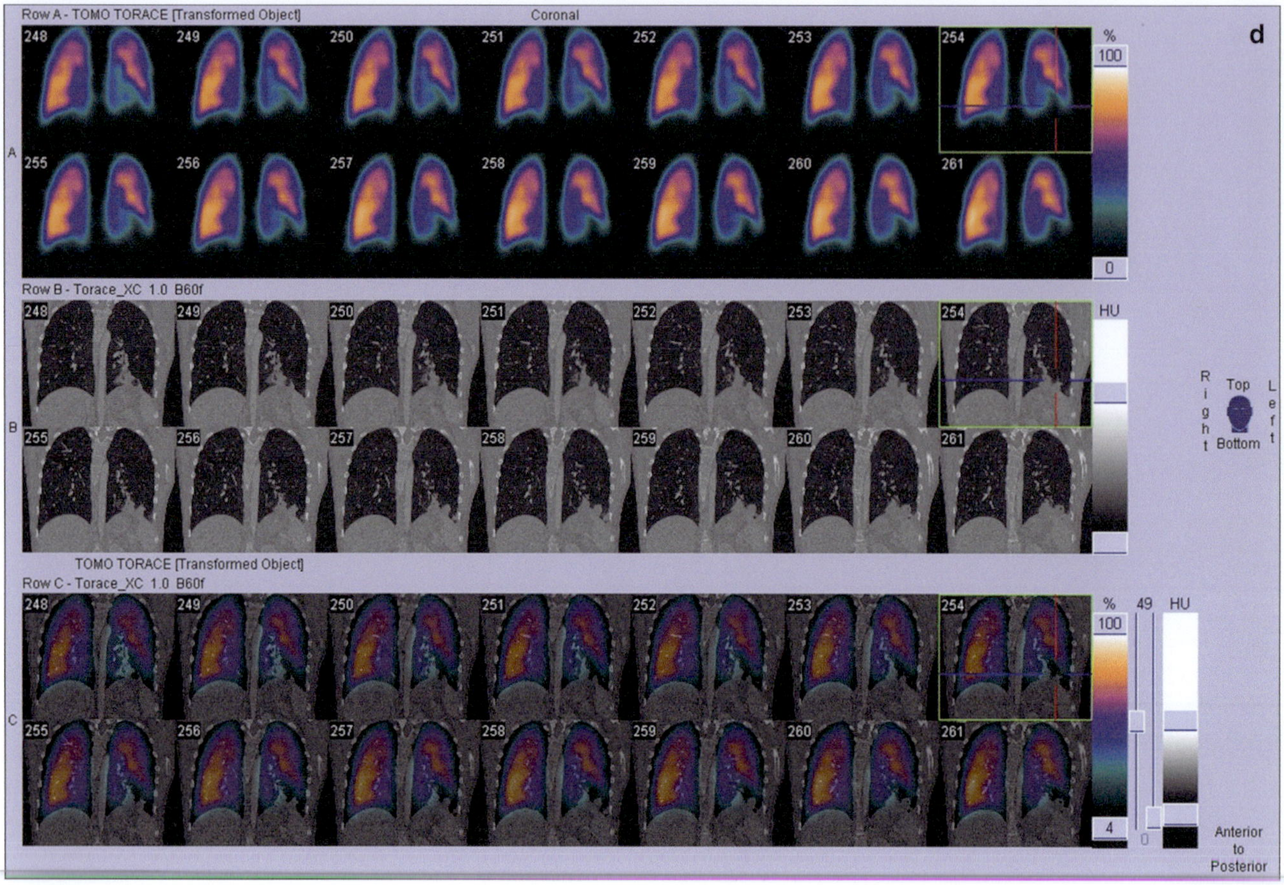

Fig. 27.16 (continued)

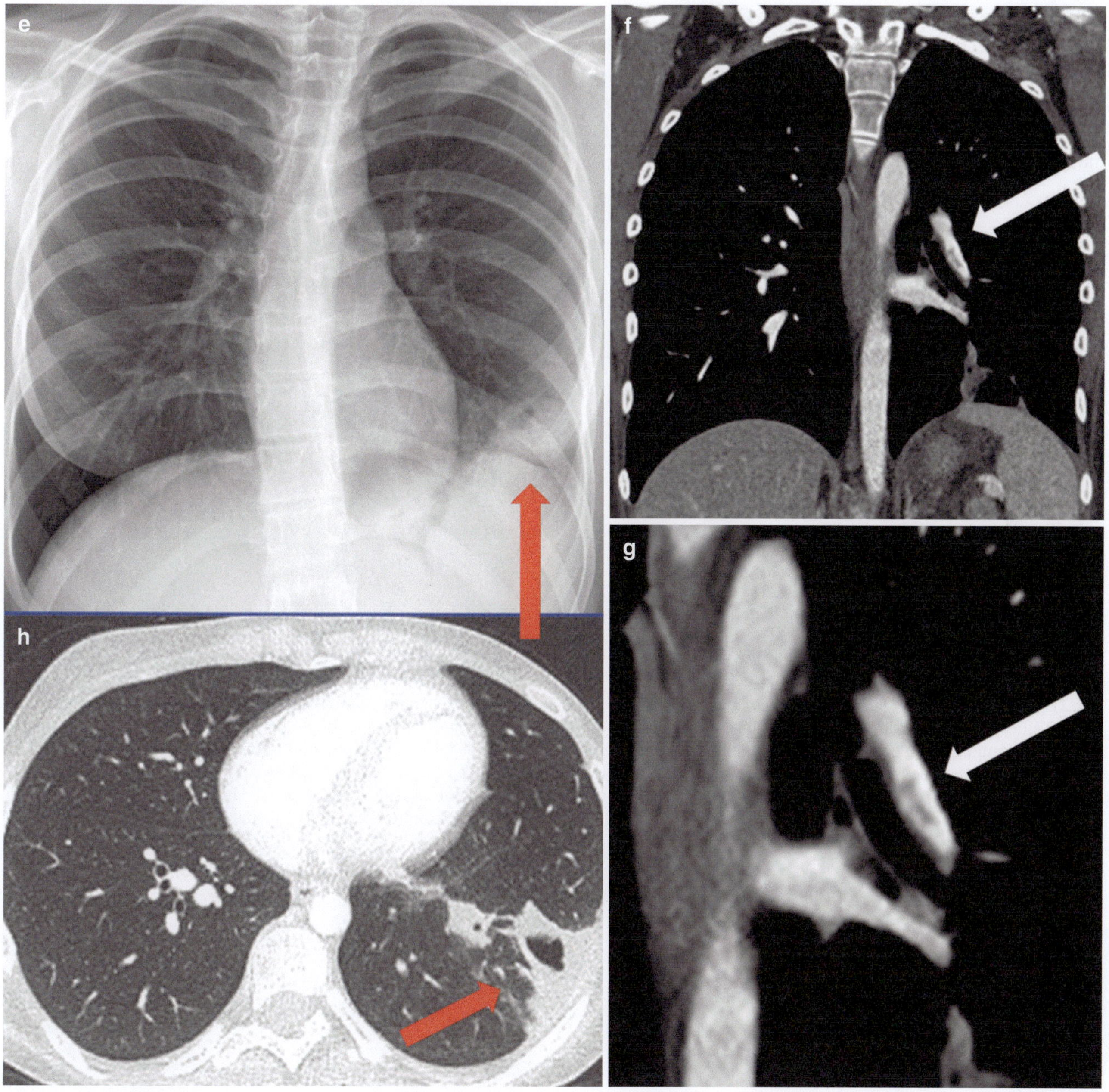

Fig. 27.16 (continued)

27.4.16 Case 27.17: A Child with COPD and Secondary Mucociliary Dyskinesia

A 7-year-old girl followed for chronic pulmonary disease and secondary dyskinesia. Early symptoms occurred to 8 months of life (frequent bronchitis and pneumonia).

She underwent nasal brushing which revealed slow pulse rate. Further examination was necessary for the framework of the pathology (Fig. 27.17).

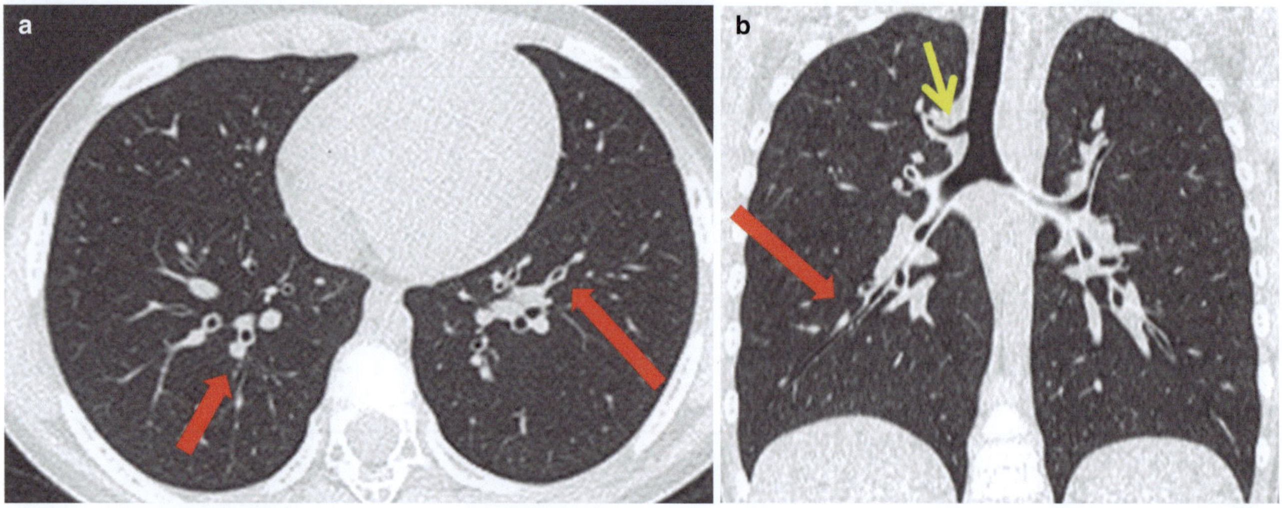

Fig. 27.17 (**a–b**) Lung ventilation scan shows patency of airways with the deposition of particles in the trachea and bronchial bifurcation, slow clearance of radioaerosol deposited in the bronchial walls with bilaterally bronchial stasis. The analysis of AT curves on bronchial regions, for the quantitative assessment of mucociliary clearance in 60 min, shows slow clearance (9 % for the left lung and 15 % for the right lung) and overall pulmonary ventilation regular. Lung ventilation scan with colloids for clearance studies must be performed far from episodes of acute infammation to avoid false positive. (**c–d**) Axial (**c**) and coronal (**d**) CT images show the presence of bronchiectasis in the lower lobes, with marked thickening of the bronchial walls (*red arrows*) and anatomical variation with right upper lobe bronchus originating from the trachea (tracheal bronchus, *yellow arrow*)

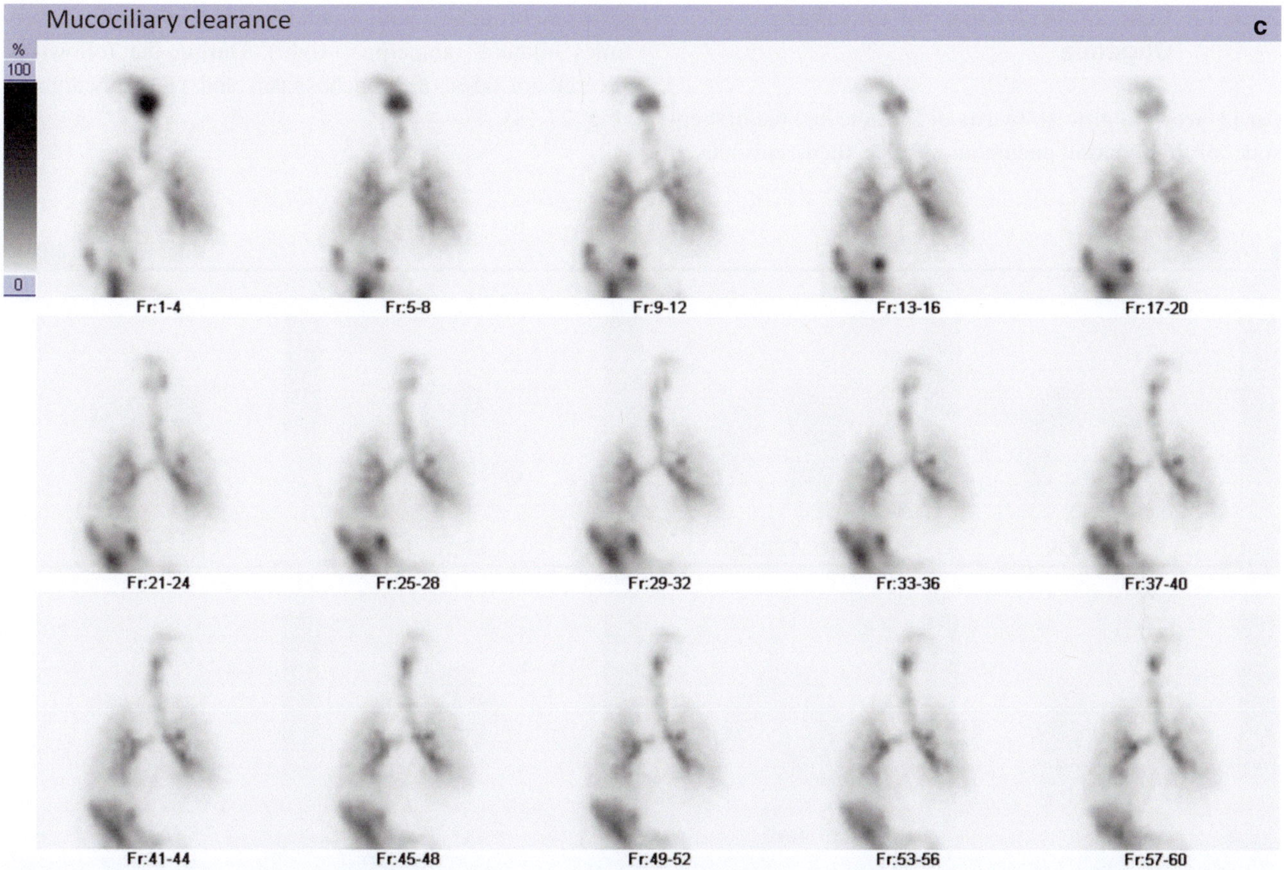

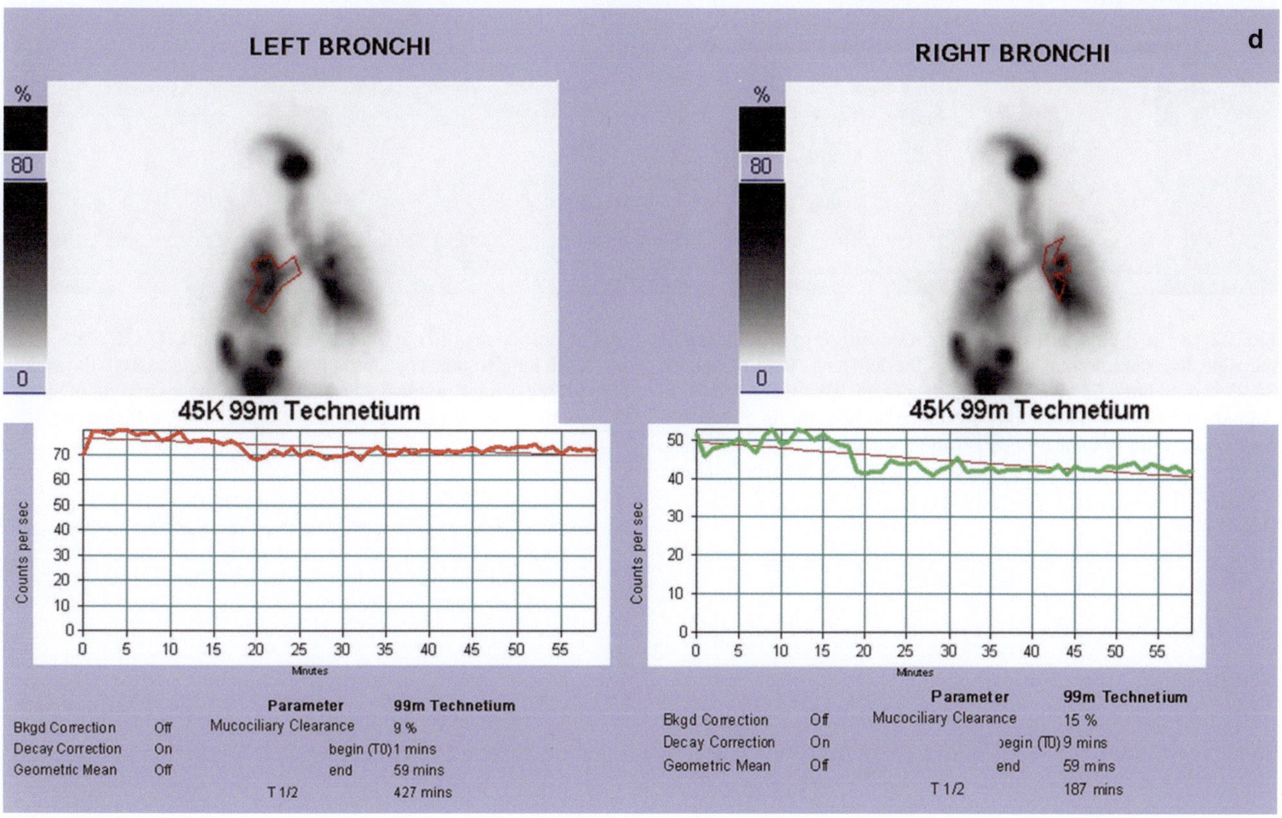

Fig. 27.17 (continued)

27.4.17 Case 27.18: A Case of Pulmonary Oligemia

An 11-year-old girl. At 2 years of life, she had the first episode of right basal pneumonia; since then, episodes of recurrent bronchitis with asthma (hisses and whistles sometimes bilateral, sometimes right). During the follow-up, several episodes of bronchospasm and right pneumonia (Fig. 27.18).

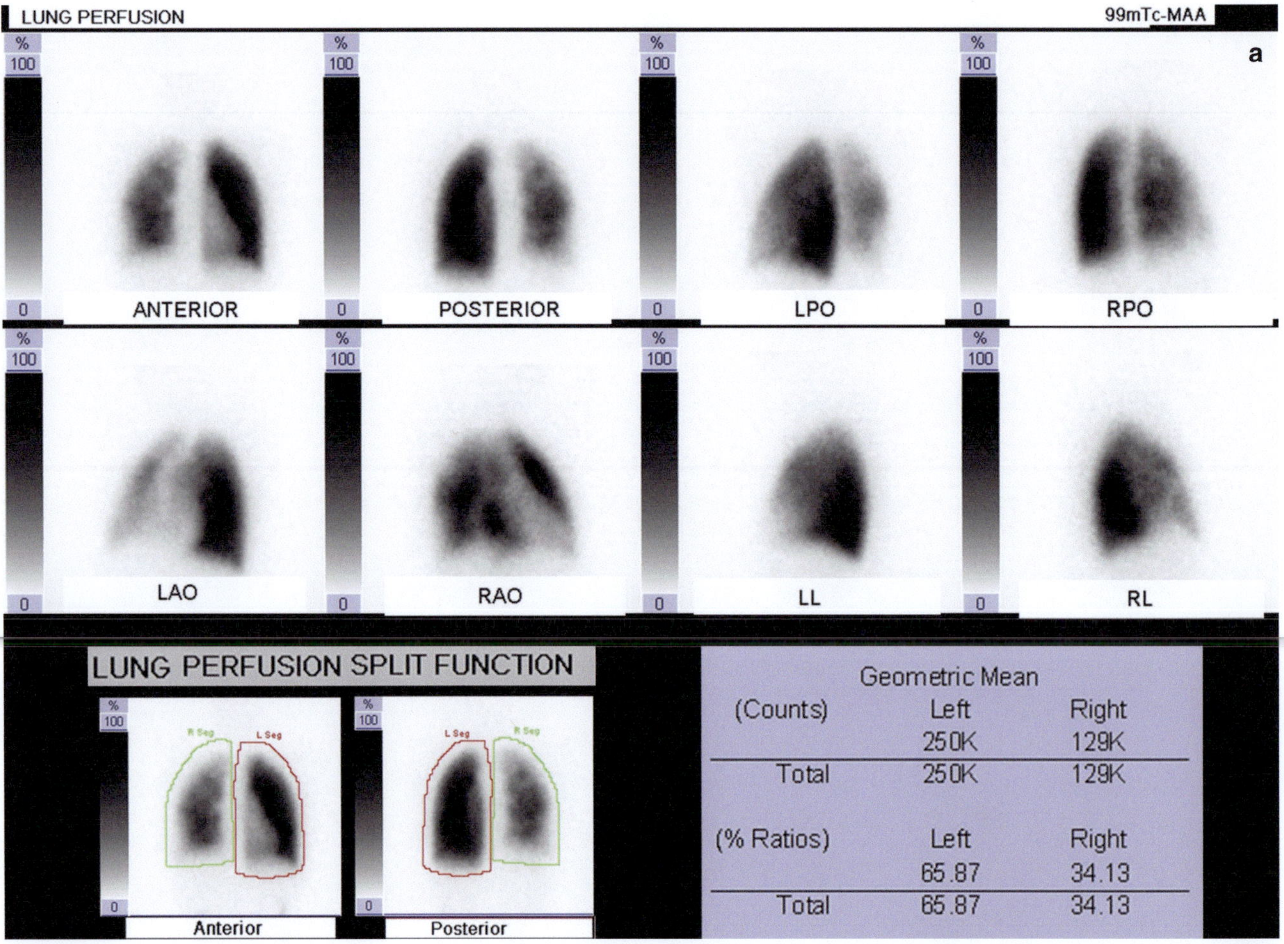

Fig. 27.18 (**a**) Lung perfusion scan shows diffuse hypoperfusion of the right lung and normal perfusion in the left lung. Rate of uptake: 34.13 % right lung; 65.87 % left lung. (**b–c**) Lung ventilation scan with colloids shows slow mucociliary clearance in the right lung with evident of stasis in several bronchi. Normal clearance in the left lung. Quantitative rate clearance: 19 % in the right lung; 51 % in the left lung. (**d–f**) Chest X-rays (**d**) and axial (**e**) and coronal (**f**) CT scans show increased lung volumes by air trapping (**c**), bronchiectasis in the middle lobe (**d**, *red arrow*), and hypodensities by air trapping in right lung with reduction of the vascular representation due to hypoperfusion (*oval*).

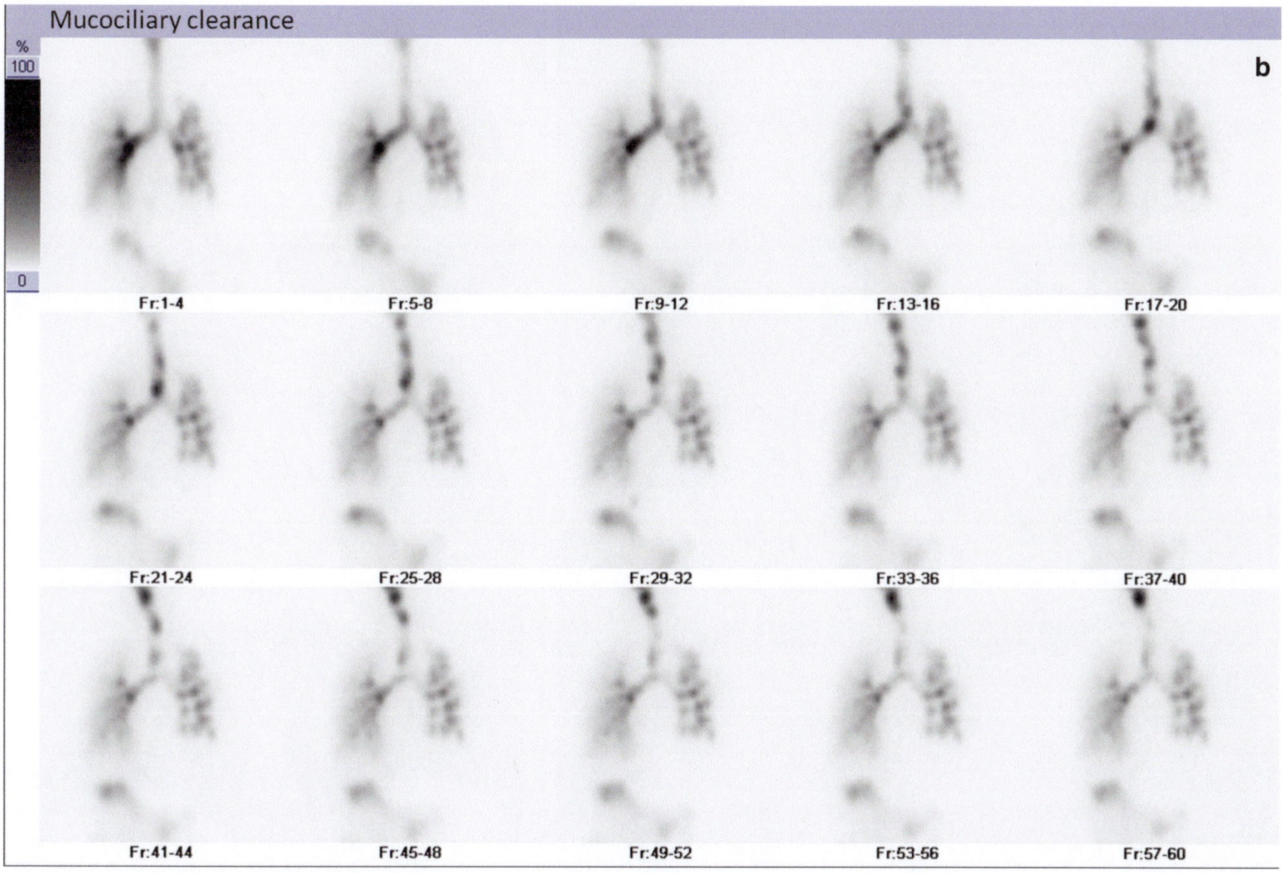

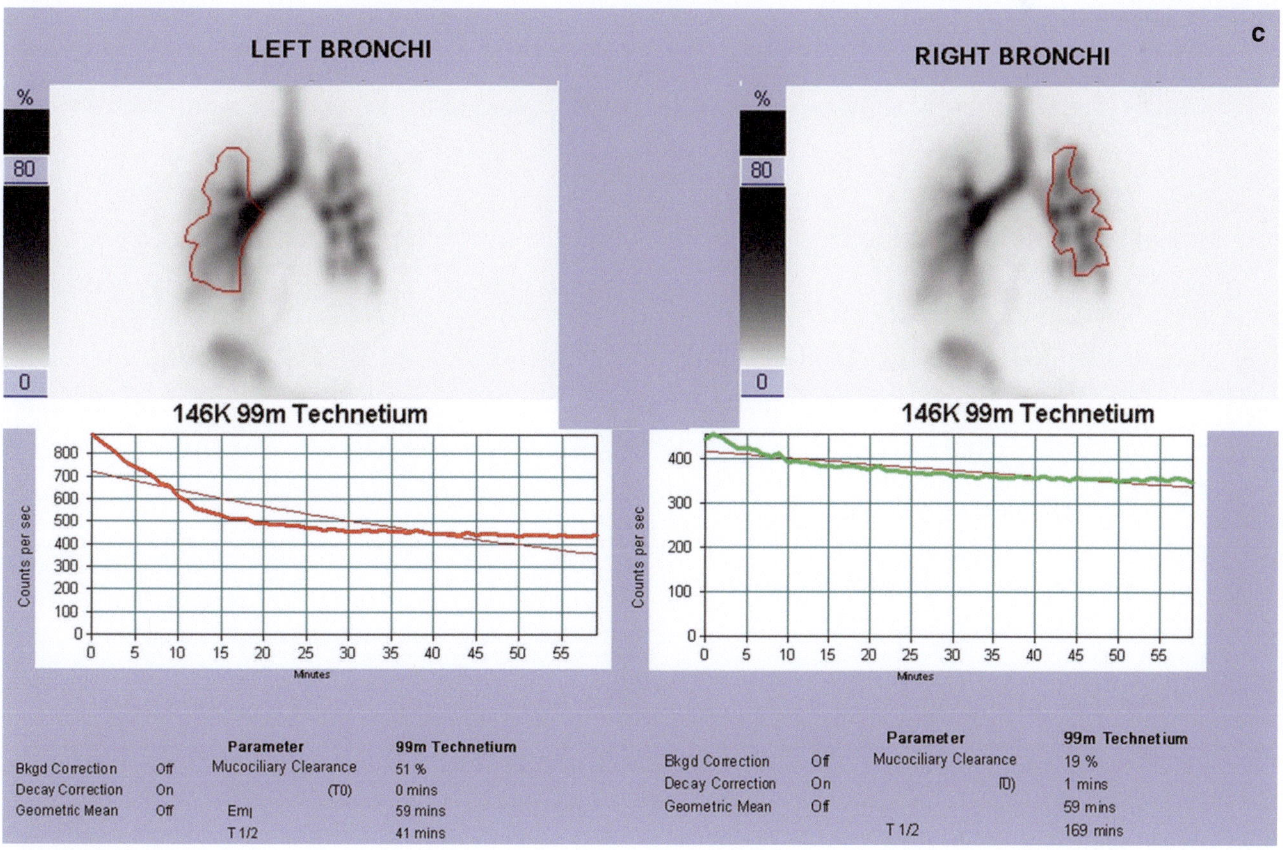

Fig. 27.18 (continued)

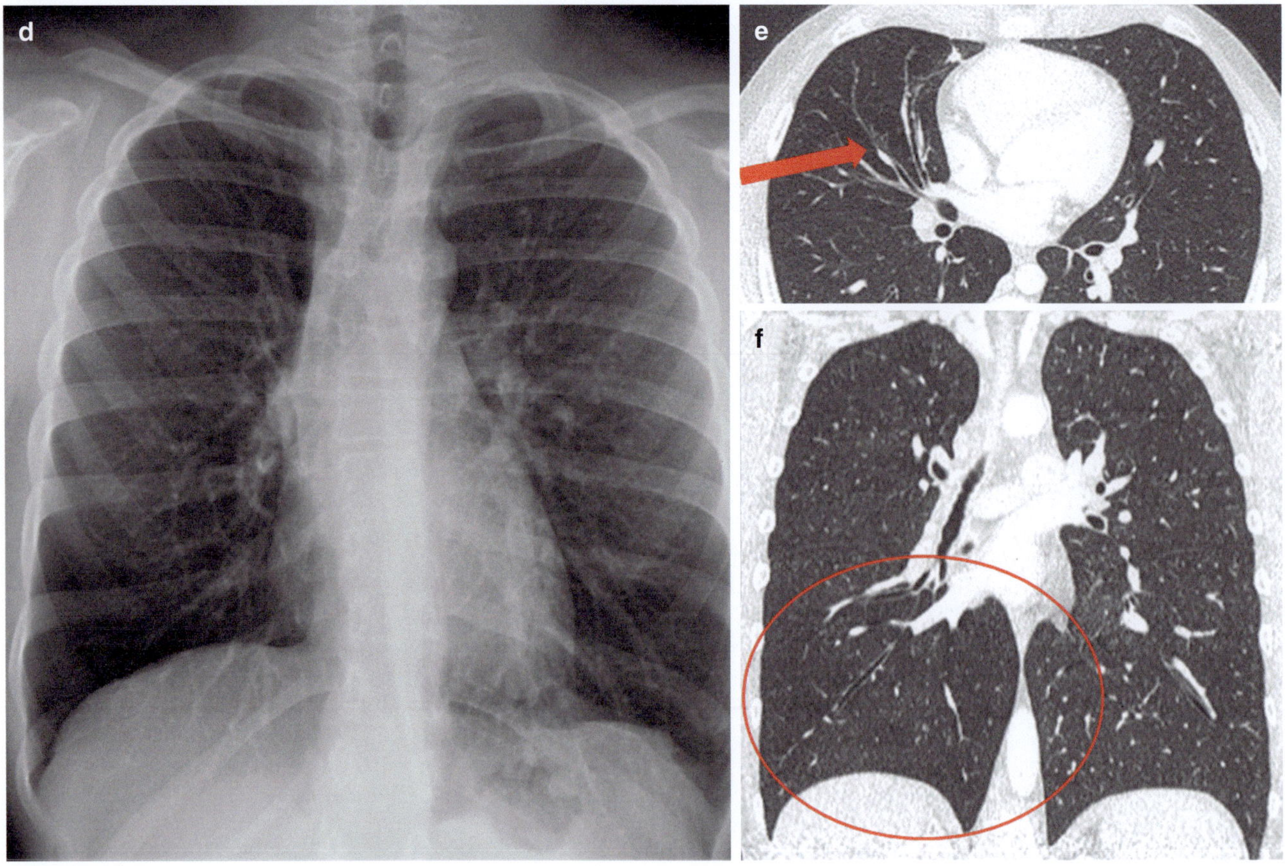

Fig. 27.18 (continued)

27.4.18 Case 27.19: A Case of Mucociliary Dyskinesia (Kartagener Syndrome)

A newborn affected by complex congenital heart disease (heart univentricular right type, CAV atrioventricular type C, mitral atresia, pulmonary atresia), submitted to cardiac surgery. When she was 3 years old, recurrent bronchitis, acute respiratory failure, and pneumonia occurred. She also presented recurring bronchospasm (Fig. 27.19)

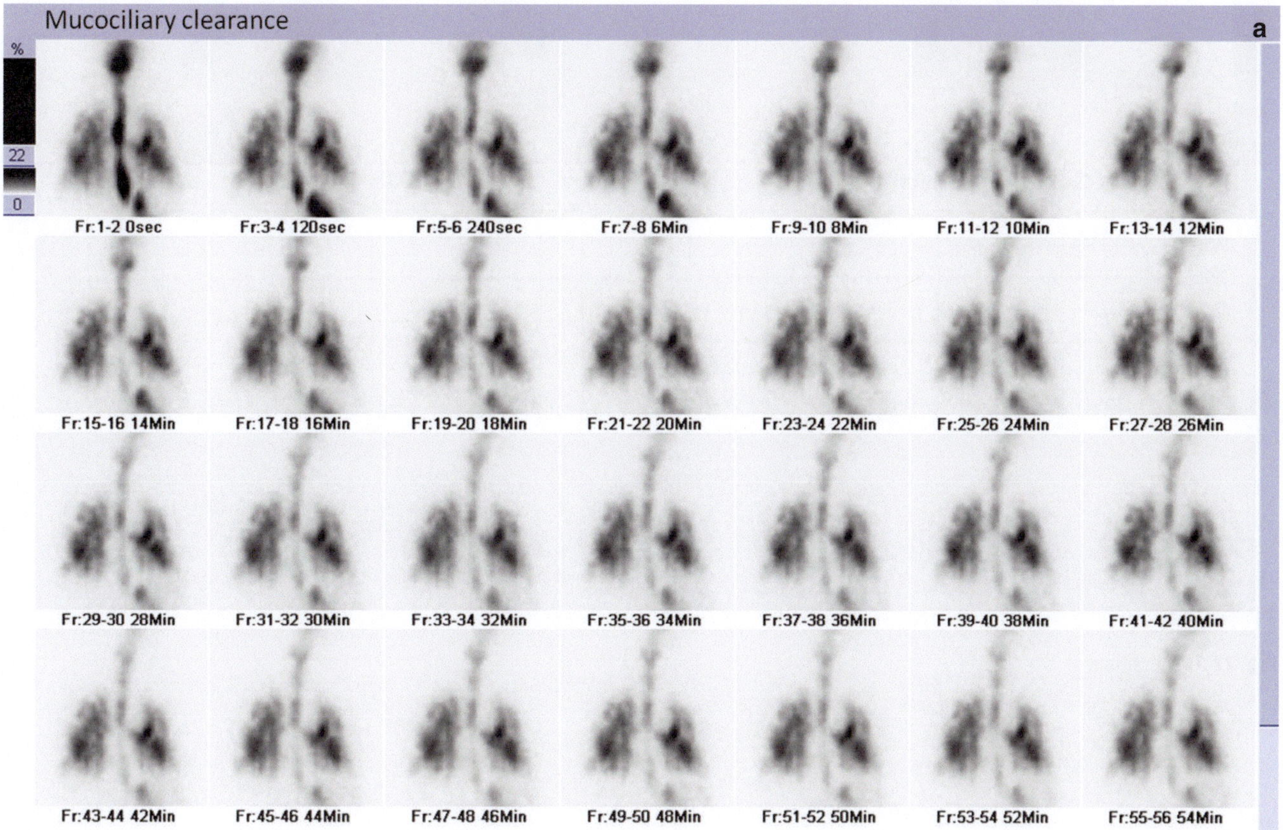

Fig. 27.19 (**a**, **b**) Lung ventilation scan with colloids shows absence of mucociliary clearance. The analysis of AT curves on bronchial regions, for the quantitative assessment of mucociliary clearance in 60 min, shows no signal reduction until the end of the study (0% of clearance for the left lung and 0% for the right lung)

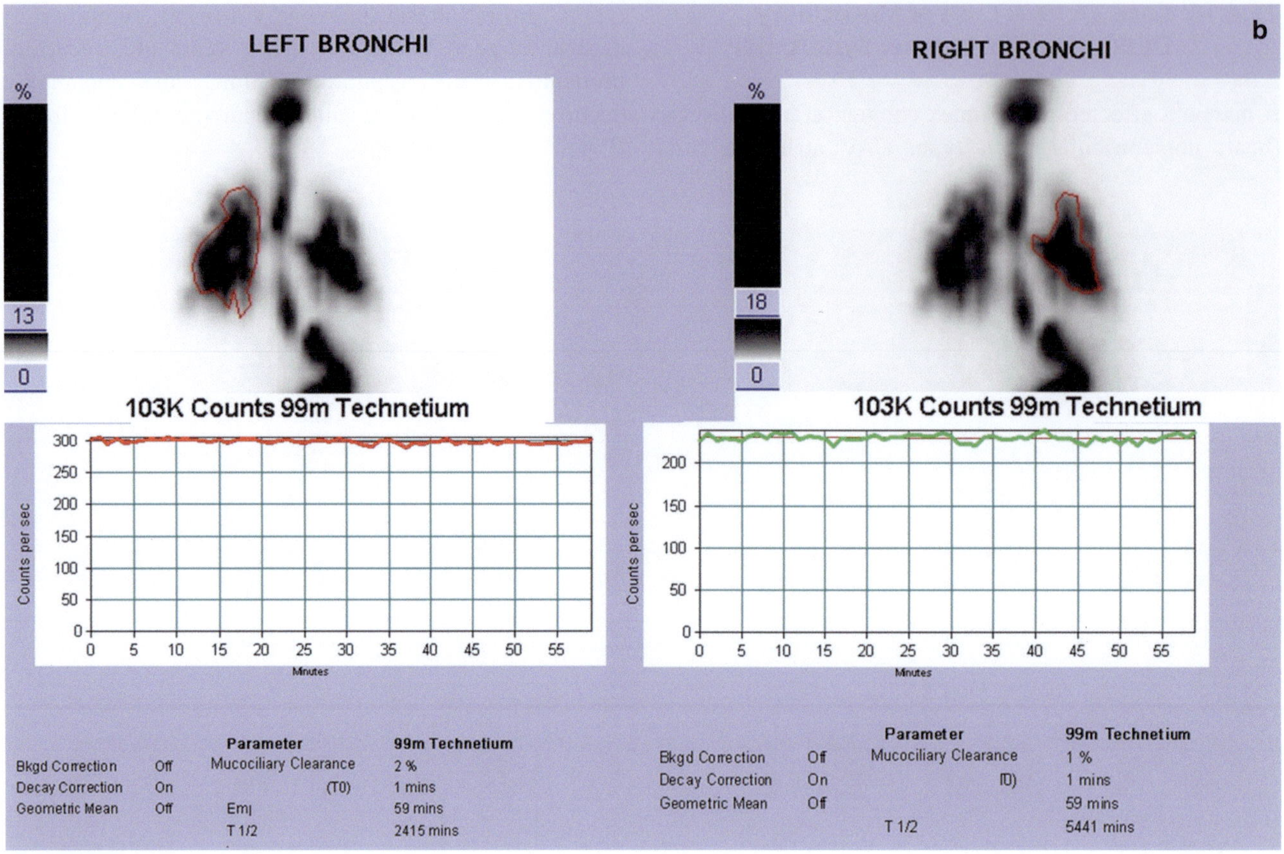

Fig. 27.19 (continued)

Further Readings

1. Ciofetta G, Piepsz A, Roca I, Fisher S, Hahn K, Sixt R, Biassoni L, De Palma D, Zucchetta P. Guidelines for lung scintigraphy in children. Eur J Nucl Med Mol Imaging 2007;34:1518–26.

MIX
Papier aus verantwortungsvollen Quellen
Paper from responsible sources
FSC® C105338

If you have any concerns about our products,
you can contact us on
ProductSafety@springernature.com

In case Publisher is established outside the EU,
the EU authorized representative is:
Springer Nature Customer Service Center GmbH
Europaplatz 3, 69115 Heidelberg, Germany

Printed by Libri Plureos GmbH
in Hamburg, Germany